GW00383824

Handbook of Disease Burdens and Quality of Life Measures

Victor R. Preedy, Ronald R. Watson (Eds.)

Handbook of Disease Burdens and Quality of Life Measures

Volume 4

With 570 Figures and 1001 Tables

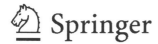 Springer

Editors:

Prof. Victor R. Preedy
Dept. Nutrition and Dietetics
Nutritional Sciences Research Division
School of Biomedical & Health Sciences
King's College London
Franklin-Wilkins Building
150 Stamford Street
London SE1 9NH
UK

Prof. Ronald R. Watson
Mel and Enid Zuckerman College of Public Health
University of Arizona
Health Science Center
1295 N. Martin
P.O. Box 245155
Tucson, AZ 85724–5155

ISBN–13: 978–0–387–78664–3

This publication is available also as:
Electronic publication under 978–0–387–78665–0 and
Print and electronic bundle under ISBN 978–0–387–78666–7
Library of Congress Control Number: 2009927296

springer.com

Printed on acid-free paper   SPIN: 11980131   2109 –5 4 3 2 1

Preface

Disease and pathologies have devastating consequences on the individual, the family unit and society in general including effect on nations or entire geographical regions. Assessing these impacts at the individual or international level has been problematical due to the diverse nature of the diseases themselves. There is also a variable response between individuals or regions. However, there is now an increasing awareness that the imposition of disease or ill health can be measured and assessed in quantitative terms. These measures of disease encompass a variety of facets: from the financial costs of treatment to the effects of a particular disease condition on the quality of life of individuals. The development and application of tools to measure these aspects have been particularly evident over the past decade. For example, suitable questionnaires developed for the general assessment of Quality of Life have now been revised and refined so that they are directly applicable to specific disease entities or even different cultures. Hitherto, there has never been a coherent publication that allocated to a single volume the many questionnaires that have been developed nor the quantitative aspects of disease in terms of finance, mortality, morbidity and quality of life measures. These aspects are addressed in The Handbook of Disease Burdens and Quality of Life Measures. It is structured into 3 main sections as follows: Part [1] Instruments and methological aspects; Part [2] Disease Burdens and Economics Impacts; Part [3] Quality of life measures and indices. The various subsections of The Handbook of Disease Burdens and Quality of Life Measures reflect the diverse nature of diseases and their impact, Sections include those pertaining to geographical aspects of disease, pathologies and metabolic disorders, early life stages and aging, cancer, cardiovascular disease, immune disorders, viral, bacterial, microbiological, infectious and parasitic diseases, psychosocial, social, behavioural, psychiatric, neurological conditions and addictions to name just a few examples. In dividing the chapters the Editors recognise the problems that this entails. Some chapters may be equally at home in more than one subsection. To a certain extent this is covered by the comprehensive coverage and excellent indexing.

Essentially, The Handbook of Disease Burdens and Quality of Life Measures represents a "one-stop-shopping" of information with suitable tables and figures. Each chapter is written by internationally or nationally recognised experts or Institutions. Each chapter is also "stand alone", self contained and well illustrated with appropriate tables and figures. The articles are written in such a way that material from one area can be readily transferable to other areas. In other words the material truly bridges the trans-disciplinary divide.

The Handbook's broad coverage and meticulous, up-to-date detail make it essential for public health researchers, medical and health practitioners, and for those involved in allocating resources and setting priorities, such as epidemiologists, sociologists, health economists, and policymakers. It is also suitable for those who specially want to broaden their knowledge-base in a rapidly expanding area of medical sciences.

Professors Victor R Preedy and Ronald Ross Watson

Table of Contents

Preface v
Contributors xxix

Volume 1

Part 1 Instruments and Methodological Aspects 1

**Part 1.1 Instruments Used in the Assessment of Disease
Impact** 1

1   **The International Classification of Functioning, Disability and Health:
A Tool to Classify and Measure Functioning** 3
G. Stucki · N. Kostanjsek · A. Cieza

2   **The Keele Assessment of Participation** 35
R. Wilkie

3   **The Global Person Generated Index** 59
F. Martin · L. Camfield · D. Ruta

4   **The Total Illness Burden Index** 73
S. Greenfield · J. Billimek · S. H. Kaplan

5   **The EQ-5D Health-Related Quality of Life Questionnaire** 87
N. Gusi · P. R. Olivares · R. Rajendram

6   **The University of Washington Quality of Life Scale** 101
S. N. Rogers · D. Lowe

7   **Comparison of Three Quality of Life Questionnaires in Urinary
Incontinence** 129
Ja Hyeon Ku · Seung-June Oh

8   **Overview of Instruments Used to Assess Quality of Life in Dentistry** 145
C. McGrath · S. N. Rogers

9   **SQOR-V: A Patient Reported Outcome Specifically Dedicated to
Chronic Venous Disorders** 161
J.-J. Guex · S. E. Zimmet · S. Boussetta · C. Taieb

10   **The Uniscale Assessment of Quality of Life: Applications to Oncology . . .179**
      E. Ballatori · F. Roila · B. Ruggeri · A. A. Bruno · S. Tiberti · F. di Orio

11   **The Bone Metastases Quality of Life Questionnaire** **195**
      X. Badia · A. Vieta · M. Gilabert

12   **The Impact of Weight on Quality of Life Questionnaire** **209**
      J. Manwaring · D. Wilfley

13   **The Quality in Later Life Questionnaire** **227**
      S. Evans

14   **The MacDQOL Individualized Measure of the Impact of Macular
      Disease on Quality of Life** **247**
      Jan Mitchell · Alison Woodcock · Clare Bradley

15   **Development and Assessment of Chinese General Quality of Life
      Instrument** **265**
      Y. Wu · G. Xie

16   **The Japanese Version of the EORTC Quality of Life Questionnaire** **285**
      G. Tóth · M. Tsukuda

Part 1.2 Contemporary Issues in Assessment **311**

17   **Calculating QALYs and DALYs: Methods and Applications to Fatal
      and Non-Fatal Conditions** **313**
      F. Sassi

18   **Accuracy of Death Certifications and the Implications for Studying
      Disease Burdens** **329**
      J. R. Pierce · A. V. Denison

19   **Completeness and Accuracy of Death Dates and the Implications
      for Studying Disease Burdens: Focus on Alternative
      Data Sources** **345**
      Min-Woong Sohn · Elissa Oh

20   **Utility Scores for Comorbid Conditions: Methodological Issues
      and Advances** **359**
      C. N. McIntosh

21   **Subjective Quality of Life Measures – General Principles
      and Concepts** **381**
      C. L. K. Lam

22   **Standard Expected Years of Life Lost as a Measure of Disease Burden:
      An Investigation of Its Presentation, Meaning and Interpretation** **401**
      R. J. Marshall

Part 2 Disease Burdens and Economic Impacts 415

Part 2.1 General Aspects, Geographical Aspects,
Pathologies and Metabolic Disorders 415

23 Health-Adjusted Life Expectancy: Concepts and Estimates 417
J. A. Labbe

**24 Individual Disability-Adjusted Life Year: A Summary Health Outcome
Indicator Used for Prospective Studies** 425
P. Zhang · M. Woodward · J. Shen · Y. Wu

**25 Integration of Quality of Life and Survival for Comparative
Risk/Outcome Assessment in Healthcare Industry** 437
J.-D. Wang · J.-S. Hwang

**26 Disability-Adjusted Life Years in Occupational Injuries and
Accidents** 447
M. Concha-Barrientos · J. Labbé Cid

27 The Income-Associated Burden of Disease in the United States 459
P. Muennig · M. Gold · E. Lubetkin · H. Jia

**28 Financial Burdens and Disability-Adjusted Life Years in Los
Angeles County** 473
G. F. Kominski · P. A. Simon · A. Y. Ho · J. E. Fielding

**29 Burden of Disease Between Two Time Frames: Mexico
Perspectives** 483
G. Rodriguez-Abrego · J. Escobedo-de la Peña · R. B. Zurita Garza · T. Ramírez-Sánchez

**30 East/West Differences in Health in Europe: Rates, Expectancies
and DALYs** 505
J. Powles · H. Gouda

31 The Burden of Neglected Diseases in Developing Countries 517
A. Boutayeb

**32 The Burden of Communicable and Non-Communicable Diseases in
Developing Countries** 531
A. Boutayeb

33 Economic Evaluation of Health Interventions: Tanzania Perspectives 547
B. Robberstad · Yusuf Hemed

34 The Burden of Disease and Injury in Serbia 587
*S. Janković · H. Vlajinac · V. Bjegović · J. Marinković · S. Šipetić-Grujicić ·
Marković-Denić · N. Kocev · M. Šantrić-Milićević · Z. Terzić-Šupić ·
N. Maksimović · U. Laaser*

35 Disease Burdens and Disability-Adjusted Life Years in Aboriginal
    and Non-Aboriginal Populations 603
    Y. Zhao

36 The Relationship Between the National Health Insurance Expenditures
    and the Burden of Disease Measures in the Iran 629
    M. Russel · H. R. Jamshidi

37 The Burden of Maternal Mortality and Morbidity in the United States
    and Worldwide 647
    C. T. Lang · J. C. King

38 The Financial Implications of Pancreas Transplant Complications 661
    J. A. Cohn · M. J. Englesbe

39 The Use of Pharmacoepidemiological Databases to Assess Disease
    Burdens: Application to Diabetes 671
    H. Støvring

40 Years of Life Lost Due to Air Pollution in Switzerland: A Dynamic
    Exposure-Response Model 685
    M. Röösli

41 Quantification of Deaths and DALYs Due to Chronic Exposure to
    Arsenic in Groundwaters Utilized for Drinking, Cooking and
    Irrigation of Food-Crops 701
    D. A. Polya · D. Mondal · A. K. Giri

Part 2.2 Early Life Stages and Aging .729

42 Disability-Adjusted Life Years in Children and Adolescents in Europe . . .731
    F. Valent · S. Di Bartolomeo

43 Disease Burden of Diarrheal and Respiratory Disorders in Children:
    Hong Kong Perspectives 751
    E. A. S. Nelson

44 Burden of Disease in Elderly Mexican Population 763
    B. Rico-Verdín · G. Rodriguez-Abrego · I. Villaseñor-Ruiz · J. L. Torres-Cosme

Volume 2

Part 2.3 Cancer 783

45 Years of Life Lost from Cancer and Applications to Research
    Funding 785
    N. G. Burnet · S. J. Jefferies · F. P. Treasure

46 Worldwide Burden of Gynecological Cancer 803
    R. Sankaranarayanan · J. Ferlay

47 Years of Life Lost from Lung, Stomach, Liver and Cervical Cancers:
    An Evaluation of the Top Cancer Killers 825
    B. Y. Goldstein · F. I. Bray · D. M. Parkin · J. W. Sellors · Z. F. Zhang

48 Burden of Cancer in Serbia 843
    H. Vlajinac · S. Sipetic-Grujicic · S. Jankovic · L. Markovic-Denic · J. Marinkovic

49 The Disease Burden of Mastectomy: Turkish Perspective and Impact
    on the Patient and Family 865
    S. Özkan · M. Özkan · V. Özmen · Z. Armay

50 The Burden of Chemotherapy Induced Nausea and Vomiting on
    Patients' Daily Lives: Italian Perspectives 885
    E. Ballatori · F. Roila · B. Ruggeri · A. A. Bruno · S. Tiberti · F. di Orio

Part 2.4 Cardiac, Vascular, Pulmonary and Dietary 899

51 Atherosclerotic Burden and Mortality 901
    J. Roquer · Angel Ois

52 Burden of Cardiovascular Diseases Among Aboriginal and Torres
    Strait Islander Peoples: Mortality, Hospitalization and Risk Factors 919
    A. G. Thrift · S. L. Gall · A. D. Brown

53 Burden of Ischemic Heart Diseases in Serbia 933
    S. Sipetic-Grujicic · H. Vlajinac · J. Marinkovic · V. Bjegovic · I. Ratkov · J. Maksimovic

54 Burden of Cerebrovascular Diseases (Stroke) in Serbia 949
    T. Pekmezovic · H. Vlajinac · S. Sipetic-Grujicic · N. Kocev · D. K. Tepavcevic ·
    L. B. Bumbasirevic

55 DALYs and Public Health Programs for Stroke: Australian Perspectives . . .965
    D. A. Cadilhac · M. L. Moodie · E. E. Lalor

56 Burden of Stroke: Indian Perspective 991
    P. M. Dalal · M. Bhattacharjee

57 Disability-Adjusted Life Years, Years of Life Lived with Disability,
    and Years of Life Lost in Stroke: Italian Perspectives 1007
    S. Mariotti

58 Burden of Ischemic Stroke and Benefits of Stroke Unit Care and
    Thrombolytic Therapy 1029
    A. Meretoja · M. Kaste · T. Tatlisumak

59   **Economic Burden of Complications During Percutaneous Coronary Intervention** 1061
M. Dewan · K. M. Jacobson · C. S. Rihal

60   **Features of Mediterranean Diet and Burden of Cardiovascular Disease** 1073
D. B. Panagiotakos · C. Pitsavos · D. P. Mikhailidis

61   **Obesity's Final Toll: Influence on Mortality Rate, Attributable Deaths, Years of Life Lost and Population Life Expectancy** 1085
K. R. Fontaine · S. W. Keith · J. A. Greenberg · S. J. Olshansky · D. B. Allison

62   **Financial Impact of Obesity** 1107
L. Barrios · D. B. Jones

63   **Burden of Disease Attributable to Obesity and Overweight: Korean Focus** 1119
Seok-Jun Yoon · Jae-Hyun Park

64   **Economic Burden of the Components of the Metabolic Syndrome** 1135
P. J. Marangos · L. J. Okamoto · J. J. Caro

65   **Zinc Deficiency and DALYs in India: Impact Assessment and Economic Analyses** 1151
A. J. Stein · M. Qaim · P. Nestel

Part 2.5   Immune Disorders, Viral, Bacterial, Microbiological, Infectious and Parasitic Diseases 1171

66   **The Impact of Infectious Diseases on the Development of Africa** 1173
A. Boutayeb

67   **Measuring the Global Burden of Tuberculosis** 1189
I. Onozaki · N. Ishikawa · D. A. Enarson

68   **Burden of Tuberculosis: Serbian Perspectives** 1211
Z. Gledovic · H. Vlajinac · T. Pekmezovic · S. Grujicic-Sipetic · A. Grgurevic · D. Pesut

69   **DALYs and Diarrhea** 1221
R. Oria · R. Pinkerton · AAM Lima · R. L. Guerrant

70   **The Burden of Rotavirus Acute Gastroenteritis in Europe** 1233
J. Bilcke · P. Van Damme · P. Beutels

71   The Economic Burden of Rotavirus Diarrhea:
     Taiwan Perspectives 1243
     Kow-Tong Chen

72   Disease Burden of Dengue Fever and Dengue Hemorrhagic Fever 1263
     J. A. Suaya · D. S. Shepard · Mark E. Beatty · J. Farrar

73   Cost-Effectiveness of a Dengue Vaccine in Southeast Asia and
     Panama: Preliminary Estimates 1281
     D. S. Shepard · J. A. Suaya

74   Burden of Sexually Transmitted *Chlamydia trachomatis*
     Infections 1297
     L. M. Niccolai · D. Berube

75   Disease Burden from Group A *Neisseria meningitidis* Meningitis in
     Hyperendemic Countries of the African Meningitis Belt 1313
     C. Suraratdecha · C. Levin · F. M. LaForce

76   DALYs in Chronic Hepatitis C : A Paneuropean Perspective 1323
     U. Siebert · A. Conrads-Frank · R. Schwarzer · B. Lettmeier · G. Sroczynski ·
     S. Zeuzem · N. Mühlberger

77   Economics and Vaccines 1335
     J. Bos · M. Postma

78   Economic Costs and Disability-Adjusted Life Years in Polio
     Eradication: A Long-Run Global Perspective .1353
     M. M. Khan

79   Financial Burdens and Disability-Adjusted Life Years in
     Echinococcosis 1373
     P. R. Torgerson

80   Measuring Japanese Encephalitis (JE) Disease Burden in Asia 1391
     W. Liu · D. Ding · J. D. Clemens · N. T. Yen · V. Porpit · Z.-Y. Xu

81   Pandemic Influenza: Potential Contribution to Disease Burden 1401
     M. Nuño

82   Prophylaxis of Healthcare Workers in an Influenza Pandemic 1419
     S. M. Moghadas

83   The Burden of Human African Trypanosomiasis 1433
     A. Shaw · J. Robays · E. M. Fèvre · P. Lutumba · M. Boelaert

84   The Economic Burden of Malaria in Nigeria and Willingness to Pay 1443
      A. Jimoh

85   Measurement of Adverse Health Burden Related to Sexual Behavior . . . 1459
      S. H. Ebrahim · M. McKenna

Volume 3

Part 2.6 Psychosocial, Social, Behavioural, Psychiatric, Neurological and Addictions 1471

86   Global Burden of Mental Health 1473
      M. Kastrup

87   Disease Burden and Disability-Adjusted Life Years Due to
      Schizophrenia and Psychotic Disorders 1493
      A. Theodoridou · W. Rössler

88   The Societal Costs of Anxiety and Mood Disorders: An
      Epidemiological Perspective 1509
      R. C. Kessler · P. S. Wang · H.-U. Wittchen

89   Estimating the Disease Burden of Combat-Related Posttraumatic Stress
      Disorder in United States Veterans and Military Service Members 1527
      M. C. Freed · R. K. Goldberg · K. L. Gore · C. C. Engel

90   Estimating the Disease Burden of Seasonal Affective Disorder 1549
      M. C. Freed · R. L. Osborn · K. J. Rohan

91   The Disease Burden of Suicide: Conceptual Challenges and
      Measurement Standards 1569
      C. A. Claassen · R. M. Bossarte · S. M. Stewart · E. Guzman · P. S. F. Yip

92   The Disease Burden Due to Epilepsy in Rural China 1591
      D. Ding · W. Z. Wang · Z. Hong

93   Alcohol Consumption and Burden of Disease: Germany and
      Switzerland 1603
      M. Roerecke · J. Rehm · J. Patra

94   Alcoholic Beverage Preference, Morbidity and Mortality 1619
      T. E. Strandberg

95   Burden of Disease Due to Alcohol and Alcohol Related Research 1633
      R. Rajendram · G. Lewison · V. R. Preedy

96   Years Life Lost Due to Smoking: A Korean Focus 1649
      S. Yoon

97   The Health and Economic Consequences of Smoking and Smoking Cessation Interventions: The Dutch Perspective 1661
M. P. M. H. Rutten-van Mölken · T. Feenstra

98   Life Years Saved, Quality-Adjusted Life Years Saved and Cost-Effectiveness of a School-Based Tobacco Prevention Program 1681
L. Y. Wang · C. Linda · R. Lowry · G. Tao

Part 2.7 Sensory and Musculoskeletal **1699**

99   Burden of Disease and Years Lived with Disability Associated with Musculoskeletal Pain 1701
M. Suka · K. Yoshida

100   Financial Burdens and Disability-Adjusted Life Years in Loss of Vision Due to Trachoma 1717
K. D. Frick

101   The Economic Burden of Rheumatoid Arthritis: Asia/Thailand Perspective 1733
M. Osiri · A. Maetzel

Part 3 Quality of Life Measures and Indices **1751**

Part 3.1 General Aspects, Pathologies and Metabolic Disorders **1751**

102   Quality of Life-Related Concepts: Theoretical and Practical Issues 1753
A. A. J. Wismeijer · A. J. J. M. Vingerhoets · J. De Vries

103   Alternative Therapies and Quality of Life 1767
J. X. Zhang

104   Leisure-Time Physical Activity and Quality of Life 1781
A. Vuillemin

105   Spa Therapy and Quality of Life 1799
G. Blasche

106   Health-Related Quality of Life and Prioritization Strategies in Waiting Lists: Spanish Aspects 1811
M. Núñez · E. Núñez · J. M. Segur

107   **Hirsutism and Quality of Life** 1825
       S. Davies

108   **Oral Health-Related Quality of Life** 1839
       U. Schütte · M. Walter

109   **Quality of Life Issues in Chronic Fatigue Syndrome** 1855
       P. G. McKay · C. R. Martin

110   **Hemoglobin Fluctuations and Correlation with Quality of Life and
       Fatigue** 1867
       G. Caocci · R. Baccoli · G. La Nasa

111   **Anemia and Quality of Life: Association with Diagnosis and
       Treatment of Anemias** 1881
       D. R. Thomas

112   **Quality of Life in Hemophilia** 1895
       S. V. Mackensen · A Gringeri

113   **Quality of Life in Amenorrhea and Oligomenorrhea** 1921
       William W. K. To

114   **Quality of Life Among Japanese Oral Contraceptive Users** 1937
       Y. Matsumoto · S. Yamabe · K. Ideta

115   **Premenstrual Syndrome and Premenstrual Dysphoric Disorder:
       Issues of Quality of Life, Stress and Exercise** .1951
       M. Kathleen B. Lustyk · W. G. Gerrish

116   **Quality of Life and Infertility** 1977
       A. Montazeri

117   **Speech Determines Quality of Life Following Total Laryngectomy:
       The Emperors New Voice?** 1989
       P. Farrand · R. Endacott

118   **Health-Related Quality of Life of Living Kidney Donors** 2003
       Ja Hyeon Ku · Hyeon Hoe Kim

119   **Quality of Life and Tryptophan Degradation** .2027
       *D. Fuchs · K. Schroecksnadel · G. Neurauter · R. Bellmann-Weiler ·
       M. Ledochowski · G. Weiss*

120   **ʟ-Carnitine Supplementation on Quality of Life and Other Health
       Measures** 2047
       G. Mantovani · A. Macciò · C. Madeddu · G. Gramignano

121   Quality of Life Among Diabetic Subjects: Indian Perspectives 2071
K. Vijayakumar · R. T. Varghese

122   Healthy Lifestyle Habits and Health-Related Quality of Life in
Diabetes 2095
C. Li · E. S. Ford

123   Quality of Life in Patients with Diabetic Foot Ulcers 2115
L. Ribu

124   Obstructive Sleep Apnea Hypopnea Syndrome and Quality of Life 2135
M. Hirshkowitz · A. Sharafkhaneh · H. Sharafkhaneh

125   Quality of Life and Pruritus 2151
J. C. Szepietowski · A. Reich

126   Quality of Life and Costs in Atopic Dermatitis .2163
R. J. G. Arnold · R. K. Kuan

127   Quality of Life in Crohn's Disease 2183
S. D. Wexner · J. C. Frattini

128   Impact of Self-Perceived Bothersomeness, Quality of Life and
Overactive Bladder 2195
Ja Hyeon Ku · Soo Woong Kim

129   Quality of Life in Men with Chronic Prostatitis/Chronic Pelvic Pain
Syndrome 2211
D. A. Tripp · J. C. Nickel

130   Quality of Life in Kidney Transplantation 2227
M. Veroux · D. Corona · V. B. Patel · P. Veroux

131   Quality of Life in Liver Cirrhosis 2239
E. Kalaitzakis

Volume 4

Part 3.2 Surgical 2255

132   Quality of Life and Functional Outcome in Pediatric Patients
Requiring Surgery: Italian Perspectives 2257
M. Castagnetti

133   Breast Reduction Surgery and Quality of Life and Clinical Outcomes . . .2271
A. Thoma · L. McKnight

134   Quality of Life and Postoperative Anesthesia in Gastrointestinal Surgery 2287
R. Kennelly · A. M. Hogan · J. F. Boylan · D. C. Winter

135   Health-Related Quality of Life After Surgery for Crohn's Disease 2305
M. Scarpa · I. Angriman

136   Postoperative Quality of Life Assessment in the Over 80's After Cardiac Surgery 2319
Christoph H. Huber

137   Quality of Life and Financial Measures in Surgical and Non-Surgical Treatments in Emphysema 2335
J. D. Miller · F. Altaf

138   Quality of Life After Revascularization and Major Amputation for Lower Extremity Arterial Disease 2353
M. Deneuville

139   Quality of Life After Laser Surgery for Eye Disorders 2379
K. Pesudovs · D. B. Elliott

Part 3.3 Early Life Stages and Aging 2395

140   Intrauterine Growth Restriction and Later Quality of Life 2397
D. Spence

141   Assessment of Quality of Life During Pregnancy and in the Postnatal Period 2411
C. R. Martin · J. Jomeen

142   Generic Quality of Life Measures for Children and Adolescents 2423
K. J. Zullig · M. R. Matthews · R. Gilman · R. F. Valois · E. S. Huebner

143   Quality of Life in Children with Cerebral Palsy 2453
A. Aran

144   Quality of Life Measures in Children with Cancer 2469
C. H. Yeh · Y.-P. Kung · Y.-C. Chiang

145   Quality of Life in Healthy and Chronically Ill Icelandic Children: Agreement Between Child's Self-Report and Parents' Proxy-Report 2483
E. K. Svavarsdottir

146   Health-Related Quality of Life in Obese Children and Adolescents 2503
M. de Beer · R. J. B. J. Gemke

147 Implementing Interventions to Enhance Quality of Life in
Overweight Children and Adolescents 2517
J. Lamanna · N. Kelly · M. Stern · S. E. Mazzeo

148 Adolescent Quality of Life in Australia 2537
A. H. Lee · L. B. Meuleners · M. L. Fraser

149 Health-Related Quality of Life Among University Students...........2555
M. Vaez · M. Voss · L. Laflamme

150 The Quality of Life and the Impact of Interventions on the Health
Outcomes of Looked After and Accommodated Young People........2579
D. Carroll · C. R. Martin

151 Quality of Life Measures During the Menopause 2593
G. D. Mishra · D. Kuh

152 Low Testosterone Level in Men and Quality of Life 2615
S. Horie

153 Measuring Quality of Life in Macular Degeneration 2633
J. Mitchell · C. Bradley

154 Quality of Life Measures in the Elderly and Later Life..............2649
S. Evans

155 Cochlear Implant Outcomes and Quality of Life in the Elderly 2667
S. R. Saeed · D. J. Mawman

156 Back Pain and Quality of Life in Elderly Women 2675
K. Zhu · R. L. Prince

157 Measuring Quality of Life at the End of Life 2687
L. A. Roscoe · D. D. Schocken

158 Quality of Life Measures in the Elderly and the Role of Social
Support in Elderly Chinese 2705
L. Zhang · R. Hunter · C. Shao

159 Quality of Life in Elderly Dyspnea Patients 2725
A. Hooshiaran · F. van der Horst · G. Wesseling · J. J. M. H. Strik · J. A. Knottnerus ·
A. Gorgels · A. Fastenau · M. van den Akker · J. W. M. Muris

160 Quality of Life and Age Urinary Incontinence Severity: Turkish
Perspectives 2745
T. M. Filiz · P. Topsever

161   Quality of Life Measures in Elderly Patients with Chronic Obstructive
      Pulmonary Disease: Japanese Perspectives 2759
      K. Kida · T. Motegi · T. Ishii · K. Yamada

Part 3.4 Cancer 2779

162   Chemotherapy for Brain Metastasis and Quality of Life 2781
      R. Addeo · G. Cimmino · S. D. Prete

163   Quality of Life Measures in Patients with Esophageal Cancer 2795
      R. Parameswaran · J. C. Clifton · J. M. Blazeby

164   Quality of Life Measures in Head and Neck Cancer 2809
      C. D. Llewellyn

165   Quality of Life in Breast Cancer Patients: An Overview of
      the Literature 2829
      A. Montazeri

166   Quality of Life with Localized Prostate Cancer: Japanese
      Perspectives 2857
      S. Namiki · L. Kwan · Y. Arai

167   Quality of Life in Men Undergoing Radical Prostatectomy for
      Prostate Cancer 2875
      M. Pearson · E. M. Wallen · R. S. Pruthi

168   Myeloproliferative Disorders and the Chronic Leukemias: Symptom
      Burden and Impact in Quality of Life 2887
      R. A. Mesa · D. P. Steensma · T. Shanafelt

169   Quality of Life in Advanced Renal Cell Carcinoma: Effect of
      Treatment with Cytokine Therapy and Targeted Agents 2905
      S. Shah · K. Gondek

170   Quality of Life for Patients Receiving Cancer Chemotherapy:
      The Japanese Perspective 2923
      H. Uramoto · J. Tsukada

171   Quality of Life Measures in Caregivers of Patients with Cancer 2935
      E. K. Grov · A. A. Dahl

172   Cancer: Influence of Nutrition on Quality of Life 2947
      M. M. Marín Caro · C. Pichard

Volume 5

Part 3.5 Cardiovascular and Pulmonary 2965

173   Quality of Life, Drugs and Diet in Hypertensive Patients 2967
      H. G. Kirpizidis

174   Measurement Issues in the Assessment of Quality of Life in Patients
      with Coronary Heart Disease 2987
      D. R. Thompson · C. R. Martin

175   Influence of Age, Sex and Episode Recurrence on Quality of Life in
      Atrial Fibrillation 2999
      M. R. Reynolds · A. S. Fein

176   Quality of Life Measures in Acute Coronary Syndromes:
      The Evaluation of Predictors in this Field of Research 3015
      R. Coelho · J. Prata

177   Home Mechanical Ventilation and Quality of Life Measures 3035
      J. L. López-Campos · W. Windisch · I. Failde

178   Quality of Life in Children with Asthma 3055
      M. L. Marsac

179   Efficacy of Environmental Interventions on Asthma-Related
      Quality of Life 3073
      J. E. Clougherty

180   Chronic Obstructive Pulmonary Disease, Lung Function and
      Quality of Life in Adult Chinese 3085
      G. Xie · A. Paice · Y. Wu

Part 3.6 Dietary and Nutritional 3097

181   Health-Related Quality of Life in Eating Disorders 3099
      C. Las Hayas · J. Á. Padierna · P. Muñoz

182   Weight-Related Stigmatization: Effects on the Quality of Life of
      Obese Adolescents 3137
      N. R. Kelly · R. W. Gow · M. Stern · S. E. Mazzeo

183   Malnutrition in Chronic Kidney Disease and Relationship to
      Quality of Life 3159
      B. Kalender

184   Nutrition and Quality of Life in Hemodialysis – the Impact of
       Nutritional Status and Quality of Life on Morbidity and Mortality
       in Hemodialysis Patients 3171
       B. Feldt-Rasmussen · T. A. Ikizler · K. Kalantar-Zadeh · J. D. Kopple

185   Nutritional Wasting in Cancer and Quality of Life: The Value of Early
       Individualized Nutritional Counseling 3189
       P. Ravasco · I. M. Grillo · M. Camilo

Part 3.7 Immune Disorders, Viral, Bacterial,
          Microbiological, Infectious and Parasitic
          Diseases 3205

186   Quality of Life Measures in HIV Low Income Women: How to Use
       Quality of Life to Design, Implement and Evaluate Programs 3207
       K. A. McDonnell

187   Quality of Life and Financial Measures in HIV/AIDS in
       Southern Africa 3223
       M. O. Bachmann · G. Louwagie · L. R. Fairall

188   Quality of Life in Immune Thrombocytopenic Purpura: China
       Perspectives 3245
       R. Yang · Z. Zhou

189   Health-Related Quality of Life in Adults with Systemic Lupus
       Erythematosus 3261
       L-S. Teh · K. McElhone · J. Abbott

190   Translation, Cultural Adaptation and Validation of Health-Related
       Quality of Life Assessment Tools: A Brazilian Perspective on
       Patients with Systemic Lupus Erythematosus 3281
       E. A. M. Freire · R. M. Ciconelli

191   Cognitive Function, Mood and Health-Related Quality of Life in
       Hepatitis C Virus-Infected Individuals 3299
       Hla-Hla Thein · G. J. Dore

192   Quality of Life in Urticaria 3327
       M. Özkan · S. Özkan · N. Kocaman Yildirim

193   Quality of Life in Group-Based Intervention Program in Inflammatory
       Bowel Disease 3339
       L. Oxelmark

Part 3.8 Psychosocial, Social, Behavioural, Psychiatric, Neurological and Addictions 3361

194 Housing and Quality of Life: An Ecological Perspective 3363
G. Nelson · S. Saegert

195 Quality of Life of Urban Slum Residents 3383
T. Izutsu · A. Tsutsumi

196 Quality of Life and Chronic Illness among Refugee Populations 3397
R. T. Mikolajczyk · A. E. Maxwell · A. Eljedi

197 Health-Related Quality of Life in Prisoners 3413
G. J. Dore

198 Quality of Life in War Veterans 3425
N. Shamspour · S. Assari

199 Post-Traumatic Stress Disorder and Quality of Life in Women 3439
C. S. Rodgers · C. B. Allard · P. Wansley

200 Relation Between Sexuality and Health-Related Quality of Life 3457
N. Shamspour · S. Assari · M. Moghana Lankarani

201 The Correlations Between the Presence of Comorbidities, Psychological Distress and Health-Related Quality of Life 3475
M. Ekici · A. Ekici

202 Quality of Life and Stigma 3489
A. Tsutsumi · T. Izutsu

203 Depressive Symptoms and Health-Related Quality of Life 3501
A. A. Dan · Z. M. Younossi

204 Quality of Life and Depression in Patient-Giver Scenarios: Reference to Amyotrophic Lateral Sclerosis 3511
A. Chiò

205 Quality of Life and Depression in Police Officers: Perspectives from Chinese in Taiwan 3541
F. H.-C Chou · M.-H. Kuo · K.-Y. Tsai

206 Health-Related Quality of Life in Obsessive-Compulsive Disorder Subjects and their Relatives [1]: Overview 3557
U. Albert · G. Maina · F. Bogetto

207   Health-Related Quality of Life in Obsessive-Compulsive Disorder
      Subjects and Their Relatives [2]: A Systematic Review and Original
      Data of Assessment of Quality of Life Measured by WHOQOL-BREF 3579
      K. Stengler

208   Quality of Life in Bipolar Disorder 3591
      B. M. Cardoso · V. V. Dias · B. N. Frey · F. K. Gazalle · F. Kapczinski ·
      M. Kauer-Sant'Anna · A. R. Rosa · J. C. Walz

209   Issues in Quality of Life Assessment in Schizophrenia 3607
      C. R. Martin · M. Fleming

210   Health-Related Quality of Life in Parents of Children with Asperger
      Syndrome and High-Functioning Autism 3625
      H. Allik · J.-O. Larsson · H. Smedje

211   Quality of Life and Neuropsychological Symptoms in Primary
      Hyperparathyroidism 3643
      T. Weber · M. Keller

212   Children with Cerebral Palsy, Psychometric Analysis and Quality
      of Life 3657
      E. Davis · E. Waters

213   Quality of Life in Dementia Patients and Their Proxies: A Narrative
      Review of the Concept and Measurement Scales 3671
      C. J. M. Schölzel-Dorenbos · P. F. M. Krabbe · M. G. M. Olde Rikkert

Volume 6

214   Quality of Life and Drug Abuse 3691
      S. Assari · M. Jafari

215   Quality of Life in HIV Positive Injecting Drug Users 3705
      M. Préau · A. D. Bouhnik · M. P. Carrieri · F. M. B. Spire

216   Quality of Life Measurement and Alcoholism: A Nursing Perspective . . . 3727
      J. H. Foster

217   Quality of Life and Psychiatric Symptomatology in Alcohol
      Detoxification 3747
      M. Ginieri-Coccossis · I. A. Liappas

218   Quality of Life in Patients Affected by Multiple Sclerosis:
      A Systematic Review 3769
      F. Patti · A. Pappalardo

219 Quality of Life in People with Lower-Limb Amputation 3785
     D. Desmond · P. Gallagher

220 Quality of Life in Spinal Cord Injury 3797
     B. Celik

221 Quality of Life in Sporadic Adult-Onset Ataxia 3809
     M. Abele

222 Quality of Life in Systemic Sclerosis 3823
     L. Mouthon · F. Rannou · A. Berezné · S. Poiraudeau

223 Quality of Life in Toenail Onychomycosis 3837
     A. Reich · J. C. Szepietowski

Part 3.9 Sensory, Musculoskeletal and Exercise 3851

224 Quality of Life Measures in the Deaf 3853
     J. Fellinger · D. Holzinger · J. Gerich · D. Goldberg

225 Hearing Aids and Quality of Life 3871
     C. E. Johnson · J. L. Danhauer

226 Cochlear Implantation and Quality of Life in Deafness 3887
     G. W. J. A. Damen · E. A. M. Mylanus · A. F. M. Snik

227 Quality of Life Measures for the Visually Impaired:
     Sub-Sahara Africa 3905
     A. Leplege · J.-F. Schemann

228 Health-Related Quality of Life in Pain Medicine: A Review of Theory
     and Practice 3917
     T. R. Vetter

229 Relationship Between Pain and Quality of Life 3933
     M. Azizabadi Farahani · S. Assari

230 Quality of Life in Ankylosing Spondylitis and Undifferentiated
     Spondyloarthropathy: Chinese Perspectives 3955
     J. R. Gu · Z. T. Liao · Z. M. Lin · R. Srirajaskanthan

231 Quality of Life Measures in Fibromyalgia 3965
     N. Gusi · Pedro R. Olivares · J. Carmelo Adsuar · A. Paice · P. Tomas-Carus

232 Quality of Life and Low Back Pain 3979
     A. Montazeri · S. J. Mousavi

233   **Disease Burden, Quality of Life and Other Measures in Polymyalgia Rheumatica** 3995
B. Dasgupta · H. M.-Kremers · E. L. Mattesson

234   **Health-Related Quality of Life in Movement Disorders** 4013
R. Dodel · A. Schrag

235   **Quality of Life Measures in Lower Limb Ischaemia** 4035
F. A. K. Mazari · T. A. Mehta · I. C. Chetter

236   **Quality of Life among Primary Caregivers of Rheumatic Patients – a South American Experience** 4053
F. Jennings · A. Jones · J. Natour

237   **Quality of Life in Conservatively Treated Lumbar Disc Disease** 4071
C. Schneider · M. Hefti · H. Landolt

238   **Quality of Life and Stress in Wheelchair-Users** 4087
M. Furlong · J. Connor

239   **Exercise and Quality of Life in Menopause** 4103
A. J. Daley · H. Stokes-Lampard · C. MacArthur

240   **Exercise and Quality of Life in COPD** 4119
J. A. Alison · Z. J. McKeough

Glossary 4133
Index 4357

Contributors

Janice Abbott
University of Central Lancashire, Preston
UK

Michael Abele
Department of Neurology
University of Bonn, Bonn
Germany

Raffaele Addeo
Oncology Unit, "S. Giovanni di Dio"
HospitaL, Frattaminore Naples
Italy

J. Carmelo Adsuar
University of Extremadura, Caceres
Spain

Marjan van den Akker
Department of General Practice, School for
Public Health and Primary Care: Caphri
Maastricht University, Maastricht
The Netherlands

Umberto Albert
Mood and Anxiety Disorders Unit
Department of Neurosciences
University of Turin, Torino
Italy

Jennifer A. Alison
Discipline of Physiotherapy, Faculty of
Health Sciences, The University of Sydney
NSW
Australia

Carolyn B. Allard
VA San Diego Healthcare System,
Department of Psychiatry,
University of California, San Diego,
CA
USA

Hiie Allik
Department of Woman and Child Health
Karolinska Institute, Child and Adolescent

Psychiatric Unit, Stockholm
Sweden

David B. Allison
Department of Biostatistics, University of
Alabama at Birmingham, UAB Station
USA

Fawaz Altaf
McMaster University, Ancaster, ON
Canada

Imerio Angriman
Department of Surgical and
Gastroenterological Science
University of Padova
Italy

Yoichi Arai
David Geffen School of Medicine (SN, YA)
Jonsson Comprehensive Cancer Center
University of California
Los Angeles (LK)
USA

Adi Aran
Shaare Zedek Medical Center
Neuropediatric Unit, Jerusalem
Israel

Zeyneo Armay
Department of Consultation Liaison
Psychiatry, University of Istanbul, Istanbul
Turkey

Renée J. G. Arnold
Department of Community and Preventive
Medicine, Mount Sinai School of Medicine,
Arnold Consultancy & Technology LLC,
New York, NY
USA

Shervin Assari
Psychology and Psychiatry Research
Department, Medicine and Health
Promotion Institute, Baqiyatallah University
of Medical Sciences, Tehran
Iran

Roberto Baccoli
Engineering and Territory Development
Physical Technical Institute
University of Cagliari
Cagliari
Italy

Max O. Bachmann
School of Medicine, Health Policy and
Practice, University of East Anglia
Norwich
UK

Xavier Badia
Health Economics and Outcomes Research
IMS Health
Spain

Enzo Ballatori
Biostatistician Freelance, AP
Italy

Limaris Barrios
Beth Israel Deaconess Medical Center
Boston, MA
USA

Stefano Di Bartolomeo
Cattedra di Igiene ed Epidemiologia –
Universitá degli Studi di Udine
Udine
Italy

Mark E. Beatty
Pediatric Dengue Vaccine Initiative
International Vaccine Institute, Seoul
Korea

Marieke de Beer
Department of Pediatrics, VU University
Medical Center, Amsterdam
The Netherlands

Rosa Bellmann-Weiler
Department of Internal Medicine
Innsbruck Medical University, Innsbruck
Austria

Alice Berezné
Department of Internal Medicine, Paris
Descartes University, Reference Center for
Necrotizing Vasculitides and Systemic
Sclerosis, Cochin Hospital, Assistance
Publique-Hôpitaux de Paris (AP-HP), Paris
France

Philippe Beutels
Center for Health Economics Research and
Modeling of Infectious Diseases (CHERMID)
Center for the Evaluation of
Vaccination (CEV), (WHO Collaborating
Center) Vaccine & Infectious Disease
Institute (VAXINFECTIO)
Antwerp University, Wilrijk (Antwerp)
Belgium

Madhumita Bhattacharjee
Lilavati Hospital, L. K. M. M. Trust Research
Centre, Bandra Reclamation, Mumbai
India

Joke Bilcke
Center for Health Economics Research and
Modeling of Infectious Diseases (CHERMID)
Center for the Evaluation of Vaccination (CEV),
Vaccine & Infectious Disease Institute
(VAXINFECTIO)
Antwerp University, Wilrijk (Antwerp)
Belgium

John Billimek
Center for Health Policy Research
University of California, Irvine, CA
USA

Vesna Bjegović
Institute of Social Medicine, School of
Medicine, University of Belgrade, Belgrade
Serbia

Gerhard Blasche
Department of Physiology, Centre of
Physiology and Pathophysiology
Medical University of Vienna, Vienna
Austria

Jane M. Blazeby
Department of Social Medicine, University
of Bristol, Bristol
UK

Marleen Boelaert
Epidemiology and Disease Control Unit
Institute of Tropical Medicine
Antwerp
Belgium

Filippo Bogetto
Mood and Anxiety Disorders Unit
Department of Neurosciences, University of
Turin
Italy

Jasper Bos
Associate Director, Merch Serono Ventures
Geneva
Switzerland

Robert M. Bossarte
Department of Psychiatry, University
Rochester, Rochester, NY
USA

Anne-Déborah Bouhnik
Southeastern Health Regional Observatory
(ORS-PACA), Research Unit UMR912,
Economic & Social Sciences Health
Systems & Societies, INSERM Marseille
France and IRD, Aix Marseille Université,
Marseille
France

Sami Boussetta
Departement Pharmaco-Economique
Pierre Fabre SA, Boulogne-sur-Seine
France

Abdesslam Boutayeb
University Mohamed Ier Oujda
Morocco

John F. Boylan
Institute for Clinical Outcomes Research
and Education (iCORE), St. Vincent's
University Hospital, Dublin
Ireland

Clare Bradley
Department of Psychology,
Royal Holloway, University of London
Surrey
UK

Freddie I. Bray
Department of Clinical- and Registry-Based
Research, Cancer Registry of Norway
Montebello, Oslo
Norway

Alex D. Brown
Centre for Indigenous Vascular and
Diabetes Research, Baker IDI Heart &
Diabetes Institute, NT
Australia

Anna A. Bruno
Dip. di Riabilitazione, Ospedale 'S
Salvatore' L'Aquila
Italy

Ljiljana B. Bumbasirevic
Institute of Neurology, Clinical Centre of
Serbia, Belgrade
Serbia

Neil Burnet
Department of Oncology, University of
Cambridge, Cambridge
UK

Dominique A. Cadilhac
National Stroke Research Institute
Heidelberg Heights, Vic
Australia

Laura Camfield
Department of International Development
Young Lives Research Group
Oxford
UK

Maria Camilo
Unidade de Nutrição e Metabolismo
Instituto de Medicina Molecular
Faculdade de Medicina da Universidade
de Lisboa
Portugal

Giovanni Caocci
Bone Marrow Transplant Centre
R. Binaghi Hospital University of Cagliari
Cagliari
Italy

Betina M. Cardoso
Alameda Victor Adalberto Kessler
Porto Alegre-RS
Brasil

J. Jaime Caro
Health Care Analytics
United BioSource Corporation
Lexington, MA
USA

Marie P. Carrieri
Research Unit "Economic & Social Sciences
Health Systems & Societies", Marseille
France and IRD, Aix Marseille Université
Marseille
France

Denise Carroll
Kibble Care and Education Centre
Paisley
Scotland

Marco Castagnetti
Section of Paediatric Urology, Urology Unit
Department of Oncological and Surgical
Sciences, University Hospital of Padova
Padua
Italy

Berna Celik
Department of Physical Medicine and
Rehabilitation, Istanbul Physical Medicine
Rehabilitation Teaching and Research
Hospital, Bahcelievler – Istanbul
Turkey

Kow-Tong Chen
Department of Public Health, College of
Medicine, National Cheng Kung University
Tainan
Taiwan

Ian C. Chetter
Academic Vascular Surgical Unit, Hull
UK

Yi-Chien Chiang
Department of Nursing, Chang Gung
Institute of Technology, Tao Yuen
Taiwan

Adriano Chio
Department of Neuroscience, ALS Center
University of Torino, Torino
Italy

Frank Chou
Department of Community Psychiatry
Kai-Suan Psychiatric Hospital, Kaohsiung
Taiwan

Rozana M. Ciconelli
Department of Medicine, Universidade
Federal de São Paulo
São Paulo
Brazil

Alarcos A. Cieza
ICF Research Branch of WHO FIC CC
(DIMDI), IHRS, Ludwig Maximilian
University, Munich, München
Germany

Gaetano Cimmino
Surgery Unit, "S. Giovanni di Dio" Hospital
Frattaminore, Naples
Italy

Cynthia A. Claassen
Department of Psychiatry, The University of
Texas Southwestern Medical Center, Dallas
TX
USA

John D. Clemens
International Vaccine Institute, Kwanak-ku
Seoul
Republic of Korea

Joanne C. Clifton
Department of Surgery, Division of
Thoracic Surgery, University of British
Columbia, British Columbia
Canada

Jane E. Clougherty
Department of Environmental Health
Harvard School of Public Health, Boston, MA
USA

Rui Coelho
Department of Psychiatry, Hospital de São
João, Porto
Portugal

Joshua A. Cohn
University of Michigan Health System
Ann Arbor, MI
USA

Marisol Concha-Barrientos
Health Department, Asociación Chilena de
Seguridad, Santiago
Chile

Jason Connor
Discipline of Psychiatry, The University of
Queensland, Mental Health Centre, Royal
Brisbane and Women's Hospital, Herston
QLD
Australia

Annette Conrads-Frank
Department of Public Health, Information
Systems and Health Technology
Assessment, UMIT - University for Health
Sciences, Medical Informatics and
Technology and ONCOTYROL Center for
Personalized Cancer Medicine
Hall i.T./Innsbruck
Austria

Daniela Corona
Organ Transplant Unit, Department of
Surgery, Transplantation and Advanced
Technologies, University Hospital of
Catania
Italy

Linda Crossett
Division of Adolescent and School Health
National Center for Chronic Disease
Prevention and Health Promotion
Centers for Disease Control and Prevention
Atlanta, GA
USA

Alv A. Dahl
The Norwegian Radium Hospital
Oslo University Hospital
Rikshospitalet, Oslo
Norway

Praful M. Dalal
Lilavati Hospital, L. K. M. M. Trust Research
Centre, Bandra Reclamation, Mumbai
India

Amanda J. Daley
Primary Care Clinical Sciences, School of
Health and Population Sciences
University of Birmingham
UK

Godelieve W. J. A. Damen
Department of Otorhinolaryngology
University Medical Centre Sint Radboud
Nijmegen
The Netherlands

Pierre Van Damme
Center for the Evaluation of Vaccination
(CEV), (WHO Collaborating Center)
Vaccine & Infectious Disease Institute
(VAXINFECTIO)
Antwerp University, Wilrijk (Antwerp)
Belgium

Amy A. Dan
Michigan State University, Environmental
Science and Policy Program
East Lansing, MI
USA

Jeffrey L. Danhauer
Department of Speech and Hearing
Sciences, University of California Santa
Barbara, Santa Barbara, CA
USA

Bhaskar Dasgupta
Department of Rheumatology, Southend
University Hospital, Essex
UK

Shan Davies
Institute of Health Research, School of
Health Science, Swansea University
Singleton Park, Swansea, Wales
UK

Elise Davis
McCaughey Centre, VicHealth Centre for
the Promotion of Mental Health and
Community Wellbeing, School of
Population Health, University of
Melbourne, VIC
Australia

Michel Deneuville
Service de Chirurgie Vasculaire et
Thoracique, University Hospital (CHU de
Pointe-à-Pitre-Abymes), Guadeloupe
French West Indies

Anne V. Denison
Texas Tech University Health Sciences
Center, Amarillo, TX
USA

Deirdre Desmond
Department of Psychology, National
University of Ireland Maynooth, Maynooth
Ireland

Misha Dewan
Drexel University College of Medicine,
Philadelphia, PA
USA

Vasco V. Dias
Bipolar Disorders Program and Molecular
Psychiatry Unit, Hospital de Clínicas
Federal University, UFRGS, Porto Alegre
Brazil
and

Bipolar Disorders Research Program,
Hospital Santa Maria, Faculty of Medicine,
University of Lisbon, (FMUL)
Portugal

Ding Ding
Department of Biostatistics and
Epidemiology, Institute of Neurology
Fudan University, WHO Collaborating
Center for Research and Training in
Neurosciences
Shanghai
China

Richard Dodel
Department of Neurology
Philipps-University Marburg, Marburg
Germany

Gregory J. Dore
National Centre in HIV Epidemiology and
Clinical Research, The University of
New South Wales, Darlinghurst
NSW
Australia

Shahul H. Ebrahim
Centers for Disease Control and
Prevention, US Department of Health and
Human Services, Atlanta, GA
USA

Aydanur Ekici
Department of Chest Diseases, Kirikkale
University, Kirikkale
Turkey

Mehmet Ekici
Department of Chest Diseases, Kirikkale
University, Kirikkale
Turkey

Ashraf Eljedi
School of Nursing, The Islamic University of
GazaGaza, Gaza Strip
Palestinian Territories

David B. Elliott
Bradford School of Optometry, University
of Bradford, Bradford, West Yorkshire
UK

Donald A. Enarson
International Union against Tuberculosis
and Lung Disease, Paris
France

Ruth Endacott
School of Nursing and Community Studies
University of Plymouth, Drake Circus
Plymouth
UK

Charles C. Engel
Department of Psychiatry Chief
Deployment Health Clinical Center, Walter
Reed Army Medical Center, Uniformed
Services University of the Health Sciences
Bethesda, MD
USA

Michael J. Englesbe
University of Michigan Health System, Ann
Arbor, MI
USA

Sherrill Evans
Centre for Social Work and Social Care
Research, School of Human Sciences
Swansea University, Singleton Park
Swansea
UK

Immaculade Failde
Area de Medicina Preventiva y Salud
Pública. E.U. Ciencias de la Salud
Universidad de Cadiz, Cadiz
Spain

Lara R. Fairall
Knowledge Translation Unit, University of
Cape Town Lung Institute and Department
of Medicine, University of Cape Town
Cape Town
South Africa

Mahdi A. Farahani
Clinical Research Department, Medicine
and Health Promotion Institute
Baqiyatallah University of Medical Sciences
Tehran
Iran

Paul Farrand
School of Psychology
University of Exeter, Exeter
UK

Jeremy Farrar
Hospital for Tropical Diseases, Oxford
University's Clinical Research Unit, Ho Chi
Minh City
Vietnam

Annemieke Fastenau
Department of General Practice, School for
Public Health and Primary Care: Caphri
Maastricht University, Maastricht
The Netherlands

Talitha Feenstra
Netherlands Institute for Public Health and
the Environment, Bilthoven
The Netherlands

Adam S. Fein
Beth Israel Deaconees Medical Center
Boston, MA
USA

Bo Feldt-Rasmussen
Division of Nephrology, Rigshospitalet
University of Copenhagen, Copenhagen
Denmark

Johannes Fellinger
Health Centre for the Deaf
Hospital St. John of God, Linz
Austria

Jacques Ferlay
Descriptive Epidemiology, Data Analysis
and Interpretation Group, International
Agency for Research on Cancer, Lyon
France

Eric M. Fèvre
Ashworth Laboratories, Centre for
Infectious, Diseases and Centre for
Infection, Immunity and Evolution
University of Edinburgh, Edinburgh
UK

Jonathan E. Fielding
Los Angeles County Department of Public
Health, Los Angeles, CA
USA

Tuncay M. Filiz
Department of Family Medicine, Kocaeli
University, Kocaeli
Turkey

Mick Fleming
Department of Health Sciences, University
of York, York
UK

Kevin R. Fontaine
Johns Hopkins University, Baltimore, MD
USA

Earl S. Ford
Behavioral Surveillance Branch, Division of
Adult and Community Health
National Center for Chronic Disease
Prevention and Health Promotion
Centers for Disease Control and Prevention
Atlanta, GA
USA

John H. Foster
Department of Health and Social Sciences
Archway Campus, Middlesex University
London
UK

Michelle L. Fraser
School of Public Health, Curtin University
of Technology, Perth, WA
Australia

Jared C. Frattini
Department of Colorectal Surgery
Cleveland Clinic Florida
Weston, FL
USA

Michael C. Freed
Deployment Health Clinical Center
Department of Psychiatry
Uniformed Services, University of the
Health Sciences Walter Reed Army
Medical Center
Washington, DC
USA

Eutilia A. M. Freire
Department of Internal Medicine
Universidade Federal da Paraíba, Paraíba
Brazil

Benicio N. Frey
Department of Psychiatry and Behavioural
Neurosciences
McMaster University, Hamilton, ON
Canada

Kevin D. Frick
Johns Hopkins Bloomberg School of Public
Health, Baltimore, MD
USA

Dietmas Fuchs
Division of Biological Chemistry, Biocenter
Innsbruck Medical University, Innsbruck
Austria

Michele Furlong
Diabetes and Endocrinology Unit, Princess
Alexandra Hospital, QLD
Australia

Seana L. Gall
Menzies Research Institute, Hobart
TAS
Australia

Pamela Gallagher
School of Nursing, Dublin City University
Dublin
Ireland

Fernando K. Gazalle
Bipolar Disorders Program and Laboratory
of Molecular Psychiatry
Hospital de Clínicas de Porto Alegre
Brazil
and
INCT Translational Medicine

Reinoud J. B. J. Gemke
Department of Pediatrics, VU University
Medical Center, Amsterdam
The Netherlands

Joachim Gerich
Department of Sociology, unit for empirical
social research, Johannes Kepler University
Linz
Austria

Winslow G. Gerrish
Department of Clinical Psychology
School of Psychology, Family and
Community, Seattle Pacific University
Seattle, WA
USA

Montserrat Gilabert
Novartis Oncology
Spain

Rich Gilman
Psychology and Special Education
Programs, Division of Developmental and
Behavioral Pediatrics, Cincinnati Children's
Hospital Medical Center
Department of General Pediatrics
University of Cincinnati Medical School
Ohio
USA

Maria Ginieri-Coccossis
Eginition Hospital, Department of
Psychiatry, Medical School, University of
Athens
Greece

Ashok K. Giri
Molecular and Human Genetics Division
Indian Institute of Chemical Biology, West
Bengal
India

Zorana Gledovic
Institute of Epidemiology, School of
Medicine, University of Belgrade,
Belgrade
Serbia

Marthe Gold
Department of Community Health and
Social Medicine, Sophie Davis School of
Biomedical Education/CUNY Medical
School, New York, NY
USA

David Goldberg
Institute of Psychiatry, King's College
London
UK

Robert K. Goldberg
Deployment Health Clinical Center
Walter Reed Army Medical Center
Washington, DC
USA

Binh Y. Goldstein
Sexually Transmitted Disease Program
Los Angeles County Department of Health,
Los Angeles, CA
USA

Kathleen Gondek
Global Health Economics, Outcomes and
Reimbursement, Bayer HealthCare
Pharmaceuticals, Montville, NJ
USA

Kristie L. Gore
Deployment Health Clinical Center,
Department of Psychiatry, USUHS Walter
Reed Army Medical Center NW
Washington, DC
USA

Anton Gorgels
Department of Cardiology, Maastricht
University Medical Centre: MUMC
Maastricht University, Maastricht
The Netherlands

Hebe Gouda
Department of Public Health and Primary
Care, Institute of Public Health, Robinson
Way, Cambridge
UK

Rachel W. Gow
Department of Psychology, Virginia
Commonwealth University
Richmond, VA
USA

Giulia Gramignano
Department of Medical Oncology
University of Cagliari, Cagliari
Italy

James A. Greenberg
Department of Health and Nutrition
Sciences, Brooklyn College of the City
University of New York, Brooklyn, NY
USA

Sheldon Greenfield
Center for Health Policy Research
University of California, Irvine, CA
USA

Anita Grgurevic
Institute of Epidemiology, School of
Medicine, University of Belgrade, Belgrade
Serbia

Isabel M. Grillo
Serviço de Radioterapia
Hospital Universitário de Santa Maria
Centro Hospitalar de Lisboa Norte Lisboa
Portugal

Alessandro Gringeri
Angelo Bianchi Bonomi Haemophilia and
Thrombosis Centre, IRCCS Maggiore
Hospital and University of Milan, Milan
Italy

Ellen K. Grov
The Norwegian Radium Hospital
Oslo University Hospital
Rikshospitalet, Oslo
Norway

Jieruo R. Gu
Division of Rheumatology, The Third
Affiliated Hospital of Sun Yat-sen
University, Guangzhou
People's Republic of China

Richard L. Guerrant
Centers for Global Health, University of
Virginia, Charlottesville, Virginia and
Federal University of Ceará, Fortaleza
Brazil

Jean-Jerome Guex
Vascular Medicine & Phlebology, Nice
France

Narcis Gusi
University of Extremadura, Cáceres
Spain

Ellen Guzman
Psychiatry Resident, Thomas Jefferson
University (Jefferson Medical College)
Philadelphia, PA
USA

Carlota Las Hayas
CIBER in Epidemiology and Public Health
Galdakao – Usansolo Hospital, Galdakao
Vizcaya
Spain

Martin Hefti
Department of Neurosurgery
Kantonsspital Aarau, Aarau
Switzerland

Yusuf Hemed
MEASURE Evaluation, Dar Es Salaam
Tanzania

Max Hirshkowitz
VAMC Sleep Center (111-i), Houston, TX
USA

Alex Y. Ho
Office of Health Assessment & Epidemiology
Los Angeles County Department of Public
Health, Los Angeles, CA
USA

Aisling M. Hogan
Institute for Clinical Outcomes Research
and Education (iCORE), St. Vincent's
University Hospital, Dublin
Ireland

Daniel Holzinger
Health Centre for the Deaf Hospital
St. John of God, Bischofstrasse Linz
Austria

Zhen Hong
Department of Biostatistics and
Epidemiology, Institute of Neurology
Fudan University, WHO Collaborating
Center for Research and Training in
Neurosciences, Shanghai
China

Afshin Hooshiaran
Institute for Education, Medical
Programme
Maastricht University, Maastricht
The Netherlands

Shigeo Horie
Department of Urology, Teikyo University
School of Medicine, Tokyo
Japan

Frans van der Horst
Department of General Practice, School for
Public Health and Primary Care: Caphri
Maastricht University, Maastricht
The Netherlands

Christoph H. Huber
Cardiovascular Surgery Division, Centre
Hospitalier Universitaire Vaudois (CHUV)
Lausanne
Switzerland

E. Scott Huebner
Department of Psychology, University of
South Carolina, Columbia, SC
USA

Jing-Shiang Hwang
Institute of Statistical Science, Academia
Sinica, Taipei
Taiwan

Kazuhisa Ideta
Department of International Cooperation
Yodogawa Christian Hospital, Osaka
Japan

T. Alp Ikizler
Vanderbilt University Medical Center
Vanderbilt University School of Medicine
Nashville, TN
USA

Takeo Ishii
Department of Pulmonary Medicine
Infection, and Oncology, Respiratory Care
Clinic, Nippon Medical School, Tokyo
Japan

Nobukatsu Ishikawa
The Research Institute of Tuberculosis
Japan Ant-Tuberculosis Association
Matsuyama, Kiyose, Tokyo
Japan

Takashi Izutsu
Department of Mental Health, Graduate
School of Medicine, The University of
Tokyo, Tokyo
Japan

Kurt M. Jacobson
Department of Cardiovascular Medicine
University of Wisconsin Hospitals & Clinics
Madison, WI
USA

Mehrdad Jafari
Department of studies in Addiction
Medicine and Health Promotion Institute
Tehran
Iran

Hamidreza Jamshidi
University of Shahidbeheshti Medical
Science University, Tehran
Iran

Slavenka Janković
Institute of Epidemiology, School of
Medicine, University of Belgrade
Belgrade
Serbia

Sarah J. Jefferies
Oncology Centre, Addenbrooke's Hospital
Cambridge
UK

Fabio Jennings
Universidade Federal de São Paulo
Rheumatology Division,
São Paulo, SP
Brazil

Haomiao Jia
School of Nursing, Mailman School of
Public Health and School of Nursing
Columbia University,
New York, NY
USA

Ayodele Jimoh
Department of Economics
University of Ilorin, Ilorin,
Kwara State
Nigeria

Carole E. Johnson
Department of Communication Disorders
Auburn University, AL
USA

Julie Jomeen
University of Hull
Hull
UK

Anamaria Jones
Universidade Federal de São Paulo
Rheumatology Division, São Paulo, SP
Brazil

Daniel B. Jones
Harvard Medical School, Beth Israel
Deaconess Medical Center, Boston, MA
USA

Evangelos Kalaitzakis
Section of Gastroenterology and
Hepatology, Department of Internal
Medicine, Sahlgrenska University Hospital
Gothenburg
Sweden

Kamyar Kalantar-Zadeh
Harold Simmons Center for Kidney Disease
Research and Epidemiology
Los Angeles BioMedical Research Institute
at Harbor-UCLA Medical Center, the David
Geffen School of Medicine at UCLA and
the UCLA School of Public Health
Torrance

Betül Kalender
Departments of Nephrology, University of
Kocaeli
Turkey

Flávio Kapczinski
Bipolar Disorders Program and Laboratory
of Molecular Psychiatry
Hospital de Clinicas de
Porto Alegre
Brazil
and
INCT Translational Medicine

Sherrie H. Kaplan
Center for Health Policy Research
University of California
Irvine, CA
USA

Markku Kaste
Department of Neurology
Helsinki University Central Hospital
University of Helsinki, Helsinki
Finland

Marianne Kastrup
Centre for Transcultural Psychiatry
Psychiatric Centre, University Hospital
Copenhagen, Rigshospitalet
Copenhagen
Denmark

Marcia Kauer-Sant'Anna
Bipolar Disorders Program and Laboratory
of Molecular Psychiatry
Hospital de Clinicas de Porto Alegre
Brazil
and
INCT Translational Medicine

Scott W. Keith
Department of Biostatistics
University of Alabama at Birmingham
Birmingham, AL
USA

Monika Keller
Department of Surgery, University Hospital
Steinhoevelstr, Ulm
Germany

Nichole R. Kelly
Department of Psychology, Virginia
Commonwealth University
Richmond, VA
USA

Rory Kennelly
Institute for Clinical Outcomes Research
and Education (iCORE), St. Vincent's
University Hospital,
Dublin
Ireland

Ronald C. Kessler
Department of Health Care Policy
Boston, MA
USA

Mahmud M. Khan
Department of Health Systems
Management, Tulane University
School of Public Health and Tropical
Medicine New Orleans, LA
USA

Kozui Kida
Department of Pulmonary Medicine
Infection, and Oncology, Respiratory Care
Clinic, Nippon Medical School, Tokyo
Japan

Hyeon Hoe Kim
Department of Urology, Seoul National
University College of Medicine, Seoul
National University Hospital Seoul
Korea

Soo Woong Kim
Department of Urology, Seoul National
University College of Medicine
Seoul National University Hospital
Seoul
Korea

Jeffrey C. King
Maternal-Fetal Medicine Department of
Obstetrics, Gynecology & Women's Health
University of Louisville College of Medicine
Louisville, KY
USA

Hristos G. Kirpizidis
Department of Cardiology, Hospital
Thessaloniki
Greece

J. Andre Knottnerus
Department of General Practice, School for
Public Health and Primary Care: Caphri
Maastricht University,
Maastricht
The Netherlands

Nazmiye Kocaman
Department of Psychiatry, Department of
Consultation Liaison Psychiatry, University
of Istanbul, Istanbul Faculty of Medicine
Çapa, Istanbul
Turkey

Nikola Kocev
Institute of Medical Statistics and
Informatics, School of Medicine, University
of Belgrade, Belgrade
Serbia

Gerald F. Kominski
Department of Health Services, UCLA
School of Public Health, Los Angeles, CA
USA

Joel D. Kopple
Division of Nephrology and Hypertension
Los Angeles Biomedical Research Institute
at Harbor-UCLA Medical Center, the David
Geffen School of Medicine at UCLA and
the UCLA School of Public Health,
Torrance, CA
USA

Nenad Kostanjsek
World Health Organization, Classification
Assessment, Surveys and Terminology
(CTS) Team, Geneva
Switzerland

Paul F. M. Krabbe
Multidisciplinary Memory Clinic Slingeland
Hospital/Alzheimer Centre Nijmegen
University Medical Centre Nijmegen
Kruisbergseweg
The Netherlands

Ja Hyeon Ku
Department of Urology, Seoul National
University College of Medicine, Seoul
National University Hospital, Seoul
Korea

Renee K. Kuan
Arnold Consultancy & Technology LLC
New York, NY
USA

Diana Kuh
MRC Unit for Lifelong Health and Ageing
Royal Free and University College
Medical School, Department of
Epidemiology and Public Health London
UK

Yi Ping Kung
School of Nursing, Chang Gung University
Tao Yuen
Taiwan

Ming Hui Kuo
Department of Occupational
Rehabilitation, Kai-Suan Psychiatric
Hospital, Kaohsiung
Taiwan

Lorna Kwan
David Geffen School of Medicine(SN, YA)
Jonsson Comprehensive Cancer Center
University of California, LA
USA

Ulrich Laaser
Section of International Public Health
University of Bielefeld, Bielefeld
Germany

Javier Labbé
Health Department, Association Chilena de
Seguridad, Santiago
Chile

Lucie Laflamme
Department of Public Health Sciences
Division of International Health, Karolinska
Institutet, Stockholm
Sweden

F. Marc LaForce
PATH, Ferney-Voltaire
France

Erin E. Lalor
National Stroke Foundation, Melbourne, Vic
Australia

Cindy L. K. Lam
Family Medicine Unit, the University of
Hong Kong
Hong Kong SAR

Jennifer Lamanna
Department of Psychology, Virginia
Commonwealth University
Richmond, VA
USA

Hans Landolt
Department of Neurosurgery Kantonsspital
Aarau
Switzerland

M. Moghana Lankarani
Department of Psychology and Psychiatry
Medicine and Health Promotion Institute
Tehran
Iran

Christopher T. Lang
Department of Obstetrics and Gynecology
The Ohio State University College of
Medicine
Columbus, OH
USA

Jan Olov Larsson
Department of Woman and Child Health
Karolinska Institute, Child and Adolescent
Psychiatric Unit, Stockholm
Sweden

Maximilian Ledochowski
Division of Nutrition Medicine, Innsbruck
Medical University, Innsbruck
Austria

Andy H. Lee
School of Public Health,
Curtin University of Technology, Perth, WA
Australia

Alain Leplege
Department of Philosophy and History of
Sciences and REHSEIS, University Paris
Diderot,
Paris
France

Beate Lettmeier
Department of Public Health, Information
Systems and Health Technology
Assessment, UMIT - University for Health
Sciences, Medical Informatics and
Technology and ONCOTYROL Center for
Personalized Cancer Medicine
Hall i.T./Innsbruck
Austria

Carol Levin
PATH, Seattle, WA
USA

G. Lewison
School of Library, Archive and Information
Studies, University College London
London
UK

Chaoyang Li
Behavioral Surveillance Branch, Division of
Adult and Community Health, National
Center for Chronic Disease Prevention and
Health Promotion, Centers for Disease
Control and Prevention, Atlanta, GA
USA

Z. T. Liao
Division of Rheumatology, The Third
Affiliated Hospital of Sun Yat-sen
University, Guangzhou
People's Republic of China

Iannis A. Liappas
Department of Psychiatry, Medical School
University of Athens
Greece

AAM Lima
Centers for Global Health, University of
Virginia, Charlottesville, Virginia and
Federal University of Ceará
Fortaleza
Brazil

Z. M. Lin
Division of Rheumatology, The Third
Affiliated Hospital of Sun Yat-sen
University, Guangzhou
People's Republic of China

Wei Liu
International Vaccine Institute
Kwanak-ku, Seoul
Republic of Korea

Carrie D. Llewellyn
Department of Primary Care & Public
Health, Brighton & Sussex Medical School
Brighton
UK

Jose L. López-Campos
Unidad Médico-Quirúrgica de
Enfermedades Respiratorias, Hospital
Universitario Virgen del Rocío.,
Seville
Spain

Goedele Louwagie
School of Health Systems and Public
Health, University of Pretoria, Pretoria
South Africa

Derek Lowe
Evidence base Practice Research Centre
(EPRC), Edge Hill University
Liverpool, UK

Richard Lowry
Division of Adolescent and School Health
National Center for Chronic Disease
Prevention and Health Promotion
Centers for Disease Control and Prevention
Atlanta, GA
USA

Erica Lubetkin
Department of Community Health and
Social Medicine, Sophie Davis School of
Biomedical Education/CUNY
Medical School
New York, NY
USA

M. Kathleen B. Lustyk
Department of Psychology
School of Psychology, Family and
Community, Seattle Pacific University
Seattle, WA
USA

Pascal Lutumba
Univérsité de Kinshasa
Democratic Republic of Congo

Christine MacArthur
Unit of Public Health, Epidemiology and
Biostatics
School of Health and Population Sciences,
University of Birmingham
UK

Antonio Macciò
Department of Medical Oncology
University of Cagliari
Italy

Sylvia V. Mackensen
Institute and Policlinics of Medical
Psychology, University Medical Centre
Hamburg-Eppendorf
Martinistr
Hamburg
Germany

Clelia Madeddu
Department of Medical Oncology
University of Cagliari
Italy

Andreas Maetzel
Amgen (Europe) GmbH, Zug, Switzerland
Department of Health Policy, Management
and Evaluation, University of Toronto
Toronto, ON
Canada

Giuseppe Maina
Mood and Anxiety Disorders Unit
Department of Neurosciences
University of Turin
Turin
Italy

Jadranka Maksimovic
Institute of Epidemiology, School of
Medicine, Belgrade University
Belgrade
Serbia

Natasa Maksimović
Institute of Epidemiology, School of
Medicine, University of Belgrade, Belgrade
Serbia

Giovanni Mantovani
Department of Medical Oncology
University of Cagliari, Cagliari
Italy

Jamie Manwaring
Department of Psychology
Washington University
St. Louis, MO
USA

Hilal Maradit-Kremers
Department of Health Sciences Research
Mayo Clinic, Rochester, MN
USA

Peter J. Marangos
Health Care Analytics
United BioSource Corporation
Bethesda, MD
USA

Monica M. Marín Caro
Geneva University Hospital, Geneva
Switzerland

Jelena Marinkovic
Institute for Medical Statistics and
Informatics, School of Medicine, Belgrade
University, Silos
Belgrade
Serbia

Sergio Mariotti
National Center for Epidemiology
Surveillance and Health Promotion, Istituto
Superiore di Sanita
Italy

Ljiljana Markovic-Denic
Institute of Epidemiology, School of
Medicine, Belgrade University, Belgrade
Serbia

Meghan L. Marsac
Department of Psychology, University of
Toledo & Children's Hospital of
Philadelphia, Philadelphia, PA
USA

Roger J. Marshall
Section of Epidemiology and Biostatistics
School of Population Health, University of
Auckland
New Zealand

Colin R. Martin
School of Health, Nursing and Midwifery
University of the West of Scotland,
Scotland
UK

Faith Martin
Department of Primary Health Care
University of Oxford
UK

Yasuyo Matsumoto
Department of International Cooperation
Yodogawa Christian Hospital, Osaka
Japan

Eric L. Mattesson
Division of Rheumatology
Mayo Clinic College of Medicine
Rochester, Minnesota
USA

Molly R. Matthews
Department of Community Medicine
School of Medicine, West Virginia
University, Morgantown, WV
USA

Deborah J. Mawman
University Department of Otolaryngology
Head-Neck Surgery, Manchester Royal
Infirmary, Manchester
UK

Annette E. Maxwell
Division of Cancer Prevention and Control
Research, School of Public Health, University
of California, Los Angeles, CA
USA

Fayyaz A. K. Mazari
Academic Vascular Surgical Unit, Alderson
House, Hull Royal Infirmary, Hull
UK

Suzanne E. Mazzeo
Department of Psychology, Virginia
Commonwealth University, Richmond, VA
USA

Karen A. McDonnell
Department of Prevention and Community
Health, George Washington University
School of Public Health and Health Services
Washington, DC
USA

Kathleen McElhone
Department of Rheumatology
Royal Blackburn Hospital, Blackburn
UK

Colman McGrath
Faculty of Dentistry, University of Hong
Kong, Hong Kong SAR
People's Republic of China

Cameron N. McIntosh
ARC Epidemiology Unit, University of
Manchester Rutherford House (Unit 4)
Manchester Science Park, Manchester
UK

Pamela G. McKay
Health Information and Research Division
Statistics Canada
Canada

Matthew McKenna
Centers for Disease Control and
Prevention, US Department of Health and
Human Services
Atlanta, GA
USA

Zoe J. McKeough
Faculty of Health Sciences, The University
of Sydney, Lidcombe
Australia

Leslie McKnight
Department of Surgery
McMaster University, Hamilton Ontario
Canada

Tapan A. Mehta
Academic Vascular Unit
University of Hull, Hull
UK

Atte Meretoja
Department of Neurology
Helsinki University Central Hospital
University of Helsinki, Helsinki
Finland

Ruben A. Mesa
Division of Hematology, Mayo Clinic
Rochester, MN
USA

Lynn B. Meuleners
School of Public Health, Curtin University of
Technology, Perth
Australia

Dimitri P. Mikhailidis
Department of Clinical Biochemistry
(Vascular Disease Prevention Clinics)
Royal Free Hospital Campus
University College London Medical School
University College London, London
UK

Rafael Mikolajczyk
Department of Public Health Medicine
School of Public Health, University of
Bielefeld, Bielefeld
Germany

John D. Miller
Department of Thoracic Surgery, Thoracic
Surgery McMaster University St. Joseph's
Hospital, Hamilton, ON
Canada

Gita D. Mishra
MRC Unit for Lifelong Health and Ageing
Royal Free and University College Medical
School, Department of Epidemiology and
Public Health, London
UK

Jan Mitchell
Department of Psychology, Royal Holloway
University of London, Surrey
UK

Seyed M. Moghadas
Institute for Biodiagnostics, National
Research Council Canada
Winnipeg, MB
Canada

Maureen P. M. H. Rutten-van Mölken
Institute for Medical Technology
Assessment, Erasmus MC, Rotterdam
The Netherlands

Debapriya Mondal
School of Earth, Atmospheric and
Environmental Sciences, The University of
Manchester
UK

Ali Montazeri
Iranian Institute for Health Sciences
Research (IHSR), Tehran
Iran

Marjory L. Moodie
Deakin Health Economics
Deakin University, Vic
Australia

Takashi Motegi
Department of Pulmonary Medicine
Infection, and Oncology, Respiratory Care
Clinic, Nippon Medical School, Tokyo
Japan

Sayed J. Mousavi
Department of Physical Therapy
Tehran University of Medical Sciences
Tehran
Iran

Luc Mouthon
Department of Internal Medicine
Paris Descartes University
Reference Center for Necrotizing
Vasculitides and Systemic Sclerosis
Cochin Hospital, Assistance
Publique-Hôpitaux de Paris (AP-HP)
Paris
France

Peter Muennig
Mailman School of Public Health, Columbia
University, New York, NY
USA

Nikolai Mühlberger
Department of Public Health, Information
Systems and Health Technology
Assessment UMIT - University for Health
Sciences, Medical Informatics and
Technology and ONCOTYROL Center for
Personalized Cancer Medicine
Hall i.T./Innsbruck
Austria

Pedro Muñoz
Department of Psychiatry
Mental Health Centre Ortuella
Ortuella, Vizcaya
Spain

Jean W. M. Muris
Research School Public Health and Primary
Care (Caphri)
Medicine and Life Sciences
Department of General Practice
Maastricht University, MD Maastricht
The Netherlands

Emmanuel A. M. Mylanus
Department of Otorhinolaryngology
University Medical Centre Sint Radboud
Nijmegen
The Netherlands

Shunichi Namiki
Department of Urology, Tohoku University
Graduate School of Medicine Sendai
Japan

Giorgia La Nasa
Bone Marrow Transplant Centre,
R. Binaghi Hospital, University of Cagliari
Cagliari
Italy

Jamil Natour
Universidade Federal de São Paulo,
Rheumatology Division São Paulo, SP
Brazil

E. A. S. Nelson
Department of Paediatrics, The Chinese
University of Hong Kong, Prince of Wales
Hospital, Shatin, Hong Kong SAR
People's Republic of China

Geoffrey Nelson
Department of Psychology, Wilfrid Laurier
University, Waterloo, ON
Canada

Penelope Nestel
Institute of Human Nutrition, Southampton
General Hospital, Southampton
UK

Gabriele Neurauter
Division of Biological Chemistry, Biocenter
Innsbruck Medical University
Innsbruck
Austria

Linda M. Niccolai
Yale School of Medicine – Epidemiology
and Public Health
New Haven, CT
USA

J. Curtis Nickel
Department of Urology, Queen's
University, Kingston, ON
Canada

Esther Núñez
Health Services. Institut Català de la Salut.
Av. Drassanes, Barcelona
Spain

Montserrat Núñez
Educational and Functional Readaptation
Unit, Rheumatology Department (ICEMEQ)
Hospital Clínic, Barcelona
Spain

Miriam Nuño
UCLA School of Public Health, Department
of Biostatistics, Los Angeles, CA
USA

Elissa Oh
Institute for Healthcare Studies
Northwestern University, Chicago, IL
USA

Seung-June Oh
Department of Urology, Seoul National
University College of Medicine, Seoul
National University Hospital, Seoul
Korea

Angel Ois
Unitat d'Ictus. Servei de Neurologia
Hospital del Mar, Barcelona
Spain

Lynn J. Okamoto
Health Care Analytics
United BioSource Corporation
Bethesda, MD
USA

Pedro R. Olivares
University of Extremadura, Cáceres
Spain

S. Jay Olshansky
School of Public Health, University of
Illinois at Chicago, Chicago, IL
USA

Ikushi Onozaki
The Research Institute of Tuberculosis,
Japan Anti-Tuberculosis Association Kiyose
Tokyo
Japan

Reinaldo Oria
Centers for Global Health, University of
Virginia, Charlottesville, Virginia and
Federal University of Cear Fortaleza
Brazil

Ferdiando di Orio
Department of Internal Medicine and
Public Health, University of L'Aquila, P.le S.
Tommasi
Italy

Robyn L. Osborn
Department of Medical and Clinical
Psychology, Uniformed Services University
of the Health Sciences Bethesda, MD
USA

Manathip Osiri
Division of Rheumatology
Department of Medicine
Chulalongkorn University
Thailand

Lena Oxelmark
Department of Neurobiology, Care
Sciences, Division of Nursing Karolinska
Institutet, Huddinge
Sweden

Mine Özkan
Department of Psychiatry
Department of Consultation Liaison
Psychiatry
University of Istanbul
Istanbul Faculty of Medicine, Çapa
Istanbul
Turkey

Sedat Özkan
Department of Psychiatry
Department of Consultation Liaison
Psychiatry, University of Istanbul
Istanbul Faculty of Medicine, Çapa
Istanbul
Turkey

Vahit Özmen
Department of Consultation Liaison
Psychiatry, University of Istanbul, Çapa
Istanbul
Turkey

Jesus Á. Padierna
Department of Psychiatry
Hospital de Galdakao Usansolo
Galdakao, Vizcaya
Spain

Demosthenes B. Panagiotakos
Department of Nutrition Science –
Dietetics, Harokopio University
Athens
Greece

Angelo Pappalardo
Department of Neurology, Multiple
Sclerosis Centre – University of Catania
Italy

Rajeev Parameswaran
Royal Devon & Exeter NHS Foundation
Trust, Exeter
UK

Jae-Hyun Park
National Cancer Control Research Institute
National Cancer Center
Goyang-si
Korea

Donald M. Parkin
Clinical Trials Service Unit and
Epidemiological Studies Unit
University of Oxford, Oxford
UK

Jayadeep Patra
Public Health and Regulatory Policies
Section, Centre for Addiction and Mental
Health, Toronto, ON
Canada

Francesco Patti
Department of Neurology, Multiple
Sclerosis Centre- University of Catania
Italy

Mathew Pearson
Division of Urologic Surgery, The University
of North Carolina at Chapel Hill
Chapel Hill NC
USA

Tatjana Pekmezovic
Institute of Epidemiology, School of
Medicine, University of Belgrade
Belgrade
Serbia

Jorge Escobedo-de la Peña
Mexican Institute of Social Security,
Regional General Hospital "Carlos
Macgregor Sanchez-Navarro"
Epidemiologic Research Unit, Mexico City
Mexico

Konrad Pesudovs
NH&MRC Centre for Clinical Eye Research
Department of Ophthalmology, Flinders
Medical Centre and Flinders University
Bedford Park, SA
Australia

Dragica Pesut
Institute of Lung Diseases and
Tuberculosis, Clinical Centre of Serbia2
Visegradska, Belgrade
Serbia

Claude Pichard
Clinical Nutrition, Geneva University
Hospital, Geneva
Switzerland

J. Rush Pierce
Department of Internal Medicine, Texas
Tech University Health Sciences Center, TX
USA

Relana Pinkerton
Centers for Global Health, University of
Virginia, Charlottesville
Virginia and Federal University of Ceará,
Fortaleza
Brazil

Christos Pitsavos
First Cardiology Clinic, Hippokration
Hospital, School of Medicine
University of Athens, Athens
Greece

Serge Poiraudeau
Department of Rehabilitation, Paris
Descartes University, Cochin Hospital
INSERM Institut Féderatif de Recherche sur
le Handicap, Paris
France

David A. Polya
University of Manchester
UK

Varinsathein Porpit
Department of Disease Control, Ministry of
Public Health, Immunization Program

Bureau of General Communicable Diseases
Bangkok
Thailand

Maarten Postma
Groningen University Institute for
Pharmacy, Department of Social Pharmacy
and Pharmacoepidemiology, University of
Groningen
The Netherlands

John Powles
Department of Public Health and Primary
Care, Institute of Public Health Cambridge
UK

Joana Prata
Department of Psychiatry, CHVNGaia/
Espinho
Portugal

Marie Préau
Research Unit UMR912, Economic & Social
Sciences, Health Systems & Societies
INSERM, Marseille, France and IRD, Aix
Marseille Université, Marseille
France

Victor R. Preedy
Department of Nutrition and Dietetics
Nutritional Sciences Division
School of Biomedical & Health Sciences
King's College London, London
UK

Salvatore D. Prete
Oncology Unit, S. Giovanni di Dio Hospital
Naples
Italy

Richard L. Prince
School of Medicine and Pharmacology
University of Western Australia
Department of Endocrinology & Diabetes
Sir Charles Gairdner Hospital, Perth, WA
Australia

Raj S. Pruthi
Division of Urologic Surgery, The University
of North Carolina at Chapel Hill
Chapel Hill, NC
USA

Matin Qaim
Department of Agricultural Economics and
Rural Development, Georg-August-
University of Goettingen, Goettingen
Germany

Teresita Ramírez-Sánchez
Mexican Institute of Social Security
Assessment Coordination, Mexico City
Mexico

Francois Rannou
Department of Rehabilitation
Paris Descartes University, Cochin
Hospital, AP-HP, INSERM Institut Féderatif
de Recherche sur le Handicap (IFR 25)
Paris

Isidora Ratkov
Institute of Epidemiology, School of
Medicine, Belgrade University, Belgrade
Serbia

Paula Ravasco
Unidade de Nutrição e Metabolismo
Instituto de Medicina Molecular
Faculdade de Medicina da Universidade
de Lisboa
Portugal

Jurgen Rehm
Dalla Lana School of Public Health
University of Toronto and Public Health
and Regulatory Policies Section
Centre for Addiction and Mental Health
Toronto, ON
Canada

Adam Reich
Department of Dermatology, Venereology
and Allergology, Wroclaw Medical
University, Wroclaw
Poland

Mathew R. Reynolds
Division of Cardiology, Beth Israel
Deaconess Medical Center, Harvard
Medical School, Harvard
USA

Lis Ribu
Oslo University College, Oslo,
Norway

Beatriz Rico-Verdín
Institute of Services of Social Security to
Civil Servants
National Medical Centre "20 de
Noviembre", Hospital Epidemiology
Division, México City
México

Charanjit S. Rihal
Cardiac Catheterization Laboratory, Mayo
Clinic, Rochester, MN
USA

Marcel G. M. Olde Rikkert
Multidisciplinary Memory Clinic Slingeland
Hospital/Alzheimer Centre Nijmegen
University Medical Centre Nijmegen
Doetinchem
The Netherlands

Jo Robays
Epidemiology and Disease Control Unit
Institute of Tropical Medicine, Antwerp
Belgium

Bjarne Robberstad
Department of Public Health and Primary
Health Care and Centre for International
Health, University of Bergen, Bergen
Norway

Carie S. Rodgers
VA San Diego Healthcare System, Mission
Valley Outpatient Services
San Diego, CA
USA

Gabriela Rodriguez-Abrego
Mexican Institute of Social Security,
Regional General Hospital "Carlos
Macgregor Sanchez-Navarro"
Epidemiologic Research Unit, Mexico City
Mexico

Michael Roerecke
Public Health and Regulatory Policies
Section, Centre for Addiction and Mental
Health, Toronto, ON
Canada

Simon N. Rogers
Evidence base Practice Research Centre
(EPRC), Edge Hill University, Liverpool
UK

Kelly J. Rohan
Department of Psychology
John Dewy Hall
The University of Vermont Burlington, VT
USA

Fausto Roila
Medical Oncology Division
Regional Hospital
Ospedale 'S. Maria della Misericordia', S
Andrea delle Fratte, Perugia
Italy

Martin Röösli
Institute of Social and Preventive Medicine
University of Bern
Switzerland

Jaume Roquer
Unitat d'Ictus. Servei de Neurologia
Hospital del Mar, Barcelona
Spain

Adriane R. Rosa
Bipolar Disorders Program, Clinical Institute
of Neuroscience, Hospital Clinic of
Barcelona
Barcelona
Spain

Lori A. Roscoe
Center for Hospice, Palliative Care &
End-of-Life Studies at USF, University
of South Florida, Tampa, FL
USA

W. Rössler
Department of General and Social
Psychiatry, University of Zürich, Zurich
Switzerland

Benedetta Ruggeri
ASUR Marche Ospedale 'Mazzoni' AP
Italy

Mehdi Russel
University of Social Welfare and
Rehabilitation, Tehran
Iran

Danny Ruta
Institute of Health Society, University of
Newcastle
UK

Shakeel R. Saeed
University College London Ear Institue
The Royal National Throat, Nose & Ear
Hospital and Royal Free Hospital
London
UK

Susan Saegert
Department of Human and Organizational
Development, Peabody College Vanderbilt
University, Nashville, Tennesse
USA

Rengaswamy Sankaranarayanan
Screening Group, International Agency for
Research on Cancer, Lyon
France

Milena Šantrić-Milićević
Institute of Epidemiology, School of
Medicine, University of Belgrade, Belgrade
Serbia

Franco Sassi
Department of Social Policy, London
School of Economics and Political Science
London
UK

Marco Scarpa
Department of Surgical and
Gastroenterological Science, Sezione di
Clinica Chirurgica I, University of Padova
Italy

Jean Francois Schemann
University Victor Ségalen – Bordeaux
Bordeaux
France

Christian Schneider
Department of Neurosurgery
Kantonsspital Aarau, Aarau
Switzerland

Douglas D. Schocken
Department of Internal Medicine Division
of Cardiovascular Disease, USF College of
Medicine and H. Lee Moffitt Cancer Center
and Research Institute, Tampa, FL
USA

Carla J. M. Schölzel-Dorenbos
Multidisciplinary Memory Clinic Slingeland
Hospital/Alzheimer Centre Nijmegen
University Medical Centre Nijmegen
Doetinchem
The Netherlands

Anette Schrag
University Department of Clinical
Neurosciences, Royal Free and
University College Medical School
London
UK

Katharina Schroecksnadel
Department of Internal Medicine
Innsbruck Medical University, Innsbruck
Austria

Ursula Schütte
Department of Prosthetic Dentistry
Technical University Dresden, Dresden
Germany

Ruth Schwarzer
Department of Public Health, Information
Systems and Health Technology
Assessment, UMIT - University for Health
Sciences, Medical Informatics and
Technology and ONCOTYROL Center for
Personalized Cancer Medicine
Hall i.T./Innsbruck
Austria

Josep M. Segur
Knee Section Orthopaedic Surgery
Department (ICEMEQ), Hospital Clínic
Barcelona
Spain

John W. Sellors
Department of Family Medicine
McMaster University, Hamilton, ON
Canada

Sonalee Shah
Global Health Economics
Outcomes and Reimbursement
Bayer HealthCare Pharmaceuticals
Montville, NJ
USA

Navvab Shamspour
Department of Psychology and Psychiatry
Medicine and Health Promotion Institute
Tehran
Iran

Tait Shanafelt
Division of Hematology, Mayo Clinic
Rochester, MN
USA

Chen Shao
Department of Urology, Xinjing Hospital
Fourth Military Medical University, Shanxi
Province
People's Republic of China

Amir Sharafkhaneh
VAMC Sleep Center (111-i), Houston
TX
USA

Hossein Sharafkhaneh
VAMC Sleep Center (111-i), Houston, TX
USA

Alexandra Shaw
AP Consultants
Andover, Hampshire
UK

Jianzhao Shen
Pharmaceutical Product Development
Wilmington, NC
USA

Donald S. Shepard
Schneider Institutes for Health Policy
Heller School, Brandeis University
Waltham, MA
USA

Uwe Siebert
Department of Public Health, Information
Systems and Health Technology
Assessment, UMIT - University for Health
Sciences, Medical Informatics and
Technology and ONCOTYROL Center for
Personalized Cancer Medicine
Hall i.T./Innsbruck
Austria
and
Institute for Technology Assessment
Department of Radiology, Massachusetts
General Hospital, Harvard Medical School/
Department of Health Policy and
Management Harvard School of Public
Health, Boston, MA
USA

Paul A. Simon
Office of Chronic Disease and Injury
Prevention, Los Angeles County
Department of Public Health
Los Angeles, CA
USA

Sandra B. Sipetic-Grujicic
Institute of Epidemiology, School of
Medicine, Belgrade University
Belgrade
Serbia

Hans Smedje
The Department of Neuroscience
Uppsala University, Child and Adolescent
Psychiatric Unit, Uppsala
Sweden

Ad F. M. Snik
Department of Otorhinolaryngology
University Medical Centre Sint Radboud
Nijmegen
The Netherlands

Min-Woong Sohn
Center for Management of Complex
Chronic Care Hines VA Hospital,
Hines, IL
USA

Dale Spence
Nursing and Midwifery Research Unit
Queen's University Belfast, Belfast
Northern Ireland
UK

Bruno Spire
Southeastern Health Regional Observatory
(ORS-PACA), Marseille
France Research Unit UMR912
"Economic & Social Sciences
Health Systems & Societies"
INSERM, Aix Marseille Université
Marseille
France

Gaby Sroczynski
Department of Public Health, Information
Systems and Health Technology
Assessment, UMIT - University for Health
Sciences, Medical Informatics and
Technology and ONCOTYROL Center for
Personalized Cancer Medicine
Hall i.T./Innsbruck
Austria

David P. Steensma
Division of Hematology, Mayo Clinic
Rochester, MN
USA

Alexander J. Stein
Institute for Prospective Technological
Studies, Sevilla
Spain

Katarina Stengler
Department of Psychiatry, University of
Leipzig, Semmelweisstr, Leipzig
Germany

Marilyn Stern
Departments of Psychology & Pediatrics
Virginia Commonwealth University
Richmond, VA
USA

Sunita M. Stewart
Department of Community Medicine
Hong Kong University
and
Department of Psychiatry, The University of
Texas Southwestern Medical Center
Dallas, TX
USA

Helen Stokes-Lampard
Primary Care Clinical Sciences, School of
Health and Population Sciences
University of Birmingham
UK

Henrik Støvring
Research Unit for General Practice
University of Southern Denmark, Odense
Denmark

Timo E. Strandberg
Department of Health Sciences/Geriatrics
University of Oulu, and Oulu University
Hospital, Unit of General Practice, Oulu
Finland

Jacqueline J. M. H. Strik
Department of Psychiatry and Psychology,
Maastricht University Medical Centre:
MUMC, Maastricht University, Maastricht
The Netherlands

Gerold Stucki
Department of Physical Medicine and
Rehabilitation, Munich University Hospital
Ludwig Maximilian University, Munich
Germany

Jose A. Suaya
Schneider Institutes for Health Policy
Heller School, Brandeis University
Waltham, MA
USA

Machi Suka
Department of Preventive Medicine
St. Marianna University School of Medicine,
Kawasaki, Kanagawa
Japan

Chutima Suraratdecha
PATH, Seattle, WA
USA

Erla K. Svavarsdottir
University of Iceland, Eirbergi
Iceland

Jacek C. Szepietowski
Department of Dermatology
Venereology and Allergology
Wroclaw Medical University, Ul.
Wroclaw
Poland

Charles Taieb
Department Pharmaco-Economique Pierre
Fabre SA, Boulogne, sur Seine
France

Guoyu Tao
Division of Sexually Transmitted Disease
Prevention, National Center for HIV
STD and TB Prevention Centers for Disease
Control and Prevention, Atlanta, GA
USA

Turgut Tatlisumak
Department of Neurology
Helsinki University Central Hospital
University of Helsinki Helsinki
Finland

Lee-Suan Teh
Department of Rheumatology, Royal
Blackburn Hospital, Blackburn
UK

Darija K. Tepavcevic
Institute of Epidemiology
School of Medicine
University of Belgrade
Belgrade
Serbia

Zorica Terzić-Šupić
Institute of Social Medicine
School of Medicine
University of Belgrade, Belgrade
Serbia

Hla-Hla Thein
National Centre in HIV Epidemiology and
Clinical Research, The University of
New South Wales, Sydney
Australia

Anastasia Theodoridou
Department of General and Social
Psychiatry, University of Zurich, Zürich
Switzerland

Achilleas Thoma
Departments of Surgery and Clinical
Epidemiology and Biostatistics
McMaster University, Hamilton Ontario
Canada

David R. Thomas
Division of Geriatric Medicine, Saint Louis
University Health Sciences Center,
Saint Louis, MO
USA

David R. Thompson
Department of Health Sciences and
Department of Cardiovascular Sciences
University of Leicester, Leicester
UK

Amanda G. Thrift
Baker IDI Heart & Diabetes Institute,
Melbourne VIC
Australia

Sergio Tiberti
Department of Internal Medicine and
Public Health, University of L'Aquila, P.le S.
Tommasi
Italy

William W. K. To
Department of Obstetrics & Gynaecology
United Christian Hospital, Kwun Tong
Hong Kong

Pablo Tomas-Carus
Department of Sports and Health
University of Evora
Portugal

Pinar Topsever
Department of Family Medicine, Kocaeli
University, Kocaeli
Turkey

Paul R. Torgerson
Institute of Parasitology, University of
Zurich, Winterthurestrasse, Zurich
Switzerland

Jose L. Torres-Cosme
National Institute of Perinatology
Public Health Division, Mexico City
Mexico

Gabor Tóth
Department of Biology and Function in the
Head and Neck (A603), Yokohama City
University Graduate School of Medicine
Yokohama
Japan

F. P. Treasure
Eastern Cancer Registration & Information
Centre, Unit C - Magog Court
Shelford Bottom, Cambridge
UK

Dean A. Tripp
Departments of Psychology
Anesthesiology, Urology
Queen's University, Kingston, ON
Canada

Kuan-Yi Tsai
Department of Community Psychiatry
Kai-Suan Psychiatric Hospital, Kaohsiung
Taiwan

Junichi Tsukada
Cancer Chemotherapy Center, University of
Occupational and Environmental Health
Japan

Mamoru Tsukuda
Department of Biology and Function in the
Head and Neck (A603), Yokohama City
University Graduate School of Medicine
Kanazawa-ku, Yokohama
Japan

Atsuro Tsutsumi
Institute of Biomedical Research and
Innovation (IBRI), Kobe
Japan

Hidetaka Uramoto
Cancer Chemotherapy Center, University of
Occupational and Environmental Health
Japan

Marjan Vaez
Department of Clinical Neuroscience
Section of Personal Injury Prevention
Karolinska Institutet, Stockholm
Sweden

Francesca Valent
Istituto di Igiene ed Epidemiologia -
Azienda Ospedaliero-Universitaria di Udine,
Udine, Italy

Robert F. Valois
Department of Community Medicine
School of Medicine, West Virginia
University, Morgantown, WV
USA

Ron T. Varghese
Department of Community Medicine
Government Medical College
Thiruvananthapuram, Kerala
India

Massimiliano Veroux
Department of Surgery, Transplantation
and Advanced Technologies
Organ Transplant Unit, University
Hospital of Catania
Italy

Thomas R. Vetter
Department of Anesthesiology, University
of Alabama School of Medicine and
Department of Health Policy and
Organization, University of Alabama at
Birmingham School of Public Health
Birmingham, AL
USA

Ana Vieta
Health Economics and Outcomes Research
IMS Health
Spain

K. Vijayakumar
Department of Community Medicine
Government Medical College
Thiruvananthapuram
India

Ignacio Villaseñor-Ruiz
Analytical Control and Coverage Extension
Commission Direction, Ministry of Health
Mexico City
Mexico

Ad J. J. M. Vingerhoets
Department of Clinical,
Developmental and Cultural Psychology
Tilburg University, Tilburg
The Netherlands

Hristina Vlajinac
Institute of Epidemiology
School of Medicine
University of Belgrade
Belgrade
Serbia

Margaretha Voss
Department of Clinical Neuroscience
Section of Personal Injury Prevention
Karolinska Institutet, Stockholm
Sweden

Jolanda De Vries
CoRPS, Department of Medical Psychology
Tilburg University, Tilburg
The Netherlands

Anne Vuillemin
EA 4003, Faculty of Medicine, Nancy
Nancy-University
School of Public Health
France

Eric M. Wallen
Division of Urologic Surgery, The University
of North Carolina at Chapel Hill
Chapel Hill NC
USA

Michael Walter
Department of Prosthetic Dentistry Faculty
of Medicine Carl Gustav Carus, Technical
University Dresden, Dresden
Germany

Julio C. Walz
Bipolar Disorders Program and Laboratory
of Molecular Psychiatry
Hospital de Clinicas de Porto Alegre
Brazil
and
INCT Translational Medicine

Jung-Der Wang
Institute of Occupational Medicine and
Industrial Hygiene, College of Public
Health, National Taiwan University
Taipei
Taiwan

Li Yan Wang
Division of Adolescent and School Health
National Center for Chronic Disease
Prevention and Health Promotion
Centers for Disease Control and Prevention
Atlanta, GA
USA

Philip S. Wang
Division of Services and Intervention
Research, National Institute of Mental
Health, Bethesda, MD
USA

Wen-Zhi Wang
Department of Neuroepidemiology
Beijing Neurosurgical Institute, Beijing
China

Patti Wansley
VA San Diego Healthcare System, Mission
Valley Outpatient Services (116A4Z), CA
USA

Elizabeth Waters
McCaughey Centre, VicHealth Centre for
the Promotion of Mental Health and
Community Wellbeing, School of
Population Health, University of
Melbourne, VIC
Australia

Theresia Weber
Department of Surgery, University Hospital
Steinhoevelstr, Ulm
Germany

Guenter Weiss
Department of Internal Medicine, Innsbruck
Medical University
Innsbruck
Austria

Geertjan Wesseling
Department of Respiratory Medicine,
Maastricht University Medical Centre:
MUMC, Maastricht University
Maastricht
The Netherlands

Steven D. Wexner
Department of Colorectal Surgery
Cleveland Clinic Florida, FL
USA

Denise Wilfley
Departments of Psychiatry, Medicine,
Pediatrics and Psychology
Washington University
St. Louis, MO
USA

Ross Wilkie
Primary Care Musculoskeletal Research
Centre, Keele University, Keele. Newcastle-
under-Lyme, Staffordshire
UK

Wolfram Windisch
Department of Pneumology, University
Hospital Freiburg, Killianstrasse 5
Freiburg
Germany

Desmond C. Winter
Institute for Clinical Outcomes Research
and Education (iCORE), St. Vincent's
University Hospital, Dublin
Ireland

Andreas A. J. Wismeijer
Department of Clinical, Developmental and
Cultural Psychology, Tilburg University
Tilburg
The Netherlands

Hans-Ulrich Wittchen
Institute of Clinical Psychology and
Psychotherapy and Centre of Clinical
Epidemiology and Longitudinal Studies
(CELOS)
Technische Universitaet Dresden
Germany

Alison Woodcock
Department of Psychology, Royal
Holloway, University of London, Egham
Surrey
UK

Mark Woodward
Department of Medicine
Mount Sinai School of Medicine
New York
USA

Yangfeng Wu
Department of Epidemiology and
Biostatistics, Peking University School of
Public Health, The George Institute, China
Beijing
China

Gaoqiang Xie
Division for CVD Prevention and Control
Network, Cardiovascular Institute and
Fuwai Hospital, Chinese Academy of
Medical Sciences and Peking Union Medical
College, Beijing
China

Zhi-Yi Xu
Shi-Ji-Tong-Le, Shangai
China

Shingo Yamabe
Department of International Cooperation
Yodogawa Christian Hospital
Osaka
Japan

Koich Yamada
Department of Pulmonary Medicine
Infection, and Oncology, Respiratory Care
Clinic, Nippon Medical School, Tokyo
Japan

Renchi Yang
Department of Hematology
Institute of Hematology and Blood
Diseases Hospital
Chinese Academy of Medical Sciences
Peking Union Medical College
Tianjin
China

Chao-Hsing Yeh
School of Nursing, University of Pittsburgh
US

Nguyen T. Yen
Department of Epidemiology, National
Institute of Hygiene and Epidemiology
(NIHE), Hanoi
Vietnam

Paul S. F. Yip
Centre for Suicide research and Prevention
The University of Hong Kong
Hong Kong
China

Seok-Jun Yoon
Department of Preventive Medicine
College of Medicine, Korea University
Seongbuk-ku, Seoul
Republic of Korea

Katsumi Yoshida
Department of Preventive Medicine
St. Marianna University School of Medicine
Kawasaki, Kanagawa
Japan

Zobair M. Younossi
Department of Preventive Medicine
St. Marianna University School of Medicine
Sugao, Miyamae-ku, Kawasaki
Kanagawa
Japan

Stefan Zeuzem
Department of Internal Medicine
Gastroenterology, Hepatology
Pneumology and Endocrinology
Johann Wolfgang Goethe-University
Frankfurt am Main
Germany

James X. Zhang
Department of Pharmacy, Virginia
Commonwealth University, VA
USA

Lei Zhang
Department of Epidemiology, Fourth
Military Medical University of PLA, Shanxi

Province
China

Puhong Zhang
Division of NCD Control and Community
Health, Chinese Center for Disease Control
and Prevention
Beijing
China

Zuo-Feng Zhang
Department of Epidemiology, UCLA School
of Public Health, Los Angeles, CA
USA

Yuejen Zhao
Department of Health and Community
Services, Northern Territory
Australia

Zeping Zhou
Department of Hematology, Institute of
Hematology and Blood Diseases Hospital
Chinese Academy of Medical Sciences
Peking Union Medical College, Tianjin
China

Kun Zhu
School of Medicine and Pharmacology
University of Western Australia
Department of Endocrinology and Diabetes
Sir Charles Gairdner Hospital
Perth, WA
Australia

Steven E. Zimmet
Dermatology & Phlebology department
Austin, TX
USA

Keith J. Zullig
Department of Community Medicine
School of Medicine, West Virginia
University, Morgantown, WV
USA

R. Beatriz Zurita Garza
Abt Associates Inc.
Bethesda, MD
USA

3 Quality of Life Measures and Indices

3.2 Surgical

132 Quality of Life and Functional Outcome in Pediatric Patients Requiring Surgery: Italian Perspectives

M. Castagnetti

1   *Introduction* 2258
1.1   From Survival to Quality of Life Assessment 2258
1.2   Quality of Life and Health-Related Quality of Life 2259
1.3   The Pediatric Setting and the Pediatric Surgical Setting 2259

2   *Examples of HRQoL Assessment in Pediatric Surgical or*
     Urological Conditions 2261
2.1   Muscle-Sparing Thoracotomy for Benign Lung Conditions 2261
2.2   Esophageal Atresia 2261
2.3   Spina Bifida 2265

3   *Considerations Based on the Studies Described* 2266
3.1   Is There a Constant Correlation Between Functional Outcome
     and HRQoL? 2266
3.2   Can Improved Surgical Outcome Only be Reached at the Price of
     Poorer HRQoL? 2266
3.3   Can Assessment of HRQoL Help in the Decision-Making? 2267
3.4   Which Instruments should be Preferred in the Evaluation of
     HRQoL in Pediatric Surgical Patients? 2267
3.5   Can Assessment of HRQoL be Based on Proxy Report? 2267
3.6   Final Considerations 2268

     Summary Points 2268

Abstract: Health related ❷ quality of life (HRQoL) is a multidimensional concept that describes the impact of a condition and the related morbidity on a person's feeling of leading a fulfilling life. Many studies in pediatric surgery and urology have so far failed to establish HRQoL and only focused on mortality and morbidity rates. By reviewing studies about HRQoL in three pediatric surgical or urological conditions, we discuss some of the most relevant points concerning the evaluation of HRQoL and its relationship with functional outcomes. The studies reviewed show that HRQoL does not necessarily parallel ❷ functional results. Studies in survivors of esophageal atresia, for instance, show that an acceptable HRQoL can be achieved even despite significant morbidity. Studies in subjects born with ❷ spina bifida, instead, show that, although surgery can achieve dramatic improvements in functional outcome in terms of urinary continence, this is not paralleled by any improvement in the HRQoL of these patients. HRQoL seems instead to improve in the caregivers. The studies reviewed also suggest that HRQoL is largely unrelated to the severity of the condition or the presence of associated anomalies. Consistently, improvement of survival of more severe neonatal conditions does not seem to be associated with a reduction in HRQoL.

In conclusion, comprehending issues that influence HRQoL allows us to offer clear expectations of outcomes after surgery to patients, families, health care professionals and policy makers in a truly patient-oriented, evidence-based manner.

List of Abbreviations: *GIQLI,* gastrointestinal quality of life index; *HRQoL,* health related quality of life; *ICQ,* illness cognition questionnaire; *PedsQL,* pediatric quality of life inventory 4.0; *QoL,* quality of life; *RSRQLI,* respiratory symptoms–related quality of life index; *SF-36,* short form – 36; *SF-12,* short form – 12™ health survey

1   Introduction

1.1   From Survival to Quality of Life Assessment

Children can be exposed to a variety of conditions requiring surgical treatment.

Over the last decades, improvements in diagnosis, management, anesthesia, peri-operative support, and surgical techniques have been paralleled by an improvement in the results of surgical treatment of many congenital and acquired pediatric surgical conditions. For instance, before 1960 less than 10% of spina bifida patients survived infancy whereas today the number exceeds 85% (Rinck et al., 1989); during the same period survival for esophageal atresia increased from about 40% to more than 95% (Louhimo and Lindahl, 1983; Ure et al., 1998).

This has caused a shift in the primary outcome measures considered for the evaluation of treatment from mere survival, to functional outcomes; and from the latter to quality of life (QoL).

QoL is of special interest for chronic diseases, and for diseases associated with a relevant risk of long-term morbidity, or in which treatment may result in a mutilation (Eiser and Morse, 2001).

Examples in children include congenital malformations such as esophageal atresia, anorectal malformations, congenital diaphragmatic hernia, or spina bifida; acquired chronic diseases such as cancer or inflammatory bowel diseases; and chronic organ failures (such as liver, kidney or bowel) requiring organ transplant (Stolk et al., 2000).

Comprehending issues that influence QoL allows us to offer clear expectations of outcomes after surgery to patients, families, health care professionals and policy makers in a truly patient-oriented, evidence-based manner.

1.2   Quality of Life and Health-Related Quality of Life

According to the World Health Organization (1995), QoL is a multidimensional concept encompassing three main domains: (1) the physical domain, which includes independence in activities of daily living and symptoms of disease; (2) the psychological domain, involving emotional, cognitive and behavioral status; and (3) the social domain, how people perceive their role and relationship with other people. Given its complexity, QoL is difficult to define and also to quantify. Therefore, a more practical approach is to restrict the assessment of QoL to the health related QoL (HRQoL), which can be defined as a multidimensional concept that includes the functional status, the psychological and social well being, the health perception and the disease and treatment-related symptoms (Guyatt et al., 1993). In other words, the impact of a chronic condition and the related morbidity on a person's feeling of leading a fulfilling life.

Initial attempts at evaluating HRQoL in pediatric surgical patients were done using ad hoc questionnaires focusing on multiple aspects of patient's life such as educational level, living arrangements, employment, and sexual relationship (Bomalaski et al., 1995; Bouman et al., 1999). Nevertheless, standardized questionnaires should be preferred. The latter can be differentiated into generic or disease-specific instruments (Patrick and Deyo, 1989). Each of the two has advantages and drawbacks. A combination of disease-specific and generic instruments can also be used, but this drastically increases the number of items to be administered.

Among the generic instruments, The Short Form – 36 (SF-36) is the most used instrument in the evaluation of adults treated as children for a congenital disease (Koivusalo et al., 2005). The pediatric quality of life inventory 4.0 (PedsQL), instead, is the most used for the evaluation of the pediatric population (Varni et al., 1999a, b, 2001, 2003). First described in 1999, it has been used in 122 studies up to January 2008 in a vast array of conditions throughout the world. Of note, of such 122 studies only 7 were in the field of pediatric surgery/urology (❷ Figure 132-1). Indeed, it appears that many studies in pediatric surgery and urology have so far failed to establish HRQoL and only presented mortality rates and crude measures of childhood morbidity (Stolk et al., 2000).

1.3   The Pediatric Setting and the Pediatric Surgical Setting

HRQoL assessment in pediatric surgical patients is unique in several respects (Eiser and Morse, 2001).

As for all the other pediatric conditions, surgical and non-surgical alike, it needs specific questionnaires devised for or adapted to children.

Such questionnaires have also to be age-specific, as the needs of children change with age and because young children have limited notions of abstract concepts and language. For very young children, questionnaires need to be devised in formats for caregiver report, as child self-report is impossible.

■ Figure 132-1

Percent of studies performed using the pediatric quality of life inventory 4.0 (PedsQL). Types of studies using the PedsQL based on a Medline/PubMed search made in January 2008. Most of the studies regard medical conditions or validation of the inventory. In only 6% of the studies, the PedsQL was used to investigate the health-related quality of life in pediatric patients with surgical or urological conditions

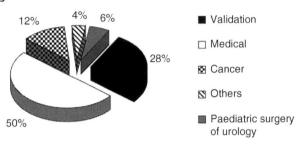

Particularly dealing with patients born with a congenital malformation, some other aspects need to be considered. To begin with, many of these patients have never experienced any previously healthy condition to compare their state of disease with. Many may have also developed ❷ coping mechanisms for their handicap.

Many of the most severe pediatric surgical patients are syndromic, which means that they have multiple concomitant malformations, which may have an impact on their HRQoL.

Finally, surgical reconstruction is often anatomical and functional. It will definitely change the patient body image and the function patients have adjusted to. Therefore, although perception of treatment-related symptoms is considered key in every HRQoL assessment, it is particularly important in surgical patients because of the irreversibility of changes suddenly caused by surgery. Furthermore, considering surgical patients, it is apparent that sometimes the need for multiple procedures rather than the condition itself can affect the quality of life, or that the HRQoL might depend more on the type of reconstructive procedure used than on the condition itself.

Herein we report the current research about HRQoL in three pediatric surgical or urological conditions, and discuss some of the most relevant points concerning the evaluation of HRQoL in pediatric surgical patients (❷ Table 132-1).

■ Table 132-1

Key questions concerning the evaluation of health related quality of life (HRQoL) in pediatric patients with surgical or urological conditions

Is there a constant correlation between functional outcome and HRQoL?
Can improved surgical outcome only be reached at the price of poorer HRQoL?
Can assessment of HRQoL help in the decision-making?
Which instruments should be preferred in the evaluation of HRQoL in pediatric surgical patients?
Can assessment of HRQoL be based on proxy report?

2   Examples of HRQoL Assessment in Pediatric Surgical or Urological Conditions

2.1   Muscle-Sparing Thoracotomy for Benign Lung Conditions

Lung resection is required in children for a variety of congenital and acquired conditions and is classically performed via a postero-lateral thoracotomy. Musculoskeletal anomalies are the major long-term complications associated with such a procedure (Jaureguizar et al., 1985). ❷ Muscle-sparing thoracotomy, video-assisted techniques, and use of mechanical stapling devices are alternatives or adjuncts proposed over time in order to reduce the invasiveness of lung resections (Mattioli et al., 1998; Rothenberg, 2000; Soucy et al., 1991).

In order to evaluate the functional outcome and the HRQoL in children undergoing a stapled lung resection via a muscle-sparing thoracotomy, Mattioli et al. (2006) performed a clinical, radiological and functional evaluation, and an assessment of HRQoL in children undergoing this operation.

Children older than 5 years and with at least 1 year of follow-up after surgery were included in the study.

Presence of asymmetry of the chest wall, rib fusion, breast and pectoral muscle maldevelopment, abnormal rib cage dynamic, winged scapula, elevation or fixation of the shoulder, and/or scoliosis was assessed by a physician not previously involved in the care of the patients assessed. Oxygen saturation was evaluated at rest and during exercise. A chest X-ray was performed in all the cases, while a CT scan only if clinically indicated. A spirometry was also offered.

An Italian version of the Short Form – 12™ Health Survey (SF-12) modified for children was used to assess HRQoL (Apolone et al., 2001). This was administered to children and their caregivers. The SF-12 is a simplified version of the SF-36, which has been proved to be reliable in the assessment of HRQoL in children.

Nineteen of the initial 52 patients with histologically proved benign lung disorders treated by a stapled lung resection via a muscle-sparing thoracotomy were eventually available for the study.

Musculoskeletal anomalies were observed in three such cases. All the patients had normal X-rays, but for the presence of a mild thickening in peri-bronchial vascular markers in three and a mild pleural thickening in two patients.

Spirometry was normal in 10 patients, obstructive in 4, restrictive in the remaining 5.

HRQoL was excellent or good in 17 out of 19 (89.5%) patients. An abnormal spirometric pattern resulted significantly more frequent in case with a poorer HRQoL (❷ *Figure 132-2*) whereas the rate of symptomatic patients was not different (❷ *Figure 132-3*).

The type of resection did not affect the outcome with a proportion of patients with excellent or very good HRQoL not statistically different in patients undergoing anatomical versus wedge resections (❷ *Figure 132-4*).

2.2   Esophageal Atresia

Long-term follow-up studies have shown that patients with esophageal atresia have morbidity from dysphagia, gastro-esophageal reflux, respiratory disorders, and problems related to associated anomalies (Anderson et al., 1992; Engum et al., 1995; Somppi et al., 1998; Ure et al., 1998).

■ Figure 132-2
Health related quality of life (HRQoL) in relation to spirometric findings. An excellent or very good HRQoL was statistically more common in patients with a normal spirometric pattern compared to patients with sufficient or poor HRQoL. Modified from Mattioli et al. Pediatr Surg Int 2006; 22: 491–495

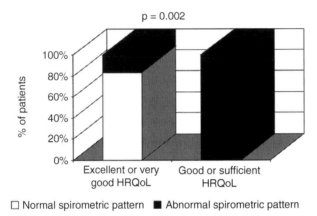

■ Figure 132-3
Health related quality of life (HRQoL) in relation to symptoms. HRQoL was not correlated to the presence of symptoms. Modified from Mattioli et al. Pediatr Surg Int 2006; 22: 491–495

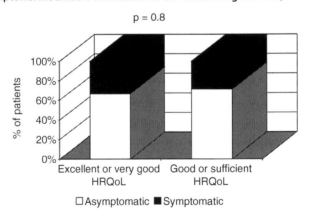

Four studies addressed the issue of HRQoL in patients with this condition using standardized and validated questionnaires (Deurloo et al., 2005; Koivusalo et al., 2005; Ure et al., 1995, 1998).

Two such studies were from the same German group that initially assessed QoL together with the functional results from eight pediatric patients after colon interposition for long-gap esophageal atresia (Ure et al., 1995), than extended the same protocol to 58 patients reassessed more than 20 years after correction of their esophageal atresia (Ure et al., 1998). Fifty patients with primary anastomosis and eight surviving patients with colon interposition were studied. The mean age was 25.3 years (range, 20–31).

■ Figure 132-4

Health related quality of life (HRQoL) in relation to the type of resection. HRQoL was not correlated to the type of lung resection. Modified from Mattioli et al. Pediatr Surg Int 2006; 22: 491–495

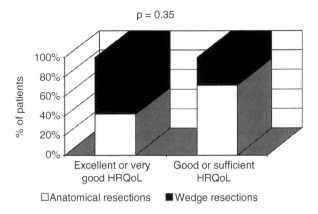

Symptoms were evaluated by a standardized interview. HRQoL assessment was performed using a combination of disease-specific and generic instruments (Eypasch et al., 1995; Selby et al., 1984; Slim et al., 1999; Spitzer et al., 1981) (❷ *Table 132-2*).

Among patients undergoing primary anastomosis, 60% suffered from respiratory symptoms, mainly attacks of cough, frequent bronchitis, and short breath; 48% reported hold up, which was instead the most frequent gastrointestinal symptom after primary anastomosis; and 22% complained gastro-oesophageal reflux symptoms such as heartburn or regurgitation.

In spite of such symptoms, HRQoL was unimpaired in these patients with a global score of 80 of 100 points, comparable to that of healthy individuals (Selby et al., 1984).

Among patients undergoing colon interposition, symptoms were more frequent. All of these patients suffered from periods of short breath. The Spitzer Index and the Gastrointestinal Quality of Life Index (GIQLI) were significantly lower compared with

■ Table 132-2

Instruments for the evaluation of HRQoL in studies on esophageal atresia patients

Study	Generic instruments	Disease-specific Instruments
Ure et al., 1995, 1998	Visual analogue scale (Selby et al., 1984)	Spitzer Index (Spitzer et al., 1981); GIQLI (Eypasch et al., 1995)
Deurloo et al., 2005	SF-36 (Validated Dutch translation) (Aaronson et al., 1998); ICQ (Evers, 2001)	GIQLI (Eypasch et al., 1995; Slim et al., 1999); 19 of the 24 items of the Esophageal Cancer Module questionnaire (Blazeby, 2003)
Koivusalo et al., 2005	SF-36 (Aalto et al., 1999); Tests of psychosocial functioning (Nurmi et al., 1995)	RSRQLI (Koivusalo et al., 2005); GIQLI (Eypasch et al., 1995; Slim et al., 1999)

SF-36: Short Form – 36; *GIQLI:* Gastrointestinal Quality of Life Index; *RSRQLI:* Respiratory Symptoms–Related Quality of Life Index; *ICQ:* Illness Cognition Questionnaire patients undergoing primary anastomosis, and the GIQLI also compared with healthy volunteers. However, the impairment in the GIQLI was exclusively caused by specific symptoms, which had no impact on physical functions, emotions, and social functions. The long-term HRQoL also in patients with colon interposition was acceptable. Besides suffering from specific symptoms these patients lead an otherwise normal life.

Deurloo et al. (2005) analyzed 97 esophageal atresia survivors, 16–48-year old. They too used a combination of generic and disease-specific questionnaires (❷ *Table 132-2*) (Aaronson et al., 1998; Blazeby et al., 2003; Evers et al., 2001; Eypasch et al., 1995; Slim et al., 1999). They found no differences in overall physical and mental health when comparing the generic HRQoL in patients who had had esophageal atresia with healthy subjects. Moreover, generic HRQoL did not appear to be influenced by the presence of concomitant congenital anomalies. Patients with concomitant congenital anomalies scored significantly lower only in the domain indigestion, which could probably reflect a focalization on the gastrointestinal system rather than the real presence of symptoms. Unfortunately, the number of patients with long-gap esophageal atresia in this study was too small to make a comparison between patients with and without long-gap esophageal atresia.

The authors conclude that after esophageal atresia correction patients generally perceive their generic and ❷ disease-specific HRQoL to be good. The presence of concomitant congenital anomalies did not influence generic HRQoL. However, a third of patients reported that the disease had had negative consequences.

Finally, Koivusalo et al. from Filland (Koivusalo et al., 2005), compared 159 esophageal atresia survivors with 400 healthy children. They used a 5-part questionnaire incorporating a combination of generic and disease-specific questionnaires (❷ *Table 132-2*) (Aalto et al., 1999; Eypasch et al., 1995; Koivusalo et al., 2005; Nurmi et al., 1995; Slim et al., 1999).

Median age was 38 (range, 24–54) years in the patients with esophageal atresia and 36 (range, 20–56) years in the control subjects (P = NS).

Respiratory symptoms were significantly more frequent and more serious in patients with esophageal atresia. Mean Respiratory Symptoms–Related Quality of Life Index (RSRQLI) scores were significantly higher in control subjects than in patients with esophageal atresia. However, in both groups, the mean RSRQLI score level was high, suggesting a low overall incidence of significant respiratory symptoms.

Mean GIQLI scores were not statistically different between patients with esophageal atresia and control subjects.

Assessment of HRQoL with the SF-36 showed that the incidence of poor quality of life in patients with esophageal atresia – including both physical and mental domains – was 14.8% (19 patients), which is within the expected incidence of 16% of the general population.

Moreover, the health problems that the patients with esophageal atresia with low HRQoL graded as most significant were related to acquired diseases ($n = 11$) – psychiatric problems ($n = 5$), acquired musculoskeletal problems (n = 3), hypertension ($n = 2$), and malignancy ($n = 1$) – or to congenital or esophageal atresia-related diseases ($n = 8$) – haircartilage hypoplasia ($n = 1$), functional gastrointestinal disorders ($n = 2$), gastro-oesophageal reflux ($n = 2$), respiratory problems ($n = 1$), vaginal atresia related vulvodynia ($n = 1$), and mental retardation ($n = 1$).

HRQoL did not differ significantly between patients with short- and long-gap types of esophageal atresia as well as among different types of esophageal reconstruction. HRQoL of patients with colon interposition was somewhat but not statistically significantly lower than in patients undergoing primary anastomosis. Functional and social problems of patients with esophageal atresia with gastric tube or colon interposition decreased significantly as the patients reached their 20s.

The Authors concluded that most adult survivors of esophageal atresia repair have a normal HRQoL. Morbidity from esophageal functional disorders and respiratory disorders with or without acquired diseases impairs HRQoL in 15% of patients with esophageal atresia.

2.3   Spina Bifida

Spina Bifida is the second most common birth defect worldwide. Patients with spina bifida can experience a variety of health problems such as ambulatory problems, faecal and urinary incontinence. Several health specialists have subjected spina bifida patients to extensive study. Here we will focus on the role of continence surgery on the final HRQoL of these patients. Indeed, it might be assumed that reconstruction for incontinent spina bifida might improve HRQoL.

MacNeily et al. (2005) performed a retrospective cohort study of 36 consecutive incontinent spina bifida cases undergoing surgery. The latter included augmentation, with or without creation of a ❯ Mitrofanoff catheterizable conduit, bladder-neck reconstruction and cecostomy. These patients were compared with a group of patients not undergoing continence surgery, but otherwise matched for age, lesion level, parental marital status, ambulatory status and shunt status.

A 5-point Likert questionnaire (❯ 5-point Likert Scale) was used for self-scoring of bladder and bowel continence. HRQoL was assessed by a validated disease-specific discriminative instrument (Parkin et al., 1997). The latter was also age specific and patients were stratified for ages, 12 years or less and 13 years or greater.

After surgery, 78% of reconstructed cases achieved urinary continence for 3 h or more with equal or superior self-reported bladder and bowel continence compared to controls. This, however, was not paralleled by a similar improvement in HRQoL. The 2-sample t testing revealed no significant difference in mean HRQoL score between those who underwent reconstruction, both in children younger than 12 years than for those older than 13.

The authors concluded that surgery may have no impact on HRQoL.

The conclusion seems supported by further two studies. Parekh et al. (2006) assessed prospectively HRQoL in 10 spina bifida patients before and up to 6 moths after continence surgery using PedsQL 4.0 (Varni et al., 1999a, 2001). Although the results of surgery were excellent, they were not paralleled by any improvement in the HRQoL of the patients. Of note, caregivers' HRQoL seems instead to increase significantly after surgery. The second study is a French cross-sectional multicentric study (Lemelle et al., 2006) attempting to determine the relationships between methods of management or urinary/faecal incontinence, methods of management, and HRQoL in 460 spina bifida patients cared for in six centers. HRQoL was evaluated by the SF-36 in adults and the VSP in children. Using both an univariate and multivariate analysis the authors found that urinary/faecal incontinence and their medical management may not play a determinant role in HRQoL of patients with spina bifida.

3 Considerations Based on the Studies Described

Evaluation of HRQoL allows us to give answer in a truly patient-oriented manner to many questions. Starting from the studies mentioned above, some key questions are addressed (❷ *Table 132-1*).

3.1 Is There a Constant Correlation Between Functional Outcome and HRQoL?

It might be hypothesized HRQoL and functional outcome/morbidity of surgery to be correlated to each other. Sometimes this is the case. In the study by Mattioli et al. (2006) about stapling lunge resections via a muscle sparing thoracotomy, the authors actually found that presence of an abnormal spirometric finding was statistically more common in patients with a poorer HRQoL. This observation however does not seem to be always true. The studies on HRQoL in patients operated on as newborns for esophageal atresia, for instance, show that although most of these patients may experience significant long-term morbidity or symptoms, their HRQoL can be expected to be normal or at least acceptable (Deurloo et al., 2005; Koivusalo et al., 2005; Ure et al., 1995, 1998).

On the contrary, the studies on the HRQoL in spina bifida patients undergoing continence surgery show that these patients, in spite of dramatic improvements in the functional outcome in terms of continence after surgery, can still perceive their HRQoL as unchanged (Lemelle et al., 2006; Macneily et al., 2005; Parekh et al., 2006).

3.2 Can Improved Surgical Outcome Only be Reached at the Price of Poorer HRQoL?

This is a key question especially in patients with congenital disease where increased survival corresponds to a survival of an increased number of patients with more severe conditions or multiple associated anomalies.

Deurloo et al. (2005) showed that this is not the case in patients with esophageal atresia. Although, a third of their patients reported that the disease had had negative consequences, generic and disease-specific QOL was generally perceived to be good, and this irrespective of the presence of concomitant congenital anomalies.

It should be said, however, that although in this study, as well as in that by Koivusalo et al. (2005), the number of patients with associated anomalies was quite high, that of severe cases with long-gap atresias was instead quite limited. Indeed, both studies assessed the long-term quality of life in adult patients that survived an operation done even more than 20 years before, therefore in an age when the worse cases usually died. Both studies (Ure et al., 1995, 1998), however, addressed the issue of as to whether cases requiring more complex reconstructions, such as colon interposition, should be expected to have a worse HRQoL. Indeed, HRQoL was found to be acceptable also in these complex cases, although they suffered a greater long-term morbidity and scored slightly lower on the HRQoL tests.

The fact that increased survival is not necessarily associated with a worse HRQoL does not seem to be peculiar of esophageal atresia. Poley et al. (2004) from Rotterdam reported similar results in patients with congenital diaphragmatic hernia and ano-rectal malformations. These patients were found to experience considerable symptomatology, but the vast majority ultimately enjoyed healthy lives.

3.3   Can Assessment of HRQoL Help in the Decision-Making?

Assessment of HRQoL in pediatric surgical patients allows for a definitive assessment of the results of surgery. This is of interest for multiple reasons. First, it allows a more accurate comparison of treatments and therefore a choice of the best one among multiple possible alternatives. Second, the improvement in survival has also led to an increase in the survival of more severe cases. In turn, this has increased the costs of intensive care assistance and for the care of patients who can have chronic morbidity. The increasing budget constraints, has evoked the question of whether the effects of a given treatment are worth the costs. There is growing political interest in evidence-based, cost-effective medicine, including pediatric surgery. Third, as these patients are generally considered at greater risk of long-term morbidity, information on their long-term HRQoL is critical for parents' counseling.

While using data about HRQoL for the decision-making, a critical attitude is mandatory. For instance, data coming from the studies in spina bifida patients seem to suggest that surgery does not affect the HRQoL of these patients. Another possible interpretation however is that, since surgery causes a change in a chronic condition, if performed late, it does not cause immediate changes in the patient HRQoL. Therefore further research in needed to check as to whether surgery should be undertaken at a younger age or a wider interval be allowed before reassessing HRQoL.

3.4   Which Instruments should be Preferred in the Evaluation of HRQoL in Pediatric Surgical Patients?

It is controversial if disease-specific questionnaires should be preferred over generic ones in the assessment of patients' HRQoL. It should be said that very few disease-specific instrument exists for pediatric patients and many studies actually adopt questionnaires devised for adult conditions (Eiser and Morse, 2001). For instance, all the mentioned studies about the HRQoL in patients operated on for esophageal atresia used as disease specific instrument a questionnaire originally devised for the evaluation of esophageal function in adult patients with esophageal cancer (Deurloo et al., 2005).

It is of note that using such instrument, Ure et al. (1998) found that some esophageal atresia patients scored even better than healthy control subjects. This is an example of how coping mechanism can work well in patients born with a congenital malformation.

On the other side, generic instruments allow for a more global evaluation of the impact of the condition on the patient life. They also enable comparison across different pediatric chronic and acute health conditions, as well as benchmarking with healthy population norms.

3.5   Can Assessment of HRQoL be Based on Proxy Report?

As mentioned before, studying pediatric conditions, because of the difficulties that small children have with notions of abstract concepts and language, it is often necessary to rely upon proxies. It is known that a variety of factors can influence a parent's rating of his or her child's HRQoL and findings reported in the literature are indeed equivocal (Canning et al., 1992; Levi and Drotar, 1999; Waters et al., 2000). Nevertheless, recent research in children (Glaser et al., 1997; Theunissen et al., 1998; Barr et al., 2000) suggests that a parent is able to report appropriate information regarding his or her child's HRQoL, especially concerning observable behaviors. There is as yet no clear evidence of whether the parents over- or under-estimate HRQoL. A number of studies indicate that parents tend to rate the child as having a poorer HRQoL than the child does him or herself, a tendency which would result in a conservative estimate of the HRQoL (Ennett et al., 1991).

With regards to the studies mentioned above, Parekh et al. (2006) evaluated HRQoL in spina bifida patients and their parents. And while there was no change in patients' HRQoL before and after surgery, they observed a significant difference in social functioning in parent report.

3.6   Final Considerations

The changing methodology of patient management should be accompanied by an increased awareness among medical providers toward patient HRQoL. In other words, patient-focused care is the key to improving HRQoL in pediatric surgery as well as other health services, and assessment of HRQoL is key for the development of a truly patient-oriented medicine.

Summary Points

- Health Related Quality of Life and functional outcomes in children with surgical conditions not necessarily coincide.
- Health Related Quality of Life can be good or acceptable in spite of significant morbidity.
- Health Related Quality of Life can be independent from the severity of the condition and the presence of associated anomalies.
- Improved survival in neonates with surgical conditions does not involve a worsening in Health Related Quality of Life.
- Proxies are generally reliable in the assessment of Health Related Quality of Life but in some cases surgery might lead to an improvement in Health Related Quality of Life more in the caregivers that in the patients.

References

Aalto AM, Aro AR, Teperi J. (1999). Rand-36 as a Measure of Health Related Quality of Life. Reliability and values in Finnish Population. STAKES research publication 101. Gummerrus, Helsinki pp. 1–78.

Aaronson NK, Muller M, Cohen PD, Essink-Bot ML, Fekkes M, Sanderman R, Sprangers MA, te Velde A, Verrips E. (1998), J Clin Epidemiol. 51: 1055–1068.

Anderson KD, Noblett H, Belsey R, Randolph JG. (1992). Surgery. 111: 131–136.

Apolone G, Mosconi P, Quattrociocchi L, Gianicolo EAL, Groth N, Ware JE Jr. (2001). Questionario sullo stato di salute SF-12. Versione italiana. Guerini e Associati Editore, Milano, pp. 1–85.

Barr RD, Chalmers D, De Pauw S, Furlong W, Weitzman S, Feeny D. (2000). J Clin Oncol. 18: 3280–3287.

Blazeby JM, Conroy T, Hammerlid E, Fayers P, Sezer O, Koller M, Arraras J, Bomalaski MD, Teague JL, Brooks B. (1995). J Urol . 154: 778–781.

Blazeby JM, Conroy T, Bottomley A, Vickery C, Arraras J, Sezer O, Moore J, Koller M, Turhal NS, Stuart R, Van Cutsem E, D'haese S, Coens C (2003). Eur J Cancer 39: 1384–1394.

Bouman NH, Koot HM, Hazebroek FW. (1999). J Pediatr Surg. 34: 399–404.

Canning EH, Hanser SB, Shade KA, Boyce WT. (1992). Pediatrics 90: 692–696.

Deurloo JA, Ekkelkamp S, Hartman EE, Sprangers MA, Aronson DC. (2005). Arch Surg. 140: 976–980.

Eiser C, Morse R. (2001). Arch Dis Child. 84: 205–211.

Engum SA, Grosfeld JL, West KW, Rescorla FJ, Scherer LR 3rd. (1995). Arch Surg. 130: 502–509.

Ennett ST, DeVellis BM, Earp JA, Kredich D, Warren RW, Wilhelm CL. (1991). J Pediatr Psychol. 16: 557–568.

Evers AW, Kraaimaat FW, van Lankveld W, Jongen PJ, Jacobs JW, Bijlsma JW. (2001). J Consult Clin Psychol. 69: 1026–1036.

Eypasch E, Williams JI, Wood-Dauphinee S, Ure BM, Schmülling C, Neugebauer E, Troidl H. (1995). Br J Surg. 82: 216–222.

Glaser AW, Davies K, Walker D, Brazier D. (1997). Qual Life Res. 6: 43–53.

Guyatt G, Feeny D, Patrick D. (1993). Ann Intert Med. 118: 622–629.

Jaureguizar E, Vaizquez J, Murcia J, Diez Pardo JA. (1985). J Pediatr Surg. 20: 511–514.

Koivusalo A, Pakarinen MP, Turunen P, Saarikoski H, Lindahl H, Rintala RJ. (2005). J Pediatr Surg. 40: 307–312.

Lemelle JL, Guillemin F, Aubert D, Guys JM, Lottmann H, Lotart-Jacob S, Mouriquand P, Ruffion A, Moscovici J, Schmitt M. (2006). Qual Life Res. 15: 1481–1492.

Levi RB, Drotar D. (1999). Int J Cancer. 83: 58–64.

Louhimo I, Lindahl H. (1983). J Pediatr Surg. 18: 217–229.

MacNeily EA, Morrell J, Secord S. (2005). J Urol. 174: 1637–1643.

Mattioli G, Buffa P, Granata C, Fratino G, Rossi G, Ivani G, Jasonni V. (1998). Pediatr Surg Int. 13: 10–13.

Mattioli G, Asquascaiti C, Castagnetti M, Bellodi S, Rossi G, Jasonni V. (2006). Pediatr Surg Int. 22: 491–495.

Nurmi JE, Salmela-Aro K, Haavisto T. (1995). Eur J Psychol Assess. 11: 108–121.

Parekh AD, Trusler LA, Pietsch JB, Byrne DW, DeMarco RT, Pope JC, Adams MC, Deshpande JK, Brock JW. (2006). J Urol .176: 1878–1882.

Parkin PC, Kirpalani HM, Rosenbaum PL, Fehlings DL, Van Nie A, Willan AR, King D. (1997). Qual Life Res. 6: 123–132.

Patrick D, Deyo R. (1989). Med Care. 27: S217–S232.

Poley MJ, Stolk EA, Tibboel D, Molenaar JC, Busschbach JJV. (2004). Arch Dis Child. 89: 836–841.

Rinck C, Berg J, Hafeman C. (1989). Adolescence. 24: 699–710.

Rothenberg SR. (2000). J Pediatr Surg. 35: 271–274.

Selby PJ, Chapman JA, Etazadi-Amoli J, Dalley D, Boyd NF. (1984). Br J Cancer. 50: 13–22.

Slim K, Bousquet J, Kwiatkowski F, Lescure G, Pezet D, Chipponi J. (1999). Gastroenterol Clin Biol. 23: 25–31.

Somppi E, Tammela O, Ruuska T, Rahnasto J, Laitinen J, Turjanmaa V, Järnberg J. (1998). J Pediatr Surg. 33: 1341–1346.

Soucy P, Bass J, Evans M. (1991). J Pediatr Surg. 26: 1323–1325.

Spitzer WO, Dobson AJ, Hall J, Chesterman E, Levi J, Shepherd R, Battista RN, Catchlove BR. (1981). J Chronic Dis. 34: 585–597.

Stolk EA, Post HA, Rutten FF, Molenaar JC, Busschbach JJ. (2000). J Pediatr Surg. 35: 588–592.

Theunissen NC, Vogels TG, Koopman HM, Verrips GH, Zwinderman KA, Verloove-Vanhorick SP, Wit JM. (1998). Qual Life Res. 7: 387–397.

Ure BM, Slany E, Eypasch EP, Gharib M, Holschneider AM, Troidl H. (1995). Eur J Pediatr Surg. 5: 206–210.

Ure BM, Slany E, Eypasch EP, Weiler K, Troidl H, Holschneider AM. (1998). J Pediatr Surg. 33: 511–515.

Varni JW, Seid M, Kurtin PS. (1999a). J Clin Outcomes Manage. 6: 33–40.

Varni JW, Seid, M, Rode CA. (1999b). Med Care. 37: 126–139.

Varni JW, Seid M, Kurtin PS. (2001). Med Care. 39: 800–812.

Varni JW, Burwinkle TM, Seid M, Skarr D. (2003). Ambulat Pediatr. 3: 329–341.

Waters E, Doyle J, Wolfe R, Wright M, Wake M, Salmon L. (2000). Pediatrics. 106: 1422–1428.

World Health Organization. (1995). Soc Sci Med. 41: 1403–1409.

133 Breast Reduction Surgery and Quality of Life and Clinical Outcomes

A. Thoma · L. McKnight

1	*Introduction*	*2272*
2	*Summary of Current Evidence*	*2273*
2.1	Meta-analysis and Systematic Reviews	2273
2.2	Randomized Controlled Trials (RCTs)	2274
2.3	Cohort Studies	2276
2.4	Case Control Studies	2278
3	*Quality of Life Measurements Used in Breast Reduction*	*2279*
4	*Generic Scales*	*2282*
4.1	Short Form 36 (SF-36)	2282
5	*Utility Measurement*	*2282*
5.1	European Quality of Life-5 Dimensions (EQ-5D)	2282
5.2	Health Utility Index Mark 2/3 (HUI 2/3)	2283
6	*Condition-Specific Scales*	*2283*
6.1	The Multidimensional Body Self Relations Questionnaire (MBSRQ)	2283
7	*Conclusions*	*2284*
	Summary Points	*2285*

Abstract: ❷ Breast hypertrophy is a common condition seen by plastic surgeons. Patients with this condition complain of upper back, neck and shoulder discomfort and sometimes chronic headaches. They also have trouble finding proper clothing and have difficulties participating in sport activities. Therefore, this condition carries important burdens in health-related quality of life (HRQL). ❷ Breast reduction surgery is the solution to this problem. However, this procedure remains controversial in some geographic jurisdictions because third party payers refuse to pay for it. Also, rather arbitrarily, some plastic surgeons refuse to perform this surgery on overweight patients with this condition. This chapter provides an up-to-date review of the breast reduction studies in which quality of life was the primary outcome measure. The studies considered in this review covered the spectrum of the level of evidence, from case series to ❷ systematic reviews. The majority of publications, however, fell into the lower levels of the evidence (i.e., cohort and ❷ case control studies). All published studies, irrespective of study design demonstrated substantial improvements in quality of life in women who undergo breast reduction surgery. The recent evidence suggests that overweight patients with breast hypertrophy benefit from breast reduction just as much as thin patients with breast hypertrophy. Additionally, the mean ❷ quality-adjusted life years (QALY) gained per patient because of the surgery was 0.12 during the 1-year follow-up period. The health-related quality-of-life (HRQL) effect of the surgery translates into an expected lifetime gain of 5.32 QALYs, which is equivalent to each patient living an additional 5.32 years in perfect health.

List of Abbreviations: *QOL*, quality of life; *HRQL*, health related quality of life; *RCT*, ❷ randomized controlled trial; *HUI 2/3*, health utilities index mark 2/3; *SF-36*, short form 36 health survey questionnaire; *STAI*, state-trait anxiety inventory; *MBSRQ*, multidimensional body-self relations questionnaire; *MPQ*, McGill pain questionnaire; *BRS*, breast-related symptoms; *GHQ12*, general health questionnaire; *STAI*, state-trait anxiety index; *RSE*, Rosenberg self-esteem scale; *SCS*, self-consciousness scale; *DAS-59*, Derriford appearance scale 59; *EQ-5D*, European quality of life-5 dimensions; *FPQ*, Finnish pain questionnaire; *FBAS*, Finnish breast-associated symptoms questionnaire; *15D*, 15D quality of life questionnaire; *HADS*, hospital anxiety and depression score; *FANLT*, functional assessment of non-life threatening conditions version 4; *EPQ-R*, Eysenck personality questionnaire-revised; *HAQ-20*, The Stanford health assessment questionnaire; *DBPT*, digital-body-photo-test; *CAPT*, color-a-person body dissatisfaction test; *SQLP*, subjective quality of life profile; *NASS*, The North American Spine Society Lumbar Spine Outcome Assessment Instrument; *BSI*, breast symptom inventory

1   Introduction

In addition to relieving clinical symptoms and prolonging survival, the primary objective of any health care intervention is the enhancement of quality of life and well-being (Berzon, 1998). The broader term of "quality of life" (QOL) can be defined as "the adequacy of people's material circumstances and to their feelings about these circumstances" (McDowell, 2006). This encompasses indicators of life satisfaction, personal wealth and possessions, level of safety, level of freedom, spirituality, health perceptions, physical, psychological, social and cognitive well-being (McDowell, 2006).

Health-related quality of life (HRQL), a sub-component of QOL, comprises all areas specific to health i.e., physical, emotional, psychological, social, cognitive, role functioning as well as abilities, relationships, perceptions, life satisfaction and well being, and refers to patients' appraisals of their current level of functioning and satisfaction with it, compared to what they perceived to be ideal (Guyatt et al., 1993; Cella et al., 1990). Impairment in HRQL is a major reason why patients seek surgical care (Thoma et al., 2008a).

Breast hypertrophy has been reported by patients to be associated with important burdens in HRQL, specifically pain, discomfort, and emotion. It also creates functional disabilities that adversely affect women because of disproportionate upper body weight. There is cumulative evidence from several studies that breast hypertrophy is associated with significant morbidity and reduced HRQL (Chadbourne et al., 2001; Jones and Bain, 2001; Chao et al., 2002; Collins et al., 2002; Miller et al., 2005; Thoma et al., 2007). Despite the growing evidence showing the salutary effect of reduction mammaplasty on women with breast hypertrophy, some insurers and government agencies set arbitrary body weight and/or tissue resection weight restrictions for coverage for reduction mammaplasty (Klassen et al., 1996; Collins et al., 2002; Kerrigan, 2005; Wagner and Alfonso, 2005; Schmitz, 2005; Thoma et al., 2007). Previous studies using a variety of instruments have reported that reduction mammaplasty had a substantial improve-ment in HRQL regardless of body weight or tissue resection weight. Collins and colleagues (2002) reported that weight loss was not an effective method of relieving the symptoms. In a recent retrospective chart review, Wagner and Alfonso (2005) found no significant difference among the various body mass index groups in terms of symptom relief or development of complication. Thoma and colleagues (2007) demonstrated that women with breast hypertro-phy of all weights benefit from reduction surgery. Women having "small" reductions (<750 g tissue resection) have been shown to have significant improvements in health related quality of life as well. We believe there is strong evidence for third party payers to change their policy and provide universal coverage for this procedure.

2 Summary of Current Evidence

Not all research evidence is judged to be of equal value. That is, different research designs have different strengths and therefore different levels of value in the decision making process (Sprague et al., 2008). For studies evaluating the best surgical treatment in descending order, we recommend the following hierarchy of evidence: ❷ meta-analysis and systematic reviews of high quality randomized controlled trials (RCTs), RCTs, cohort studies, case-control studies, case series, expert opinions, and in vitro and animal studies (Sprague et al., 2008). This ranking has an evolutionary order, moving from simple observational methods at the bottom through to increasingly sophisticated and statistically refined study designs at the top level of evidence. Many of the publications in the breast reduction surgery literature fall into the lower levels of the evidence.

2.1 Meta-analysis and Systematic Reviews

In a well done systematic review the findings of all high quality studies pertaining to a particular clinical question are evaluated together to provide more valid information than any one study can (Haines et al., 2008). In a meta-analysis, the results of the primary studies that meet the standards for inclusion in a review are mathematically pooled to give a result that is more precise because of the overall increase in numbers of study participants contributing data (Haines et al., 2008). Systematic reviews and meta-analyses of the effectiveness of treatments can be performed based on RCTs and/or observational studies. However, RCTs are the traditional study design of choice for primary studies used in meta-analyses, as they are the most likely to be valid (Haines et al., 2008).

There have been two systematic reviews performed on the breast hypertrophy literature (Chadbourne et al., 2001; Jones and Bain, 2001). Chadbourne and colleagues (2001) performed a systematic review and subsequent meta-analysis of the breast hypertrophy literature from 1985–1999. Twenty nine studies were identified that examined physical breast symptoms and QOL in reduction mammaplasty patients. The authors were able to pool data from 15 studies on physical symptoms (headache, neck, shoulder, lower back and breast pain, shoulder grooving, numbness in hand and intertrigo). They found an improvement in all physical symptoms post-operatively. Only four studies administered specific QOL scales to assess QOL. Due to a lack of data, only psychological and physical functioning domains could be analyzed, revealing a risk difference (95% confidence interval) of 0.46 (0.00–1.00) and 0.58 (0.44–0.71) respectively.

Jones and Bain (2001) conducted a similar systematic review of breast hypertrophy articles from 1966–1997. Of the 17 publications identified, all reported physical breast symptoms and ten studies examined QOL (four using validated QOL scales) in reduction mammaplasty patients. Although the reporting outcomes varied greatly among studies, a substantial improvement in physical breast symptoms was reported in all studies. The measurement and reporting of quality of life was inconsistent among studies and was therefore difficult to analyze. However, all studies reported an improvement of psychological well-being after surgery. The authors were not able to perform a meta-analysis due to a lack of data on the subject.

Neither systematic review identified any randomized controlled trials in the breast hypertrophy literature from 1966 to 1999. Randomized controlled trials are considered the most scientifically rigorous study design.

2.2   Randomized Controlled Trials (RCTs)

RCTs offer the maximum protection against bias and are generally regarded as the most scientifically rigorous study design to evaluate the effect of a surgical intervention (Sprague et al., 2008). This type of study offers the maximum protection against biases in the choice of treatment as it facilitates blinding and reduces selection bias, and it balances both known and unknown prognostic factors across treatment groups. Lack of randomization predisposes a study to potentially important imbalances in baseline characteristics between two study groups (Sprague et al., 2008). In breast reduction RCTs have evaluated the use of drains (Rayatt et al., 2005; Collis et al., 2005), lung function (Iwuagwu et al., 2006a), complication rates (Cruz-Korchin and Korchin, 2003), pain management (Bell et al., 2001; Culliford et al., 2007) and upper limb nerve conduction (Iwuagwu et al., 2005). However, very few RCTs in breast hypertrophy have examined QOL (❷ *Table 133-1*).

Iwuagwu and colleagues (2006b,c) randomized patients to early surgery (surgery within 3 weeks of initial visit) or late surgery (surgery within 4–6 month of initial visit). QOL was measured using several validated patient reported questionnaires at the initial visit and 16 weeks after surgery (early surgery group, n = 36) and 16 weeks after initial visit (late surgery group, n = 37). Patients randomized to reduction mammaplasty had significant improvements in depression, pain, anxiety, extroversion and emotional stability.

■ Table 133-1
Randomized Controlled Trials (RCTs) examining quality of life (QOL) in breast hypertrophy patients

Authors	Intervention	Comparative intervention	Outcomes	Time horizon	Conclusions
Saariniemia et al., 2007	Breast reduction surgery, n = 40	Breast hypertrophy women not undergoing surgery, n = 42	Quality of life, pain, breast related symptoms	6 months	Statistically significant and clinically important improvements in all scores of the SF-36, FPQ, FBAS, 15D post-operatively
Iwuagwu et al., 2006b	Delayed surgery (Surgery within 2 weeks of initial visit), n = 36	Early surgery (Surgery within 4–6 months of initial visit), n = 37	Anxiety and depression	4–6 months	Statically significant increase in the proportion of HADS normal scores in both anxiety and depression scores in the early treatment group
Iwaugwu et al., 2006c	Delayed surgery (Surgery within 2 weeks of initial visit), n = 36	Early surgery (Surgery within 4–6 months of initial visit), n = 37	Quality of life and emotional stability	4–6 months	Early surgery groups experienced statistically significant improvements in: All domains of the FANLT and SF-36, Pain, anxiety and depression domains of the EuroQOL, Extroversion and emotional stability of EPQ-R
Freire et al., 2007	Delayed surgery (n = 50)	Early surgery (n = 50)	Pain and functional capacity	6 months	Early surgery groups experienced statistically significant improvements in the following HAQ-20 domains: getting dressed, getting up, walking, maintaining personal hygiene, reaching, and grasping objects Neck, shoulder and lower back pain using visual analogue pain scale

This table summarizes the outcomes of RCTs published in the breast reduction literature. *EQ-5D* European quality of life-5 dimensions; *SF-36* short form 36 health survey questionnaire; *FPQ* Finnish pain questionnaire; *FBAS* Finnish breast-associated symptoms questionnaire; *15D* 15D quality of life questionnaire; *HADS* hospital anxiety and depression score; *FANLT* functional assessment of non-life threatening conditions version 4; *EPQ-R* Eysenck personality questionnaire-revised; *HAQ-20* The Stanford health assessment questionnaire

Freire et al., (2007) conducted a similar study. One hundred consecutive patients were randomized to early (immediate surgery, n = 50) or late surgery (surgery 6 months after the initial assessment, n = 50). Quality of life was measured using a ❷ generic health scale and a visual analogue pain scale 6 months after the initial visit. Women who underwent surgery experienced significant improvements in neck, shoulder and lower back pain and an increase overall quality of life.

Friere et al., (2007) used a lottery randomization system which is not an adequate method. The method of randomization is so crucial to the validity of the study that it needs to be done correctly and be transparent. Using even or odd birth year or alternate chart number or lottery are inadequately concealed and are prone to selection bias. The use random number tables or computer programs to generate the sequences are correct ways to randomize patients (Thoma et al., 2008b).

A computer randomization system was used in a recent Finnish study by Saariniemia and colleagues (2007). Breast hypertrophy patients were randomized to receive breast reduction surgery (n = 40) or receive no surgical treatment (n = 42). Quality of life was measured using a combination of validated general health, pain specific and breast symptom questionnaires at the initial visit and 6 months later. Statistically significant and clinically important improvements in all quality of life, pain and breast related symptoms were observed in the surgical group post-operatively.

2.3   Cohort Studies

❷ Prospective cohort studies involve the identification and follow-up of individual patients who have received a treatment of interest. Although, prospective cohort studies are considered lower level evidence, they have generated an abundance of important data on the HRQL in patients undergoing breast reduction surgery. Since the last systematic review of the literature (Chadbourne et al., 2001), several new prospective cohort studies have been published (❷ *Table 133-2*).

In a recent study, we assessed and measured the HRQL experienced by breast reduction patients using four reliable and validated QOL measures (Thoma et al., 2005, 2007). Consecutive patients with breast hypertrophy completed self-reported outcome measurement tools at one week and one day pre-surgery and 1, 6, and 12 months post-surgery. We found an improvement in all health-related quality-of-life measures from before surgery to 1 month after surgery regardless of patient body mass index and tissue resection weight. The improvement from 1 month after surgery was maintained to 1 year after surgery for all health-related quality-of-life instruments.

Spector and Karp, (2007) found similar results in a cohort of 171 women who underwent reduction mammaplasty. Quality of life was assessed using a custom-made 5 point likert scale per-operatively and at 1 and 3 years post-operatively. Patients reported improvements in buying clothes, participating in sports and running. These results were similar to an earlier studied performed by Blomqvist and colleagues (2000, 2004). Quality of life of 49 women was assessed using a validated scale and 3 custom made 10 point Likert scale questionnaires pre-operatively and 1 and 3 years post-operatively. Statistically significant improvements in overall quality of life and pain were observed at 1 year and maintained 3 years post-operatively. A limitation of these studies was the use of non-validated instruments to assess quality of life.

◘ Table 133-2

Cohort studies examining quality of life (QOL) in women undergoing breast reduction surgery

Authors	Population	Outcomes	Outcomes assessment scales	Time horizon	Conclusions
Thoma et al., 2007	52 women undergoing reduction mammaplasty	HRQL, breast symptoms, body image and self-esteem	HUI 2/3, SF-36, BRS, MBSRQ	1 year	Mean scores for HUI 2/3, SF-36, BRS, MBSRQ increased postoperatively.
Spector and Karp, 2007	59 women, breast resection of <1000 g	Breast related symptoms	Questionnaire designed by the authors (non-validated)	3–12 months	Significant improvement in breast related symptoms post-operatively
Borkenhagen et al., 2007	40 women undergoing reduction mammaplasty	Body image	Digital-body-photo-test (DBPT) and color-a-person body dissatisfaction test (CAPT)	6 months	DBPT and CAPT Scores for dissatisfaction were significantly lower post-operatively
Spector et al., 2006	102 women undergoing reduction mammaplasty	Breast related symptoms	Questionnaire designed by the authors (non-validated)	3–6 months	Significant improvement in breast related symptoms post-operatively
Chahraoui et al., 2006	20 women undergoing reduction mammaplasty	Quality of life, anxiety, psychological distress	SQLP, GHQ12, STAI	4 months	Statistically significant improvements in GHQ12 sleep disorders and difficulties in enjoying their activities domains and SQLP pain, physical appearance, material life, intellectual capacities and inner life domains post-operatively
Miller et al., 2005	56 women undergoing reduction mammaplasty	Quality of life, Breast related symptoms, self-esteem	SF-36, Symptom inventory questionnaire, RSE	6 months	Significant improvements all domains of SF-36, RSE and Symptom Inventory Questionnaire post-operatively

☐ Table 133-2 (continued)

Authors	Population	Outcomes	Outcomes assessment scales	Time horizon	Conclusions
Blomqvist et al., 2000, 2004	49 women undergoing reduction mammaplasty	Pain, breast related symptoms, quality of life	SF-36, 10-point pain scale and 10-point breast related symptoms scale developed by the authors (non-validated)	3 years	Significant improvements in pain and breast related symptoms and all SF-36 domains post-operatively
Chao et al., 2002	55 women undergoing reduction mammaplasty	Physical functioning and quality of life	SF-36, EuroQOL, MBSRQ, MPQ, BRS, NASS Lumbar spine outcome assessment instrument	6 months	Significant improvements in pain (MPQ) and physical functioning (NASS) post-operatively
Behmand et al., 2000	69 women undergoing reduction mammaplasty	Quality of life and breast related symptoms	SF-36, a health-related quality-of-life questionnaire, and the BSI	9 months	Significant improvements in all domains of the SF-36 and BSI post-operatively

This table summarizes the outcomes of prospective cohort studies published in the breast reduction surgery literature. *HUI 2/3* health utilities index mark 2/3; *SF 36* short form 36 health survey questionnaire; *BRS* breast-related symptoms; *MBSRQ* multidimensional body-self relations questionnaire; *DBPT* digital-body-photo-test; *CAPT* color-a-person body dissatisfaction test; *GHQ12* general health questionnaire; *SQLP* subjective quality of life profile; *RSE* Rosenberg self-esteem scale; *MPQ* McGill pain questionnaire; *NASS* The North American Spine Society Lumbar Spine Outcome Assessment Instrument; *BSI* breast symptom inventory

The benefits of breast reduction surgery have been observed as early as 4–6 months post-operatively. Chahraoui et al., (2006) found significant improvements anxiety 4 months post-operatively in 20 women who underwent breast reduction surgery. Statistically significant improvements in physical disability, pain 6 months post-operatively in 55 women were reported by Chao and colleagues (2002). Breast related symptoms, self-esteem and general quality of life improved substantially 6 months post-operatively in a cohort of 56 women (Miller et al., 2005).

A limitation of prospective cohort studies is that they are prone to selection bias. To prevent selection bias, the comparison groups in an observational study should be as similar as possible except for the factors under study. Previous research has reported that observational studies tend to show larger treatment effects than RCTs and may show a greater benefit than what actually exists. However, some investigators argue that well-constructed observational studies lead to similar conclusions as RCTs (Sprague et al., 2008).

2.4   Case Control Studies

A ❷ case-control study is a type of observational study which begins with the identification of individuals who already have the outcome of interest, (referred to as the cases), and a suitable control group without the outcome event (referred to as the controls).

Collins and colleagues (2002) evaluated the quality of life, breast related symptoms, body image, self esteem and pain in women who underwent breast reduction surgery and two control groups: (1) Women with bra size greater than D, "hypertrophy group" (2) Women with bra size less than D "normal group." Quality of life was assessed using validated instruments at the initial visit and again in the surgical group 6–9 months post-operatively. Control subjects were matched for age; however, hypertrophy and operative groups had significantly higher BMI than that of normal controls. Women who underwent surgery rated their appearance significantly higher post-operatively compared to their initial assessment. Also, women in the surgical group experience significant improvements in quality of life and lower pain post-operatively. Pain post-operatively was similar to pain reported by both controls. Multiple regression analysis revealed improvement in outcomes was not associated with age, weight of resected tissue, BMI or bra cup size pre-operatively.

Quality of life, body image and self-esteem were assessed in women suffering from breast hypertrophy (n = 71) and women who had underwent breast reduction surgery in the last two years (n = 94) (Hermans et al., 2005). Groups were matched for age and body mass index. Women in the operative group had significantly better quality of life, lower pain and physical disability and anxiety compared to the non-operative control groups. The non-operative control group demonstrated significantly higher insecurity, shame and unattractiveness (❯ Table 133-3).

3   Quality of Life Measurements Used in Breast Reduction

Traditionally QOL has been measured by complication rates, photographs and surgical assessments. However, these outcome measures are not sufficient to assess patient quality of life. Validated, reliable and responsive patient questionnaires specific to breast reduction surgery are the best method of measuring breast surgery outcomes. Validity refers to the ability of the questionnaire to measure what is intended to be measured. The ability of the questionnaire to produce consistent and reproducible results determines its reliability. The instrument must be sensitive enough to measure changes as a result of the surgical intervention, termed responsiveness.

A wide variety HRQL instruments, generic and disease or ❯ condition specific, have been applied to the area of breast hypertrophy and reduction mammaplasty (❯ Table 133-4). Generic HRQL instruments allow HRQL to be compared among patients with different types of diseases but may not be sensitive enough to detect small differences in patient groups with specific disabilities (Thoma et al., 2008a). Generic HRQL instruments provide an overall assessment of HRQL, with questions covering many health-related domains such as physical, social, emotional, and cognitive functioning, mental health, pain and general health. These include both descriptive health status questionnaires (i.e., Short Form 36 Health Survey Questionnaire (SF-36)), and health ❯ utility measures (i.e., European Quality of Life-5 Dimensions (EQ-5D)). Utilities measures provide preference-weighted outcome measures that represent patients' preferences for a given health state relative to death (represented by 0) or perfect health (represented by 1). There are various methods of measuring utilities including the visual analogue scale, the standard gamble, the time trade-off, and standardized questionnaires including the EQ-5D and the Health Utilities Index (HUI) (Thoma et al., 2008a).

Disease-specific (condition-specific) HRQL measures consist of questions focusing on specific symptoms and impairments relevant to a particular disease state or surgical intervention (Thoma et al., 2008a). Evidence from other clinical settings has shown that the generic

◻ Table 133-3

Cohort studies examining quality of life in breast hypertrophy patients

Authors	Population	Outcomes	Outcomes assessment scales	Time horizon	Conclusions
Hermans et al., 2005	Non-operative breast hypertrophy control group (n = 71) and operative group who had breast reduction surgery 2 years prior (n = 94)	Quality of Life, Physical Appearance, Body Image and Self-Esteem	SF-36, EQ-5D, RSE, SCS, DAS-59, Visual Analogue Scale used to subjectively measure breast appearance	2 years	Non-operative group had scored significantly higher in DAS-59 domains: insecurity, pain, shame, and unattractiveness. Operative group had significantly higher self-esteem score (RSE), significantly lower anxiety (SCS), significantly higher SF-36 scores in 7/8 domains, improved pain and physical disability (EQ-5D)
Collins et al., 2002	Group 1: Hypertrophy control group with bra cup sizes > D (n = 88); Group 2: Control group with bra cup sizes <D (n = 96); Group 3: Operative group (n = 179)	Quality of life, pain, breast related symptoms	SF-36, EuroQOl, MBSRQ, and the MPQ, BRS	?	After surgery, the operative subjects improved significantly from pre-surgical means in all domains of the SF-36. After surgery, pain was significantly lower and similar to that of our controls

This table summarizes the outcomes of case control studies published in the breast reduction surgery literature. *RSE* Rosenberg self-esteem scale; *SCS* self-consciousness scale; *DAS-59* Derriford appearance scale 59; *EQ-5D* European quality of life-5 dimensions; *SF-36* short form 36 health survey questionnaire; *MBSRQ* Multidimensional Body-Self Relations Questionnaire; *MPQ* McGill pain questionnaire; *BRS* Breast-Related Symptoms

instruments may be as efficient as the disease-specific ones. However, breast hypertrophy patients have unique breast related and psychological symptoms that may not be captured by only using a generic instrument. A recommendation was made by Guyatt et al., (1993) to include a generic, a disease (condition) specific instrument and a utility measurement in the evaluation of medical interventions. There has been a wide variety of well-developed instruments to assess psychological functioning in breast hypertrophy patient (❱ *Table 133-5*).

■ Table 133-4

Generic scales used to assess the benefit of breast reduction surgery

Instrument	Author, Year
Short form 36 health survey questionnaire (SF-36)	Thoma et al., 2007
	Iwuagwu et al., 2006
	Hermans et al., 2005
	Miller et al., 2005
	Thoma et al., 2005
	Blomqvist and Brandberg, 2004
	Collins et al., 2002
	Behmand et al., 2000
	Klassen et al., 1996
General health questionnaire	Chahraoui et al., 2006
	Klassen et al., 1996
Stanford health assessment questionnaire	Freire et al., 2007
Functional assessment of non-LIFE threatening conditions version 4 (FANLT)	Iwuagwu et al., 2006

This table lists the generic scales that have been used to assess quality of life in breast hypertrophy patients

■ Table 133-5

Instruments used to assess psychological functioning in breast reduction surgery patients

Instrument	Author, Year
Rosenberg self esteem scale	Hermans et al., 2005
	Miller et al., 2005
	Klassen et al., 1996
Hospital anxiety and depression (HAD) scale	Iwuagwu et al., 2006
Eysenck personality questionnaire	Iwuagwu et al., 2006
State-trait anxiety inventory	Chahraoui et al., 2006
Derriford appearance scale 59	Hermans et al., 2005

This table lists the psychological functioning scales that have been used to assess quality of life in breast hypertrophy patients

A recent systematic review of quality of life instruments used in breast surgery conducted by Pusic et al., (2007) identified several breast surgery specific questionnaires including: The Multidimensional Body Self Relations Questionnaire (MBSRQ), and Breast Related Symptoms Questionnaire (BRS). Only the BRS has been developed specifically for breast reduction patients. However, very few studies have used breast specific scales to assess QOL after reduction mammaplasty.

4   Generic Scales

Several different generic instruments have been used to assess the quality of life in breast reduction patients (❷ *Table 133-4*). The most commonly used instrument is the Short Form 36.

4.1   Short Form 36 (SF-36)

The SF-36 is a multipurpose, short form health survey with 36 questions consisting of eight domains: Physical function (10 items), role physical (4 items), bodily pain (2 items), general health (5 items), vitality (4 items), social functioning (2 items), role emotional (4 items), and mental health (5 items) (Ware, 1996). The two summary measures of the SF-36 are the physical component summary and the mental component summary. The scores for the multifunction item scales and the summary measures of the SF-36 vary from 0 to 100, with 100 being the best possible score and 0 being the lowest possible score. There is no principle for calculating the magnitude that constitutes a clinically important difference on the Short Form 36 subscales. A 10-point change in scores has been suggested as a rule of thumb with which to apply on 100-point quality-of-life scales (Thoma et al., 2007).

5   Utility Measurement

Utility scores of HRQL derived from responses to generic single index instruments such as the Health Utility Index (HUI) and European Quality of Life-5 Dimensions (EQ-5D) have the required measurement properties for calculating quality-adjusted life years (QALYs). QALYs are the measure of effectiveness in cost-utility analysis. This outcome measure incorporates both changes in quantity of life (i.e., reduction of mortality) and quality of life (i.e., reduction in morbidity) into a standard "metric."

$$QALY = (duration\ of\ health\ state) \times (utility\ of\ health\ state) + (future\ remaining\ life\ expectancy - duration\ of\ health\ state) \times (utility\ of\ successful\ reconstruction)$$

QALYs are used in economic analyses to calculate the Incremental Cost-Utility Ratio (ICUR). ICUR determines if the "novel" procedure is cost-effective, when compared to an "old procedure" or not (Thoma et al., 2008b). The ICUR represents the marginal cost per marginal unit of utility (effectiveness) and is calculated as follows:

$$ICUR = \Delta C / \Delta U = (Mean\ Cost\ "intervention" - Mean\ Cost\ free\ "comparative\ intervention")/ (Mean\ QALY\ "intervention" - Mean\ QALY\ "comparative\ intervention")$$

This ratio, which integrates costs and effectiveness, tells us whether we should adopt the novel procedure. The result is represented as cost per QALY. In simple words, it tells us how much it costs to prolong the life of a patient by one extra year in perfect health. The higher the ICUR, the greater the incremental cost for an additional healthy year of life.

5.1   European Quality of Life-5 Dimensions (EQ-5D)

The EQ-5D was created in 1990 by an international and interdisciplinary team (The EuroQOL Group, 1990). It consists of five dimensions of health (1) mobility, (2) self-care, (3) usual activities, (4) pain/discomfort, (5) anxiety/depression. Each dimension comprises three levels (1) no problems, (2) some/moderate problems, (3) extreme problems (◗ *Table 133-6*).

◘ Table 133-6

Utility measurement scales used to assess quality of life in breast reduction surgery patients

Instrument	Author, Year
EuroQOL	Iwuagwu et al., 2006
	Hermans et al., 2005
	Collins et al., 2002
Health utilities index mark 2/3 (HUI 2/3)	Thoma et al., 2007

This table lists the utility scales that have been used to assess quality of life in breast hypertrophy patients

5.2   Health Utility Index Mark 2/3 (HUI 2/3)

The Health Utility Index is a family of comprehensive, reliable, responsive, and valid multi-attribute utility instruments. The HUI is a well-known health status and quality of life assessment instrument developed as an indirect method of measuring utilities (preferences) in clinical trials and other studies (Torrance et al., 1996; Furlong et al., 2001; Feeny et al., 2002). The HUI is a comprehensive, reliable, responsive, and valid multi-attribute utility instrument.

Responses to the questionnaire are converted using standard algorithms to levels of the Health Utilities Index Mark 2 (HUI2) and Mark 3 (HUI3) multi-attribute health status classification systems. The attribute levels are combined with published scoring functions to calculate utility scores of overall HRQL. The Health Utilities Index Mark 2 and Mark 3 health status classification systems are complementary. Together, they provide descriptive measures of ability or disability for health state attributes and descriptions of comprehensive health status. The minimum clinically important difference in Health Utility Index means is 0.03 for health-related quality of life and 0.05 for single-attribute utility scores (◗ *Table 133-6*).

6   Condition-Specific Scales

6.1   The Multidimensional Body Self Relations Questionnaire (MBSRQ)

The MBSRQ was designed to assess quality of life after breast reconstruction surgery. It is a well-validated self-report inventory for the assessment of self-attitudinal aspects of the body-image construct. The MBSRQ is a 69-item self-report inventory for the assessment of self-attitudinal aspects of the body-image constructs (Cash et al., 1990). The MBSRQ is intended for use with adults and adolescents over the age of 15 years (Cash et al., 1990). Two forms of the Multidimensional Body Self Relations Questionnaire are available, the full version and the Multidimensional Body Self Relations Questionnaire Appearance Scales. The full, 69-item version consists of seven factor subscales: (1) appearance evaluation, (2) appearance orientation, (3) fitness evaluation, (4) fitness orientation, (5) health evaluation, (6) health orientation, and

(7) illness orientation. There are also three multiple item subscales: (1) the body areas satisfaction scale, (2) the overweight preoccupation scales, and (3) the self-classified weight scale. In breast reduction patients, the most relevant subscales are likely the appearance evaluation and the appearance orientation. Measuring body image Scores vary from 1 to 5. A high score indicates emphasis on one's looks, attention to one's appearance, and engaging in extensive grooming behaviors. A low score indicates apathy about one's appearance, one's looks are not especially important, and not expending much effort to "look good." High scorers feel mostly positive and satisfied with their appearance; low scorers have a general unhappiness with their physical appearance.

A recent systematic review by Pusic and colleagues (2007) identified questionnaires developed and validated for use in cosmetic and reconstructive breast surgery. Only seven questionnaires specific to breast surgery were found:

1. Dow Corning questionnaire (Cash et al., 2002)
2. McGhan (McGhan Medical Corporation, 1995)
3. Breast Implant Replacement Study (BIRS) (LipoMatrix, Inc., unpublished)
4. Breast Evaluation Questionnaire (BEQ) (Anderson et al., 2006)
5. Breast-Related Symptoms Questionnaire (BRSQ) (Anderson et al., 2006)
6. Michigan Breast Reconstruction Outcomes Study – Satisfaction questionnaire (MBROS-S) (Kerrigan et al., 2001)
7. Michigan Breast Reconstruction Outcomes Study – Body Image Questionnaire (MBROS–BI) (Kerrigan et al., 2002)

Of the seven, only one, the Breast-Related Symptoms Questionnaire (BRSQ), had undergone adequate development and validation in breast surgery patients. The BRSQ lists 13 breast-related symptoms with five levels and the respondent indicates how much of the time she has the symptoms: upper back pain, difficulty finding bras and clothes, headaches, breast pain, lower back pain, rashes under breasts, bra strap grooves, difficulty participating in sports, neck pain, shoulder pain, hard time running, pain in hands, arm pain. From this question-naire, two scores are derived. The first score is the breast symptom summary score (BSS score), which is calculated by taking the mean scores of all 13 items. The BSS score varies from 0 to 100, with a high score corresponding to fewer and less severe breast symptoms. For the second score, seven items of the 13-item scale are used to provide the physical symptom count.

7   Conclusions

All published studies, irrespective of study design, have demonstrated substantial improve-ments in QOL in women who undergo reduction mammaplasty. A plethora of instruments have been used to assess quality of life in breast reduction patients. However, very few studies have used breast specific scales, specifically the BSRQ. A combination of generic, breast specific and utility instruments should be used in future studies examining quality of life in these patients.

High quality research evidence is needed now to compare the multitude of breast reduc-tion techniques used (i.e., inferior pedicle, vertical scar techniques) and perform cost-effectiveness analysis to identify which techniques are cost-effective (Thoma et al., 2008b).

Summary Points

- Breast reduction surgery is the most common plastic surgery procedure for breast hypertrophy.
- Some insurers and government agencies set arbitrary body weight and/or tissue resection weight restrictions for coverage for breast reduction surgery.
- A wide variety health related quality of life instruments, generic and disease or condition specific, have been applied to the area of breast hypertrophy.
- Various study designs have been used to assess quality of life in breast reduction surgery patients. Most falling into lower level research evidence (observational studies).
- All published studies, irrespective of study design or quality of life measurement tool, have demonstrated substantial improvements in quality of life in women who undergo breast reduction surgery.

References

Anderson RC, Cunningham B, Tafesse E, Lenderking WR. (2006). Plast Reconstr Surg. 118: 597.

Behmand RA, Tang DH, Smith DJ, Jr. (2000). Ann Plast Surg. 45(6): 575–80.

Bell RF, Sivertsen A, Mowinkel P, Vindenes H. (2001). Acta Anaesthesiol Scand. 45: 576–82.

Berzon RA. (1998). Understanding and using health-related quality of life instruments within clinical research. In: Staquet MJ, Hays RD, Fayers PM (eds.) Quality of Life Assessment in Clinical Trials: Methods and Practice. Oxford University Press, Oxford.

Blomqvist L, Eriksson A, Brandberg Y. (2000). Plast Reconstr Surg. 106: 991–997.

Blomqvist L, Brandberg Y. (2004). Plast Reconstr Surg. 114: 49–54.

Borkenhagen A, Röhricht F, Preiss S, Schneider W, Brähler E. (2007). Ann Plast Surg. 58: 364–370.

Cash TF, Duel LA, Perkins LL. (2002). Plast Reconstr Surg. 109: 2112.

Cash TF, Pruzinsky T. (1990). Body Images: Development, Deviance, and Change. The Guilford Press, New York.

Cella DF, Tulsky DS. (1990). Oncology (Williston Park). 5: 29–38.

Chadbourne EB, Zhang S, Gordon MJ, Ro EY, Ross SD, Schnur PL, Schneider-Redden PR. (2001). Mayo Clin Proc. 76: 503–510.

Chahraoui K, Danino A, Benony H, Frachebois C, Clerc AS, Malka G. (2006). J Psychosom Res. 61: 801–806.

Chao JD, Memmel HC, Redding JF, Egan L, Odom LC, Casas LA. (2002). Plast Reconstr Surg. 110: 1644–1652.

Collins ED, Kerrigan CL, Kim M, Lowery JC, Striplin DT, Cunningham B, Wilkins EG. (2002). Plast Reconstr Surg. 109: 1556–1566.

Collis N, McGuiness CM, Batchelor AG. (2005). Br J Plast Surg. 58: 286–289.

Cruz-Korchin N, Korchin L. (2003). Plast Reconstr Surg. 112: 1573–1578.

Culliford AT, IV, Spector JA, Flores RL, Louie O, Choi M, Karp NS. (2007). Plast Reconstr Surg. 120: 840–844.

Feeny D, Furlong W, Torrance GW, Goldsmith CH, Zhu Z, DePauw S, Denton M, Boyle M. (2002). Med Care. 40: 113–128.

Freire M, Neto MS, Garcia EB, Quaresma MR, Ferreira LM. (2007). Plast Reconstr Surg. 119: 1149–1156.

Furlong WJ, Feeny DH, Torrance GW, Barr RD. (2001). Ann Med. 33: 375–384.

Guyatt GH, Feeny DH, Patrick DL. (1993). Ann Intern Med. 118: 622–629.

Haines T, McKnight L, Duku E, Perry L, Thoma A. (2008). Clin Plast Surg. 35: 207–214.

Hermans BJ, Boeckx WD, De Lorenzi F, van der Hulst RR. (2005). Ann Plast Surg. 55: 227–231.

Iwuagwu OC, Bajalan AA, Platt AJ, Stanley PR, Drew PJ. (2005). Ann Plast Surg. 55: 445–448.

Iwuagwu OC, Platt AJ, Stanley PW, Hart NB, Drew PJ. (2006a). Plast Reconstr Surg. 118: 1–6.

Iwuagwu OC, Walker LG, Stanley PW, Hart NB, Platt AJ, Drew PJ. (2006b). Br J Surg. 93: 291–294.

Iwuagwu OC, Stanley PW, Platt AJ, Drew PJ, Walker LG. (2006c). Scand J Plast Reconstr Surg Hand Surg. 40: 19–23.

Jones SA, Bain JR. (2001). Plast Reconstr Surg. 108: 62–67.

Kerrigan CL. (2005). Prospective study of outcomes after reduction mammaplasty (Discussion). Plast Reconstr Surg. 115: 1032.

Kerrigan CL, Collins ED, Striplin D, et al. (2001). Plast Reconstr Surg. 108: 1591.

Kerrigan CL, Collins ED, Kim HM, et al. (2002). Med Decis Making. 22: 208.

Klassen A, Fitzpatrick R, Jenkinson C, et al. (1996). BMJ. 313: 454.

McDowell I. (2006). Measuring Health: A Guide to Rating Scales and Questionnaires, 3rd ed. Oxford University Press, Oxford.

McGhan Medical Corporation. (1995). Saline-Filled Mammary Implant Augmentation Clinical Study Protocol (Unpublished archival document). ASPS Archives, Arlington Heights, IL.

Miller BJ, Morris SF, Sigurdson LL, Bendor-Samuel RL, Brennan M, Davis G, Paletz JL. (2005). Plast Reconstr Surg. 115: 1025–1031.

Pusic AL, Chen CM, Cano S, Klassen A, McCarthy C, Collins ED, Cordeiro PG. (2007). Plast Reconstr Surg. 120: 823–837.

Rayatt SS, Dancey AL, Jaffe W. (2005). Plast Reconstr Surg. 115: 1605–1608.

Saariniemia KM, Sintonen H, Kuokkanen HO. (2008). Scand J Plast Reconstr Surg Hand Surg. 42: 194–198.

Schmitz D. (2005). Insurers tighten restrictions for reduction mammaplasty. Plast Surg News. 1.

Spector JA, Karp NS. (2007). Plast Reconstr Surg. 120: 845–850.

Spector JA, Rebecca K, Culliford AT, IV, Karp NS. (2006). Plast Reconstr Surg. 117: 374–381.

Sprague S, McKay P, Thoma A. (2008). Clin Plast Surg. 35: 195–205.

The EuroQOL Group. (1990). Euro QOL – a new facility for the measurement of health-related quality of life. Health Policy 16: 199–208.

Thoma A, Cornacchi SD, Lovrics PJ, Goldsmith CH. (2008a). Can J Surg. 51: 215–224.

Thoma A, Sprague S, Temple C, Archibald S. (2008b). Clin Plast Surg. 35: 275–284.

Thoma A, Sprague S, Veltri K, Duku E, Furlong W. (2005). Health Qual Life Outcomes. 3: 44.

Thoma A, Sprague S, Veltri K, Duku E, Furlong W. (2007). Plast Reconstr Surg. 120: 13–26.

Torrance GW, Feeny DH, Furlong WJ, Barr RD, Zhang Y, Wang Q. (1996). Med Care, 34: 702–722.

Wagner DS, Alfonso DR. (2005). Plast Reconstr Surg. 115: 1034.

Ware JE, Jr. (1996). The SF-36 health survey. In: Spilker B. (ed.) Quality of Life and Pharmacoeconomics in Clinical Trials, 2nd ed. Lippincott-Raven Press, Philadelphia, PA, pp. 337–345.

134 Quality of Life and Postoperative Anesthesia in Gastrointestinal Surgery

R. Kennelly · A. M. Hogan · J. F. Boylan · D. C. Winter

1	*Introduction*	*2288*
2	*Post Operative Anesthetic Modalities*	*2289*
2.1	Systemic Analgesia	2289
2.2	Regional Anesthesia	2290
2.2.1	Intraspinal	2290
2.2.2	Peripheral Nerve Blockade	2291
3	*Post Operative Pain*	*2291*
3.1	Systemic Morphine (PCA) Versus Epidural Analgesia	2291
3.2	Systemic Morphine (PCA) Versus Intrathecal Morphine	2296
3.3	Peripheral Nerve Block in Gastrointestinal Surgery	2296
4	*Patient Outcome*	*2296*
5	*Quality of Life*	*2297*
6	*Concluding Remarks*	*2301*
	Summary Points	*2302*

Abstract: Gastrointestinal surgery impacts considerably on quality of life particularly in the post operative period. The magnitude of this effect is governed by the systemic response to surgery and minimally invasive techniques have allowed for considerable advances in this area. Traditionally, the role of the anaesthetist was limited to pain control. Adequate analgesia is essential for rapid rehabilitation after surgery and is a major factor contributing to patient satisfaction. However, ❷ anesthesia may have a further influence by favorably modulating the systemic response, expediting recovery and improving quality of life.

Various anesthetic regimens have been utilized in gastrointestinal surgery. Intraspinal techniques have shown promising results in comparison with more conventional intravenous analgesics but evidence of improved outcome is scarce.

Multimodal post operative care has an undoubted positive impact on patient outcome however the influence of the anesthetic component is difficult to ascertain. Some recent trials have indicated that epidural anesthetic techniques improve QOL in the post operative period when compared to more traditional anesthetic techniques. While these results are encouraging, further clinical trials are needed assessing impact of anesthesia on quality of life before recommendations can be made.

List of Abbreviations: *CEI*, continuous epidural infusion; *CGQL*, Cleveland global quality of life questionnaire; *GI*, gastrointestinal; *IV*, intravenous; *MASTER*, Multicentred Australian Study of Epidural Anesthesia; *NSAID*, ❷ non-steroidal anti-inflammatory drugs; *PCA*, patient controlled analgesia; *PCEA*, patient controlled epidural analgesia; *QOL*, quality of life; *RCT*, randomized controlled trial; *SF 8*, Short form 8 questionnaire; *SF 36*, Short form 36 questionnaire; *VAS*, visual analogue scale

1   Introduction

Quality of Life (QOL) and other patient-outcome studies may reveal important differences between treatment options from the perspective of the patient (Coffey et al., 2002; Flynn et al., 2003; Kalbassi et al., 2003; Kell et al., 2003; Winter et al., 2004). These patient centered, evidence-based data are important for planning interventions, including post-operative analgesia. Major surgery imposes pain, physical, mental and physiological stresses that translate into diminished QOL (Wu et al., 2003). The focus on ❷ perioperative management is driven by the concept that modulation of these stressors can impact favorably on postoperative morbidity and therefore improve QOL. It is known that the type of surgical intervention is a major determinant impacting on QOL (az De et al., 2003) and increased understanding of the role of the operation has given rise to interest in muscle sparing incisions and minimally invasive surgical techniques. This concept has formed the basis for numerous investigations into the modulation of inflammatory markers in open vs. laparoscopic procedures (Hill, 2006; Schietroma et al., 2004; Schietroma et al., 2007). The overall impression is that reduction of size of incision reduces the inflammatory stress response.

Similarly the role of anesthesia as a purely analgesic intervention is now being questioned. Certainly pain control is essential and remains the most important endpoint when assessing anesthetic techniques however the impact of anesthesia on the metabolic and endocrine consequences of major surgery is now an area of active research (Holte and Kehlet, 2002b). It is important to remember that it is the integration of analgesic care with a perioperative recovery program which emphasizes ❷ minimally invasive surgery, conservative IV fluid titration, minimal use of nasogastric intubation and early oral intake and rapid mobility that has brought about the recent advancements in perioperative patient management. Bearing this in mind the anaesthetist has an integral role to play in perioperative patient care. There are numerous pharmaceutical combinations and drug delivery mechanisms present in the modern day anesthetic armentarium. All of these have been used to varying affect in the postoperative setting. The aim of this chapter is to examine the evidence in the published literature of the effectiveness of these modalities in gastrointestinal surgery with particular emphasis on patient outcome and quality of life.

2   Post Operative Anesthetic Modalities

2.1   Systemic Analgesia

Opioid analgesia has been the mainstay of post operative analgesia and indeed is the model against which all techniques are measured. The original method of delivering post operative analgesia involving nurse controlled administration has largely been replaced by patient controlled analgesia (PCA) pumps (❷ *Figure 134-1*). A PCA device provides as needed bolus analgesia to the patient. There is a timed lock out function preventing overdose. PCA has been available for almost 25 years and is accepted as the optimum method of systemic opioid delivery after major surgery. It provides good pain control and increases patient satisfaction (Nitschke et al., 1996). However, side effects such as sedation and nausea and vomiting are common and opiate induced respiratory depression can result in poor patient outcome.

◻ Figure 134-1

Patient Controlled Analgesia Device. These devices allow the patient to self administer intravenous anesthetic agents such as opioid medication

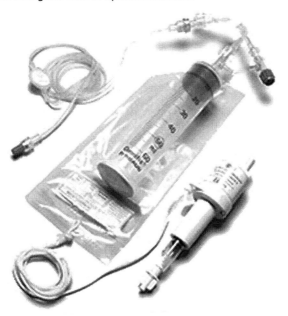

2.2 Regional Anesthesia

2.2.1 Intraspinal

Intraspinal techniques involve the instillation of anesthetic agents (opioids or local anesthetic or a combination) into the epidural (extradural) space or the subarachnoid (intrathecal) space. Due to the anatomy of the spinal cord, intrathecal or spinal anesthesia is only possible below the level of the conus medullaris and therefore is only relevant to low colorectal and perineal procedures. Epidural anesthesia can be used as an anesthetic solution for upper and lower gastrointestinal surgery (❷ *Figure 134-2*). Intraspinal anesthesia is widely used

❑ Figure 134-2

Anatomy of Lumbar Spine, magnetic resonance image (MRI). Arrows identify anatomy of the spinal cord including the specific sites where intraspinal anesthesia is administered (a) **Conus medullaris: end of spinal cord** (b) **Epidural space** (c) **Subarachnoid space** (d) **Point of entry for epidural catheter**

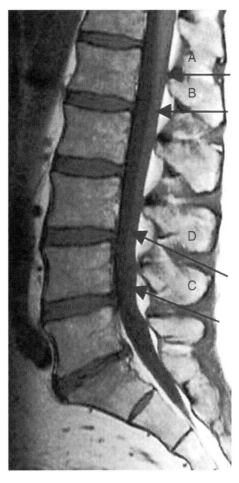

and delivers excellent pain relief (Block et al., 2003; Gwirtz et al., 1999). Opioid related side effects tend to be less frequent due to the smaller dose required to provide an analgesic effect however ❷ pruritus and nausea and vomiting, motor block and urinary retention can occur and can cause reduced patient satisfaction (Wu et al., 2001).

2.2.2 Peripheral Nerve Blockade

Paravertebral, intercostal nerve blockade and interpleural instillation of anesthetic agents can be employed to achieve local pain control in the post operative period following esophagect-omy (Richardson and Cheema, 2006). More experimental mechanisms of peripheral blockade relevant to abdominal surgery have been described (McDonnell et al., 2007). Evidence of the impact of these techniques on patient outcome and quality of life will be addressed.

3 Post Operative Pain

Many studies have been performed comparing the analgesic effects of differing post operative anesthetic regimes. As a rule, visual analogue scales (VAS) are used to assess pain from the patient's perspective. The patient is asked to mark their level of pain on a 100 mm line where 0 equals no pain and 100, the worst pain ever experienced (❷ *Figure 134-3*). It must be

◘ Figure 134-3
Visual Analogue Pain Score. This is a common device employed to assess pain from the patient's perspective

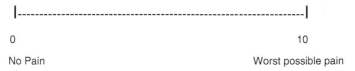

remembered that although pain impacts on QOL it is not the only contributory factor. The measurement of QOL requires application of patient questionnaires that have been psychometrically validated allowing for the condition and the context i.e., the post operative setting. VAS is useful for measurement of trends of pain control only. To extrapolate this data as a surrogate marker of QOL is a gross over simplification only apparent when the VAS is compared with a typical validated QOL instrument (❷ *Figure 134-4*). All things considered however, pain control is an integral factor in maintaining QOL and therefore deserves attention.

3.1 Systemic Morphine (PCA) Versus Epidural Analgesia

The efficacy of epidural analgesia in comparison with patient controlled systemic analgesia was examined by ❷ meta-analysis (Block et al., 2003). A total of 100 randomized controlled trials

■ Figure 134-4

Short Form 36 questionnaire (SF-36). An instrument for assessment of quality of life, validated in the postoperative setting

1. In general, would you say your health is:	
Excellent	1
Very good	2
Good	3
Fair	4
Poor	5

2. **Compared to one year ago**, How would your rate your health in general **now**?	
Much better now than one year ago	1
Somewhat better now than one year ago	2
About the same	3
Somewhat worse now than one year ago	4
Much worse now than one year ago	5

The following items are about activities you might do during a typical day. Does **your health now limit you** in these activities? If so, how much?

(Circle One Number on Each Line)

	Yes, Limited a Lot	Yes, Limited a Little	No, Not limited at All
3. **Vigorous activities**, such as running, lifting heavy objects, participating in strenuous sports	[1]	[2]	[3]
4. **Moderate activities**, such as moving a table, pushing a vacuum cleaner, bowling, or playing golf	[1]	[2]	[3]
5. Lifting or carrying groceries	[1]	[2]	[3]
6. Climbing **several** flights of stairs	[1]	[2]	[3]
7. Climbing **one** flight of stairs	[1]	[2]	[3]
8. Bending, kneeling, or stooping	[1]	[2]	[3]
9. Walking **more than a mile**	[1]	[2]	[3]
10. Walking **several blocks**	[1]	[2]	[3]

☐ Figure 134-4 (continued)

11. Walking **one block**	[1]	[2]	[3]
12. Bathing or dressing yourself	[1]	[2]	[3]

During the **past 4 weeks**, have you had any of the following problems with your work or other regular daily activities **as a result of your physical health**?

(Circle One Number on Each Line)

	Yes	No
13. Cut down the amount of time you spent on work or other activities	1	2
14. **Accomplished less** than you would like	1	2
15. Were limited in the **kind** of work or other activities	1	2
16. Had **difficulty** performing the work or other activities (for example, it took extra effort)	1	2

During the **past 4 weeks,** have you had any of the following problems with your work or other regular daily activities **as a result of any emotional problems** (such as feeling depressed or anxious)?

(Circle One Number on Each Line)

	Yes	No
17. Cut down the **amount of time** you spent on work or other activities	1	2
18. **Accomplished less** than you would like	1	2
19. Didn't do work or other activities as **carefully** as usual	1	2

20. During the **past 4 weeks,** to what extent has your physical health or emotional problems interfered with your normal social activities with family, friends, neighbors, or groups?

(Circle One Number)

Not at all 1

Slightly 2

Moderately 3

Quite a bit 4

Extremely 5

◻ **Figure 134-4 (continued)**

21. How much **bodily** pain have you had during the **past 4 weeks**?

(Circle One Number)

None 1

Very mild 2

Mild 3

Moderate 4

Severe 5

Very severe 6

22. During the **past 4 weeks,** how much did **pain** interfere with your normal work (including both work outside the home and housework)?

(Circle One Number)

Not at all 1

A little bit 2

Moderately 3

Quite a bit 4

Extremely 5

These questions are about how you feel and how things have been with you **during the past 4 weeks**. For each question, please give the one answer that comes closest to the way you have been feeling.

How much of the time during the **past 4 weeks** . . .

(Circle One Number on Each Line)

	All of the Time	Most of the Time	A Good Bit of the Time	Some of the Time	A Little of the Time	None of the Time
23. Did you feel full of pep?	1	2	3	4	5	6
24. Have you been a very nervous person?	1	2	3	4	5	6
25. Have you felt so down in the dumps that nothing could cheer you up?	1	2	3	4	5	6
26. Have you felt calm and peaceful?	1	2	3	4	5	6

■ Figure 134-4 (continued)

27. Did you have a lot of energy?	1	2	3	4	5	6
28. Have you felt downhearted and blue?	1	2	3	4	5	6
29. Did you feel worn out?	1	2	3	4	5	6
30. Have you been a happy person?	1	2	3	4	5	6
31. Did you feel tired?	1	2	3	4	5	6

32. During the **past 4 weeks,** how much of the time has your **physical health or emotional problems** interfered with your social activities (like visiting with friends, relatives, etc.)?

(Circle One Number)

All of the time 1

Most of the time 2

Some of the time 3

A little of the time 4

None of the time 5

How TRUE or FALSE is <u>each</u> of the following statements for you.

(Circle One Number on Each Line)

	Definitely True	Mostly True	Don't Know	Mostly False	Definitely False
33. I seem to get sick a little easier than other people	1	2	3	4	5
34. I am as healthy as anybody I know	1	2	3	4	5
35. I expect my health to get worse	1	2	3	4	5
36. My health is excellent	1	2	3	4	5

were included in the study. Epidural techniques provided significantly better pain relief over parenteral delivery with a combination of opioid and local anesthetic providing the best results. A further meta-analysis comparing a patient controlled epidural (PCEA) and a continuous infusion (CEI) (Wu et al., 2005) showed a significant reduction in side effects in the PCEA group with comparable analgesia.

3.2   Systemic Morphine (PCA) Versus Intrathecal Morphine

Intrathecal anesthesia, unlike epidural, is administered as a once only dose.

Trials comparing this technique to PCA have reported improved analgesia in the immediate post operative period in the intrathecal group and reduced parenteral morphine consumption (Beaussier et al., 2006; Devys et al., 2003). It is important to note that regardless of these findings there was no difference in incidence of adverse reactions and side effects, nor was there any difference in length of hospital stay.

From these studies it can be concluded that intrathecal opioid improves pain scores in the first post operative day in gastrointestinal surgery. The lack of improvement in patient outcome and increased exposure to side effects associated with spinal analgesia would suggest that its effect on patient QOL is questionable.

3.3   Peripheral Nerve Block in Gastrointestinal Surgery

The mainstay of treatment for esophageal cancer is surgery. It is performed either through a combined ❷ thoracotomy and upper abdominal incision or ❷ laparotomy and ❷ trans hiatal resection with a small proportion of centers performing minimally invasive procedures (Bottger et al., 2007; Luketich et al., 2003). There is much discussion regarding the best surgical approach and the role of minimally invasive techniques and there is no doubt that the surgical stress response is modulated to a large extent by these variables. Much research has been conducted into the optimum methods for achieving pain control and preliminary results are promising (McDonnell et al., 2007; Richardson et al., 1995, 1999) No comparison has yet been made with epidural analgesia or intrathecal techniques and so no conclusions can be drawn as to the comparative impact these may have on patient satisfaction.

From the current literature it can be concluded that epidural analgesia provides the best pain control in gastrointestinal surgery. A combination of opioid and local anesthetic is the preferred anesthetic regimen for use via the epidural route. Peripheral nerve blocks and intrathecal administration provide good pain relief in the first postoperative day and can be used in conjunction with parenteral morphine. As previously discussed, pain control is important in maintaining patient quality of life however it is not the whole story. Patient morbidity and mortality (known collectively as patient outcome) have a large part to play.

4   Patient Outcome

Gastrointestinal surgery is associated with significant morbidity and mortality which impact on quality of life. Most complications are common to all procedures but their prevalence is variable and depends on the site of surgery. Pulmonary complications can occur in any patient post operatively however they are more common in esophageal procedures. A recent survival analysis of a large cohort of esophagectomy patients found that the development of pneumonia was the single greatest factor impacting on mortality (Atkins et al., 2004).

❷ Paralytic ileus occurs to some extent in all intra-abdominal procedures (Delaney et al., 2006). Many studies have looked at the effect of anesthetic regimes on rates of specific complications, the results are conflicting. A large meta-analysis at the start of the new millennium examined the use of epidural analgesia over the previous 30 years (Rodgers et al., 2000). It concluded that epidural analgesia significantly reduced both morbidity and mortality. Unfortunately this work related to a heterogeneous population undergoing all types of operations with widely varying postoperative management plans. These same categorical results have yet to be repeated in the field of gastrointestinal surgery. Two recent reviews (Ballantyne et al., 1998; Holte and Kehlet, 2002a) stated that epidural analgesia reduced pulmonary complications in major abdominal procedures however the majority of the data used to reach this conclusion in both reviews was at least twenty years old and so did not allow for the advances in perioperative management outside the control of the anesthetist. The MASTER anesthesia trial study group (Rigg et al., 2002), found no difference in major morbidity or mortality when comparing epidural analgesia to the more traditional parenteral opioid regime save for a small increase in respiratory failure in the parenteral group.

Bearing this in mind, patient outcome as a primary end point has not provided us with very many answers regarding the best anesthetic regimen to use in the post operative setting in gastrointestinal surgery.

5   Quality of Life

Patient outcome is an objective measure of patient wellbeing. It is important to distinguish, however, between outcome and patient reported quality of life when scrutinizing the literature. There is a paucity of data examining the impact of post operative anesthesia on quality of life from the patient's perspective. It is often assumed that reduction in postoperative complications correlates with improved QOL and logical as this may seem, evidence is needed to support this corollary. Sporadic inclusion of QOL as a secondary endpoint occurs but these studies are often underpowered to draw meaningful conclusions for lesser study objectives (Liu and Wu, 2007).

Even as there is little in the published literature regarding the effect of anesthesia on QOL, there is far less concerning gastrointestinal surgery.

Unlike traditional outcome measures, post operative quality of life and patient satisfaction can be influenced by such wide ranging factors as gender, age, patient expectations and anxiety preoperatively (Kalkman et al., 2003). QOL cannot be assessed retrospectively as is possible with morbidity or mortality (Wu et al., 2006) (due to recall bias) making QOL a difficult end point for any study demanding real time collection of data and close follow up. As previously mentioned, the heterogeneous nature of many studies and the wide variety of perioperative management strategies create great difficulty in ascertaining the contribution of anesthetic choice to patient quality of life. Even the timing of anesthetic interventions is a possible confounder in the comparison of the effect of different regimes on QOL (Ochroch et al., 2002). Zutshi et al. (2005) examined the differential effect of thoracic epidural vs. intravenous PCA analgesia on QOL post colonic resection. All patients were recruited to fast track perioperative management with anesthetic regime representing the only test portion of the care pathway. QOL was assessed using the SF 36 questionnaire at 30 days. Interestingly, no difference in QOL was found between the two groups (❷ *Table 134-1*). These results must be qualified by the fact that the primary endpoint for this study was patient length of stay and is underpowered to draw conclusions regarding QOL. The reported QOL data is, therefore, subject to a type 1 error.

Our own investigations have shown that post operative epidural analgesia improves QOL in patients undergoing ❷ aero digestive surgery (Winter et al., 2007). Patients were randomized

❏ Table 134-1

Comparison of outcome for Short Form-36 component scores, Cleveland Global Quality of Life Scores (CGQL), satisfaction survey, and recovery of normal activity for PCA and epidural patients between PCA and epidural

	PCA	Epidural	Wilcoxon
	Median (Q1, Q3)	Median (Q1, Q3)	P value
Discharge			
Mental component scale	46.9 (38.0, 57.1)	53.6 (37.5, 59.5)	0.38
Physical component scale	41.1 (34.4, 45.8)	32.3 (27.3, 41.1)	0.06
CGQOL	0.63 (0.5, 0.8)	0.40 (0.4, 0.6)	0.043
Happiness	10.0 (9.0, 10.0)	10.0 (9.0, 10.0)	0.73
Hospital satisfaction	9.0 (8.0, 10.0)	9.0 (7.0, 10.0)	0.70
Surgery satisfaction	10.0 (8.0, 10.0)	10.0 (9.0, 10.0)	0.81
Activity percent	50.0 (25.0, 50.0)	40.0 (10.0, 50.0)	0.51
Day 10			
Mental component scale	52.8 (42.6, 58.3)	56.0 (43.6, 58.0)	0.53
Physical component scale	30.1 (25.0, 42.6)	32.0 (28.6, 36.9)	0.91
CGQOL	0.60 (0.5, 0.8)	0.50 (0.3, 0.7)	0.15
Happiness	9.0 (8.0, 10.0)	8.0 (6.0, 9.0)	0.32
Hospital satisfaction	8.5 (4.0, 9.0)	8.0 (7.0, 10.0)	0.42
Surgery satisfaction	9.0 (9.0, 10.0)	9.0 (8.0, 10.0)	0.71
Activity percent	50.0 (30.0, 50.0)	40.0 (25.0, 50.0)	0.38
Day 30			
Mental component scale	49.2 (36.4, 60.2)	43.6 (31.9, 50.8)	0.16
Physical component scale	35.8 (30.1, 42.8)	37.5 (32.8, 42.6)	0.74
CGQOL	0.75 (0.6, 0.8)	0.60 (0.4, 0.8)	0.063
Happiness	9.0 (7.5, 10.0)	8.0 (7.0, 10.0)	0.59
Hospital satisfaction	9.0 (5.0, 9.5)	8.0 (5.5, 9.0)	0.57
Surgery satisfaction	9.0 (8.0, 9.0)	9.0 (7.0, 10.0)	0.86
Activity percent	70.0 (55.0, 80.0)	57.5 (35.0, 75.0)	0.35

Reprinted from Zutshi M. et al., Am J Surg. 189. ((Copyright 2005), with permission from Elsevier, Figures are medians with 1st and 3rd quartiles). Patient cohort = 34. Control: n = 20. Test group: n = 14 to receive either PCA delivered systemic opioid or thoracic epidural infusion of local anesthetic/opioid combination. Using the validated instruments short form questionnaire 8 (SF-8) and short form questionnaire 36 (SF-36), we showed that thoracic epidural provided superior QOL at all time points (❷ *Figure 134-5*). A questionnaire designed to assess the patient's self caring ability from a nursing perspective showed that epidural analgesia allowed increased mobility and independence despite the extra equipment. Patient satisfaction was also assessed and this mirrored the QOL results. VAS was applied as a measure of pain as a secondary endpoint and pain scores closely correlated with patient reported QOL. A randomized trial of open colon resection patients found similar improvements in QOL as a result of epidural anesthesia (Carli et al., 2002). Using the SF-36, better scores were noted immediately post operatively and persisted for 6 weeks. There was a concomitant improvement in pain scores, mobility and a faster return of bowel function (❷ *Table 134-2*).

Notwithstanding these findings, it would be simplistic to claim that anesthesia is the sole variable that has significant impact on QOL in the post operative patient. Simple interoperative variability such as differences in placement of intercostal sutures has been shown to have a significant impact on post operative pain. Differences in surgical access such as muscle sparing thoracotomy and minimally invasive techniques play a large role in post operative recovery by modulating the surgical stress response. How and ever, there is little doubt that anesthetic management can greatly influence the patient experience in the post operative setting (❷ *Table 134-3*).

■ **Figure 134-5**
Mean physical and mental quality of life scores for epidural and PCA groups. Data from Prof. Winter (unpublished results). Values represent means with 95% confidence intervals. Increasing scores indicate increasing quality of life. Total patient cohort = 60. Control group: n = 30. Test group: n = 30. PCS and MCS indicate physical and mental scores on the quality of life scoring instruments. [†] P value < 0.001. *SF-8* Short form 8 questionnaire; *SF-36* Short form 36 questionnaire

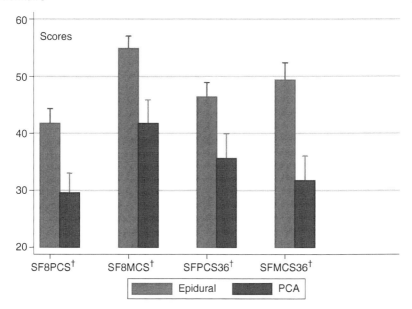

◘ Table 134-2

Difference from Baseline Values of Functional Exercise Capacity and Health-related Quality of Life at 3 and 6 Weeks after Surgery

	PCA Group (n = 31)		Epidural Group (n = 32)		
	Mean	SD	Mean	SD	Significant Effect
6-minute walking test (m)					
3 wk	−62.9	74.5	−32.0	62.6	Time x group; P = 0.0005
6 wk	−21.7	48.3	−5.0	59.0	–
Physical health					
3 wk	−13.5	10.0	−11.2	11.3	Time x group; P = 0.0001
6 wk	−5.5	9.7	−3.8	10.4	–
Mental health					
3 wk	−3.1	12.6	−5.0	11.6	Group; P = 0.002
6 wk	−3.3	13.9	−8.7	12.7	–
SF-36 subscales					
Physical functioning					
3 wk	−29.4	24.3	−23.7	25.1	Time x group; P = 0.0001
6 wk	−10.5	17.3	−6.9	26.0	–
Role – physical					
3 wk	−63.4	44.9	−36.3	58.4	Group; P = 0.0109
6 wk	−50.0	54.3	−9.7	51.5	Time x group; P = 0.0003
Role – emotional					
3 wk	−22.62	50.56	−6.45	51.94	Group; P = 0.0023
6 wk	−26.44	54.47	−19.36	44.54	–
Bodily pain					
3 wk	−19.8	33.4	−12.1	30.8	Time x group; P = 0.0001
6 wk	−0.1	26.1	−5.4	31.5	–
General health					
3 wk	−4.2	18.5	−2.9	19.8	Time x group; P = 0.0022
6 wk	−0.1	18.7	−3.9	17.1	–
Vitality					
3 wk	−17.3	21.5	−1.6	25.8	Group; P = 0.0093
6 wk	−4.5	17.1	−8.2	22.4	Time x group; P = 0.0001

◘ Table 134-2 (continued)

	PCA Group (n = 31)		Epidural Group (n = 32)		
Social functioning					
3 wk	−25.0	30.6	−11.3	26.5	Group; P = 0.0223
6 wk	−16.8	33.1	−5.6	40.2	Time x group; P = 0.0078
Mental health index					
3 wk	−4.7	26.2	−5.6	22.8	Group; P = 0.0496
6 wk	−0.7	26.7	−13.8	22.8	Time x group; P = 0.0084

Figures represent mean with standard deviation (SD). Increasing numbers indicate improved quality of life P values shown for significant results. Patient cohort = 63. Control group: n = 31. Test group: n = 32. PCA patient-controlled analgesia; SF-36 Short Form 36; Wk Week)

◘ Table 134-3

A summary of randomised controlled trials (RCTs) examining the effect of post operative anesthesia on Quality of Life (QOL) in gastrointestinal surgery

Author	n	Type of surgery	Anesthetic regimes Control	Test	Quality of Life Instrument(s)	Findings
Carli et al Ref 7	63	Abdominal	IV PCA n = 31	Thoracic Epidural n = 32	SF-36 assessed preoperatively and at 3 and 6 weeks post surgery	Significant improvement in QOL in epidural group at all time points
Winter et al Ref 31	60	Thoracic	IV PCA n = 30	Thoracic Epidural n = 30	SF-8 (24 hours post surgery) and SF-36 (day 7 post surgery)	Significant improvement in QOL inepidural group
Zutshi et al Ref 37	34	Abdominal	IV PCA n = 20	Thoracic Epidural n = 14	SF-36 and CGQL assessed preoperatively and day 10 and day 30 post surgery	No difference detected

IV PCA Intravenous patient controlled analgesia; SF-36 Short form 36 questionnaire; SF-8 Short form 8 questionnaire; CGQL Cleveland global quality of life questionnaire

6   Concluding Remarks

Patient wellbeing relies on many factors including intraoperative, perioperative and genetic variables and anesthesia is central to these processes. While traditional calculation of morbidity may not reflect this reality, patient centered measures of QOL highlight the importance of appropriate anesthesia in the postoperative period. Intraspinal anesthesia and particularly epidural delivery results in optimum pain relief and patient satisfaction. Large scale prospective trials will clarify the exact benefit of different modalities of anesthetic delivery on patient mobility, psychological well being and overall quality of life.

Summary Points

- The major factor impacting on patient outcome in gastrointestinal surgery is the systemic response to injury.
- A multidisciplinary approach (anesthesia, surgery, nursing staff and physiotherapy) is needed to optimize patient outcome.
- Pain, patient outcome and quality of life are discrete measurements of patient management and are not interchangeable.
- Intraspinal analgesia provides good pain relief and can have an opioid sparing effect however, the side effect profile can be poor.
- It is not definitively shown that intraspinal analgesia shortens inpatient stay or reduces complication rates or shortens length of hospital stay.
- There are very little data regarding the impact of anesthesia on post operative quality of life.

References

Atkins BZ, Shah AS, Hutcheson KA, Mangum JH, Pappas TN, Harpole DH Jr, D'Amico TA. (2004). Ann Thorac Surg. 78(4): 1170–1176.

az De LA, Oteiza MF, Ciga MA, Aizcorbe M, Cobo F, Trujillo R. (2003). Br J Surg. 90(1):91–94.

Ballantyne JC, Carr DB, deFerranti S, Suarez T, Lau J, Chalmers TC, Angelillo IF, Mosteller F. (1998). Anesth Analg. 86(3): 598–612.

Beaussier M, Weickmans H, Parc Y, Delpierre E, Camus Y, Funck-Brentano C, Schiffer E, Delva E, Lienhart A. (2006). Reg Anesth Pain Med. 31(6): 531–538.

Block BM, Liu SS, Rowlingson AJ, Cowan AR, Cowan JA Jr, Wu CL. (2003). JAMA. 290(18): 2455–2463.

Bottger T, Terzic A, Muller M, Rodehorst A. (2007). Surg Endosc. 21(10): 1695–1700.

Carli F, Mayo N, Klubien K, Schricker T, Trudel J, Belliveau P. (2002). Anesthesiology. 97(3): 540–549.

Coffey JC, Winter DC, Neary P, Murphy A, Redmond HP, Kirwan WO. (2002). Dis Colon Rectum. 45(1): 30–38.

Delaney CP, Senagore AJ, Viscusi ER, Wolff BG, Fort J Du, W, Techner L, Wallin B. (2006). Am J Surg. 191(3): 315–319.

Devys JM, Mora A, Plaud B, Jayr C, Laplanche A, Raynard B, Lasser P, Debaene B. (2003). Can J Anaesth. 50(4): 355–361.

Flynn MJ, Winter DC, Breen P, O'Sullivan G, Shorten G, O'Connell D, O'Donnell A, Aherne T. (2003). Eur J Cardiothorac Surg. 24(4): 547–551.

Gwirtz KH, Young JV, Byers RS, Alley C, Levin K, Walker SG, Stoelting RK. (1999). Anesth Analg, 88(3): 599–604.

Hill AG. (2006). Br J Surg. 93(4): 504–505.

Holte K, Kehlet H. (2002a). Minerva Anestesiol. 68(4): 157–161.

Holte K, Kehlet H. (2002b), Clin Nutr. 21(3): 199–206.

Kalbassi MR, Winter DC, Deasy JM. (2003). Dis Colon Rectum. 46(11): 1508–1512.

Kalkman CJ, Visser K, Moen J, Bonsel GJ, Grobbee DE, Moons KG. (2003). Pain. 105(3): 415–423.

Kell MR, Power K, Winter DC, Power C, Shields C, Kirwan WO, Redmond HP. (2003). Ir J Med Sci. 172(2): 63–65.

Liu SS, Wu CL. (2007). Anesth Analg. 105(3): 789–808.

Luketich JD, velo-Rivera M, Buenaventura PO, Christie NA, McCaughan JS, Litle VR, Schauer PR, Close JM, Fernando HC. (2003). Ann Surg. 238(4): 486–494.

McDonnell JG, O'Donnell B, Curley G, Heffernan A, Power C, Laffey JG. (2007). Anesth Analg. 104(1): 193–197.

Nitschke LF, Schlosser CT, Berg RL, Selthafner JV, Wengert TJ, Avecilla CS. (1996). Arch Surg. 131(4): 417–423.

Ochroch EA, Gottschalk A, Augostides J, Carson KA, Kent L, Malayaman N, Kaiser LR, Aukburg SJ. (2002). Anesthesiology. 97(5): 1234–1244.

Richardson J, Cheema S. (2006). Br J Anaesth. 96(4): 537.

Richardson J, Sabanathan S, Jones J, Shah RD, Cheema S, Mearns AJ. (1999). Br J Anaesth. 83(3): 387–392.

Richardson J, Sabanathan S, Mearns AJ, Shah RD, Goulden C. (1995). Br J Anaesth. 75(4): 405–408.

Rigg JR, Jamrozik K, Myles PS, Silbert BS, Peyton PJ, Parsons RW, Collins KS. (2002). Lancet. 359(9314): 1276–1282.

Rodgers A, Walker N, Schug S, McKee A, Kehlet H, van ZA, Sage D, Futter M, Saville G, Clark T, Macmahon S. (2000). BMJ. 321(7275): 1493.

Schietroma M, Carlei F, Cappelli S, Pescosolido A, Lygidakis NJ, Amicucci G. (2007). Hepatogastroenterology. 54(74): 342–345.

Schietroma M, Carlei F, Franchi L, Mazzotta C, Sozio A, Lygidakis NJ, Amicucci G. (2004). Hepatogastroenterology. 51(60): 1595–1599.

Winter DC, Dozois EJ, Pemberton JH. (2007). Curr Drug Ther. 2: 75–77.

Winter DC, Murphy A, Kell MR, Shields CJ, Redmond HP, Kirwan WO. (2004). Dis Colon Rectum. 47(5): 697–703.

Wu CL, Cohen SR, Richman JM, Rowlingson AJ, Courpas GE, Cheung K, Lin EE, Liu SS. (2005). Anesthesiology. 103(5): 1079–1088.

Wu CL, Naqibuddin M, Fleisher LA. (2001). Reg Anesth Pain Med. 26(3): 196–208.

Wu CL, Naqibuddin M, Rowlingson AJ, Lietman SA, Jermyn, RM, Fleisher LA. (2003). Anesth Analg. 97(4): 1078–1085.

Wu CL, Rowlingson AJ, Herbert R, Richman JM, Andrews RA, Fleisher LA. (2006). J Clin Anesth. 18(8): 594–599.

Zutshi M, Delaney CP, Senagore AJ, Mekhail N, Lewis B, Connor JT, Fazio VW. (2005). Am J Surg. 189(3): 268–272.

135 Health-Related Quality of Life After Surgery for Crohn's Disease

M. Scarpa · I. Angriman

1 *Surgery for Crohn's Disease: for Whom, Why, When and How* *2306*

2 *Why Measure Quality of Life after Surgery for Crohn's Disease* *2308*

3 *Preoperative HRQL: Concerns about Surgery* *2310*

4 *Early Postoperative HRQL* *2311*

5 *Long-Term Postoperative HRQL* *2314*

   Summary Points *2317*

Abstract: Crohn's disease cannot be healed but just taken into remission. Intestinal obstruction and fistulization, lack of response to medical management and perianal disease are the most frequent indication for intestinal surgery.

Why is it necessary to measure quality of life after surgery for Crohn's disease? Firstly, morbidity and mortality provide a partial and, very often, incomplete picture of outcome. Secondarily, nowadays, indications for surgery for Crohn's disease are broader and not limited to life saving procedures but in many cases they include chronic conditions such as failure of medical therapy, or poor quality of life on it self. Finally, quality of life is a more patient orientated measure of outcome that can give the patients' point of view about the procedure that is proposed.

HRQL is a multi-dimensional concept which includes several dimensions based on biological and symptom variables. Disease-related worries and concerns about the disease on itself and its therapy reflect one of these dimensions and they are considered to be a major determinant of HRQL in patients with IBD. In fact, concerns about having surgery and having an ostomy bag have a relevant impact on HRQL of Crohn's disease patients and having surgery increases concerns about body stigma.

The early impact of surgery on HRQL is an important component of the patient's decision regarding immediate and future surgery and understanding his or her recovery. Obviously, HRQL is expected to improve after operative procedures. In effect, in most of the studies, a significant improvement in HRQL early in the postoperative period was observed. Improvement, apparently, occurred irrespective of the disease activity measured with CDAI, the indication for surgery, type of procedure (abdominal or perineal), and history of previous surgery.

On the contrary, the long-term impact of surgery on HRQL is more controversial. Some studies, mainly those performed with generic questionnaires, reported an improved HRQL while other (those performed with disease specific instruments) described a decreased HRQL. According to these authors, HRQL, apparently, depends mainly on the long-term disease activity.

1   Surgery for Crohn's Disease: for Whom, Why, When and How

As well explained in the previous chapter, Crohn's disease is a chronic, transmural inflammatory disease of the gastrointestinal tract of unknown ethiology that can involve any part of the alimentary tract from the mouth to the anus but most commonly affects the small intestine and colon. Its most common clinical manifestations are abdominal pain, diarrhoea, and weight loss and it can be complicated by intestinal obstruction or localized perforation with fistula formation.

Nowadays, either medical therapy or surgical treatments are palliative: Crohn's disease cannot be healed but just taken into remission; in fact, operative therapy can provide effective symptomatic relief for those patients with complications from Crohn's disease and can produce a reasonable long-term benefit. The great part of patients with Crohn's disease requires surgery some time during the course of their illness. In patients with more than 20 years of disease, the cumulative probability of surgery is estimated to be 78%. The indications for operation are limited to complications that include intestinal obstruction, intestinal perforation with fistula formation or abscess, free perforation, gastrointestinal bleeding, urologic complications, cancer, and perianal disease (Delaney and Fazio, 2001). Since there is no curative intent, surgery should be specifically directed to the complication and only the segment of bowel involved in the complicating process should be resected. In fact, wide resections give no further benefit and can lead to the short bowel syndrome.

Intestinal obstruction and perforation are the main intestinal complications of Crohn's disease and therefore the most frequent indication for intestinal surgery. Obstruction is usually caused by chronic fibrotic lesions, which eventually narrow the lumen of the bowel, producing partial or near-complete obstruction. Free perforations into the peritoneal cavity leading are a rare presentation in patients with Crohn's disease. More commonly, fistulas occur between the sites of perforation and adjacent organs, such as loops of small and large intestine, the urinary bladder, the vagina, the stomach, and sometimes the skin, usually at the site of surgical scar such as the site of the previous appendectomy or laparotomy (Delaney and Fazio, 2001). Localized abscesses often occur near the sites of perforation. Rarely, Crohn's colitis may result in toxic megacolon. Perianal disease (fissure, fistula, stricture, or abscess) can occur in up to 48% of patients and it can affect their sexual life. Perianal disease may be the sole presenting feature in 5% of patients and may precede the onset of intestinal disease. Extra intestinal manifestations of Crohn's disease may be present in 30% of patients and the most common ones are skin lesions, such as erythema nodosum and pyoderma gangrenous, arthritis and joint pain, uveitis and iritis, hepatitis and pericholangitis, and aphthous stomatitis. These extra intestinal manifestations can heavily affect quality of life but they may persist after surgery. Finally, long-standing Crohn's disease predisposes to cancer of both the small intestine and colon. Recent evidence indicates that the risk of cancer in Crohn's disease of the colon is at least as great as that in ulcerative colitis and this could be a major concern for patients. Common indications for surgery in Crohn's disease patients are shown in ❯ *Figure 135-1*.

Intestinal obstruction is the most common indication for surgical therapy in patients with Crohn's disease. Surgery is required in case of complete obstruction and in patients with partial obstruction whose condition does not resolve with non operative management. The treatment of choice of intestinal obstruction caused by Crohn's disease is segmental resection

◾ Figure 135-1

Indications for surgery in patients with Crohn's disease (personal data Scarpa and Angriman, 2008)

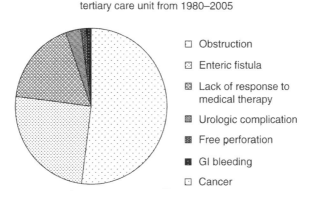

Indication for surgery in 312 patients in a
tertiary care unit from 1980–2005

☐ Obstruction

▨ Enteric fistula

▩ Lack of response to
medical therapy

▦ Urologic complication

▦ Free perforation

◼ GI bleeding

☐ Cancer

of the involved segment with primary re-anastomosis. In selected patients with obstruction caused by strictures (either single or multiple), one option is to perform a strictureplasty that effectively widens the lumen but avoids intestinal resection (Delaney and Fazio, 2001). Strictureplasty has the most application in those patients in whom multiple short areas of narrowing are present over long segments of intestine, in those patients who have already had several previous resections of the small intestine, and when the areas of narrowing are due to fibrous obstruction rather than acute inflammation. This procedure preserves intestine and is associated with complication and recurrence rates comparable to resection and re-anastomosis. The role of laparoscopic surgery for patients with Crohn's disease has not been clearly defined. In appropriately selected patients, for example those with single or multiple stenosis, localized abscesses, simple intra-abdominal fistulas, and peri-anastomotic recurrent disease, this technique appears feasible and safe and clearly improves body image of these patients.

Indications for surgery also include a lack of response to medical management or complications of Crohn's colitis, which include obstruction, hemorrhage, perforation, and toxic megacolon. Depending on the diseased segments, operations commonly include segmental colectomy with colo-colonic anastomosis, subtotal colectomy with ileo-rectal anastomosis, and in patients with extensive perianal and rectal disease, total proctocolectomy with Brooke ileostomy. A particularly troubling problem after proctocolectomy in patients with Crohn's disease is delayed healing of the perineal wound. Although controversial, continence-preserving operations, such as ileoanal pouch anastomosis or continent ileostomies (Kock pouch) are proscribed for patients with Crohn's colitis because of the high rate of recurrence of Crohn's disease in the pouch. The treatment of perianal disease should be conservative.

Even if surgery for Crohn's disease provide patients with often significant symptomatic relief it is not curative and recurrence rates are reported as high in most series (Wolff, 1998). Endoscopic evidence of recurrence is detected in approximately 70% of patients within 1 year of surgery and reoperation, rates are 25–30% at 5 years and 40–50% at 20 years. Approximately 45% of patients will ultimately require a second operation, of which only 25% will require a third operation. Despite the risk of recurrence, many patients who have had surgery for Crohn's disease wish that they had had their operation sooner. The overwhelming majority of such patients report relief of symptoms after surgery, restoration of a feeling of well-being and the ability to eat normally, and a reduction in the need for medical therapy.

2   Why Measure Quality of Life after Surgery for Crohn's Disease

As exhaustively described in the previous chapter, Crohn's disease affect quality of life since it is a chronic illness with many relapses and symptoms that interfere with daily activities of patients (Kirshner, 1980), who are often young and with a subsequently long life expectancy (Guassora et al., 2000). Patients with Crohn's disease generally experience worse quality of life than those with ulcerative colitis (Casellas et al., 2001). As would be expected, quality of life is worse during relapse than remission, but even when in remission studies have found patients' quality of life is poorer than that of healthy controls (Casellas et al., 2001; Drossman et al., 1989). Quality of life in Crohn's disease is adversely affected by smoking and taking steroids and it is worse in women (Blondel-Kucharski et al., 2001). In such a scenario, the measurement of health related quality of life (HRQL) is particularly relevant in these patients. But why is it even more necessary to measure quality of life after surgery in these patients?

The first reason is that traditional outcome measures for assessing surgical procedure such as morbidity and mortality provide a partial and, very often, incomplete picture. In the first half of the twentieth century these measures were appropriate because most gastrointestinal surgical procedures were associated with high complication and operative mortality rates. In the first cohort of patients who underwent abdominoperineal resection, for example, the operative mortality was 32% while today the accepted operative mortality is under 5%. In such a scenario, obviously, survival was the main measure to assess a surgical procedure's success and, consequently, the decision to adopt an operative technique was largely based on operative mortality and on long-term survival (McLeod, 1999). Today, operative mortality rates for intestinal surgery for Crohn's disease is under 1% [personal data], so, fortunately, operative mortality is of limited use as an outcome measure to discriminate between two surgical techniques or determine the value of a surgical technique as compared with medical therapy (McLeod, 1999). Therefore, HRQL can be used to integrate the traditional outcome measure to assess therapeutic efficacy of a surgical procedure in patients with CD (Irvine, 1994) and to identify treatment strategies that are preferable from the point of view of patients. Furthermore, quality of life represents an indispensable index to evaluate the success of a procedure not only in the short run but also in a longer period of time (Casellas et al., 1999; McLeod and Baxter, 1998).

A second reason is that, nowadays, indications for surgery for Crohn's disease are broader. They are not limited to life saving procedures such as in case of intestinal bleeding, peritoneal sepsis or obstruction but in many cases they include chronic conditions such as failure of medical therapy, or poor quality of life on it self. The adoption of laparoscopic approach has largely minimized the disability associated with surgery, thus, in some cases, surgery may be considered as an alternative to medical therapy. In such situation, where the indication for surgery is poor quality of life, it is thus essential that quality of life should be measured before and after the procedure to determine whether the therapeutic intervention has been worthwhile (McLeod, 1999). Finally, the goal of surgery in Crohn's disease is not to cure the disease but to improve quality of life, and thus surgical procedures should be evaluated in terms of their impact on HRQL of these patients.

The third reason for measuring quality of life in patients with Crohn's disease after surgery is because it is a more patient orientated measure of outcome that can give the patients' point of view about the procedure that is proposed (McLeod, 1999). Although physiologic outcomes are easier to measure, they may not necessarily correlate with patients' perception of their status. Physiologic outcomes provide information to the clinicians but may be of limited interest to patients and often correlate poorly with well being (McLeod, 1999). For example, after reconstructive surgery for ulcerative colitis surgeons have generally tended to assess outcome in terms of stool frequency. However, evidence suggests that this criterion does not correlate well with patients' perceived quality of life and satisfaction with the outcome of their surgery (McLeod, 1999). Furthermore, the heterogeneity of Crohn's disease manifestations make it difficult to use a single symptom to measure disease severity, so many indexes, such as the Crohn's Disease activity Index or the Perianal Crohn's Disease Activity Index, have been developed to assess function or disease activity. Anyway, measurement of functional status alone is of limited value because only the physical domain is assessed in these indexes and other domains, such as the psycho-social, which have an impact on quality of life, are not included.

Several studies investigated the impact of surgery on the HRQL of CD patients submitted to intestinal surgery (Casellas et al., 2000; Delaney et al., 2003; Maartense et al., 2006;

Scarpa et al., 2007a; Scott and Hughes, 1994; Thaler et al., 2005; Thirlby et al., 1998, 2001; Tillinger et al., 1999; Yazdanpanah et al., 1997). Some studies were focused on the early post operative outcome or on the comparison between the preoperative and the post operative HRQL (Casellas et al., 2000; Delaney et al., 2003; Maartense et al., 2006; Scott and Hughes, 1994; Tillinger et al., 1999; Yazdanpanah et al., 1997). All these studies demonstrate that, although undergoing surgery seems to be a major preoperative concern (Drossman et al., 2001; Canavan et al., 2006), in the months immediately following surgery patients affected by CD show a significant increase of their HRQL (Casellas et al., 2000; Delaney et al., 2003; Maartense et al., 2006; Scott and Hughes, 1994; Tillinger et al., 1999; Yazdanpanah et al., 1997). Fewer studies assessed the HRQL outcome after a long-term follow up and most of them did it either with a disease specific questionnaire or a generic tool. Therefore, the different studies obtained different results, making this point the most controversial one (Casellas et al., 2000; Scarpa et al., 2007a; Thaler et al., 2005; Thirlby et al., 2001). In fact, the authors of the Seattle University, using a modified version of the generic Short Form 36 (SF36), claimed that the quality of life of CD patients after ileo-colic resection was improved in long term follow up (Thirlby et al., 1998, 2001). On the contrary, the other authors who used respectively Gastro Intestinal Quality of Life Index (GIQLI), Inflammatory Bowel Disease Questionnaire (IBDQ) and Padova Inflammatory Bowel Disease Quality of Life (PIBDQL) score, reported a long term decrease of HRQL in these patients (Casellas et al., 2000; Scarpa et al., 2007a; Thaler et al., 2005).

Therefore, the analysis of quality of life after surgery for Crohn's disease is mandatory if we want to answer correctly to the main question that patients ask when they are proposed the operation: "How will I feel after the operation; what will my life be like?" These sorts of questions are even more crucial if we propose operation to patients just for poor quality or for failure of medical therapy.

3   Preoperative HRQL: Concerns about Surgery

HRQL is a multi-dimensional concept which includes several dimensions based on biological and symptom variables. Disease-related worries and concerns about the disease on itself and its therapy reflect one of these dimensions and it is considered to be a major determinant of HRQL in patients with IBD (Hjortswang et al., 1999). Descriptive research into the concerns of patients with IBD has been advanced by the development of the Rating Form of IBD Patients' Concerns (RFIPC) by Drossman et al. (1991), which quantifies the degree of concerns with specific issues related to IBD. Different studies in various samples of IBD patients revealed a high concordance in the ranking of worries assessed by the RFIPC (De Rooy et al., 2001; Maunder et al., 1999; Moser et al., 1995). These major concerns are similar across different cultures (Levenstein et al., 2001). Thus, it is important for clinicians to be aware of them so that they take them in account when Crohn's disease patients have to be counseled for a surgical therapy.

In a recent German study which used RFIPC, the top ranked concerns were as follows: effects of medication, having an ostomy bag, uncertain nature of disease, being a burden on others, energy level, loss of bowel control, having surgery, achieving full potential, attractiveness, developing cancer, and feelings about the body (Mussell et al., 2004). In these patients population the concern about having surgery was at the sixth place. The ranking of concerns was consistent with that reported in previous studies (De Rooy et al., 2001; Moser et al., 1995) and in a cross-cultural validation study (Levenstein et al., 2001). These results for the RFIPC total score and the sub-scores were also similar to those reported from another outpatient study that used the same German questionnaire (Moser et al., 1995).

Nevertheless, in a French study, the concern of having surgery was at the second place of the in the ranking of the concerns. In fact, this study reported that the most important fears expressed by the patients affected by Crohn's disease (noted on a scale from 0 – no fear – to 100 – maximal fear –), were: "lack of energy" (65.0%), "having an intestine operation" (64.6%), "having an ostomy bag" (63.8%) and "the unpredictable nature of the disease" (62.8/100) (Etienney et al., 2004).

On the contrary, according to a recent British study (Canavan et al., 2006), the most important concerns for patients were the uncertain nature of the disease, adverse effects of medication, having to use an ostomy bag, low-energy levels and the possible need for surgery which was only at the fifth place (Drossman et al., 1989; Levenstein et al., 2001). Disease-related concerns and anxieties regarding body image were rated highest in all subgroups, whilst sexual concerns were lowest (Canavan et al., 2006). These concerns did not change with disease duration but changed before and after the therapy: patients who had surgery reported a worse QoL, showed the highest level of concern regarding body image whereas the greatest concerns of patients who had not undergone surgery were about disease complications (Canavan et al., 2006).

Among the individual concerns that were greatest across all patient groups, the possible need for an ostomy bag seem to have a great impact on their quality of life (Canavan et al., 2006). In fact, this concern has also been rated amongst the most important in other studies of patients with Crohn's disease (Blondel-Kucharski et al., 2001; Drossman et al., 1989; Levenstein et al., 2001). It is possible that concerns about ostomy bags could be reduced by better patient education about the likely need for such surgery and what it would entail.

In conclusion, concerns about having surgery and having an ostomy bag have a relevant impact on HRQL of Crohn's disease patients and having surgery increases concerns about body stigma. Nevertheless, a high percentage of patients who actually had operations for CD felt they would be willing to go through surgery again (Delaney et al., 2003) and, also the study by Scott et al. reported that patients with CD with a previous ileocolic resection would have liked to have had their operation earlier (Scott and Hughes, 1994). Therefore, as the possibility of future surgery could be a major concern for these patients, the results of these two studies may help CD patients to understand that surgical intervention can contribute to improvement in HRQL and it may be possible to reduce level of concern regarding body stigma by counseling patients about their surgery preoperatively. Ranking of need of surgery and need of ostomy bag among worries assessed by the RFIPC in different studies is shown in ❯ Table 135-1.

4 $\quad$ Early Postoperative HRQL

The early impact of surgery on HRQL is an important component of the patient's decision regarding immediate and future surgery and understanding his or her recovery. Obviously, HRQL is expected to improve after operative procedures. However, in CD patients, the role of surgical treatment is merely symptom control rather than cure of disease, and patients are discharged form the surgical ward still on medications that can produce a confounding effect. So, surgery is sometimes perceived as a detrimental step, and this perception may result in

◻ Table 135-1

Ranking of need of surgery and need of ostomy bag among worries assessed by the RFIPC in different studies

Study	Year	Patients	Country	Most important concern	"Possible need for surgery" ranking	"Having an ostomy bag" ranking
Blondel-Kucharski et al.	2001	231	France	having an ostomy bag	Fourth	First
Etienney et al.	2004	141	France	energy level	Second	Third
Mussell et al.	2004	47	Germany	effect of medications	Sixth	Second
Canavan et al.	2006	221	UK	uncertain nature of the disease	Fifth	Third

procrastination on the part of the patient and the clinician, with prolonged continuation of (sometimes) inappropriate non surgical care (Delaney et al., 2003).

Several studies have reported the effect of surgery for CD on HRQL, although many have been retrospective and based on small numbers of patients. A critical review from the group of Toronto evaluated earlier studies on the effect of surgery on HRQL in patients with IBD (Maunder et al., 1995). They evidenced that the earlier studies were uncontrolled and used semi quantitative measures of HRQL so they were scarcely conclusive (Bechi and Tonelli, 1982; Lindhagen et al., 1983; Scott and Hughes, 1994). Other studies were found to be retrospective comparison between current and preoperative function (Cooper et al., 1986; Meyers, 1983). Nevertheless, successive retrospective studies reported an improved HRQL in patients undergoing surgery for CD (Casellas et al., 2000; Meyers et al., 1980; Nissan et al., 1997), and a comparable improvement in HRQL, irrespective of the procedure performed (Broering et al., 2001).

Some prospective studies investigated the effect of surgery and other treatment on HRQL as measured by various instruments after 3 months in the postoperative period. Thirlby and colleagues measured HRQL of a group of 36 CD patients with the Health Status Questionnaire and they reported an improvement 3 months after surgery (Thirlby et al., 1998), while Yazdanpanah and associates observed a significant improvement of the HRQL in 26 patients undergoing surgery at 3 and 6 months in the postoperative period (Yazdanpanah et al., 1997). Another prospective study from the University of Vienna measured HRQL by Crohn's Disease Activity Index, Time Trade-Off technique, Direct Questioning of Objectives and the RFIPC in 16 patients at three 1-month intervals in the postoperative period and found it to be improved significantly at 3 and 6 months after surgery (Tillinger et al., 1999). However, after 24 months, the long term improvement of the quality of life was reported only for the 12 patents with CD in remission. Thus, it is difficult to attribute the good quality of life to surgery instead of disease activity.

Three prospective studies specifically investigated the effect of surgery on early postoperative HRQL of CD patients. Blondel-Kucharski and colleagues reported that recent surgery impaired HRQL but it is not clear from their report what the mean duration of follow up after surgery when measurement of HRQL occurred (Blondel-Kucharski et al., 2001). In addition, the sample size of their study population in whom the early postoperative change in HRQL was measured was quite small. In the another study, from the Cleveland Clinic, the effect of surgery were prospectively evaluated on early postoperative HRQL using CGQL, which had initially been validated in patients with ulcerative colitis undergoing restorative proctocolectomy and, alter, it had been validated for CD patients (Delaney et al., 2003; Kiran et al., 2003). In this study, a significant improvement in CGQL early in the postoperative period was observed. Improvement, apparently, occurred irrespective of the disease activity measured with CDAI, the indication for surgery, type of procedure (abdominal or perineal), and history of previous surgery (Delaney et al., 2003). A greater improvement in CGQL in the postoperative period occurred in female patients and those who did not have any complications in the first month of postoperative period. Although the reason for the greater improvement in the latter group is obvious, there was no apparent reason why women benefited more than men, especially as both had similar preoperative CGQL scores (Delaney et al., 2003). As expected, patients who had complications within a month of surgery (irrespective of whether it was major or minor) had a smaller improvement in CGQL than those who had no complication. Patients who were on steroids at the time of surgery had a significantly better improvement than those who were not on steroids. Finally they concluded that HRQL after surgery for CD, as measured by CGQL, seem to improve a month after operation (Delaney et al., 2003). However this result is influenced by the scarce discriminative ability of CGQL which is a generic questionnaire and, therefore, their conclusion might sound a little optimistic (Scarpa et al., 2007b).

Finally, the group of Amsterdam compared laparoscopic assisted and open ileocolic resection for primary Crohn's disease in a randomized controlled trial (Maartense et al., 2006). Sixty patients were randomized for laparoscopic-assisted or open surgery. Primary outcome parameter was postoperative quality of life during 3 months of follow-up, measured by SF-36 and GIQLI questionnaire. And their conclusion was that generic and diseases specific quality of life measured was not different for laparoscopic-assisted compared with the open ileocolic resection (Maartense et al., 2006).

Prospective studies investigating short term HRQL after surgery for Crohn's disease are shown in ❷ *Table 135-2*.

◻ Table 135-2
Prospective studies assessing short term HRQL after surgery for CD

Study	Year	Patients	Country	Follow up	Questionnaire	HRQL after surgery
Yazdanpanah et al.	1997	26	France	3–6 months	SF36, RFIPC	improved
Thirlby et al.	1998	36	USA	3 months	HSQ	improved
Tillinger et al.	1999	16	Austria	3–6 months	RFIPC, TTO	improved
Blondel-Kucharski et al.	2001	231	France	0–3–6–9–12 months	SF36, RFIPC	impaired
Delaney et al.	2003	172	USA	1 months	CGQL	improved
Maartense et al.	2006	62	Netherlands	1–2–3 months	SF36, GIQLI	improved

5   Long-Term Postoperative HRQL

It is generally reckoned that the impairment of HRQL in Crohn's disease is substantial, it is worse in disease relapses and it is more severe than in ulcerative colitis (Guyatt et al., 1989) but in the literature the analysis of long term HRQL outcome after bowel surgery for Crohn's disease did not lead to a definite conclusion. On one side there are Thirlby et al., who reported that the quality of life after bowel resection for Crohn's disease was equal to norms for general population after a median follow up of 16 months (Thirlby et al., 2001). This could possibly be explained by the speculation to those patients with chronic illness experience better HRQL as the duration of their disease increases because their expectations of health decrease (Alison et al., 1997). On the other side Thaler et al. and Casellas et al., who used respectively GIQLI and IBDQ, reported a long term decrease of HRQL in these patients respectively 42 and 34 months after surgery (Casellas et al., 2000; Thaler et al., 2005). This could be explained considering that the model described above probably does not fit Crohn's disease well because the condition often follows a remitting and relapsing pattern and the response shift model may be more suitable for diseases that remain constant over many years or gradually deteriorate.

However, there is also a different and more technical possible explication of this discrepancy. In a recent paper, we demonstrated that the difference in the conclusions of different HRQL studies on the same subjects may be due to the different type of questionnaire used (Scarpa et al., 2007b). In fact, in a further study, we observed a similar discrepancy between the results of generic Cleveland Global Quality of Life which seemed to indicate a HRQL similar to healthy controls and those of disease specific Padova Inflammatory Bowel Disease Quality of Life (PIBDQL) which showed significantly worse HRQL of CD patients compared to healthy subjects (Scarpa et al., 2007a). These results are shown in ❷ *Figures 135-2* and ❷ *135-3*.

The CGQL score consists in three items (current quality of life, current quality of health and current energy level) each on a scale of 0–10 (0, worst; 10, best) (Fazio et al., 1999). The CGQL was created to assess HRQL in patients affected by ulcerative colitis after restorative proctocolectomy and then was successfully used in Crohn's disease HRQL analysis (Kiran et al., 2003) and its translation in Italian language was validated in one of our previous paper (Scarpa et al., 2007b).

The PIBDQL score was developed for patients affected by ulcerative colitis and Crohn's disease (Martin et al., 1995; Scarpa et al., 2004). This tool, predisposed to be self-administered, consists of 29 multiple choice questions which explore: intestinal symptoms (8 questions), systemic symptoms (7 questions), emotional function (9 questions) and social function (5 questions). The possible answers for each question were graduated on a four point scale and the maximal score was 87 (0, best; 87, worst).

The question of whether a generic non specific questionnaire or a disease specific measure for HRQL should be used in patients with Crohn's disease has not been conclusively solved (Thaler et al., 2005). Generic tools have the advantage that they can be used for comparison between different health conditions and can be easily managed and disease-specific questionnaires can be used in intra-group comparison, such as seriated evaluation to assess the success of a therapy, and are usually more discriminative (Scarpa et al., 2007b). Probably, the optimal study should include both type of questionnaires to draw any conclusion and the single questionnaire should not be considered separately but should be analyzed in the full context.

Furthermore, in our study the postoperative follow up was medially of 46 months (Scarpa et al., 2007a), similarly to those of the studies of Thaler et al. (2005) and Casellas et al. (2000).

■ Figure 135-2

Quality of life in 96 patients with Crohn's disease after ileocolonic resection after a 47.1 (40.7–53.5, 95% CI) months follow up compared to that of 69 healthy controls as measured with a generic quality of life questionnaire (CGQL). No significant difference was observed between the two groups with the exception of the current quality of health that resulted lower in Crohn's disease patients (p < 0.05) (Scarpa et al., 2007a)

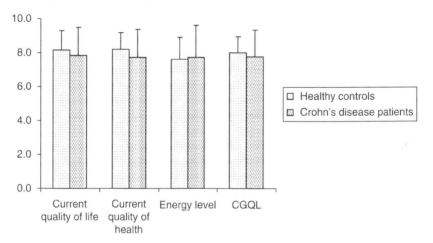

Long-term generic quality of life after ileocolonic resection for Crohn's disease

■ Figure 135-3

Quality of life in 63 patients with Crohn's disease after ileocolonic resection after a 43.7 (36.6–50.9, 95% CI) months follow up compared to that of 81 healthy controls as measured with a disease specific quality of life questionnaire (PIBDQL). All the scores resulted significantly higher, worse, in Crohn's disease patients (p < 0.01) (Scarpa et al., 2007a)

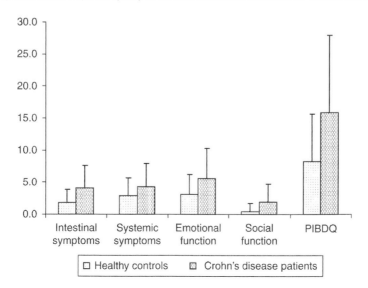

Long-term disease specific quality of life after ileocolonic resection for Crohn's disease

On the contrary, the patients in the study of Thirlby et al. had a median follow up of 16 months. In our opinion, this short "long-term" follow up could account for another part of the discrepancy above described. Patients in the first months after surgery fully enjoy a restored health compared the poor preoperative HRQL (Casellas et al., 2000; Delaney et al., 2003; Maartense et al., 2006; Scott and Hughes, 1994; Tillinger et al., 1999; Yazdanpanah et al., 1997) and, probably, 16 months after they are still in the "long wave" of the post operative enthusiasm (Scarpa et al., 2007a). After 3 years, or more, from surgery the frank positive effect of the surgical removal of the diseased bowel on HRQL appear to be greatly faded (Casellas et al., 2000; Thaler et al., 2005). After the post-surgical positive peak HRQL of Crohn's disease patients appears to return to a low plateau where only the current health status really matters. In fact, results form our study showed that the HRQL appear to be significantly related only to current disease activity expressed either by CDAI scores or with number of daily bowel movements (Scarpa et al., 2007a). Also Casellas et al. demonstrated that HRQL is strictly related to clinical disease activity and that the remission is the main predictor of good HRQL irrespective of the means (surgery or medical treatment) used to achieve it (Casellas et al., 2000). Similarly, Andersson et al. concluded that, in patients with colonic Crohn's disease, health related quality of life seems to be more dependent of present symptoms than type of previous surgery or the need for immunosuppressive medication as aggressive disease as well as previous colonic surgery lacked predictive value (Andersson et al., 2003).

McLeod et al. showed that surgical treatment significantly improves the HRQL of patients with severe Ulcerative Colitis but the improvement was independent of the very different surgical procedure employed (conventional ileostomy, Kock pouch or ileal reservoir). HRQL appeared to be a function of therapeutic efficacy rather than of the surgical procedure used (McLeod et al., 1991). This is even truer if we consider the different type of surgery for Crohn's disease. Our results demonstrated that there is no difference in terms of long term HRQL between patients submitted to open surgery and patients who underwent laparoscopy assisted ileocolic resection. This result confirmed those reported by Maartense et al. in the short term follow up and by Thaler et al. in the long term (Maartense et al., 2006; Thaler et al., 2005). Furthermore not only cosmetic impact of scar sparing surgery (laparoscopy) seemed to play little role in long term HRQL outcome (Dunker et al., 1998) but also bowel sparing surgery (strictureplasty) failed to demonstrate a long term improvement of HRQL (Broering et al., 2001). Disease activity is the most important factor for health related quality of life which underlines the need to use all available measures, medical or surgical, to bring these patients into clinical remission (Andersson et al., 2003).

In conclusion the analysis of long term HRQL after surgery for Crohn's disease with generic questionnaires showed an apparently normal quality of life with a good energy level but with an impaired quality of health. In fact, disease specific questionnaire evidenced a significant impairment of bowel and systemic symptom domains with important consequences on the emotional and social functions. Therefore, HRQL appears to be significantly related only to current disease activity independently form the surgical technique or access.

Our studies showed that generic and disease-specific questionnaires give different results so, in our opinion, HRQL should be analyzed with both type of questionnaires at the same time (Scarpa et al., 2007a, b). Generic questionnaire are useful tool to compare the HRQL between different illnesses whereas disease-specific questionnaire are the most useful tools to make intra-group comparison such as seriated evaluations of the success of a therapy.

Long term quality of life outcome after surgery for Crohn's disease in the different studies is resumed in ❷ *Table 135-3*.

◻ Table 135-3

Long term HRQL after surgery for CD

Study	Year	Patients	Country	Follow up	Questionnaire	HRQL after surgery
Thirlby et al.	2001	56	USA	16 months	SF36	Similar to healthy subjects
Thaler et al.	2005	37	USA	42 months	GIQLI	Lower than healthy subjects
					SF36	Lower than healthy subjects
Casellas et al.	2000	29	Spain	34 months	IBDQ	Lower than healthy subjects
Scarpa et al.	2007a	• 96	Italy	46 months	PIBDQL	Similar to healthy subjects
		• 63			CGQL	Lower than healthy subjects

Summary Points

- The goal of surgery in Crohn's disease is not to cure the disease but to improve quality of life.
- HRQL can be used to integrate the traditional outcome measure to assess therapeutic efficacy of a surgical procedure in patients with Crohn's disease.
- Need of surgery and need of ostomy bag are among the most important concerns of Crohn's disease patients.
- Generic and disease-specific questionnaires give different results so, HRQL of Crohn's disease patients should be analyzed with both type of questionnaires at the same time.
- Almost all the authors, agree that HRQL of Crohn's disease patients improves after surgery in the early postoperative period.
- The analysis of long term HRQL after surgery for Crohn's disease with generic questionnaires showed an apparently normal quality of life.
- Disease specific questionnaires evidenced that long term HRQL after surgery for Crohn's disease is significantly related only to current disease activity independently form the surgical technique or access.

References

Alison PJ, Locker D, Feine JS. (1997). Soc Sci Med. 45: 221–230.

Andersson P, Olaison G, Bendtsen P Myrelid P, Sjodahl R. (2003). Colorectal Dis. 5: 56–62.

Bechi P, Tonelli L. (1982). Int Surg. 67: 325–328.

Blondel-Kucharski F, Chircop C, Marquis P, Cortot A, Baron F, Gendre JP, Colombel JF. (2001). Groupe d'Etudes Thérapeutique des Affections Inflammatoires Digestives (GETAID) Am J Gastroenterol. 96: 2915–2920.

Broering DC, Eisenberger CF, Koch A, Bloechle C, Knoefel WT, Dürig M, Raedler A, Izbicki JR. (2001). Int J Colorectal Dis. 16: 81–87.

Canavan C, Abrams KR, Hawthorne B, Drossman D, Mayberry JF. (2006). Aliment Pharmacol Ther. 23: 377–385.

Casellas F, Lopez-Vivancos J, Badia X, Vilaseca J, Malagelada JR. (2001). Eur J Gastroenterol Hepatol. 13: 567–572.

Casellas F, López-Vivancos J, Badia X, Vilaseca J, Malagelada JR. (2000). Am J Gastroenterol. 95: 177–182.

Casellas F, López-Vivancos J, Vergara M, Malagelada J. (1999). Dig Dis.17: 208–218.

Cooper JC, Jones D, Williams NS. (1986). Ann R Coll Surg Engl. 68: 279–282.

Delaney CP, Kiran RP, Senagore AJ, O'Brien-Ermlich B, Church J, Hull TL, Remzi FH, Fazio VW. (2003). J Am Coll Surg. 196: 714–721.

Delaney CP, Fazio VW. (2001). Surg Clin North Am. 81: 137–158.

De Rooy EC, Toner BB, Maunder RG, Greenberg GR, Baron D, Steinhart AH, McLeod RS, Cohen Z. (2001). Am J Gastroenterol. 96: 1816–1821.

Drossman DA, Leserman J, Li ZM, Mitchell CM, Zagami EA, Patrick DL. (1991). Psychosom Med. 53: 701–712.

Drossman DA, Patrick DL, Mitchell CM, Zagami E, Applebaum MI. (1989). Dig Dis Sci. 34: 1379–1386.

Dunker MS, Stiggelbout AM, van Hogezand RA, Ringers J, Griffioen G, Bemelman WA. (1998). Surg Endosc. 12: 1334–1340.

Etienney I, Bouhnik Y, Gendre JP, Lemann M, Cosnes J, Matuchansky C, Beaugerie L, Modigliani R, Rambaud JC. (2004). Gastroenterol Clin Biol. 28: 1233–1239.

Fazio VW, O'Riordain MG, Lavery IC, Church JM, Lau P, Strong SA, Hull T. (1999). Ann Surg. 1230: 575–586.

Guassora AD, Kruuse C, Thomsen OO, Binder V. (2000). Scand J Gastroenterol. 35: 1068–1074.

Guyatt G, Mitchell A, Irvine EJ, Singer J, Williams N, Goodacre R, Tompkins C. (1989). Gastroenterology. 96(3): 804–810.

Hjortswang H, Almer S, Strom M. (1999). Eur J Gastroenterol Hepatol. 11: 1099–1104.

Irvine EJ. (1994). Gastroenterology. 106: 287–296.

Kiran RP, Delaney CP, Senagore AJ, O'Brien-Ermlich B, Mascha E, Thornton J, Fazio VW. (2003). Am J Gastroenterol. 98(8): 1783–1789.

Kirshner J. (1980). JAMA. 243: 557–563.

Levenstein S, Li Z, Almer S, Barbosa A, Marquis P, Moser G, Sperber A, Toner B, Drossman DA. (2001). Am J Gastroenterol. 96: 1822–1830.

Lindhagen T, Ekelund G, Leandoer L, Hildell J, Lindström C, Wenckert A. (1983). Acta Chir Scand. 149: 415–421.

Maartense S, Dunker MS, Slors JF, Cuesta MA, Pierik EG, Gouma DJ, Hommes DW, Sprangers MA, Bemelman WA. (2006). Ann Surg. 243: 143–149.

Martin A, Leone L, Fries W, Naccarato R. (1995). Ital J Gastroenterol. 27: 450–454.

Maunder RG, Toner B, de Rooy E, Moskovitz D. (1999). Can J Gastroenterol. 13: 728–732.

Maunder RG, Cohen Z, McLeod RS, Greenberg GR. (1995). Dis Colon Rectum. 38: 1147–1161.

McLeod RS (1999). Adv Surg. 33: 293–309.

McLeod RS, Baxter NN. (1998). World J Surg. 28: 375–381.

McLeod RS, Churchill DN, Lock AM. (1991). Gastroenterology. 101: 1307–1313.

Meyers S. (1983). Mt Sinai J Med. 50: 190–192.

Meyers S, Walfish JS, Sachar DB, Greenstein AJ, Hill AG, Janowitz HD. (1980). Gastroenterology. 78: 1–6.

Moser G, Tillinger W, Sachs G, Genser D, Maier-Dobersberger T, Spiess K, Wyatt J, Vogelsang H, Lochs H, Gangl A. (1995). Eur J Gastroenterol Hepatol. 7: 853–858.

Mussell M, Bocker U, Nagel N, Singer MV. (2004). Eur J Gastroenterol Hepatol. 16: 1273–1280.

Nissan A, Zamir O, Spira RM, Seror D, Alweiss T, Beglaibter N, Eliakim R, Rachmilewitz D, Freund HR. (1997). Am J Surg. 174: 339–341.

Scarpa M, Ruffolo C, D'Incà R, Filosa T, Bertin E, Ferraro S, Polese L, Martin A, Sturniolo GC, Frego M, D'Amico DF, Angriman I. (2007a). Inflamm Bowel Dis. 13(4): 462–469.

Scarpa M, Ruffolo C, Polese L, Martin A, D'Incà R, Sturniolo GC, D'Amico DF, Angriman I. (2007b). Arch Surg. 142(2): 158–165.

Scarpa M, Angriman I, Ruffolo C, Ferronato A, Polese L, Barollo M, Martin A, Sturniolo GC, D'Amico DF. (2004). World J Surg. 58(2): 122–126.

Scott NA, Hughes LE. (1994). Gut. 35: 656–657.

Thaler K, Dinnewitzer A, Oberwalder M, Weiss EG, Nogueras JJ, Wexner SD. (2005). Colorectal Dis. 7: 375–381.

Thirlby RC, Sobrino MA, Randall JB. (2001). Arch Surg. 136: 521–527.

Thirlby RC, Land JC, Fenster LF, Lonborg R. (1998). Arch Surg. 133: 826–832.

Tillinger W, Mittermaier C, Lochs H, Moser G. (1999). Dig Dis Sci. 44: 932–938.

Yazdanpanah Y, Klein O, Gambiez L, Baron P, Desreumaux P, Marquis P, Cortot A, Quandalle P, Colombel JF. (1997). Am J Gastroenterol. 92: 1897–1900.

Wolff BG. (1998). World J Surg. 22: 364–369.

136 Postoperative Quality of Life Assessment in the Over 80's After Cardiac Surgery

Christoph H. Huber

1	*Introduction*	*2320*
2	*Original Data*	*2321*
2.1	Coronary artery Bypass Grafting in Combination with Aortic Valve Replacement ($n = 41$)	2322
2.2	Outcome of Cardiac Surgery in patients over 80	2323
2.2.1	Early Outcomes	2323
2.3	Mortality (Cumulative Survival in Brackets)	2323
2.4	QoF after Cardiac Surgery in the Patients over 80	2323
2.4.1	The Scoring Classification	2323
2.4.2	Nottingham Health Profile	2325
2.4.3	Short Form-36	2325
2.4.4	Sickness Impact Profile	2326
2.4.5	Seattle Angina Questionnaire	2326
2.4.6	Advantages of the SAQ versus SF-36	2326
2.4.7	Original Data	2326
2.5	Methodological Considerations	2328
2.6	Gender Difference	2330
2.7	Surgical Therapy of Ischemic Heart Disease in the Elderly	2330
2.8	Aortic Valve Surgery	2330
2.9	Survival and QoL Impacting Factors	2331
2.10	Financial Impact on Healthcare Resources	2332
2.11	Final Considerations	2332
	Summary Points	*2332*

Abstract: ❷ Heart disease is the leading cause of death in the industrialized nation, and 25% of patients over the age of 80 are functionally limited by their underling cardiovascular condition. Coronary artery diseases have a prevalence of 18–20% in the elderly. There are principally no differences in treatment options and surgical indications in this age group compared to the younger population. Cardiac surgery is a very effective therapy to improve functional status of patients with coronary artery and heart valve disease. In this chapter the impact of heart surgery on Quality of Life (QoL)in this very challenging age segment is summarized.

Recent studies confirm the important gain of QoL with a very acceptable mortality in patients over 80 years after heart surgery. These extremely satisfying results should be confronted with the rather reserved referral practice, often withholding old patients for long from cardiac surgery.

List of Abbreviations: *AVR,* ❷ Aortic valve replacement; *BMI,* Body mass index; *CABG,* ❷ Coronary artery bypass grafting; *CAD,* Coronary artery disease; *CCS,* Canadian Cardiovascular Society grading; *COPD,* Chronic obstructive airway disease; *CPB,* Cardiopulmonary bypass; *EC,* Erythrocyte concentrate; *IABP,* Intra aortic balloon pump; *ICU,* Intensive care unit; *IDDM,* Insuline-dependent diabetes mellitus; *LIMA,* Left internal mammary artery graft; *LVEF,* Left ventricular ejection fraction; *MI,* Myocardial infarction; *NHP,* ❷ Nottingham Health Profile; *NIDDM,* Non-insulin-dependent diabetes mellitus; *NYHA,* New York Heart Association grading; *PAD,* Peripheral arterial disease; *QoL,* Quality of life; *SAQ,* ❷ Seattle Angina Questionnaire; *SF36,* Short form 36; *SIP,* ❷ Sickness Impact Profile

1   Introduction

Life expectancy at birth is increasing leading to a growing older population. From 1982, life expectancy at birth has increased in Switzerland, the UK, and the US from 76.3, 75.7, and 75.5 years to 79.9, 77.9, and > 77 years, respectively. By 2022, life expectancy will reach 82.0 years in Switzerland, 80.8 years in the UK, and 80.2 in the US. In the Western European population, 16% is over 65 years old, in the US 13%, and in Switzerland 15% compared to 7% in the world population.

It is estimated that the US population will include more than 25 million persons of at least 80 years of age by 2050 (Spencer, 1989). At present, 5% of the Swiss population is aged 80 years and above, and this percentage continues to rise. Life expectancy at the age of 80 in Switzerland reaches an additional 6.6 years for male and another 7.8 years for female habitants.

Heart diseases are the number one cause of death in the industrialized nations. More than 25% of the population 80 years and above (Statistical Abstract of the United States/1994 (114th edn.), 1994) are functionally limited by their underling cardiovascular disease, and the prevalence of coronary artery disease is 18–20% in the US and Europe. Many patients in this age group are long withheld from cardiac surgery because of "too advanced age" from a surgical therapy point of view, and remain severely symptomatic despite maximum medical therapy. Nevertheless, as a result of information campaigns based on the surprisingly good results of recent studies suggesting a very acceptable mortality and morbidity, more and more patients over 80 are referred to the cardiac surgeon.

This ongoing trend is well reflected in the increased patient population over 80 years undergoing heart surgery at our institution. The numbers have steadily increased from 4.3%

in 2000 to 5.5% in 2002 and to 6.4% in 2004. Interestingly, in the last 3 years the percentage of patients over 80 years has shown accelerated growth with 8.7% in 2006 and 10.8% in 2007.

A further decline in mortality and morbidity is mostly due to advances in operative techniques, myocardial protection strategies, and per-operative care. Cardiac surgery can nowadays be performed safely in patients of 80 years and older with good mid-term results.

With the advance of elderly surgical candidates and increasing healthcare costs, quality of life (QoL) particularly in this age segment has become a major area of interest. The commonly used objective indicators for risk–benefit analysis such as survival rates, and return to normal activity are of lesser concern in the older patient population as, for example, return to self-care and the more subtle QoL indicators. Outcome assessment requires data collection focusing also on the personal perception of his or her health, physical well-being, and mental state. "Not just the absence of death but life with the vibrant quality that was associate[d] with the vigour of youth" (Elinkton , 1966) described QoL best. Many studies have reported on the QoL after a cardiac surgery (Rothenhausler et al., 2005; Thornton et al., 2005) and an increasing number on the surgical results in patient over 80 (Craver et al., 1999; Kirsch et al., 1998), but only very few recent studies have combined QoL assessment with objective surgical outcomes of octogenarians undergoing heart surgery (Goyal et al., 2005).

2   Original Data

The author has reviewed a single-center experience spanning from 1999 to 2003. A total of 136 consecutive octogenarians underwent either isolated coronary artery bypass grafting (CABG), isolated aortic valve replacement (AVR) or combined CABG/AVR (Huber et al., 2007). Objective data were obtained from the patients' records.

Information on QoL of the 120 surviving patients and causes of deaths were obtained via telephone interviews during a 2-month period by a single investigator. The surviving patient himself was questioned in the first line; relatives, patient's general practitioners or cardiologists, and hospital autopsy records served to acquire additional information.

A modified Seattle Angina Questionnaire was completed in 100% of the survivors, and the preoperative patients characteristics are summarized in ❯ Table 136-1.

In the CABG group consisting of 61 patients, unstable angina pectoris was the most common symptom. Forty-two patients (69%) had a CCS of III or more and 27 (44%) presented with a history of myocardial infarction, in 11 patients less than 14 days before and in 16 patients more than 2 weeks before surgery. Only five patients (8.2%) presented with an LVEF of equal to or less than 35%.The LVEF was 59 ± 13%. In 53 patients (87%), three-vessel and in seven patients (11%) two-vessel disease was present. Left main stem disease was diagnosed in 25 patients (41%). Multiple revascularization included quintuple CABG in seven cases (11%), quadruple in 25 cases (41%), and triple in 23 cases (38%), whereas two-vessel revascularization was performed six times (10%). In 47 patients (77%), the left anterior descending artery was bypassed with LIMA graft, and eight patients (13%) got a radial artery graft. The operation time was 168 ± 40 min and the bypass time was 77 ± 29 min. Mean aortic cross-clamp time was 46 ± 18 min.

Aortic valve replacement was performed 34 times for aortic stenosis. Most patients presented with severe dyspnea; 62% were in NHYA ≥ III and LVEF was 60.4 ± 14%. In 16 cases (47%) concomitant aortic insufficiency grade I or II was noted. Stented bioprosthesis were implanted in 25 cases (74%), stentless in 1 case (3%), and a mechanical valve in 8 cases

◘ Table 136-1

Preoperative patient characteristics

Variables	All (*n* = 136) No. of patients (%)	CABG (*n* = 61) No. of patients (%)	AVR (*n* = 34) No. of patients (%)	CABG/AVR (*n* = 41) No. of patients (%)
Males	80 (59)	39 (64)	15 (44)	26 (63)
Age	82.3 ± 2.1	82.0 ± 1.8	82.6 ± 2.0	82.5 ± 2.6
NYHA or CCS ≥III	90 (66)	43 (70)	21 (62)	26 (63)
Hypertension	83 (61)	38 (62)	15 (44)	30 (73)
Dyslipidemia	70 (51)	33 (54)	14 (41)	23 (56)
Pos. family history	34 (25)	14 (23)	6 (18)	14 (34)
NIDDM/IDDM	14 (10)	(10)	(9)	5 (13)
	/ 2 (1.5)	/2 (3.3)	0	0
Creatinine≥120 μmol/l	26 (19)	10 (16)	7 (21)	9 (22)
COPD	21 (15)	7 (11)	7 (21)	7 (17)
Tobacco abuse	33 (24)	23 (38)	4 (12)	6 (15)
PAD	19 (14)	10 (16)	4 (12)	5 (12)
Atrial fibrillation	26 (19)	7 (11)	10 (29)	9 (22)
Previous MI	35 (26)	27 (44)	2 (6)	6 (15)
Anticoagulation	14 (10)	8 (13)	5 (15)	1 (2.4)

BMI Body mass index, *CAD* Coronary artery disease, *CCS* Canadian Cardiovascular Society, *COPD* Chronic obstructive airway disease, *MI* Myocardial infarction, *IDDM* Insulin dependent diabetes mellitus, *NIDDM* Non insulin dependent diabetes mellitus, *LVEF* Left ventricular ejection fraction, *NYHA* New York Hear Association, *PAD* Peripheral arterial disease

(24%). Mean cardiopulmonary bypass time was 76 ± 28 min, and mean aortic cross-clamp time 53 ± 14 min. Overall operation time was 152 ± 37 min.

2.1 Coronary artery Bypass Grafting in Combination with Aortic Valve Replacement (*n* = 41)

Six (15%) patients had left main disease, 10 (24%) presented with triple vessel CAD, and 35 (87%) had either double- or single-vessel CAD. Twenty (48%) patients had single vessel revascularization, 14 (34%) has double, and 11(27%) had triple or more. Thirteen (31%) LIMAs and 3 (7.3%) radial arteries were harvested. Stented bioprostheses were implanted in 34 cases (83%), stentless bioprostheses in 1 (2.4%), and a mechanical valve in 13 (31%). Mean cardiopulmonary bypass time for combined AVR and CABG was 90 ± 35 min, and mean aortic cross-clamp time was 62 ± 19 min. The overall operative time was 169 ± 41 min.

2.2 Outcome of Cardiac Surgery in patients over 80

2.2.1 Early Outcomes

The most frequent postoperative complication in all groups was arrhythmias with atrial fibrillation in 29 patients (21%). Permanent pacemaker became necessary in two patients only (1.5%).

Four patients (3.0%) suffered per-operative myocardial infarction after combined AVR/CABG, but none required IABP support in this group. Twenty-seven patients (20%) needed inotropic drugs to wean from CPB, and in 21 cases (15%) inotropes had to be continued for more than 24 h. Prolonged mechanical ventilation (>2 days) was necessary in eight cases (5.9%). The average length of stay in the intensive care unit (ICU) was 2.7 ± 1.6 days, and five atients (3.7%) stayed for more than 1 week. Temporary dialysis was required in two cases (1.5%), but in both the renal function recovered completely. Eight patients (5.9%) underwent reintervention: in six cases (4.4%) for persistent bleeding and in two cases (1.5%) because of deep sternal wound infection.

Five patients (3.7%) suffered from permanent neurologic impairment and three (2.2%) recovered fully from a transient neurologic impairment. Hospital stay was 14.2 ± 10.1 days, with six patients (4.4%) staying for more than 25 days (range 5–110). In ❷ *Table 136-2*, the early complications (<30 days) are listed in relation to the type of surgery.

2.3 Mortality (Cumulative Survival in Brackets)

In-hospital death occurred in six cases (4.4%). One month after surgery, 130 patients (95%) were alive. Survival rate at 1, 3, and 5 years was 93, 90, and 73% respectively. The highest mid-term survival rate was recorded in the isolated AVR, with 31 patients (75%) alive. In contrast, combined operations with CABG/AVR showed the lowest 5-year survival, with 35 patients alive (65%). The CABG group survival positioned itself between AVR and CABG/AVR groups, with 54 patents alive, corresponding to a cumulative 5-year-survival of 70% (see ❷ *Figure 136-1*).

Causes of the 16 deaths over 5 years were mostly of non-cardiac origin. Fatal pneumonia caused death in five cases (31.3%). In two patients (12.5%) cerebro-vascular accidents, in three (18.8%) septicaemia, in one (6.3%) mesenterial infarction, in one (6.3%) cerebral haemorrhage, and in one female patient (6.3%) euthanasia led to death. In five cases (31.3%) a cardiac cause has been found to be the cause of death. ❷ *Table 136-3* shows a comparison of intervention-linked cumulative survival in octogenarians after cardiac surgery.

2.4 QoF after Cardiac Surgery in the Patients over 80

2.4.1 The Scoring Classification

QoF measures are accepted outcome measures well nestled into clinical research, but seldom routinely used in clinical practice (Higginson and Carr, 2001). It might have been Florence Nightingale to first introduce QoF assessment as routine clinical care outcome measure (Rosser, 1985). The term "quality of life," popularized after a presidential commission to

■ Table 136-2

Postoperative complications

Variable	All (n = 136) No. of patients (%)	CABG (n = 61) No. of patients (%)	AVR (n = 34) No. of patients (%)	CABG/AVR (n = 41) No. of patients (%)
Inotropic drug support required	27 (19.9)	9 (14.8)	9 (26.4)	9 (22.0)
IABP	1 (0.7)	1 (1.6)	0	0
ICU (days)	2.7 ± 1.6	2.8 ± 1.5	2.6 ± 1.2	2.7 ± 2.1
Prolonged ventilation (>24 h)	8 (5.9)	4 (6.6)	3 (8.8)	3 (7.3)
Duration of inotropes (h)	13.5 ± 29.0	8.3 ± 22.3	17.6 ± 33.0	0.75 ± 1.4
No. of intraoperative EC	1.5 ± 2.0	1.4 ± 1.8	1.8 ± 2.2	1.5 ± 2.0
No. of postoperative EC	1.0 ± 5.1	1.4 ± 7.4	0.9 ± 2.0	0.5 ± 1.2
Transient neurologic impairment	3 (2.2)	1 (1.6)	0	2 (4.9)
Permanent neurologic impairment	5 (3.7)	4 (6.6)	1 (2.9)	0
Myocardial infarction	4 (2.9)	0	0	4 (9.8)
Temporary dialysis	3 (2.2)	1 (1.6)	1 (2.9)	1 (2.4)
Antibiotic treatment (>48 h)	26 (19.1)	5 (8.2)	11 (32.4)	10 (24.4)
Deep sternal infections needing reoperation	2 (1.5)	0	2 (5.9)	0
Reoperation for bleeding	6 (4.4)	2 (3.3)	2 (5.9)	2 (4.8)
Atrial fibrillation	29 (21.3)	8 (13.2)	10 (29.4)	11 (26.8)
Permanent pacemaker	2 (1.5)	0	2 (5.9)	0
Hospital stay mean time (days)	14.2 ± 10.1	14.1 ± 13.5	13.8 ± 5.9	14.8 ± 6.2
No. of drugs at discharge	5	5	5	5

Early complications (<30 days) in relation to the type of surgery and additionally assessed postoperative variables
EC Erythrocyte concentrate, *IABP* Intra Aortic Balloon Pump, *ICU* Intensive care unit

John F. Kennedy, defined health-related QoL assessment as an achievable goal for 2000 (William, 1991).

Even though objective indicators are straightforward to assess, QoL might be more vague to quantify, as it is highly dependent on the subjective judgment by the patient. Measuring tools have been constructed to normalize, objectivise, and to eventually allow comparison between disease-specific populations (Campbell et al., 1976). Of the approximately ten instruments, the most commonly used QoL assessment tools for heart disease include the SF36 used in about 20% of studies, the Nottingham Health Profile (NHP) used in about 40% of the ischemic heart disease studies, the Sickness Impact Profile (20% of studies), and the Seattle Angina Questionnaire (SAQ) (20% of studies) (Dempster and Donnelly, 2000).

◻ Figure 136-1

Kaplan–Meyer survival curves, comparing CABG, AVR, and the combined procedures in patients over 80 years of age. Unit on the time axis is expressed in days and unit on the survival axis is expressed in percentage

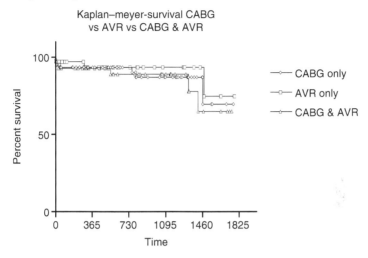

◻ Table 136-3
Cumulative survival

Operation	30-day survival	1-year survival	3-year survival	5-year survival
All operations (n = 136)	95 ± 1.7% (7)	93 ± 2.0% (9)	90 ± 2.1% (12)	73 ± 7.9% (16)
Isolated CABG (n = 61)	95 ± 2.7% (3)	93 ± 3.2% (4)	87 ± 5.3% (6)	70 ± 16.1% (7)
Isolated AVR (n = 34)	97 ± 2.8% (1)	94 ± 4.3% (2)	94 ± 4.3% (2)	75 ± 17.1% (3)
AVR and CABG (n = 41)	92 ± 4.0% (3)	92 ± 4.0% (3)	88 ± 5.3% (4)	65 ± 15.2% (6)

Table shows a comparison of intervention linked cumulative survival in octogenarians after cardiac surgery. In brackets: cumulative absolute numbers of occurred death within every survival interval

2.4.2 Nottingham Health Profile

The NHP is divided in the first part into 38 itemscovering six scales including mobility, pain, energy, sleep, emotional reaction and social isolation. The second part investigates disease impact on daily life including work, homecare, social life, sexual activity, holidays, and interests.

2.4.3 Short Form-36

The ❷ Short Form-36 (SF-36) is a multipurpose, short-form health survey with 36 questions and perhaps is the most commonly used healthcare measuring tool. It yields an 8-scale profile of functional health and well-being scores as well as psychometrically based physical and mental health, investigating physical and social functioning, role limitations of physical or emotional origin, vitality, mental health, physical pain, and overall health condition.

2.4.4   Sickness Impact Profile

The SIP is a large 136-item instrument grouped into 12 scales. SIP can be subdivided into two clusters including the physical dimension (three scales) and the psychosocial dimension (four scales) and the remaining five scales.

2.4.5   Seattle Angina Questionnaire

The SAQ regroups 19 items measuring five specific scales: physical limitations, anginal stability, anginal frequency, treatment satisfaction, and disease perception targeting a specific disease and treatment group.

2.4.6   Advantages of the SAQ versus SF-36

In the authors' study, the use of a modified SAQ instead of the SF-36 questionnaire (Immer et al., 2004, 2005) was motivated by the increased age, the specific disease, and treatment characteristics of the analyzed patient population. The SF-36 is known to be a generic measure, as opposed to one that targets a specific age, disease, or treatment group. The SAQ (Dougherty et al., 1998; Spertus et al., 1995) as opposed to the SF-36 is a shorter 19-item questionnaire. The fewer number and the simple nature of the questions were found to be more suitable to address the very old patient population. All question investigating anginal-related outcomes were supplemented with the symptom of dyspnea in order to address aortic valve disease as well (see ❯ Table 136-4). This modification is by itself not validated, but it does not interfere with the angina assessment and provides a simple tool to measure valve-related QoL perception.

2.4.7   Original Data

Mean follow-up period was 890 days (range from 69 to 1853). Information was collected by telephone interviews. One-hundred and 30 patients left the hospital, and at follow-up 120 patients were alive. A validated SAQ including two additional questions regarding dyspnea was used to assess the QoL (see ❯ Table 136-4). This modified 11-item multiple choice instrument examines mobility and activity, cardiac symptoms perception, disease perception, treatment satisfaction as well as emotional well-being, and enjoyment of life. In order to allow for assessment of valve pathologies, dyspnea as an additional symptom was added to the questions regarding chest pain.

QoL improved considerably after cardiac surgery. Overall, 97 patients (81%) were not at all or only slightly disabled in their daily activities (see ❯ Figure 136-2). Physical exercise was not limited or only a little limited in 84 cases (70%). Symptoms decreased post cardiac surgery in 112 patients (93%), only 2 patients (1.7%) felt worse than before operation, and 6 patients (5%) described unchanged symptoms (see ❯ Figure 136-3). Eighty-six patients (72%) were free of angina or dyspnea, while eight (6.6%) remained moderately to severely symptomatic. In the CABG group, 42 patients (77.7%) did not have to take nitroglycerin anymore, and overall 93 patients (77%) were very satisfied and another 21 patients (17.4%) were satisfied

◘ Table 136-4

Modified Seattle Angina Questionnaire

No	Question (Q)/Answer options (A)
1.	Q: How limited are you in your daily activities inside your flat/house?
	A: severely limited/moderately limited/limited/little limited/not limited
2.	Q: How limited are you moving up stairs or walk up a little hill?
	A: severely limited/moderately limited/limited/little limited/not limited
3.	Q: Compare your Angina or dyspnea today and before the operation?
	A: lot more/somewhat more/unchanged/less/much less
4.	Q: Over the past 4 weeks, on average, how many times have you had angina or dysnpea?
	A: Four times or more a day/ 1–3 times day/three or more times a week/less than once a week/ never in the last 4 weeks.
5.	Q: Over the past 4 weeks, on average, how many times have you taken nitroglycerin?
	A: Four times or more a day/ 1–3 times day/three or more times a week/less than once a week/ never in the last 4 weeks.
6.	Q: How bothersome is it for you to take your pills as prescribed?
	A: very/moderately/little/not at all/no drugs prescribed
7.	Q: How satisfied are you that everything possible is being done to treat your heart?
	A: not satisfied/somewhat satisfied/satisfied/Very satisfied
8.	Q: How satisfied are you with the overall treatment of your heart disease?
	A: very dissatisfied/somewhat dissatisfied/little dissatisfied/satisfied / very satisfied
9.	Q: Over the last 4 weeks, how much has your angina or dyspnea interfered with your enjoyment of life?
	A: strongly interfered/somewhat interfered/little interfered/not interfered
10.	QQ: If you had to spend the rest of your life with your actual discomfort, how would you feel about this?
	A: very dissatisfied/somewhat dissatisfied/little dissatisfied/satisfied / very satisfied
11. (a)	Q: (a) How often do you worry that you may have a heart attack or die suddenly?
(b)	A: can't stop/often/from time to time/rarely/never
	Q: Q: (b) Where do you live?

Questionnaire used for quality of life assessment via telephone interview

by the previous treatment. Only six patients (5%) felt not satisfied enough to take their prescribed medication. Furthermore, 112 patients (93.4%) were very reassured to have continuous, full access to medical treatment (see ❯ *Figure 136-4a*).

Interference of cardiac disease with daily enjoyment of life was described by only 9 patients (7.5%), whereas 111 patients (92.5%) had no reduction in their QoL. Sixty-nine patients (58%) were very optimistic to conserve their present activity of life. Thirty-three patients (27.7%) did think about recurrence of their heart disease from time to time, but only 17 patients (14.2%) were anxious more frequently about having a heart attack or die suddenly (❯ *Figure 136-4b*). In contrast, 30 patients (45%) undergoing aortic valve replacement with or without concomitant

☐ Figure 136-2

The percentage and absolute numbers of patients having answered question 1 and 2 with no or little limitations in their daily activities

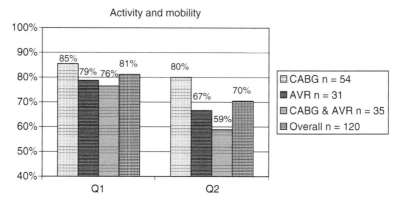

☐ Figure 136-3

Percentage and absolute numbers of patients having answered question 3 with much less or less angina or dyspnea and question 4 with angina or dyspnea less than once a week or never in the last 4 weeks

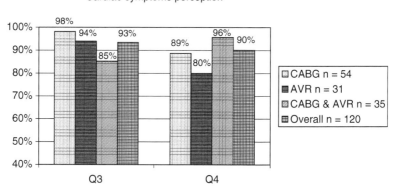

CABG worried at least once a day of dying, versus 6 patients (11.1%) after isolated coronary artery bypass surgery.

And finally, 116 patients (97%) at follow-up lived in their own homes and preserved a high degree of self-care.

2.5   Methodological Considerations

Since the mid-1980s, the per- and postoperative survival in octogenarians after cardiac surgery has steadily increased to become highly acceptable nowadays (Alexander et al., 2000). Patients 80 years and older represent a very distinct population from the younger

■ Figure 136-4
(a) Percentage and absolute numbers of patients having answered question 7 and 8 with satisfied or very satisfied with their treatment. (b) The percentage and absolute numbers of patients having answered question 9 and 10 with little interference or no interference and satisfied or very satisfied about their emotional well-being, and question 8 with satisfied or very satisfied with their treatment as well as question 11 with rarely or never worrying about a heart attack or sudden death event

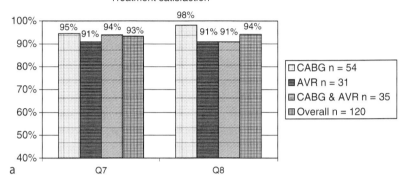

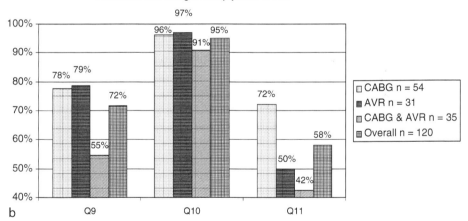

cardiac patients (Fruitman et al., 1999). Measurement of morbidity and mortality provide only a small amount of information about the patient's postoperative physical, functional, emotional, and mental well-being.

Little is known about the postoperative symptom perception in patients 80 years and older after a cardiac surgery. The author analyzed the postoperative QoL in 120 consecutive octogenarians post CABG, AVR, or a combination of both procedures. Mean follow-up was about 2½ years, and none of the surviving patients was lost at follow-up. The QoL of 54 patients after CABC surgery, of 31 patients after AVR, and of 35 patients after combined procedures was compared.

The initial assessment was based on the two main cardiac functional symptoms: chest pain and dyspnea. As older patients are known to have advanced symptoms at presentation for surgery, NYHA class III and IV are a more common finding in octogenarians than they are in younger patients (Goyal et al., 2005; Hunt et al., 2000). Alexander et al. (Rothenhausler et al., 2005) described NYHA class III to IV heart failure being present in 16.6% compared to 9.8% in patients younger than 80 years. Fruitman and coworkers (Fruitman et al., 1999) have also shown a significant, higher presence of NYHA IV in octogenarians.

Questions 1–5 of the SAQ address either one or both symptoms. In CABG patients, unstable angina pectoris was the presenting symptom, with more than two-thirds of the patients being in a CCS $\geq$ III. Near-equal distribution was found for dyspnea in patients undergoing AVR, with 62% being in NYHA $\geq$ III. In the combined CABG/AVR group, dyspnea was the leading symptom (see ❷ Table 136-1). In contrast, LVEF (59 $\pm$ 14%) did not differ from the values in younger collectives possibly because of a selection bias in this older patient segment. Despite a lower than average prevalence of COPD 18, prolonged ventilation (>24 h) for respiratory failure affected 6–9% of the patients (see ❷ Table 136-2). Very similar results have been reported previously (Goyal et al., 2005). This might reflect the diminished physiologic reserves and a more pronounced tendency to fluid retention.

2.6   Gender Difference

Gender difference decreases with age progression. Forty-one percent of patients were women, as opposed to 20–30% described in younger population (Avery et al., 2001; Rothenhausler et al., 2005). The underling study did not identify either a trend for higher female or male in-hospital mortality as described by others. Therefore, female gender may be a weaker risk factor in elderly compared to younger women.

The higher difference of pre- and postoperative symptoms in this older patient subgroup is a further argument for the benefit of early operative treatment in patients over 80 years.

2.7   Surgical Therapy of Ischemic Heart Disease in the Elderly

Some studies have suggested that severe three-vessel diseases are less prevalent at very advanced age (Goyal et al., 2005), a fact the authors oft the study could not confirm, as 78% of the CABG patients presented with triple-vessel CAD and 42% had left main disease. Independent of age, the primary target of surgical therapy for ischemic heart disease is complete revascularization, reflected in the high number of triple or quintuple CABGs (79%).

Arterial grafts such as LIMA are less frequently used as bypass grafts in the elderly (Goyal et al., 2005; Kolh et al., 2001), even though the authors favor the principle of the LIMA as the graft of choice in CABG patients for all ages and therefore should not be withheld from octogenarians as demonstrated by a 77% LIMA and 13% radial artery use for revascularization of the left coronary artery territory.

2.8   Aortic Valve Surgery

The choice of the prosthetic aortic valve is a trade-off between the lower life expectancy for patients 80 years and older and the higher risk of complications from oral anticoagulation medication. Tissue valves are therefore implanted in 80% of the patients. Twenty percent of patients got a mechanical valve motivated by ongoing oral anticoagulation medication. Most frequent indication for anticoagulation was for atrial fibrillation, present in 25% of patients undergoing aortic valve surgery.

2.9   Survival and QoL Impacting Factors

Survival rates are very acceptable. Three years after surgery 124 patients (90%) were alive, and after 5 years of operation 120 patients (73%) (see ❷ *Table 136-3*). These survival rates are comparable to or slightly higher than the ones described in other studies (Akins et al., 1997; Asimakopoulos et al., 1997; Craver et al., 1999; Kirsch et al., 1998; Melby et al., 2007; Rosengart et al., 2002; Rothenhausler et al., 2005; Tsai et al., 1994), and show good early and mid-term postoperative results justifying not withholding cardiac surgery from the increasing elderly and very old population.

However, longevity is not the primary goal in patients over 80; therefore, good operative outcomes imply not only safety and survival but also the gain of comfort in daily life. The marked improvement of the NYHA functional class as well as improvement of the CCS class that we found (72% free of angina or dyspnea) has also been reported previously (Kumar et al., 1995; Sundt et al., 2000; Thornton et al., 2005). Nevertheless, only marginal attention had been paid in most studies to the improvement of the emotional well-being, treatment satisfaction, and disease perception. The results of the present study in octogenarians demonstrate a remarkable improvement in the QoL and a significant improvement in the patient's functional status after cardiac surgery.

Activity and mobility improved in ischemic and valvular disease, with nearly 80% of the patients feeling no or only very little limitation in their daily activity (see ❷ *Figure 136-2*). The improvement in exercise tolerance is less homogenously distributed, with 80% of CABG patients reporting virtually free of limitation and only 59% of the patients in the combined procedures group. This difference in exercise tolerance is reflected again in the symptom perception by the patient. Ninety-eight percent of the CABG patients, compared to 85% of CABG and AVR patients, felt considerable improvement of their angina or dyspnea compared to their preoperative clinical condition. The vast majority (93%) of all the octogenarians felt much better after surgery (see ❷ *Figure 136-3*). In all types of operations, more than 90% of the patients were moderately satisfied or very satisfied with the overall treatment of their heart disease. And, it is note worthy that nearly 100% of the CABG patients as well as 91% of the AVR or CABG and AVR patients felt pleased to have access to full medical treatment, despite their advanced age (see ❷ *Figure 136-4a*). Over 95% of the patients at follow-up lived in their own homes and enjoyed a high degree of autonomy. Similar results have been found by Fruitman et al. (1999), Kumar et al. (1995), Heijmeriks et al. (1999), Rumsfeld et al. (2001), and Yun et al. (1999).

It is noteworthy that 21% of the CABG/AVR patients and 12% of the AVR patients worry at least daily about a heart attack or about sudden death as compared to less than 4% in the isolated CABG group. A possible explanation might be that the more advanced the disease stage, the higher the incidence of so-called near death experiences in patients with aortic stenosis after syncope resulting from a delayed referring practice. This particular emotional dimension might improve if patients with aortic stenosis are operated on earlier independent of their age.

The average octogenarians after heart surgery take 5.3 pills, but 75–80% feel only a little or not at all deranged by the daily medication.

2.10   Financial Impact on Healthcare Resources

Happier and healthier octogenarian come at an increased cost. Looking at the economical dimension of patients over 80 undergoing heart surgery does result in 20–27% higher hospital costs as reported (Peterson et al., 1995). Avery et al. attributed the increase of total direct hospital cost in octogenarians to a more severe risk profile and to longer consecutive ICU and hospital stay (6). However, emphasis on early extubation and timely aggressive mobilization after surgery also has successfully decreased the overall intubation time and length of stay of this elderly patient population in ICUs to 2.8 days (see ❷ *Table 136-2*). This is between the previously reported 6.8 days (4), or 5.1 days (Goyal et al., 2005) and the 1.7–1.1 days of Dalrymple-Hay et al. (1999). The hospital stay of 14.5 days is in the range of previously published values (11). In contrast, with the increased in-hospital cost are the excellent postoperative recovery and gain in QoL, providing back the potential of self-care, which might also be largely compensated by reduced consecutive disease-associated costs compared to medical treatments alone with frequent re-hospitalization for repetitive congestive heart failure and invalidating cardiac symptoms (Sollano et al., 1998).

2.11   Final Considerations

Selected patients of 80 years and older after cardiac surgery show a remarkable QoL and a considerable increase in their emotional well-being (see ❷ *Figure 136-4b*), as well as an important increase in their functional status with a satisfactory medium-term, 5-year survival (see ❷ *Figure 136-1*) at a reasonably low risk. The stunning recovery from being a bedridden patient to a self-caring patient is a further very important advantage after cardiac surgery in this challenging age group. Therefore, in selected octogenarians, early operative treatment should not be withheld, and the adoption of an early referral might further increase the patient's postoperative benefits.

Summary Points

- Twenty-five percent of patients over the age of 80 are functionally limited by their underling cardiovascular condition.
- Heart surgery is a very effective therapy to improve the survival and functional status of patients with coronary artery and heart valve disease in all age groups.
- In heart surgery patients of increased age and decreased life expectancy, QoL represents an important end point.
- Ninety-three percent of selected patients of 80 years and older show a remarkable QoL and a considerable increase in their emotional well-being after heart surgery.
- Earlier and more aggressive surgical therapy substantially increases outcome of heart surgery in octogenarians and should not be withheld until a progressed-disease stage.
- Adoption of an earlier referral practice might further increase the postoperative benefits of patients.

References

Spencer G. (1989). US bureau of Census: Projections of the Population of the United States by Age, Sex and Race:1988 to 2080. Washington, DC: US Government Printing Office. Current Population Reports, Series P-25, No 1018.

Statistical Abstract of the United States/1994 (114th edn.) (1994). Washington DC: Department of Commerce, US Bureau of the Census, 84.

Elinkton JR. (1966). Ann Inter Med. 64: 711–714.

Rothenhausler HB, Grieser B, Nollert G, Reichart B, Schelling G, Kapfhammer HP. (2005). Gen Hosp Psychiatry. 27(1): 18–28.

Thornton EW, Groom C, Fabri BM, Fox MA, Hallas C, Jackson M. (2005). J Thorac Cardiovasc Surg. 130 (4): 1022–1027.

Kirsch M, Guesnier L, LeBesnerais P, Hillion ML, Debauchez M, Seguin J, Loisance DY. (1998). Ann Thorac Surg. 66(1): 60–67.

Craver JM, Puskas JD, Weintraub WW, Shen Y, Guyton RA, Gott JP, Jones EL. (1999). Ann Thorac Surg. 67(4): 1104–1110.

Goyal S, Henry M, Mohajeri M. (2005). ANZ J Surg. 75 (6): 429–435.

Huber CH, Goeber V, Berdat P, Carrel T, Eckstein F. (2007). Eur J Cardiothorac Surg. 31(6): 1099–2105.

Higginson IJ, Carr AJ. (2001). BMJ. 322(7297): 1297–1300.

Rosser RM. (1985). A History of the Development of Health Indices. In: Smith GT (ed.) Measuring the Social Benefits of Medicine. Office of Health Economics, London.

William JI. (1991). Theoretic Surg. 6: 152–157.

Campbell A, Converse PE, Rodgers WL. (1976). The Quality of American Life. Russel Sage Foundation, New York, pp. 1–583.

Dempster M, Donnelly M. (2000). Heart. 83(6): 641–644.

Immer FF, Althaus SM, Berdat PA, Saner H, Carrel TP. (2005). Eur J Cardiovasc Prev Rehabil. 12(2): 138–143.

Immer FF, Lippeck C, Barmettler H, Berdat PA, Eckstein FS, Kipfer B, Saner H, Schmidli J, Carrel TP. (2004). Circulation. 110(11 Suppl 1): II250–II255.

Spertus JA, Winder JA, Dewhurst TA, Deyo RA, Prodzinski J, McDonell M, Fihn SD. (1995). J Am Coll Cardiol. 25(2): 333–341.

Dougherty CM, Dewhurst T, Nichol WP, Spertus J. (1998). J Clin Epidemiol. 51(7): 569–575.

Alexander KP, Anstrom KJ, Muhlbaier LH, Grosswald RD, Smith PK, Jones RH, Peterson ED. (2000). J Am Coll Cardiol. 35(3): 731–738.

Fruitman DS, MacDougall CE, Ross DB. (1999). Ann Thorac Surg. 68(6): 2129–2135.

Hunt JO, Hendrata MV, Myles PS. (2000). Heart Lung. 29(6): 401–411.

Avery GJ 2nd, Ley SJ, Hill JD, Hershon JJ, Dick SE. (2001). Ann Thorac Surg. 71(2): 591–596.

Kolh P, Kerzmann A, Lahaye L, Gerard P, Limet R. (2001). Eur Heart J. 22(14): 1235–1243.

Akins CW, Daggett WM, Vlahakes GJ, Hilgenberg AD, Torchiana DF, Madsen JC, Buckley MJ. (1997). Ann Thorac Surg. 64(3): 606–614; discussion 614–615.

Rosengart TK, Finnin EB, Kim DY, Samy SA, Tanhehco Y, Ko W, Lang SJ, Krieger KH, Isom OW. (2002). Am J Med. 112(2): 143–147.

Tsai TP, Chaux A, Matloff JM, Kass RM, Gray RJ, DeRobertis MA, Khan SS. (1994). Ann Thorac Surg. 58 (2): 445–50; discussion 450–451.

Melby SJ, Zierer A, Kaiser SP, Guthrie TJ, Keune JD, Schuessler RB, Pasque MK, Lawton JS, Moazami N, Moon MR, Damiano RJ Jr. (2007). Ann Thorac Surg. 83(5): 1651–1656; discussion 1656–1657.

Asimakopoulos G, Edwards MB, Taylor KM. (1997). Circulation. 96(10): 3403–3408.

Kumar P, Zehr KJ, Chang A, Cameron DE, Baumgartner WA. (1995). Chest. 108(4): 919–926.

Sundt TM, Bailey MS, Moon MR, Mendeloff EN, Huddleston CB, Pasque MK, Barner HB, Gay WA Jr. (2000). Circulation. 102(19 Suppl 3): III70–III74.

Heijmeriks JA, Pourrier S, Dassen P, Prenger K, Wellens HJ. (1999). Am J Cardiol. 83(7): 1129–1132, A9.

Rumsfeld JS, Magid DJ, O'Brien M, McCarthy M Jr, MaWhinney S, Scd, Shroyer AL, Moritz TE, Henderson WG, Sethi GK, Grover FL, Hammermeister KE. (2001). Ann Thorac Surg. 72 (6): 2026–2032.

Yun KL, Sintek CF, Fletcher AD, Pfeffer TA, Kochamba GS, Mahrer PR, Khonsari S. (1999). Ann Thorac Surg. 68(4): 1314–1320.

Peterson ED, Cowper PA, Jollis JG, Bebchuk JD, DeLong ER, Muhlbaier LH, Mark DB, Pryor DB. (1995). Circulation. 92(9 Suppl): II85–II91.

Dalrymple-Hay MJ, Alzetani A, Aboel-Nazar S, Haw M, Livesey S, Monro J. (1999). Eur J Cardiothorac Surg. 15(1): 61–66.

Sollano JA, Rose EA, Williams DL, Thornton B, Quint E, Apfelbaum M, Wasserman H, Cannavale GA, Smith CR, Reemtsma K, Greene RJ. (1998). Ann Surg. 228 (3): 297–306.

137 Quality of Life and Financial Measures in Surgical and Non-Surgical Treatments in Emphysema

J. D. Miller · F. Altaf

1	*Introduction*	*2337*
1.1	Importance of Measuring QOL as an Outcome in COPD Patients	2338
2	*QOL Measurements Tools*	*2339*
2.1	What Is the Minimal Important Clinical Difference (MICD) of QOL Instrument?	2339
3	*Economic Measures*	*2342*
3.1	Calculating Cost per QALY (CUI): An Example	2343
4	*Impact of Medical Intervention on QOL in COPD Patients*	*2343*
4.1	Inhaled Corticosteroids (ICS)	2343
4.2	Bronchodilators	2344
4.2.1	B2 Agonists	2344
4.2.2	Anticholinergics	2344
4.2.3	Combination Therapy	2344
4.2.4	Pulmonary Rehabilitation (PR)	2345
4.2.5	Oxygen	2346
5	*Impact of Surgical Intervention on QOL in COPD Patients*	*2347*
6	*Financial Impact of Medical and Surgical Intervention in COPD Patients*	*2349*
	Summary Points	*2350*

Abstract: The cost of health care is continuing to escalate world wide. More people are living longer and often with more challenging medical conditions. The personal and societal cost for survival is growing yearly.

Medical and surgical advances, unfortunately, have not been able to stop this growing financial burden. Occasionally new surgical interventions can favorably affect the overall health care cost. If an intervention can create a healthier patient with fewer health care needs, society may experience an overall saving. Such was the early hope for ❷ Lung Volume Reduction Surgery (LVRS).

If LVRS can save productive lives and reduce a patients' ongoing need for medicines, such as oxygen therapy, there may be an overall financial gain to society. If, however, LVRS differs costs into the future as well as add the new surgical costs clearly there will be no overall saving. In this later instance the gain to a patients' well being must be weighed against the cost of the intervention. Lastly when there is no overall gain for the patient and no saving to society it is clear that we should not invest in the intervention.

This chapter reviews the tools used to evaluate a patients health-related quality of life (❷ HRQOL) and reviews the world literature evaluating health gains and losses following LVRS. The cost of LVRS to society will be reviewed and compared with other medical and surgical interventions with an emphasis on other treatments for advanced ❷ emphysema.

We begin with a general outline of the definition of Quality of Life (QOL), and a review of the research tools in use to evaluate QOL. These tools can be designed to assess a patients' quality of life specifically as it related to a particular disease state such as chronic obstructive lung disease (❷ COPD) (a disease specific QOL measure), or it can be designed as a broader tool assessing QOL as ones' general health impacts on their perception of well being.

The two major short-comings of a QOL measure is its subjective nature (individual preference based) and its inability to include one of the worst health related outcomes, death. Traditionally a subject who has died is not able to report on their QOL and is omitted from further assessment and is not included in the group assessment. Only patients who are able to complete the questionnaire at the give time are included in that time's overall group score. Health Utilities, however, is a societal preference based score and ascribes the value zero for death. It therefore can be used as a tool to follow a group of patients over time and include loss of life in the overall scoring of health quality for that group.

Healthcare economists can use ❷ health utility (HU) scores of a study group over time as a measure of that groups' overall health for that time period. It is reported in units called Quality Adjusted Life Years (❷ QALYs). A comparison between research groups allows the investigator an opportunity to assess the gain or loss of health. This difference is also reported in quality adjusted life years (QALYs). Knowing the gain or loss in QALYs and the cost difference between two groups allows the economist to report the cost per QALY. The cost per QALY is a value of a very general nature and allows for comparison of interventions of various types to one and other.

This chapter will outline in more detail each of these measures and tools and discuss their application to the financial assessment of LVRS.

List of Abbreviations: *COPD*, chronic obstructive pulmonary disease; *CRDQ*, Chronic Respiratory Disease Questionnaire; *CUA*, cost utility assessment; *CUI*, cost utility index; *DLCO*, Carbon monoxide diffusion capacity; *FEV1*, forced expiratory volume in one second; *HRQOL*, health-related quality of life; *HUI*, ❷ health utility index; *ICER*, The incremental cost-utility ratio; *ISOLDE*, inhaled steroid in obstructive lung disease; *LTOT*, long-term oxygen therapy; *LVRS*, lung volume reduction surgery; *MICD*, minimal important clinical difference; *MRC*, Modified Medical Research Council Dyspnea Index; *NETT*, National Emphysema Treatment Trial; *NHP*, Nottingham Health Profile; *Pao2*, peripheral arterial oxygen content; *PFSDQ*, Pulmonary Function Status and Dyspnea Questionnaire; *PFSS*, pulmonary function status scale; *PR*, ❷ pulmonary rehabilitation; *QALYs*, quality adjusted life years; *QOL*, quality of life; *QWB*, Quality of Well-Being Questionnaire; *SF-36*, Short Form 36 questionnaire; *SGRQ*, St. George's Respiratory Questionnaire; *SIP*, sickness impact profile; *SOLQ*, Seattle Obstructive Lung Disease Questionnaire

1   Introduction

Chronic obstructive pulmonary disease (COPD) is chronic progressive and disabling long-term lung diseases that include chronic bronchitis (irreversible narrowing of small bronchi causing airflow limitations) and emphysema (abnormal enlargement of the air spaces distal to the terminal bronchioles accompanied by destruction of their walls causing air trapping and inefficient exchange of gases across to and from the blood). It is a preventable disease that is caused primarily by cigarette smoking. As the disease naturally progress, patients become progressively short of breath and disabled affecting their life in general. Because treatments options has not succeeded in general to reverse the disease progression, interventions that result in improving symptomatology and ❷ quality of life tools (QOL) of theses patients are of prime importance.

Several definitions of QOL has been proposed, simply it can be identified as an individual's satisfaction or happiness with life in domains he or she considers important OR *subjective feeling that one's life overall is going well.* Thus, quality of life is, by definition, a subjective concept, dependent on cultural perspectives and values.

Several domains and variables are included in QOL assessment, These domains might be psychological and social; physical and mental health; emotional and cognitive dimensions, for example, happiness and satisfaction with life; the ability to function bodily, sexually, socially and occupationally; objective status in terms of finances, working conditions, family conditions. . . . etc.

Numerous taxonomies of life domains have been proposed based on studies of general populations of both well and ill people. A typical taxonomy is that of Flanagan (1978), which categorizes 15 dimension of life quality, into five domains, as shown below (❷ *Table 137-1*). These factors and domains act and interact in multiple diminutions in determining one's quality of life (Testa and Simonson, 1996).

The concept of HRQOL encompasses the impact of the individual's health on his or her ability to perform activities of daily living deemed to be important. Generally speaking, assessment of HRQL represents an attempt to determine how variables within the dimension of health (e.g., a disease or its treatment) relate to particular dimensions of life that have been determined to be important.

◼ Table 137-1

Flanagan's domains of QOL

Physical and material well-being
Material well-being and financial security
Health and personal safety
Relations with other people
Relations with spouse
Having and rearing children
Relations with parents, siblings, or other relatives
Relations with friends
Social, community, civic activities
Helping and encouraging others
Participating in local and governmental affairs
Personal development, fulfillment
Intellectual development
Understanding and planning
Occupational role career
Creativity and personal expression
Recreation
Socializing with others
Passive and observational recreational activities
Participating in active recreation

As this model includes five domains, other models have included more/different domains and items in an attempt to be reflective of the true person QOL. *QOL* quality of life

1.1   Importance of Measuring QOL as an Outcome in COPD Patients

More and more studies are including QOL measures as a primary out come in patients with COPD for several reasons

- QOL measures are used to quantify the impact of the condition and to compare the effects of lung diseases with the other chronic medical problems.
- QOL measures can be used to evaluate changes resulting from therapeutic interventions especially when the results of various therapeutic interventions has failed to show survival benefits in patients with sever COPD.
- For prognostication. Previous studies showed correlation between measures for QOL and mortality independent of disease severity. In one study (Domingo-Salvany et al., 2002), in addition to the FEV1, both SGRQ and SF-36 scores were an independent predictors of mortality in a cohort of COPD patients.
- QOL measures are necessary as a central component of cost/effectiveness analysis (Kaplan and Ries, 2005).

2   QOL Measurements Tools

There are several generic and disease-specific instruments that can be used to objectively measure QOL in patients with COPD, each incorporating various aspects of physical, psychological, and social function.

1. Generic QOL instruments: general measures that respond to broad changes in patient's health state and have the advantage of being a common assessment tool so it can compare QOL across several diseases.
2. Disease-specific QOL instruments: are instruments that are designed to have greater sensitivity to minimal clinical changes in variables that are specific to a particular disease (e.g., COPD) which will thereafter affect the score of that instrument.

Each QOL instrument is a questionnaire that has unique domains and items that address specific health related issues; each candidate answers these questionnaires and is subsequently assigned a score for each domain as well as a total score. These scores can be used to assess a study group before and after an intervention, or to compare QOL between study groups.

A good QOL instrument must be valid (ability of the instrument to actually measure what it claims to measure), responsive (ability of the instrument to detect clinically significant changes) and reliable (repeated measurements in the same setting yields very similar results), giving these facts, several measures for dyspnea and QOL have been thoroughly verified methodologically in COPD patients.

2.1   What Is the Minimal Important Clinical Difference (MICD) of QOL Instrument?

The Minimally Important Clinical Difference (MICD) is the smallest difference in the score of the QOL instrument that informed patients or physicians perceive as important, either beneficial or harmful. An intervention that led to a change in health reflected by that MCID-score would lead the patient or clinician to consider a change in the management. It is possible for QOL score changes to have statistically significant difference and yet not have meaningful clinical implications.

Unfortunately, there is no "gold standard" methodology of estimating the MICD, A possible and widely used, but weak, technique would be to approach a group of experts and ask them whether the particular score looks like a reasonable measure of what is important to patients, as they perceive it (But not as the patient perceive it).Understanding the MICD will help in interpreting the impact of the intervention and in helping the authors in estimating sample size and defining who are the responders (whom they reached MICD).

Basic concepts regarding few of these instruments are illustrated in ❷ Table 137-2.

The American Thoracic Society maintains a website (www.atsqol.org) that summarizes QOL measures that can be used in outcomes research for lung disease. The site lists measures by disease and offers references on their use.

3. Quality-adjusted life years (QALYs), are the units of quality of life over time (number of years lived). Each year in perfect health is assigned the value of 1.0 QALYs. Death for a full year would have a value of 0. If a patient is alive but not in a perfect health, for example blind or be confined to a wheelchair, then the QALYs would have a value between 0 and 1.

◼ Table 137-2

Commonly used QOL measures in COPD patients

Instruments	Conduction and estimated time	Domains and/or categories	Item, n	QOL improve as score (increase/ decrease)	MICD
Generic					
Nottingham Health Profile (NHP) (Hunt et al., 1985)	Self; 5–10 min	Energy, pain, sleep, social isolation, emotional reactions, physical mobility	38	Decrease	Not determined
Medical Outcomes Study Short Form 36-Item Health Survey (SF-36) (Ware and Sherbourne, 1992)	Self or interviewer; 5 min	Physical functioning; role limitations due to physical health problems; bodily pain; social functioning; general mental health; role limitations due to emotional problems, vitality, energy or fatigue; general health perceptions	36	Increase	(5–12.5) points change of score
Sickness Impact Profile (SIP) (Bergner et al., 1976; Bergner et al., 1981)	Self or interviewer; 20–30 min	Domains:physical and psychosocial Categories: sleep and rest, eating, work, home management, recreation and pastimes, ambulation, mobility, body care and movement, social interaction, alertness behavior, emotional behavior, communication	136	Decrease	Not determined
Disease-specific					
Chronic Respiratory Disease Questionnaire (CRDQ) (Guyatt et al., 1987)	Interviewer; 15–25 min	Dyspnea, fatigue, emotional function, mastery	20	Increase	(0.5) points change of score

◘ Table 137-2 (continued)

Instruments	Conduction and estimated time	Domains and/or categories	Item, n	QOL improve as score (increase/ decrease)	MICD
Pulmonary Functional Status and Dyspnea Questionnaire (PFSDQ) (Lareau et al., 1994)	Self; 15 min	Domains functional status, dyspnea Categories: self care, mobility, home management, eating, recreation, social	164	Decrease	Not reported
St. George's Respiratory Questionnaire (SGRQ) (Jones et al., 1992)	Self or interviewer; 10 min	Symptoms, activity, impacts	76	Decrease	4% improvement in separate domains or total score
Seattle Obstructive Questionnaire (SOLQ) (Tu et al., 1997)	Self; 5–10 min	Physical function, emotional function, coping skills, treatment and satisfaction	29	Increase	Not determined

Different scaling and scoring system has been developed for each domain instrument, total score can be then evaluated which reflect the QOL status of the candidate. *CRDQ* Chronic Respiratory Disease Questionnaire; *MICD* minimal important clinical difference; *NHP* Nottingham Health Profile; *PFSDQ* Pulmonary Function Status and Dyspnea Questionnaire; *PFSS* Pulmonary function status scale; *SF-36* Short Form 36 questionnaire; *SGRQ* St. George's Respiratory Questionnaire; *SIP* sickness impact profile; *SOLQ* Seattle Obstructive Lung Disease Questionnaire

◘ Table 137-3
Calculating QALYs

	Years lived (a)	Health state as measured by health utility tool (b)	QALYs gained (= a × b)
Intervention A	4	0.75	3 QALYs
Intervention B	4	0.5	2 QALYs

Intervention A will generate additional QALYs (1 year of perfect life) in comparison to intervention B. QALYs: quality adjusted life years

The values between 0 and 1 are usually determined by using a QOL measure called a, health utility. Several health utilities are in practice and include: Standard Gamble, Time Tradeoff and the standardized instruments of the Quality of Well-Being Questionnaire (QWB), the *Health Utility Index (HUI) and the European Quality of Life tools* (Yusen et al., 2002). Calculating QALY is illustrated in ● *Table 137-3*.

The Canadian LVRS Study Group used HUI as a measure of QALYs. The HUI is a 15 min self administered generic instrument questionnaire that is used for classification of health status.

Health status is valued according to a multi-active, multi-attribute utility function estimated from preference scores obtained from random sample from the general public. The scoring function assigns a single summary score at an interval between 0.00 (deceased) and 1.0 (perfect health).

3   Economic Measures

Economists have developed different techniques to compare treatments in term of cost and outcome. Several measures have been used to compare the financial impact of different treatments.

1. Cost effectiveness or value-for-money, is a technique used to compares the relative expenditure (costs) and outcomes (effects) of two or more interventions. Although it is the most commonly used, it only measures a single outcome, such as life-years gained or patients cured, as the basis of comparing treatments.

2. Cost utility analysis (CUA), is a technique used to compare the relative expenditures (costs) and outcomes (effects) of two or more interventions where the outcomes are measured in terms of years of full health gained or lost (multiple outcomes) using a measures such as QALYs. The cost utility index (CUI) is expressed as the costs required to generate a year of perfect health (one QALY) using the intervention being studied.

A CUA has the generalizability needed to compare various treatment options with one and other. Several registries are now common and are available to compare various interventions including drugs, prostehetics and surgery thus provide health care policy makers with a common unit of cost for health gain for each intervention to determine how to allocate health care funds.

In Canada, cost-effectiveness threshold of $20,000/QALY is considered within most healthcare budgets while treatments that cost more than $100,000/QALY are considered to be outside budget limits, these limits differ between countries as their health budgets and health care values differ. An arbitrary figure of $20,000–50,000 dollars per QALY has commonly been applied as the threshold (❯ Table 137-4).

Cost-effectiveness Analysis Registry of various interventions for various diseases can be found at www.tufts-nemc.org/cearegistry/

3. The incremental cost-utility ratio (ICER) is the ratio between the difference in costs and the difference in QALYs both interventions produced.

◻ Table 137-4

A sample of cost-effectiveness analysis registry

Intervention	Cost/QALY (US dollars)
Mammographic screening/colon cancer screening	10,000–25,000
Implantable cardioverter-defibrillator	30,000–85,000
Dialysis in end stage renal disease	50,000–100,000
LVRS	100,000–300,000
Left ventricular assist device	500,000–1,400,000

The last three interventions would not be considered good value for money (cost effective). LVRS: lung volume reduction surgery

◻ Table 137-5

Calculating cost per QALY in dollars

	Intervention A	Intervention B	Difference (or increment)
Mean costs of treatment per patient (not average)	7,000	4,000	3,000 (a)
Mean utility (QALYs) per patient (not average)	0.7	0.5	0.2 (b)
Incremental cost per QALY (ICER) (= a/b)			15,000

Intervention A will coast 15,000 dollars per one full functional year gained by the intervention. *QALY* quality adjusted life years

3.1 Calculating Cost per QALY (CUI): An Example

Estimates of utility, costs and incremental cost per QALY have been calculated using an updated version of a cost-utility model proposed by Hutton et al. (1996). Cost per QALY estimates should be incremental rather than average since incremental method will present the additional costs and health gains over time for each intervention. Thus it closely reflects the impact of in the real world; especially in COPD patients where long terms follow up is a standard, helping of choosing one intervention over another. A simple example of calculating coast per QALY is illustrated below in ❯ *Table 137-5*.

4 Impact of Medical Intervention on QOL in COPD Patients

Published guidelines on COPD state that the goals of pharmacologic therapy should be to control symptoms, improve health status, and reduce the frequency of COPD exacerbations (O'Donnell et al., 2003). Bronchodilators are the mainstay of pharmacotherapy for patients with COPD. They are effective in treating symptoms and improving exercise capacity but do not alter disease progression. On the other hand, inhaled corticosteroids (ICS) have beneficial effects in a subset of patients with chronic, stable COPD. They reduce the frequency of exacerbations in those patients with advanced disease (FEV1 $\leq$50% of predicted) who experience, on average, at least 1 exacerbation per year.

Below will discuss the impact of different medical interventions on QOL in patients with COPD. Few studies have looked at the effect of these treatments in comparison to placebo while the others have looked at the effect of treatment combinations in comparison to placebo or single treatment strategy.

4.1 Inhaled Corticosteroids (ICS)

Looking at the effect of ICS on QOL, few studies have looked their effects in comparison to placebo in randomized controlled trials

- (ISOLDE) trial (Burge et al., 2000) used the SGRQ as a measure of QOL showed that patients on ICS showed a slower decline in health status compared with those on placebo, although statistically significant these were less than the MICD that is required with the SGRQ.
- In a recent review (Yang et al., 2007) of randomized trials, rate of change in SGRQ in units/year was analyzed in five long-term studies (2,507 patients), showed a slowing in the rate of decline of quality of life in ICS group compared to placebo.

4.2   Bronchodilators

4.2.1   B2 Agonists

Few studies compared inhaled B2 agonists (long and short acting) to placebo

- QOL improved with formoterol (long acting ❷ B2 agonist) over 12-week treatment in a randomized controlled trial comparing it with placebo (Dahl et al., 2001), formoterol showed statistically significant improvement in SGRQ of a difference that exceeded the MICD.
- In a review of studies comparing B2 agonists with placebo in COPD patients (Appleton et al., 2006), Twenty-four studies (6,061 participants) were included, this review demonstrated improvement in SGRQ total score and domains including symptoms, activity and impact over a period of 12 months in treatment arm versus placebo arm.

4.2.2   Anticholinergics

Few studies has looked at the effect of ❷ anticholinergics to placebo

- In a randomized-controlled double-blinded studies, tiotropium significantly improved dyspnea scores and the SGRQ total score when compared with placebo (Brusasco et al., 2003; Donohue et al., 2002).

4.2.3   Combination Therapy

Long-acting B2 agonists and ICS have both been recommended in guidelines for the treatment of chronic obstructive pulmonary disease. Their co-administration in a combined inhaler may facilitate adherence to medication regimens, and improve efficacy. Two types of combined inhaler exist currently (B2 agonist and ICS): budesonide/formoterol (Symbicort), and fluticasone/salmeterol (Advair or Seretide).

Several studies have looked at the effect of combined therapy against *placebo* or *single* therapy in randomized controlled way, recent reviews has looked at these studies looking primarily at exacerbation rate and mortality benefits as well as HRQOL secondarily.

- Looking at 11 studies (6,427 participants) were two different combination preparations (fluticasone/salmeterol and budesonide/formoterol) were tested against placebo, both treatments led to significant improvement in QOL measured by CRDQ (Nannini et al., 2007a).
- On the other hand, another review looked at the studies that compare above treatments versus long acting B2 agonists alone, this review included ten studies, a total of 7,598 patients, showed an improvement of QOL measured by the CRDQ and SGRQ (Nannini et al., 2007c).
- On a third review of randomized controlled studies comparing above combination therapies against ICSs alone, seven studies, a total 5,708 patients, showed an improvement of QOL measured by SGRQ (Nannini et al., 2007b).

As above stated, the combined effect of both B2 agonists and ICS on QOL is better than placebo and/or each medication alone.

Adding anticholinergics to B2 agonists and ICS (triple combination) has had an added effect; A recent randomized controlled trial (Aaron et al., 2007) looking at combined medical treatments (Tiotropium, salmeterol and inhaled ❷ steroids fluticasone) showed an improvement of QOL measured by SGRQ and CRDQ in patients who received the combination.

In summary, ICS and bronchodilators (B2 agonists and anticholinergics) improve QOL in COPD patients but this effect gets more evident as one therapy is added to another but it must be emphasized that this should be interpreted cautiously since these measures of QOL may not reach their minimal clinically significant score. In that context clinical studies should report their results of QOL measures only when they reach their minimal clinically significant score and should attribute their results to the most affected domains.

4.2.4   Pulmonary Rehabilitation (PR)

As defined recently by The American Thoracic Society and the European Respiratory Society: PR is an evidence-based, multidisciplinary, and comprehensive intervention designed for patients with chronic respiratory diseases who are symptomatic and often have decreased daily life activities.

Many rehabilitation strategies have been developed for patients with disabling COPD. Programs typically include components such as patient assessment, exercise training, education, nutritional intervention, and psychosocial support. Studies suggest that best results are achieved with programs of 6–10 weeks' duration that involve 6–8 patients per class.

Looking at its effect on QOL

- A recent review (Lacasse et al., 2006) involving 31 randomized studies showed statistically and clinically significant improvements in different QOL measures and their domains including dyspnea, fatigue, emotions, and patient control over disease.
- A recent meta analysis (Cambach et al., 1999) showed significant improvements of QOL measured by CRDQ and all of its domains.

Based on theses studies and other studies, American College of Chest physicians guidelines recommendations were as following

1. A program of exercise training of the muscles of ambulation is recommended as a mandatory component of pulmonary rehabilitation for patients with COPD. Grade of recommendation, 1A.
2. Pulmonary rehabilitation improves the symptom of dyspnea in patients with COPD: Grade of recommendation, 1A.
3. Pulmonary rehabilitation improves HRQOL in patients with COPD. Grade of recommendation, 1A.

Home-based PR programs, which provide greater flexibility, have recently been compared in several studies with conventional hospital-based programs. Despite few limitations in these studies, improvements in exercise capacity, symptoms, and QOL have been demonstrated with home-based PR (Na et al., 2005).

As of now one can conclude that there is strong evidence support the fact of improvement of QOL as a result of pulmonary rehabilitation, more studies are needed to look at the benefit of home based PR programs since it may improve compliance, which may impact the outcome, and decrease the coast.

4.2.5   Oxygen

The basic goal of long term oxygen therapy (LTOT) in patients with chronic stable COPD is to maintain peripheral arterial oxygen content values (Pao2) $> / = 60$ mm mercury. Long term therapy currently targets patients with sever COPD and clinically significant chronic respiratory failure, which is defined as a Pao2 $< / = 55$ mm mercury, or as a Pao2 $< / = 60$ mm mercury and either cor pulmonale (right ventricular failure due to pulmonary hypertension) or hematocrit $> / = 55\%$.

Oxygen therapy for patients with chronic, stable COPD is generally administered via nasal prongs at 1–6 L/min, from a cylinder or concentrated oxygen, using one or more of the following approaches: (1) long term oxygen therapy (LTOT) (2) use with exercise (3) use during sleep (4) use during air travel and (5) use as needed for symptoms of dyspnea independent of activity. Of these, LTOT (defined as therapy for >15 h/d) has been shown to have beneficial effects on exercise capacity, mental capacity, cardiopulmonary hemodynamics, and survival in patients with severe COPD with hypoxemia and chronic respiratory failure.

Giving that survival benefit, LTOT was targeted in many studies in regard to QOL with variable results. As some studies showed some improvement in QOL, others did not due to financial constrains, decrease in patient mobility and damaging of social relationships as will as a disturbing noise and nasal/ear discomfort associated with the use of nasal tubes.

- In one study (Okubadejo et al., 1996) comparing 19 patients that met the criteria for LTOT with 18 less hypoxic patients with better baseline SGRQ scores over a period of 6 months; no change in QOL using SGRQ has been found in patients with severe COPD using an oxygen concentrator.
- A recent observational study conducted in Brazil (Tanni et al., 2007) looked at the effect of LTOT in hypoxemia patients after transitioned from cylinder to concentrated oxygen, this study resulted in clinically significant improvement in SGRQ total scores mainly manifested on symptoms and impact domains, worth mentioning this result was not observed in non hypoxemic patients (pao2 > 60 mm mercury at rest).

Looking at oxygen during exercise training of pulmonary rehabilitation, a review published recently including five randomized trials (Nonoyama et al., 2007), a comparison was done between supplemental oxygen compared to control (compressed air or room air) during the exercise-training component of a pulmonary rehabilitation in COPD patients whom they did not meet criteria for long-term oxygen therapy (see above) showed no significant differences in QOL.

Looking at Ambulatory oxygen, a randomized controlled study conducted on 41 patients, whom they are hypoxic on exercise only, over a 12 weeks period using a cylinder oxygen tanks. Improvements were seen in all domains of the CRDQ for cylinder O2 compared with cylinder air but at study completion, (41%) of responders did not want to continue therapy, with 11 citing poor acceptability or tolerability (Eaton et al., 2002).

Finally as of oxygen therapy, LTOT proven survival benefits justify the use of this treatment modality but wither patients should expect an improvement in HRQOL is still not well defined but as technology advances smaller, portable and quieter devices with longer supplement period may give more freedom which may improve the overall QOL though financial restrains will be a limiting factor. Ambulatory and exercise oxygen therapy are not justified based on QOL results alone and one could not conclude that these interventions would necessarily improve QOL.

5   Impact of Surgical Intervention on QOL in COPD Patients

Several surgical procedures has be implemented for the treatment of sever COPD including bullectomies, autonomic denervation, Lung volume reduction surgery (LVRS), endobronchial valve implantation and lung transplantation. Of those the most that has been studies are (LVRS) and lung transplantation which is beyond the scope of discussion in this chapter.

Because LVRS has been developed as a surgery to palliate disabling symptoms of emphysema, many studies now have included QOL outcomes along with the commonly measured physiologic and functional outcomes. Many symptom scales and disease-specific and general instruments of QOL have been used for evaluating emphysema patients before and after LVRS. Case-control studies and randomized studies have shown a consistent improvement in symptoms related to emphysema and general QOL tools validating the use of LVRS as a palliative therapy for selected patients with emphysema (❷ Table 137-6).

In a recent review of randomized studies (Tiong et al., 2006), 1,663 patients were included of a total of eight studies, 73% of the study group recruited from NETT study. This study showed Improvement in SGRQ in LVRS group in excess of minimum clinically important difference as will as improvement in all four domains of the CRDQ at 12 and 24 months as well as in SF-36.

As there is improvement in QOL measures during the early period after LVRS this usually decline over years and may even get worse than baseline in subset of patients who received LVRS. This has been illustrated in the recent long term update of NETT (Fishman et al., 2003; Naunheim et al., 2006) looking at 1,218 patients with the longest follow up period of 5 years looking at SGRQ as a measure of QOL. This study has showed

- Clinically significant improvement in QOL (>8 unit decrease in the SGRQ) occurred in 40%, 32%, 20%, 10%, and 13% of LVRS patients in comparison to the medical group of 9%, 8%, 8%, 4%, and 7% at 1, 2, 3, 4, and 5 years after randomization of all patients

☐ Table 137-6

Major studies reporting health-related quality-of-life assessments after lung volume reduction surgery

Author	Study type	N	N follow-up (mo)	Instruments	Outcomes
Cooper et al. (1995)	Case-controlled	20	6	MRC	Improved
				FF-36	
Brenner et al. (1997)	Case-controlled	145	6	MRC	Improved
Anderson (1999)	Case-controlled	20	12	QOLS	Improved
Moy et al. (1999)	Case-controlled	19	6	SF-36	Improved
Hamacher et al. (2002)	Case-controlled	39	24	MRC	Improved
				SF-36	
Appleton et al. (2003)	Case-controlled	29	51	MRC	Improved
Ciccone et al. (2003)	Case-controlled	250	52	MRC	Improved
				SF-36	Improved
Lofdahl et al. (2000)	Randomized	28	12	SGRQ	Improved
Pompeo et al. (2003)	Randomized	60	6	MRC	Improved
Geddes et al. (2000)	Randomized	48	12	SF-36	Improved
Goldstein et al. (2003)	Randomized	55	12	CRDQ	Improved
NETT (Fishman et al., 2003; Naunheim et al., 2006)	Randomized	1218	60	CRDQ	Improved
				SGRQ	Improved
				QWB	Improved
Hillerdal et al. (2005)	Randomized	106	12	SGRQ	Improved
				SF-36	Improved
Miller et al. (2006)	Randomized	62	24	CRDQ	Improved
				SF-36	Improved
				HUI	Improved

CRQ Chronic Respiratory Disease Questionnaire; *MRC* Modified Medical Research Council Dyspnea Index; *HUI* Health utility index; *NETT* National Emphysemia Treatment Trial Research Group; *SF-36* Medical Outcomes Study Short-Form Health Survey; *SGQR* St. George's Respiratory Questionnaire; *SF-36* Medical Outcomes Study Short-Form Health Survey; *QWB*: Quality of Well-Being Questionnaire

(p < 0.001, years 1–3; p < 0.005, year 4). Patients who had Upper-lobe-predominant and low baseline exercise capacity were the most to benefit from this procedure, on the other hand, this benefit was not obvious in high risk patients (FEV1 < 20% and carbon monoxide diffusion capacity (DLCO) <20 and homogeneous emphysema on computed tomography).

• The mean changes from the post rehabilitation baseline in SGRQ among enrollees in both the medical and LVRS cohorts was quite variables. On average for the whole patients, LVRS patients experienced initial improvement in SGRQ where medical patients deteriorated and fell below their baseline values. Despite that the mean changes from baseline favored survivors in the LVRS group throughout the duration of follow-up but this was deteriorating over time for both cohorts falling below the baseline for high risk group whom they received LVRS.

As this landmark study illustrated, patient's QOL in general improve early post operatively but unfortunately deteriorate gradually over years. It is obvious that low risk patients have a better QOL than medical cohort and the majority of survivors will have a better QOL in comparison to their baseline over 5 years periods which justify the benefit of surgery in this cohort of patients. On the other hand the majority of high risk patients and patients with non upper lobe predominant disease survivors will have worse than their baseline SGRQ score by third year post operatively though still doing better than the medical cohort, this may not justify doing the procedure in this set of patients using QOL as a sole reason especially in the absence of survival benefit.

From a different angle, our group has studied the effect of LVRS looking primarily at quality adjusted life years (QALYs) using HUI (see above) (Miller et al., 2006). The HUI difference between intervention arms over the 2 years of the study is expressed in quality-adjusted life years (QALYs) gained.

- The LVRS patients were found to have 0.21 more QOL than best medical group patients over a 2-year time horizon.
- The difference between the groups at 2 years in all four domains of the CRDQ achieved statistical significance and MICD.
- Eight of 10 domains of the SF-36 achieved the ❷ MCID at 2 years, but only one achieved statistical significance.

Giving above data, LVRS will offer a transient improvement of QOL but as time progress the benefits start to decrease attributed to the chronic progressive nature of the disease, this decline is noticed earlier and faster (quicker worsening of QOL) in high risk patients (see above) and patients with good baseline exercise capacity and lower lobes predominant disease in comparison to patients with upper lobes predominance and poor baseline exercise capacity which may justify the conduct of this procedure in this set of patients.

6   Financial Impact of Medical and Surgical Intervention in COPD Patients

Patients with COPD have chronic progressive diseases, limited therapeutic options have been proved to only slow the progression of the disease rather than reverse or at most arrest its progression. As this disease progress it affects patient's life in variety of aspects including clinical deterioration, as this happen patients continue to seek medical attention for long period as the disease progress. Both medical and surgical options for these patients are coasty and need a long term follow up which increase the burden on the health system. In absence of survival benefits of the treatment options and due to the chronic nature of the disease, solutions that would alter patient's quality of life and decrease the coast will be at most important.

Few studies have looked at the cost effectiveness of surgical treatment versus medical treatment in patients with COPD.

- Our group has looked at the incremental cost-effectiveness of LVRS compared with best medical therapy alone over a 2-year time horizon (Miller et al., 2006), this was defined as the ratio of the difference between treatment groups in mean costs to the difference in quality-adjusted life years (cost per QALY, ICER, see above) using HUI as a measure. Dividing the incremental mean cost of LVRS patients ($28,119) by their incremental QALYS (0.21) results in an incremental cost-effectiveness ratio of $133,900 per QALY gained for patients treated with LVRS. (N.B: Lung transplantation costs $137,000–294,000 per QALY gained).

- A recent follow up of the coast effectiveness of LVRS over medical treatment of NETT study using QWB as a utility measure (Ramsey et al., 2007) confirmed a cost difference of $140,000 per QALY gained in patients treated with LVRS at 5 years. In subgroup analysis, the cost-effectiveness of LVRS in patients with upper-lobe emphysema and low exercise capacity was $77,000 per QALY gained at 5 years. This difference was attributed mainly to the higher QALY rather than a lower coast in comparison to the high risk patients.

As a result LVRS is relatively poor cost-effectiveness overall though in a sub group of patients with upper-lobe, low exercise capacity, it appears that rates of cost-effectiveness might be considered a good value for the level of expenditure required. Giving that, Cost/QALYs should not be used in isolation and many other factors should be considered in treatment decision making in COPD patients.

Summary Points

- Medical and surgical treatments of COPD patients have failed to reverse or arrest the progression of the disease and improve survival. This made any intervention that will improve the QOL of these patients of at most important.
- QOL is an individual's satisfaction or happiness with his/her life that can be objectively measured by several QOL tool (questionnaires) that include different domains of life, these tools can be general or specific to certain disease as their domains change.
- The effect of any intervention in BOTH improving QOL and number lived years (QALYs) can be measured by health utility tools.
- The decision to choose any medical intervention by health agencies depend on BOTH its effect (QALYs) and cost of each intervention (cost/QALYs). The best intervention is the one that cost less for better QALYs gained.
- Registry data can be used to compare the effect (cost/QALYs) of different interventions. These data can help in allocation of financial resources to the neediest interventions in that community.
- Bronchodilators and ICS inhalation therapy improve QOL especially if they combined together.
- Community pulmonary rehabilitation improve QOL.
- LTOT may improve QOL and that will be more observed as technology advances to provided smaller containers at lower cost.
- LVRS is a palliative procedure that has not clearly showed improvement in survival in COPD patients but it did improve QOL in comparison to medically treated patients at higher coast.
- Although LVRS improve QOL, this is unfortunately a temporary effect and QOL continue to decline over time up to baseline or even worse giving the progressive nature of this disease.

- LVRS is poor cost effective intervention, especially in certain set of patients though the decision to proceed with this intervention should not be based solely on this fact since this procedure may prove cost effective as longer follow up results come out.

References

Aaron S, Vandemheen M, Fergusson D, Maltais F, Bourbeau J, Goldstein R, Balter M, O'Donnell D, McIvor A, Sharma S, Bishop G, Anthony J, Cowie R, Field S, Hirsch A, Hernandez P, Rivington R, Road J, Hoffstein V, Hodder R, Marciniuk D, McCormack D, Fox G, Cox G, Prins H, Ford G, Bleskie D, Doucette S, Mayers I, Chapman K, Zamel N, FitzGerald M. (2007). Ann Intern Med. 146: 545–555.

Anderson KL. (1999). Am J Crit Care. 8: 389–396.

Appleton S, Adams R, Porter S, Peacock M, Ruffin R. (2003). Chest. 123: 1838–1846.

Appleton S, Poole P, Smith B, Veale A, Lasserson TJ, Chan MM, Cates CJ. (2006). Cochrane Database Syst Rev. Issue 3. Art. No: CD001104.

Bergner M, Bobbitt RA, Carter WB. (1981). Med Care. 19: 787–805.

Bergner M, Bobbitt RA, Pollard WE. (1976). Med Care. 14: 57–67.

Brenner M, McKenna RJ, Gelb AF. (1997). Chest. 112: 916–923.

Brusasco V, Hodder R, Miravitlles M. (2003). Thorax. 58: 399–404.

Burge PS, Calverley PM, Jones PW. (2000). BMJ. 320: 1297–1303.

Cambach W, Wagenaar RC, Koelman TW. (1999). Arch Phys Med Rehabil. 80: 103–111.

Ciccone AM, Meyers BF, Guthrie TJ. (2003). J Thorac Cardiovasc Surg 125: 513–525.

Cooper JD, Trulock EP, Triantafillou AN. (1995). J Thorac Cardiovasc Surg. 109: 106–116.

Dahl R, Grerst LA, Nowak D. (2001). Am J Respir Crit Care Med. 164: 778–784.

Domingo-Salvany A, Lamarca R, Ferrer M. (2002). Am J Respir Crit Care. Med 166: 680–685.

Donohue JF, van Noord JA, Bateman ED. (2002). Chest. 122: 47–55.

Eaton T, Garrett JE, Young P, Fergusson W, Kolbe J, Rudkin S, Whyte K. (2002). Eur Respir J. 20: 306–312.

Fishman A, Martinez F, Naunheim K, Piantadosi S, Wise R, Ries A, Weinmann G, Wood DE. (2003). N Engl J Med. 348: 2059–2073.

Flanagan JC. (1978). Am Psychol. 33: 138–147.

Geddes D, Davies M, Koyama H. (2000). N Engl J Med. 343: 239–245.

Goldstein RS, Todd TRJ, Guyett G. (2003). Thorax. 58: 405–410.

Guyatt GH, Berman LB, Townsend M. (1987). Thorax. 42: 773–778.

Hamacher J, Buchi S, Georgescu CL. (2002). Eur Respir J. 19: 54–60.

Hillerdal G, Lofdahl CG, Strom K, Skoogh BE, Jorfeldt L, Nilsson F. (2005). Chest. 128: 3489–3499.

Hutton J, Brown R, Borowitz M. (1996). Pharmacoeconomics. 9(Suppl 2): 8–22.

Hunt SM, McEwen J, McKenna SP. (1985). J R Coll Gen Pract. 35: 185–188.

Jones PW, Quirk FH, Baveystock CM. (1992). Am Rev Respir Dis. 145: 1321–1327.

Kaplan RM, Ries AL. (2005). J Cardiopulm Rehabil. 25: 321–331.

Lacasse Y, Goldstein R, Lasserson TJ, Martin S. (2006) Cochrane Database Syst Rev. Issue 4. Art. No.: CD003793.

Lareau SC, Carrieri-Kohlman V, Janson-Bjerklie S. (1994). Heart Lung. 23: 242–250.

Lofdahl CG, Hillerdal G, Strom K. (2000). Am J Respir Crit Care Med. 161: A585.

Miller JD, Malthaner RA, Goldsmith CH, Goeree R, Higgins D, Cox PG, Tan L, Road JD. (2006). Ann Thorac Surg 2006 81: 314–321.

Moy ML, Ingenito EP, Mentzer SJ, Evans RB, Reilly JJ Jr. (1999). Chest 115: 383–389.

Na JO, Kim DS, Yoon SH. (2005). Monaldi Arch Chest Dis. 63: 30–36

Nannini L, Cates CJ, Lasserson TJ, Poole P. (2007a). Cochrane Database Syst Rev. Issue 4. Art. No.: CD003794.

Nannini LJ, Cates CJ, Lasserson TJ, Poole P. (2007b). Cochrane Database Syst Rev. Issue 4. Art. No.: CD006826.

Nannini LJ, Cates CJ, Lasserson TJ, Poole P. (2007c). Cochrane Database Syst Rev. Issue 4. Art. No.: CD006829.

Naunheim K, Wood D, Fishman A. (2006). Ann Thorac Surg. 82: 431–443.

Nonoyama ML, Brooks D, Lacasse Y, Guyatt GH, Goldstein RS. (2007). Cochrane Database Syst Rev. Issue 4. Art. No.: CD005372.

O'Donnell DE, Aaron S, Bourbeau J, Hernandez P, Marciniuk D, Balter M, Ford G, Gervais A,

Goldstein R, Hodder R, Maltais F, Road J. (2003). Can Respir J. 10(Suppl): 11A–65A.

Okubadejo AA, Paul EA, Jones PW, Wedzicha JA. (1996). Eur Respir J. 9: 2335–2339.

Pompeo E, Marino M, Notroni I, Matteucci G, Mineo TC. (2003). Ann Thorac Surg. 70: 948–954.

Ramsey S, Shroyer L, Sullivan S, Wood D. (2007). Chest. 131: 823–832.

Tanni SE, Vale SA, Lopes PS, Guiotoko MM, Godoy IL, Godoy IR. (2007). J Bras Pneumol. 33: 161–167.

Testa MA, Simonson DC. (1996). N Engl J Med. 334: 835–840.

Tiong LU, Davies HRHR, Gibson PG, Hensley MJ, Hepworth R, Lasserson TJ, Smith B. (2006). Cochrane Database Syst Rev. Issue 4. Art. No.: CD001001.

Tu S, McDonell M, Spertus J. (1997). Chest. 112: 614–622.

Ware JE Jr, Sherbourne CD. (1992). Med Care. 30: 473–483.

Yang IA, Fong KM, Sim EHA, Black PN, Lasserson TJ. (2007). Cochrane Database Syst Rev. Issue 4. Art. No.: CD002991.

Yusen RD, Morrow LE, Brown KL. (2002). Semin Thorac Cardiovasc Surg. 14: 403–412.

138 Quality of Life After Revascularization and Major Amputation for Lower Extremity Arterial Disease

M. Deneuville

1	Introduction	2354
1.1	HRQOL Tools in LEAD	2355
2	Generic Questionnaires	2355
3	Disease-Specific Instruments	2358
3.1	The Vascular Quality of life Questionnaire (VascuQol)	2359
3.2	Other and Alternative Measures	2360
4	Impact of Revascularization on HRQOL	2360
5	Impact of Revascularization for Intermittent Claudication on HRQOL	2362
6	Impact of Revascularization for Critical Limb Ischemia	2365
7	Impact of Limb Amputation on HRQOL	2370
8	Current limitations/Future Outlook of QOL Assessment of Patients with LEAD	2373
9	Conclusion	2375
	Summary Points	2375
	Appendix	2376

Abstract: Lower extremity arterial disease (❯ LEAD) is not a curable disease and ❯ revascularization procedures have little or no effect on the overall life expectancy. Hence, treatment should be aimed primarily at alleviating symptoms, controlling risk factors and improving health-related quality of life (HRQOL). LEAD is associated with impaired HRQOL not only in physical domains but also in social function, emotional and mental health. LEAD is commonly associated with many risk factors each being capable to deteriorate HRQOL independently.

In contrast to the well-developed body of publications on surgical outcomes, prospective data on patient-oriented outcomes after revascularization are still lacking with a total volume of publications currently below 40.

The available data provide some evidence that successful revascularization immediately improves the HRQOL in patients suffering from ischemic claudication with a lasting benefit on physical functioning for at least 12 months while a trend toward return to baseline values in mental health, emotional and vitality domains is commonly observed. Surprisingly, patients with unsuccessful revascularization with minimal increase in lower limb blood flow still experience some improvement in pain, emotional reactions and family relationships in the first year. In the most severe form of LEAD (critical limb ischemia), an immediate and lasting benefit on HRQOL is seen after successful revascularization although less pronounced than in claudicants. However, despite long-term limb salvage and optimal graft functioning, patients successfully revascularized remain functionally disabled when compared to age-matched subjects, nevertheless they report similar well-being. After major limb amputation, some improvement in HRQOL can be expected through pain relief and the maintenance of mobility either with prosthetic rehabilitation or wheel chair ambulation.

The measurement of HRQOL is clearly needed at baseline and after vascular operations but its future role in the decision making process is yet to be defined.

List of Abbreviations: *ABI,* ❯ ankle brachial index; ❯ *CLI,* critical limb ischemia; *ET,* ❯ endovascular therapy; *HRQOL,* health-related quality of life; ❯ *IC,* intermittent claudication; *LEAD,* lower extremity arterial disease; *OVS,* open vascular surgery; *PTA,* percutaneous transluminal angioplasty; *TASC,* Trans-Atlantic Inter-Society Consensus; *VBG,* venous bypass graft

1   Introduction

Lower extremity arterial disease (LEAD) is a common illness in adults over 50 years. It is currently established that LEAD is likely to indicate an extensive and severe degree of systemic atherosclerosis with a markedly increased risk of coronary and cerebro-vascular acute events. In population studies, the risk of limb amputation is lower than 1–2% in contrast with a high cardiovascular mortality, ranging from 5 to 10%/year (ACC/AHA, 2006; Novgren et al., 2007).

The available data clearly indicates that the general health status and quality of life of patients affected by LEAD are both significantly impaired compared to subjects without LEAD in age-matched general populations in the USA (Gibbons et al., 1995; Holtzman et al., 1999), Germany (Engelhardt et al., 2006), Spain (Hernandez-Osma et al., 2002), UK (Pell, 1995; Basil, 2006) and northern Europe (Klesvgard et al., 2001; Hallin et al., 2002).

Self-perceived limitations in their physical activities truly exist in patients with LEAD when compared with other vascular conditions (aortic aneuvrysm, carotid stenosis) which are generally asymptomatic (Hallin et al., 2002). In addition, LEAD is also associated with substantial impairment in other HRQOL domains including social function, emotional and mental health (Pell, 1995, Khaira et al., 1996; Breek et al., 2002). Many risk factors commonly associated with LEAD are each being capable to deteriorate HRQOL independently (Cherr et al., 2007; Aquarius et al., 2007; Rajagopalan et al., 2006).

Revascularization is mainly indicated in patients complaining of lifestyle limitations in their walking abilities (i.e., intermittent claudication, IC) or in limb-threatening conditions such as critical limb ischemia (CLI) or acute ischemia. However, most studies after revascularization reported little or no effect on survival when compared to the overall life expectancy in LEAD. Therefore, the goals of revascularization should be mainly geared toward relief of symptoms and improvement of HRQOL increasing life expectancy should be reached only with an aggressive medical treatment and life style modifications.

The outcome of vascular surgery is traditionally assessed by means of technical endpoints that include patency, limb salvage and survival rates, all relevant for the surgeons who perform the procedures (Novgren et al., 2007; ACC/AHA, 2006). However, the patient is more interested in answers to basic concerns like improved mobility, maintained or regained ability to engage in family or social activities, relief of pain and preservation of the body wholeness among many aspects of HRQOL.

Surprisingly, patient-oriented measurements were not considered in the assessment of vascular surgery until the early 90's, more than forty years after the first bypass grafting and 25 years after the development of balloon angioplasty.

Clearly, HRQOL measurements have been neglected for too many years and must now be regarded as an important factor in every-day clinical practice (Novgren et al., 2007; ACC/AHA, 2006). However, despite of a significant increase in the volume of publications in the last 10–15 years, there is still a limitation of data. The emerging role of HRQOL measurements in both the decision making for the surgical interventions in LEAD as well as the post interventional outcome is yet to be defined.

This chapter will review and discuss the available data on HRQOL in patients with LEAD eligible for surgical treatment.

1.1 HRQOL Tools in LEAD

Before 1999, few studies were published using many different instruments to measure HRQOL. Interpretation of the available data was limited by the variety of instruments used, the various bias that included small number of patients studied, high rate of nonresponders, survey design and/or inclusion criteria which more likely excluded the most severe patients. Earlier studies used internationally recognized generic questionnaires or instruments adapted from them. Over the last 8 years, such disease-specific tools aimed at HRQOL assessment in LEAD were designed, validated and used in several large prospective studies for evaluating the different degree of severity of LEAD (Chong et al., 2002; Morgan et al., 2001).

2 Generic Questionnaires

❯ The Short Form-36 (SF-36) has been used most widely, and since a large component of this questionnaire measures physical function, this instrument has proved to be more suitable for patients with IC (Wann-Hansson et al., 2004) and has been recommended by the TASC as the preferred generic health outcome measure in lower limb ischemia. However, most studies using the SF-36 have shown that it tends to behave as a functional scale responding best within its physical domain (Currie et al., 1995; Bosch et al., 1999; Deutschmann et al., 2007). The RAND-36 questionnaire is very similar (Bosh et al., 1999).

❯ *Figure 138-1–138-3* compares the average scores reported in the largest studies on IC and CLI by using generic (SF-36 and NHP) and disease-specific (VascuQOL) questionnaires.

❯ The Nottingham Health Profile (NHP) has been the second most frequently used generic tool in LEAD. It has been developed first as a measure of perceived stress relating to potentially disabling conditions. The NHP is a two-part instrument. The first part comprises 38 yes-no items investigating the patient's degree of distress within the domains of physical mobility (8 items), pain (8 items), sleep (5 items), energy (3 items), social isolation (5 items), and emotional reactions (9 items). The answers give a range of possible scores in each domain from zero (no problem at all in the domain) to 100 (all problems present).

The second part consists of seven yes-no statements about the frequency of daily living problems with paid employment, housework, family relationships, social life, sex life, hobbies and holidays. The result is presented as a percentage of affirmative responses. The second part is seldom used in LEAD (Klevsgård et al., 2001) and less appropriated to CLI.

When compared to SF-36 (Klevsgård et al., 2002; Wann-Hansson et al., 2004), the NHP scores were more skewed and less homogenously distributed. However, it seemed more sensitive in detecting within-patients changes after revascularization for both IC and CLI and to better discriminate among levels of ischemia. Those patients have more problems with mobility and pain which are better screened in the NHP domains of bodily pain and social functioning that contain respectively 8 and 5 items while SF-36 contains only 2.

□ Figure 138-1

Short Form-36: comparison of the mean scores (range:0–100) in claudicants (seven pooled studies) versus CLI (five pooled). *PF* physical functioning; *RP* role physical; *BP* bodily pain; *GH* general health; *RE* role emotional; *VI* vitality; *MH* mental health; *SF* social functioning

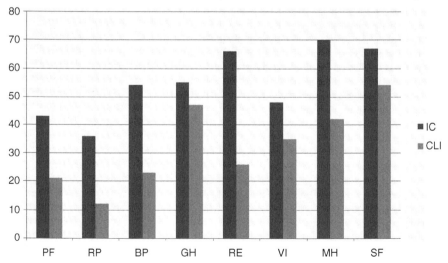

■ Figure 138-2
Nottingham Health Profile: comparison of the mean scores (range:0–100) in claudicants (four pooled studies) versus CLI (five pooled). Phys mob: physical mobility; Emo reac: emotional reaction; Soc isol: social isolation

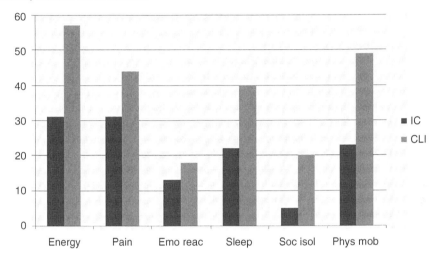

■ Figure 138-3
Vascular Quality of life Questionnaire (VascuQOL): comparison of the mean scores (range:0–7) in claudicants (two pooled studies) versus CLI (two pooled)

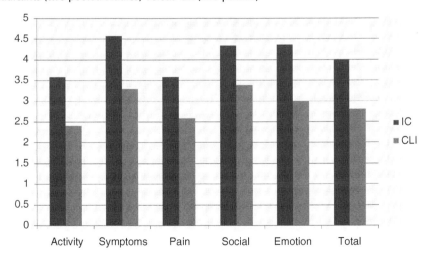

❯ The EuroQOL is administered in two parts. The first part consists of a simple questionnaire of 5 questions regarding mobility, self-care, usual activities, pain/discomfort and anxiety/depression, with each with three possible levels of severity corresponding to "absence of problem" (level 1), some problems" (level 2) and "extreme problems" (level 3). The responses classify the subject into one of 243 different profiles and produce a single numeric index of health status. The EuroQOL also incorporates a visual analogue scale (VAS) on which patients are requested to rate their self-perceived health status on a scale from the worst imaginable (0) to the best (100). The VAS index generated is friendly and easy to read.

EuroQOL was used in two large multicenter randomized studies, the Dutch BOA (Bypass, Oral anticoagulants, or Aspirin) study in the Netherlands (Tangelder et al., 1999) and the Bypass versus angioplasty in severe ischemia of the leg trial performed in UK (Basil, 2005).

❯ The WHOQOL-100 is an instrument from the World Health Organization. It consists of 100 questions with 24 facets in six domains. Dutch investigators from the University of Leiden used an abbreviated version with only three domains: physical health, level of independence and social relationships (Breek et al., 2002; Aquarius et al., 2007).

The ❯ Ql-index Spitzer was developed in Canada and USA to measure HRQOL in patients with cancer. The index includes five dimensions: involvement in own occupation, activities of the daily living, perception of own health support of friends and family and outlook of life. Each domain is scored 0, 1 or 2 with a best possible score of 10. This generic index has been used only in three of the earlier studies of HRQOL in patients with CLI at Sao Paulo, Brazil (Albers et al., 1992).

❯ The Functional status Questionnaire comprises five domains: general health (1 item), activities of the daily living (6 items), social activities (3 items) and mental well being (5 items). This tool was used only in one study (Gibbons et al., 1995) designed to evaluate the functional outcome and the return to well-being after infrainguinal revascularizations.

3   Disease-Specific Instruments

These tools are supposed to be more accurate and responsive to detect changes in the level of the disease severity within patients before and after therapy.

Most of the various attempts made at developing a specific questionnaire for LEAD were in fact limited to HRQOL measurements in patients suffering from IC.

The ❯ Walking Impairment Questionnaire (WIQ) was among the first developed. In a small series of fourteen patients after bypass surgery for IC, the functional improvement measured with the WIQ was not predicted from the routine noninvasive testing (Regensteiner et al., 1993).

This 15-items questionnaire investigates four domains of walking ability: pain, distance, speed and stair climbing. The distance summary score reflects a patient's rating of four degrees of difficulty in walking up to seven distances, ranging from indoor to five blocks. An important limitation is that the WIQ does rely on the patient's estimate of walking distance previously proved to be inaccurate. Similar inaccuracy is likely to affect speed appreciation. In addition, patients may be variously concerned by stair climbing disability.

Therefore, the WIQ is a condition-specific scale which is more able to detect impairment and changes in patients with a relatively preserved level of function, rather than being a HRQOL measure.

Nevertheless, the WIQ is well validated to use in patient with IC and has been used in several studies as an adjunct to generic HRQOL measures (Feinglass et al., 2000).

The ❯ CLAUS-S was initially developed in Germany to investigate pharmacological intervention in claudicants. The original version listed 80 items which required 18 min to score were found unsuitable for clinical practice. A revised version was restricted to

47 items grouped into five domains, including seven specific subgroups, which each generate a score: daily life, pain, social life, disease-specific anxiety and mood. Until 2002, this questionnaire translated in French, Dutch and Flemish had no published validation for its English version.

Recently, the questionnaire was assessed for validity and responsiveness together with two generic (SF-36, EuroQOL) and two other disease-specific instruments in a small prospective study at the Hull Royal Infirmary (Metha et al., 2006). In that study, CLAUS-S failed to fully capture mild (pain domain only) and moderate (pain and everyday life) improvements in QOL of patients treated for IC. In term of responsiveness, the CLAUS-S appeared to be equivalent to the SF-36. The authors concluded that the extra time, effort and resources involved in administering the CLAUS could be questioned. However, this tool was used recently in the Oslo Balloon Angioplasty versus Conservative Treatment Study (Nylaende et al., 2007).

The ❷ Intermittent Claudication Questionnaire (ICQ) was recently developed at the Imperial College of Medicine and University of Oxford to measure HRQOL of patients with claudication. (Chong et al., 2002). It consists of 16 questions exploring limitations due to leg pain during daytime activities (8 items), at work, hobbies, social life and errands (4 items), emotional impact (3 items) and pain severity (1 item). Each question has a 5 point adjectival scale except the latter which has 6.

The instrument produces a single score on a scale from 0 to 100, where 0 is the best possible and 100 is the worst possible health rate. This questionnaire was initially piloted in 20 patients, and then administered to 124 stable claudicants. It was found to be friendly with an average completion time lower than 4 min. Responsiveness of the ICQ was assessed in 60 patients treated conservatively and 40 patients treated with PTA. To our best knowledge, ICQ was not used since the initial report from the promoters (Chong et al., 2002).

The ❷ Sickness Impact profile, IC (SIPic) was derived from the generic questionnaire SIP that assesses sickness related behavior. It is a simple instrument that consists of 12 items. The SIPic score is simply the sum of the total number of the dysfunctional items endorsed, ranging from 0 to 12 (Metha et al., 2006).

3.1   The Vascular Quality of life Questionnaire (VascuQol)

This disease-specific questionnaire was designed at the King College in London (Morgan et al., 2001) to cover the whole spectrum (IC to CLI) of patients with LEAD.

It contains 25 items subdivided into 5 dimensions: pain (4 items), symptoms (4 items), activities (8 items), social (2 items) and emotional (7 items). Each question has a 7-point response option ranging from 1 (worst score possible) to 7 (best score). Each domain is scored 1–7 and a final total score 1–7 is obtained by summing all the items scores divided by 25.

A relevant point regarding self-reported walking distance in this questionnaire was to incorporate a qualitative response to grade the changes in their walking ability instead of absolute measurement of the walking distance which proved to be inaccurate.

The validity and responsiveness of VascuQol were tested twice comparatively with different generic (SF-36, EuroQOL) or disease-specific (CLAUS-S, SIPic) QOL instruments in patients with claudication (De Vries et al., 2005; Mehta et al., 2006). In both studies, VascuQol was proved to be the most responsive and the only tool that could detect both mild and moderate clinical improvement.

The authors recommended the VascuQol as the preferred questionnaire in future trials and clinical follow-up, but, to our best knowledge, VascuQol has been only used in one large prospective multicentre study (Nguyen et al., 2006).

3.2   Other and Alternative Measures

Several researchers, mainly in the earlier period of HRQOL investigations in the field of vascular surgery, designed "home-made tools" to selectively investigate specific conditions like night time pain, foot and toe pain at rest, calf muscle cramping, swelling of legs, unhealed sores or ulcers (Gibbons et al., 1995).

Johnson et al. (1997) had constructed an "environment scoring system" to assess the suitability of the patients' home situation. In the same study, the authors also used different generic or condition-specific instruments to measure pain (visual analogue scale/ Burford thermometer), mobility (graded scale), depression and anxiety (Hospital anxiety and Depression scale), independent activities of daily living/self care (Barthe's score) and lifestyle (Frenchay index).

In addition to the generic questionnaires RAND-36 and EuroQol-5D, Bosh et al. (1999) added several valuational measures like time-tradeoff, Standard-gamble and health rating scale. In the latter, patients were asked to rate their current state of health on a scale from 0 to 100. In the ❷ time-tradeoff, patients were asked how many years they would trade in exchange for full health rather than living a full life expectancy in his/her current health status. In the ❷ standard-gamble, patients were asked what risk of death they would willingly take to improve their current state up to full health.

Alternatively, several authors used a different approach for assessing QOL either because they felt usual questionnaires could be difficult to administrate, nonvalid or inappropriate in specific communities, like Caribbean patients (Deneuville, 2006). The domains of ❷ maintenance of ambulation and ❷ independence in the residential and living status were pragmatically assessed in a real-world belief that these endpoints represent also major concerns for the patients with LEAD seeking surgical care and, therefore, major determinants in their quality of life (Nicoloff et al., 1998; Taylor et al., 2005; Kalbaugh et al., 2006; Deneuville, 2006).

4   Impact of Revascularization on HRQOL

It has been first argued that revascularization provided the best possible chance for rehabilitation and improvement of the quality of life but the scientific proof of these statements remained unavailable many years after the introduction of OVS and ET.

When reporting standards for OVS were originally established, a successful arterial reconstruction was defined as patency of the conduit (permeability rates), increased limb perfusion (ABI) and for CLI, limb salvage. It was assumed that these relevant objectives from a technical/surgeon-oriented point of view would correlate with the unstated ultimate goals which are improvement or maintenance of lower limb function, ambulation and perhaps survival.

Over the years, however, a growing body of evidence indicated that optimal technical results were not always translated to improved function or increased survival.

First, despite significant decrease in post operative morbidity, revascularization procedures are commonly associated with complications perceived as minor from the surgeon's point of view but yet impairing the patient's quality of life.

Decreased sexual ability is commonly an area of concern and dissatisfaction for patients after aortoiliac surgery (Hallin et al., 2002). Infrainguinal VBGs, notably for CLI, are associated with a 11–32% incisional wound complication rate (Novgren et al., 2007; Goshima et al., 2004; Basil, 2005). Healing of ischemic tissue loss occurs in average 15–20 weeks after surgery (Novgren et al., 2007) and requires reoperation in the first 3 months in almost half of the patients (Goshima et al., 2004). Taken together, wound complications and tissue loss may result in a readmission rate up to 50% in the first 3 months, not taking into consideration the pain, discomfort and anxiety experienced for the outpatients during wound management. Another area of concern after infrainguinal VBGs is the surveillance requirement and the subsequent revision of stenosis or failing bypass in 20–40% of cases at 3–5-year follow-up (TASC II). An ideal outcome defined as patent graft without revision, healed wounds and independence in living and ambulation was seen in only 14% of patients (Nicoloff et al., 1998).

Redo surgery (secondary patency) is generally associated with a lesser improvement in HRQOL than in patient with primary surgical success (Tangelder et al., 1999; Klevsgård et al., 2001).

Indeed, the adverse outcomes as observed after OVS are significantly reduced after endovascular procedures. Since its creation in 1964 by Dotter et al., the use of PTA and its later refinements (ET) have increased exponentially in the management of LEAD. The rapid and widespread acceptance of ET in the clinical practice is supported by intuitive and generally accepted advantages. Those include low procedural morbidity and mortality, early technical success exceeding 90% (Novgren et al., 2007) for most lesions, the speed with which the intervention can be performed and the reduced hospital stay. However, higher immediate failure rate (20%) and redo at 12 months (27%) are commonly reported (Chetter et al., 1999; Feinglass et al., 2000; BASIL, 2005).

Undertaken in the UK, the BASIL study was a randomized controlled trial to compare the two treatment strategies in CLI. Among 452 selected patients, 228 were assigned to receive a bypass-first and 224 a PTA-first strategy. The primary endpoint was amputation (of the trial limb) free survival. The trial ran for 5.5 years. At the end of follow up, 55% of patients were alive without amputation, 16% had lost the trial limb with 8% subsequently dead following the amputation and 29% of patients died with their intact limb. The authors concluded that the two strategies were associated with broadly similar outcomes in terms of amputation free-survival but, in short-term, surgery was associated with a higher morbidity and was more expensive than PTA. However, after 2 years, the data analysis strongly suggested that surgery provides a significantly reduced risk of future amputation, death or both.

Both strategies improved similarly the HRQOL at 3 months (Euro5D and SF-36 physical component summary scores), a result that was largely sustained during follow-up. A weak but not significant trend toward better HRQOL was seen in the bypass group.

Second, it was found that there is a functional decline in several patients groups with specific morbidities despite successful revascularization. In a large cohort of 841 patients followed in an average of 24 months after revascularization for CLI (endovascular procedures, 35%, open surgery, 62% or both), Taylor et al. reported that the main independent predictors of dismal functional outcome and survival were an impaired ambulatory capacity before surgery and the presence of dementia. Those patients did not only experience a 1.5 to threefold risk of death but also a twofold to threefold risk of ambulatory deterioration and a sixfold risk of losing their independent living when compared to referent controls. Patients with dementia or walking disabilities at presentation had a decreased survival and poor functional results even when compared with the cohort of patients who lost their limb (Taylor et al., 2005). In the same line, Gibbons found that patient's perceptions of good function and well being at baseline were predictive of satisfactory function and well being after revascularization (Gibbons et al., 1995). Klevsgård et al. observed that improvement of HRQOL was associated with the patient's sense of coherence (Klevsgård et al., 2001).

Third, several studies reported counterintuitive improvement of HRQOL after failed OVS (Tangelder et al., 1999) or PTA (Klevsgård et al., 2001).

Finally, functional impairment in patients with LEAD is far from being confined to hemodynamic abnormalities in the lower limb blood flow. With little doubt, lower limb integrity serve as a major governor of the patient's physical ability. Likewise, occlusive disease in other vascular beds, target-organ complications of risk factors and the effect of aging have adverse and cumulative effects on the lower extremity function. Those include hip and knee arthritis, overweight, muscle weakness and hemiparesis, breathlessness, angina pectoris, vertigo or decreased visual acuity.

Previous population-based studies had shown that 29% of people aged over 65 had mobility-related disability and 11% were living in institutions. In a prospective cohort study of 1122 subjects of 71 years or older in age living in the community and without self-reported disability at baseline, 19% had mobility-related disability at 4-year follow-up and 10% disability in activities of daily living (Guralnik et al., 1995). Back, hip or knee joint disease is present in 23–40% of patients with LEAD (Breek et al., 2002; Rucker-Whitaker et al., 2005), a wide majority of whom being retired (Paaske, 1995).

Those figures cannot be ignored in a realistic attempt of improving lower extremity function in patients with LEAD.

5   Impact of Revascularization for Intermittent Claudication on HRQOL

In Western countries, according to large population-based studies, IC affects approximately 5–12% of the population over 55 years. Annual mortality rate in these patients is as high as 5–10%, mainly caused by atherothrombotic events in the coronary and cerebral vascular beds.

Data of the natural course of IC in nonwhite populations are scarce but indicate differences in prevalence, mode of presentation (Rucker-Whitaker et al., 2005) and comorbidities (Deneuville et al., 2008).

The available literature clearly indicate that most of the deterioration of HRQOL perceived by claudicants are attributable to the limitation in the patient's daily routine physical activities, interference with social activities, problems at work and limitations of other activities as a result of impaired physical health (Pell et al., 1995, Khaira et al., 1996; Breek et al., 2002).

Currently, surgery is indicated for individuals with a vocational or lifestyle disability due to IC (ACC/AHA 2006; Novgren et al., 2007).

From the pathophysiological point of view, the restoration of an adequate arterial blood flow in the lower limb during exercise has been regarded for many years as the primary endpoint. Indeed, a considerable amount of surgical reports have repeatedly proven that revascularization for IC does increase arterial blood flow as documented by a significant rise in ABI at rest and after exercise (Currie et al., 1995; De Vries et al., 2005).

Surprisingly, it had been shown that ABI changes correlate poorly with improvement in HRQOL. This finding was consistently present whatever the generic (Currie et al., 1995) or disease specific domains and indices tested (Chong et al., 2002; De Vries et al., 2005; Mehta et al., 2006). In that line, of particular relevance, most studies comparing PTA and OVS for IC indicate similar improvement despite objectively higher increase in ABI -in an average of 0.3–0.4- after OVS (Regensteiner et al., 1993; Currie et al., 1995; Feinglass et al., 2000) while less significant changes 0.1–0.2 following ET (Whyman et al., 1996; Mehta et al., 2006).

By contrast, objective measurement of improved walking ability (ie, treadmill testing or 6-minute walk test) have better correlation with improvement in HRQOL (Regensteiner et al., 1993; Metha et al., 2006). Klevsgård et al. (2001) reported significant improvement in the NHP's dimensions of pain, physical mobility, energy and emotional reactions after successful revascularization in claudicants in whom treadmill walking distance also improved compared to patients without increased walking distance at 12-months follow-up.

This suggests that walking ability is more important for the claudicant that total lower limb blood flow and that reduction in walking ability has a much greater impact than increase in ABI.

There is little doubt that successful revascularization immediately improves the HRQOL in claudicants with a lasting benefit for at least 12 months. This consistent finding is also observed either with a patent graft (Regensteiner et al., 1993; Feinglass et al., 2000; Klevsgård et al., 2001) or PTA (Whyman et al., 1996; Chetter et al., 1999; Bosch et al., 1999; Kalbaugh et al., 2006, Deutschmann et al., 2007; Nylaende et al., 2007).

❯ *Table 138-1* summarizes the results from four randomized controlled trials (Whyman et al., 1996; Bosch et al., 1999; Nylaende et al., 2007; Sabeti et al., 2007), eleven prospective observational studies, three of which being aimed at validation (Chong et al., 2002) or comparaison of HRQOL questionnaires (De Vries et al., 2005; Metha et al., 2006).

A considerable improvement is commonly observed in all dimensions of the NHP (Klevsgård et al., 2001), at least in the physical functioning SF-36 scores (Chetter et al., 1999; Kalbaugh et al., 2006; Deutschmann et al., 2007, Nylaende et al., 2007), all the domains assessed by RAND-36 questionnaire (Bosh et al., 1999), the EuroQOL visual analogue scale (Chetter et al., 1999) and the EuroQoL-5D scores (Bosh et al., 1999; De Vries et al., 2005). Valuational measures (like time trade-off, health utilities index) are also improved (Chetter et al., 1999; Bosh et al., 1999).

Regarding disease-specific questionnaire, all four HRQOL instruments showed a significant improvement compared to the baseline values after revascularization, mainly with PTA. This finding was consistently independent of the tool used, the WIQ (Regensteiner et al., 1993), the Intermittent Claudication Questionnaire (Chong et al., 2002), the CLAU-S (Metha et al., 2006; Nylaende et al., 2007), the SIPic (Metha et al., 2006) and the VascuQol. However, the latter was the most responsive instrument to detect small changes after treatment when compared with the other disease-specific and generic questionnaires (De Vries et al., 2005; Metha et al., 2006).

An additional proof of the benefits from revascularization is the significant deterioration of HRQOL in significant restenosis not followed by a successful re intervention (Deutschmann et al., 2007) and in symptomatic nontreated occlusions (Tangelder et al., 1999; Deutschmann et al., 2007).

The most pronounced effects of PTA can be expected within the immediate postinterventional period (Chetter et al., 1999; Bosch et al., 1999; Kalbaugh et al., 2006; Deutschmann et al., 2007) while a trend toward return to baseline values in several domains is commonly

◼ Table 138-1

Studies investigating the quality of life (QOL) after open vascular surgery (*) and/or endoluminal therapy (§) for intermittent claudication

Main author, year	Study design	Patients	Attrition %	Follow-up (months)	QOL tool	Improvement in QOL
Regensteiner, 1993, Denver, Colorado	PS	14*	0	3	WIQ	Walking distance and speed
Currie, 1995, Bristol, UK	PM	186 (34*, 74§)	8	12	SF-36	Pain, physical function * Versus § same results
Whyman, 1996[a], Edinburgh, UK	RC	62 (30§)	–	6	NHP	Pain only better results after § Versus medical treatment
Chetter, 1999, Leeds, UK	PS	108 §	12	6	SF-36 EuroQOL	All domains except general health, emotional downward trend at 6 m
Bosch, 1999[b], The Netherlands	RC	254 §	6	24	RAND-36 EuroQOL	All dimensions physical domains, pain and EuroQol most sensitive
Feinglass,2000, Chicago, Illinois	PM	526 (60*,40§)	18	19	SF-36 restricted WIQ	Pain, physical function/higher improvement after * Versus §
Klevsgard, 2001, Lund, Sweden	PM	84 (*, § ND)		12	NHP	All domains
Klevsgard, 2002, Lund, Sweden	PS	40 (25* 15§)	–	1	SF36 NHP	Pain, vitality, physical function all domains NHP
Chong, 2002, London, UK	PS	100 (40§)	–	3	ICQ multiple	ICQ most sensitive better results after § Versus medical treatment
De Vries, 2005, The Netherlands	PS	243 (*, § ND)	13	6	multiple	VascuQol most responsive
Metha, 2006, Hull, UK	PS	70	0	6	multiple	All domains VascuQol most responsive
Kalbaugh, 2006, Greenville, S Carol	PS	54§	ND	12	SF-36	Physical function, role physical, pain
Deutschmann, 2007, Graz, Austria	PS	130§	37	12	SF-36	Same results + social function at 6 m

◨ Table 138-1 (continued)

Main author, year	Study design	Patients	Attrition %	Follow-up (months)	QOL tool	Improvement in QOL
Nylande, 2007[c], Oslo, Norway	RC	56 (28§)	ND	24	SF-36 Claus-S	Physical function benefits not sustained at 24 m better results § Versus optimal medical treatment
Sabeti, 2007[d] Vienna, Austria	RC	104§	ND	12	SF-36	ND

[a]Balloon angioplasty vs medical treatment (unsupervised exercise)
[b]Primary vs optional stent implantation in the iliac artery
[c]Balloon angioplasty + OMT vs optimal medical treatment (OMT) alone
[d]Primary vs optional stent implantation in the femoral superficial artery
ND no data; PS Prospective cohort, single centre, RC randomized controlled, PM Prospective cohort, multicenter

observed at follow-up. This was true for SF-36 mental health, emotional and vitality domains at 1-year (Kalbaugh et al., 2006). In the OBACT study, the reduction in pain during activity and pain severity (CLAUS-S) which was seen at 6 and 12 months disappeared after 2 years (Nylaende et al., 2007).

However, for the largest (Bosh et al., 1999) or more recent studies (Nylaende et al., 2007), the positive effects of PTA on physical functioning lasted at least for 2 years.

Surprisingly, patients with unsuccessful revascularization with minimal increase in ABI (Feinglass et al., 2000; Klevsgård et al., 2001) still experienced some improvement in pain, emotional reactions and family relationships in the first year. In the sample of the Dutch BOA study (Tangelder et al., 1999), all eight domains of the SF-36 as well as EuroQOL scores were roughly similar in patients with asymptomatic graft occlusions and in those with patent grafts, with a tendency of lower values in the physical domain in the first group. In selected patients, Klevsgård et al. (2001) reported that 35% of bypass grafts and 28% of PTA performed were unable to increase ABI by more than 0.15. As mentioned by Feinglass et al., poor performances than in published academic series may unfortunately be more representative of results across the broad range of practice.

In studies comparing the effect of revascularization on HRQOL in claudicants vs CLI, claudicants consistently outperformed patients undergoing treatment for CLI in nearly all domains (Kalbaugh et al., 2006; Deutschmann et al., 2007).

These findings provide some evidence that revascularization, especially with ET, could be of benefit in a significant number of claudicants traditionally treated conservatively.

6   Impact of Revascularization for Critical Limb Ischemia

CLI faces the vascular surgeons as one if not the most difficult challenge. CLI is commonly associated with severe multilevel occlusions of the lower limb arteries and an adaptation failure in the microcirculation. As CLI generally occurs in elderly patients, all age-related nonvascular conditions (notably hip or knee arthritis, muscle deconditioning or vertigo) are likely to impair the lower extremity function more severely than in claudicants. Likewise, various clustering of complications from both known risk factors and atherosclerosis in other vascular beds may adversely impact far beyond the ability to walk (❯ Table 138-2).

It is universally accepted that CLI has a profound detrimental effect on HRQOL. A highly consistent finding in the literature is the significantly lower HRQOL scores in patients with CLI vs claudication independently of the instrument used (De Vries et al., 2005; Tangelder et al., 1999; Klevsgård et al., 2001, 2002; Kalbaugh et al., 2006; Deutschmann et al., 2007). ❯ Figures 138-1–138-3 summarize the mean scores from the generic instruments SF-36 and NHP and from the disease-specific questionnaire VascuQOL in pooled samples of patients from various surgical studies of IC and CLI.

From the technical point of view, revascularization in CLI provides fairly good results with 5-year limb salvage rates exceeding 70–75% (Taylor et al., 2006; ACC/AHA, 2006; Novgren et al., 2007). OVS is required more often in CLI due to the multilevel occlusive lesions.

The concept of limb salvage relies on an intuitive expectation of preserving a life-style and a sense of well-being that would be lost with limb amputation. Although mortality after OVS for CLI is currently low (1–2%, TASC, 2007), systemic or neurologic complications after operation are common, up to 10–15% (Gibbons et al., 1995; Tangelder et al., 1999, BASIL, 2005).

Furthermore, the expenditure of effort to attain limb salvage is considerable, notably in patients with tissue loss. A critical period of 15–20 weeks (Novgren et al., 2007; Goshima et al., 2004) with reoperation, re admission due to delayed healing of surgical wounds/tissue loss and/or redo surgery has profound detrimental effects on the mental and emotional health (Tangelder et al., 1999, N'Guyen, 2006).

The late outcomes in patients operated for CLI are disappointing. The 5-year survival rate after revascularization (Taylor et al., 2006; ACC/AHA, 2006) is low (42–50%) with little or no effect of surgery.

Gibbons et al. (1995) reported that less than half (47%) of 156 patients in whom an infrainguinal revascularization had been performed for CLI reported being "back to normal" after 6 months despite optimal technical results of graft patency (93%) and limb salvage (97%).

Similarly, Seabrook et al. (1999) have shown that despite long-term limb salvage and optimal graft functioning, patients successfully revascularized for CLI remained functionally disabled when compared to age-matched subjects without LEAD, nevertheless they reported similar well-being. In that case-control study, 70 patients with VBGs performed for limb salvage (mean ABI of 0.93, normal flow velocities and no evidence of flow disturbances or morphological defects), with a mean follow-up of 45 months were compared with age and gender-matched controls with normal ABI and no history of vascular occlusive disease. Less than half of patients (47%) reported that they had no problems with the revascularized limb and only 27% were able to report that the operated leg was better than the opposite unoperated leg.

Adverse symptoms when ambulating were reported by 38% of the patients and at rest by 36%. Patients had significant decreased in their functional ability to walk for various distances, perform household tasks including those requiring mild energy level and bath. Patients exhibited also significantly less independence in activities of daily living and reported a

◻ Table 138-2

Comparison of patient's demographics in large series of critical limb ischemia versus claudication

	Critical limb ischemia						Claudication		
	Gibbons N = 318	Taylor N = 841	BASIL N = 452	Deneuville N = 501	PREVENT N = 1404	Feinglass N = 526	DeVries N = 348	Chong N = 224	Aquarius N = 200
Age (mean)	66	68	67% >70 year	75	69	69	64	70	63
Sex ratio male/female	1.65	1.31	>70 years	0.84	1.77	4.1	3.48	1.87	2.07
Diabetes %	81	54	42	62	64	16	18	22	16
Smokers (current) %	70 (21)	67 (41)	80 (36)	26 (15)	73 (ND)	28 (ND)	93 (ND)	90 (ND)	66 (ND)
Stroke, %	15	ND	21	14	20	ND	ND	ND	ND
ESRD, %	18	13	ND	12	12	ND	4	ND	4
CHF, %	14	ND	ND	24	ND	47	10	ND	32
CAD, %	41	57	36	18	46		36	ND	ND
Vasc surgery, %	62	36	33		28	ND	–	ND	ND
Amputation, %	5	ND	ND	2	ND	ND	ND	ND	ND
Home independent	ND	96	ND	97	ND	ND	ND	ND	ND
Ambulatory	70	79	ND	84	ND	NA	NA	NA	NA
With assistance	20	17	ND	9	ND	NA	NA	NA	NA
Wheelchair	4	3	ND	4	ND	NA	NA	NA	NA
Bedridden	3	ND	ND	3	ND	NA	NA	NA	NA
Tissue loss, %	74	59	74	72	75	NA	NA	NA	NA

ESRD end stage renal disease; *CAD* coronary arterial disease; *CHF* congestive heart failure; *Amputation* previous major amputation; *Vasc surgery* previous vascular surgery; *ND* no data; *NA* not applicable significant greater need of using cane indoors or walker and wheelchair outdoors. Only 37% of the patients (vs. 67 in controls) left their home as part of their daily life activities which is likely to explain differences in the domains of social functioning, the patient's group were being more limited than controls to visit friends or relatives, attend religious services or other social events.

Despite the presence of persistent symptoms, 91% of patients stated that they were "glad they had the bypass operation" and that "the discomfort and time in the hospital" was worthwhile. Furthermore, there was no significant difference in the general health perception between patients and controls.

All of the studies analyzed except one (Hernandez-Osma et al., 2002) reported significant, immediate and lasting benefit on HRQOL after successful revascularization for CLI (◗ Table 138-3).

PREVENT III is, to our best knowledge, the largest study investigating HRQOL following revascularization in patients with CLI. This multicenter (83 North American sites), double-blind, randomized trial was primarily aimed to evaluate the efficacy (versus placebo) of intraoperative treatment of venous grafts with edifoligide (thought to inhibit venous stenosis due to smooth muscle cell proliferation) to prevent graft failure in patients undergoing infrainguinal VBGs for CLI. The trial was negative for this primary endpoint.

As part of PREVENT III, the effect of infrainguinal VBGs was prospectively assessed by using the VascuQOL in 1404 patients at baseline, 3 and 12 months after surgery. The overall results expand on most findings from earlier studies investigating the changes of HRQOL after OVS for CLI.

The mean VascuQOL scores increased in all five domains, resulting in significant changes from baseline to 3-month follow-up. At 1-year, the improvement observed was maintained with an additional modest benefit (mean increase, 15%).

As expected, patients free from any graft-related events (stenosis >70%, thrombosis, reoperation) experienced the highest increase in HRQOL scores which is in agreement with the results reported after successful revascularization from previous studies (Chetter et al., 1999; Klevsgard et al., 2001; Thorsen et al., 2002; Tangelder et al., 1999).

Despite successful graft revision, patients with graft-related events had lower HRQOL scores at 12 months than patients free from any graft-related events. This finding is in accordance with previous studies (Tangelder et al., 1999; Klevsgard et al., 2001) reporting significant increase in pain and sleep disturbances after redo revascularization while another study showed no impact on HRQOL (Thorsen et al., 2002).

Some improvement from baseline was still seen after failed revascularization, notably in the domain of pain, a finding reported by previous authors (Chetter et al., 1998; Klevsgard et al., 2001), especially in case of aymptomatic occlusion (Tangelder et al., 1999). In PREVENT-III, multivariate analysis showed that diabetes was also related to a reduced gain in HRQOL after 1-year, a finding in accordance with other studies (Holtzman et al., 1999; Engelhardt et al., 2006).

Unfortunately, the robustness of findings from PREVENT III is threatened by the high number of survey nonresponders (48%) who were more likely to be diabetics, nonwhite patients or patients with graft-related events. Amputation had the greatest effect on 12-month nonresponse (88%) precluding any meaningful measurement of the effect of amputation.

Currently, the available literature strongly indicates that revascularization does improve HRQOL in patients suffering CLI, although the magnitude of that improvement is not consistent among studies.

◻ Table 138-3

Studies investigating the quality of life (QOL) after open vascular surgery (*) and/or endoluminal therapy (§) for critical limb ischemia

Main author	Study design	Patients	Attrition %	Follow-up (months)	QOL tools	Improvement in QOL
Albers, 1992, Sao Paulo, Brazil	PS	61 (14*)	21	12	Generic QL-index	Improved, similar after * Versus medical therapy
Thompson, 1995, Leicester, UK	RS	112 (86*)	35	16–18	Self made	Depression, mobility, social functioning no difference between 1st or 2nd patent grafts
Paaske, 1995, Aarhus, Denmark	PS	153*	33	18–36	Self made	Physical mobility only
Gibbons, 1995, Boston, USA	PM	250*	37	6	Generic composite	Daily living, vitality, mental well-being
Johnson, 1997, Sheffield, UK	PS	150 (44*,26§)	27	12	Generic composite	Pain, mobility, self-care, depression (only after*)
Chetter, 1998, Leeds, UK	PS	55*	22	12	Generic SF36	Physical and social functioning, pain, vitality
Seabrook, 1999, Milwaukee, USA	Case-control	70*	–	45	Generic Derived SF-36	Optimal bypass: lower versus controls
Holtzman, 1999, Minneapolis, USA	RS	166 (104*,61§)	–	12–84	Generic SF12, SF36	Lower improvement in diabetics/older patients
Tangelder, 1999, The Netherlands	RC	405*	9	21	Generic EuroQOL SF-36	Highest in patent grafts and asymptomatic occlusion
Tretinyak, 2001, Milwaukee, USA	PS	46*	ND	3	Generic SF36	Physical functioning
Klevsgard, 2001, Lund, Sweden	PS	62 (ND*/§)	14	12	Generic NHP	Pain, sleep, mobility
Hernandez, 2002, Barcelona, Spain	PS	52 (30*)	43	12	Generic SF36	No changes, trend to degradation
Thorsen, 2002, Copenhagen, DK	PS	60*	20	12	Generic NHP	Pain, sleep
Klevsgard, 2002	PS	40 (34* 6§)	–	1	Generic SF36/NHP	Pain, social isolation, physical mobility NHP more responsive

138

□ Table 138-3 (continued)

Main author	Study design	Patients	Attrition %	Follow-up (months)	QOL tools	Improvement in QOL
BASIL trial, 2005, UK	RC	452 (228* 224§)	2	60	EuroQol SF-36	All domains EuroQoL physical and mental component SF-36
Deneuville, 2006, Guadeloupe, FWI	RS	175*	17	42	Self made	Ambulation, daily living, self care > amputees
Kalbaugh, 2006, Greenville, USA	PS	30§	ND	12	SF-36	Pain only
Engelhardt, 2006, Augsburg, Germany	PS	86*	14	6	SF-36	All domains lower in diabetics
PREVENT III, 2006, USA, Canada	RC	1404*	48	12	VascuQOL	All domains lower in diabetics and graft related events
Deutschmann, 2007, Graz, Austria	PS	60§	37	12	SF-36	Physical function, pain (social function at 6 m)

+BOA Dutch Bypass Oral anticoagulants or Aspirin study. Comparison oral anticoagulants versus aspirin in the prevention of infrainguinal bypass grafts occlusion; *BASIL* Bypass versus Angioplasty in Severe ischemia of the Leg. Comparison of infrainguinal bypass grafts versus balloon angioplasty in the treatment of CLI; *PREVENT III* Comparison of edifoligide versus placebo to prevent vein graft failure after infrainguinal bypass grafts in the treatment of CLI

RS retrospective, single centre; *PS* prospective cohort, single centre; *PM* prospective cohort, multicentre; *RC* randomized controlled

While most studies identified significant improvement in the domains of pain, sleep (Thorsen et al., 2002; Kalbaugh et al., 2006), few authors reported a marked benefit in physical functioning (Chetter et al., 1998; Klevsgard et al., 2001; Engelhardt et al., 2006). The increase in mobility remained generally modest and limited to activities not requiring some initiative. (Jonhson et al., 1997; Seabrook et al., 1999). The effect on social functioning (Chetter et al., 1998), anxiety and depression (Jonhson et al., 1997) was variable among studies.

However, there is still no evidence on how HRQOL measurements in everyday practice could modify the current decision making process (see section VI).

7   Impact of Limb Amputation on HRQOL

Several condition-specific instruments have been developed to measure and assess HROL in the prosthetic practice which were recently reviewed (Gallagher and Desmon, 2007).

This section rather focuses on the available data of HRQOL after limb amputation related to LEAD which is known to be predominant in Western countries.

◘ Table 138-4

Studies investigating the quality of life (QOL) after major amputations of the lower limb

Main author	Study design	Patients A1 (A2)	Able to walk %	Follow-up (months)	QOL tools	Changes/baseline
Albers, 1992, Sao Paulo, Brazil	PS	16 (+6)	43	12	Generic QL-index	Unchanged trend: worsening in A2
Pell, 1993, Edinburgh, UK	Case control	149	42	–	NHP	Lesser QoL versus controls driven by mobility
Thompson, 1995, Leicester, UK	RS	17 (+7)	ND	16–18	Self made	Scores A1 = A2
Johnson, 1997, Sheffield, UK	PS	46 (+ND)	ND	12	Generic composite	Improved pain, anxiety unchanged self-care deteriorated life style A2
Chetter, 1998, Leeds, UK	PS	(11)	63	12	Generic SF36	Improved pain, vitality, social function, mental
Holtzman, 1999, Minneapolis,USA	RS	(28)	36	12–84	Generic SF12, SF36	ND
Tangelder, 1999, The Netherlands	RC	36 (+38)	ND	21	EuroQOL SF-36	Deterioration all domains except pain worsening in A2
Deneuville, 2006, PAP, FWI	RS	78 (+35)	34	42	Self made	Deteriorated daily living, mobility Scores A1 = A2
PREVENT III, 2006	RC	(125)	ND	12	VascuQOL	Unconclusive 88% nonresponse

A1 primary amputation, A2 secondary amputation (following failed revascularization)
RS retrospective, single centre; PS prospective cohort, single centre; PM prospective cohort multicentre; RC randomized controlled; ND no data

Prospective data on HRQOL after limb amputations for LEAD are scarce in the literature and reflect a generally poor outcome (❯ *Table 138-4*).

Several studies (Johnson et al., 1997; Chetter et al., 1998; Tangelder et al., 1999) indicate that amputation carries a significant improvement of pain. Chetter et al. reported that amputees had higher SF-36 scores in the psychosocial domains than patients with a patent revascularization. According to the authors, this favorable outcome is mainly explained by pain relief and realization that the problem of life as an amputee can be overcome.

HRQOL studies in dysvascular amputees suggest a strong link between mobility and other physical and nonphysical domains. Among the very first publications in that field, Pell et al. published a large retrospective survey of 149 amputees still alive at a median interval of 38 months after operation. Assessed by using NHP, amputees had significantly the worst scores for all domains compared with age and sex matched controls. After stepwise logistic regression analysis, physical mobility was the only health domain for which the difference between amputees and controls remained independently significant (Pell, 1993). This finding confirms the intuitive statement that impaired mobility account for much of the social isolation and emotional disturbances experienced by amputees.

This finding is relevant because the maintenance of mobility, although best reached after prosthetic rehabilitation can be also obtained through wheel chair ambulation. In addition, dysvacular amputees are characterized by low rates of rehabilitation.

In a recent large retrospective review of 553 amputees, Taylor et al. (Taylor et al., 2005) reported a maintenance of ambulation rate of 51% at 2-year follow-up, which is in accordance with the findings from other modern (Nehler et al., 2003; Holtzman et al., 2004; Deneuville, 2006) or earlier studies (Pell, 1993). Nehler et al. reported that, despite an aggressive rehabilitation program, less than one fourth of patients were able to walk out of their homes at 10 and 17 months, and that many patients ambulated indoors only in a limited fashion with an assistance device (Nehler et al., 2003).

These apparently disappointing results reflect the poor general condition of patients requiring limb amputation performed in the ultimate course of CLI. Thus, as discussed in the previous section, various impairments commonly associated clearly preclude any attempt at rehabilitation.

Yet, unsuccessful prosthetic rehabilitation is not synonym of complete loss of ambulation. In older patients or in whom rehabilitation failed after above knee amputation (60–70%), an independent ambulation indoors may be maintained with assistance devices/ wheelchair and even outside with the use of wheelchair/adapted motor vehicle (Nehler et al., 2003; Taylor et al., 2005). Although no specific data on HRQOL in such sample of patients is currently available, pain relief and maintenance of ambulation probably have a favorable impact. Indeed, the degree of handicap may depend upon environmental adaptation at home and outside – car equipment and urban facilities.

By contrast, younger healthy amputees with below-knee amputation achieve functional results similar to that might be expected after successful revascularization (Chetter et al., 1998; Nehler et al., 2003; Taylor et al., 2005; Deneuville, 2006) and experience fairly good HRQOL.

There is conflicting data about the effect on HRQOL of secondary amputations performed after failed bypass. Several studies reported dramatic impact on HRQOL in all domains except pain (Tangelder et al., 1999) or severe and lasting limitations of physical functioning despite relatively fair rehabilitation rates (Chetter et al., 1998). By contrast, other studies showed little (Albers et al., 1992) or no difference between primary amputees (without revascularization) and those with amputations performed subsequently to a failed bypass (Johnson et al., 1997; Deneuville, 2006).

Intuitively, failed attempts at limb salvage are likely to have detrimental effects during the entire process of major surgery often lasting several weeks. In addition of marked physical decline, this period also result in profound psychological deterioration. Several patients may decline an immediate amputation which will be subsequently required for life-threatening complications. According to Chetter et al. (1998) patients with nonredeemable occluded graft who declined amputation not only return to the dismal HRQOL experienced before operation but also demonstrated further deterioration in psychosociological domains of the SF-36. This is may be expected as they all the effort and pain had been experienced in vain.

This undesirable sequence must certainly be avoided through a more appropriate selection of patients possibly based on pre operative HRQOL measurements.

8   Current limitations/Future Outlook of QOL Assessment of Patients with LEAD

The current data analysis on HRQOL measurements in LEAD identifies several limitations and pitfalls.

First, in most research studies, patients with communication difficulties and nonvascular disease in the lower limbs restricting their walking ability are generally excluded in an effort to increase consistency. The percentage of excluded patients ranged from 7 to 21% (Gibbons et al., 1995; Klevsgard et al., 2002; Thorsen et al., 2002; Hernandez-Osma et al., 2002; De Vries et al., 2005). The improvement of HRQOL reported in those favorable samples of selected patients are likely to be the upper limit expected.

Second, the number of nonresponders which is at least 14–20% of the sample studied (Klevsgard et al., 2002; Thorsen et al., 2002; De Vries et al,, 2005) exceeds 50% in some occasions (Gibbons, 2005; Deutschmann et al., 2007; N'Guyen, 2006). Furthermore, nonresponders are more likely to have surgical complications and to be current smokers (Gibbons, 2005). In the prospective study PREVENT-III, the rate of nonresponders at 12 months was 52%. Therefore, the lack of data acquisition is likely to lessen, if not negate, the improvement in HRQOL which was identified after VGB.

These drawbacks raise the question of the generalization of data of HRQOL studies for all patients considered for surgical treatment of LEAD.

Third, there is clearly a link between LEAD and depressed mood, found in up to 30% of patients. It has been suggested that revascularization could improve depression symptoms (Johnson et al., 1997). By contrast, recent studies identified depression (Cherr et al., 2007) as a factor of adverse outcome after revascularization and distressed personality as an independent predictor of less improvement in HRQOL (Aquarius, 2007). Likewise, Thorsen et al. (2002) found that dissatisfied patients who experienced failed surgery with or without subsequent limb amputation, unhealed tissue loss or diabetic neuropathy had greater distress preoperatively in the domains of emotional reactions, social isolation and energy. The poor perceived HRQOL for those patients could not be only explained by the presence of comorbidities, a finding suggesting that preoperative poor perceived health is an independent predictor of revascularization failure (Thorsen et al., 2002). In the same line, it has been previously shown that the disease severity did not have significant effect on mental health and emotional role (Pell et al., 1995).

Breek et al. found in claudicants that risk factors and comorbidities adversely affect HRQOL in nonphysical components. With more comorbid diseases, patients had lower scores on the facets of overall health, general health, energy, fatigue and showed more dependence on medications and treatment (Breek et al., 2002). These intuitive findings are in accordance with other studies showing additional negative effects of diabetes (Holtzman et al., 1999;

Engelhardt et al., 2006; N'Guyen, 2006) and end stage renal failure (Rajagopalan et al., 2006) on HRQOL in patients with LEAD.

Furthermore, the addition of patient-perceived HRQOL as an outcome measure may influence a trend toward more operations in those patients underscoring their HRQOL and placing unrealistic expectations in surgery. This profile is likely to be found in subjects with behavior counterproductive for long-term outcome (i.e., reluctant to required lifestyle changes like smoking cessation). Feinglass et al. reported that among 277 claudicants patients treated conservatively, 40% were engaged in regular physical exercise while in patients oriented to OVS and PTA, only 15 and 9%, respectively, agreed in such program (Feinglass et al., 2000). The devastating effects of failed revascularization in younger patients with more virulent form of atherosclerosis and forcefully seeking for surgery are well-known outcome in every-day practice. If possible, surgery should be avoided below 50 years (ACC-AHA guidelines 2005).

Therefore, the complex interaction between depressed mood and chronic illness associated with LEAD is an important HRQOL parameter that is needed to be addressed in future studies.

Current data strongly suggest the benefits of including HRQOL as an additional outcome measure in treatment of LEAD.

The first step should clearly be directed toward large data collection on the HRQOL status of patients at baseline and regularly after treatment in prospective studies and in the clinical setting.

Therefore, an international standardization should be recommended. There is some evidence that the Vascular Quality of Life Questionnaire (De Vries et al., 2005; Metha et al., 2006; N'Guyen, 2006) is the best candidate to assess HRQOL in the whole spectrum of LEAD. In selective researchs on the impact of treatment in claudicants, the TASC II (Novgren et al., 2007) recently recommended to use a validated, disease-specific health status questionnaire; or the physical functioning domain of a validated generic health status questionnaire.

The second step should be a direct application of baseline HRQOL measurements in the decision-making process.

For instance, patient-based initial assessment could support a more aggressive approach for claudicants (Feinglass et al., 2000, Taylor et al., 2005). The "conservative" or "best medical" treatment commonly fails because the demand placed on the patient is unaffordable and unrealistic. A new concept in the treatment of vocational or lifestyle limiting IC could be aimed at improving QOL with first-intent endovascular therapy to increase the patient's performance during exercise therapy and training and encourage him/her to enroll more efficiently in smoking cessation programs and lifestyle changes.

Failure to improve HRQOL, patient's awareness and compliance to all therapies during this more favorable period with high benefit/risk balance and focused lesion highly amenable to endovascular therapy should be seen as a missed opportunity.

Regarding the optimal method of assessing interventions in CLI, the role of HRQOL is more questionable. The aim to return healthy individual to their place in the society is unrealistic. Treatment should attempt to maintain the QOL at the premorbid level.

Possibly, HRQOL measurements may help to address a difficult issue is the decision-making; who will be best served by primary amputation and who will cope well with all the demanding process of revascularization.

Further investigations in the field of decision making analysis (Brothers et al., 2007) are also needed to highlight whether HRQOL measurements are equally efficient alone or integrated in such models.

9   Conclusion

Revascularization has positive effects on various domains of HRQOL in patients with severe forms of LEAD. The highest improvement in physical function is obtained in claudicants, an effect lasting for at least two years after successful OVS or PTA, while more limited improvement are generally observed in the domain of pain in patients treated for CLI.

Despite a growing number of publications in the last ten years, prospective data are still lacking in many medical and surgical aspects of HRQoL in patients with LEAD. The measurement of HRQOL is clearly needed at baseline and after OVS and ET but the future role of patient-oriented outcome in the decision making process is yet to be defined.

This critical issue is of particular relevance in the projected progression of LEAD related to type II diabetes mellitus all over the world and graving in most industrialised countries.

Summary Points

- LEAD is associated with impairment not only in physical domains but also social function, emotional and mental health in most generic and disease-specific questionnaires assessing HRQOL.
- LEAD is commonly associated with many risk factors (i.e., diabetes mellitus, metabolic syndrome, obesity, end stage renal failure) each being capable to deteriorate HRQOL independently.
- Successful revascularization immediately improves the HRQOL in claudicants with a lasting benefit on physical functioning for at least 12 months while a trend toward return to baseline values in mental health, emotional and vitality domains is commonly observed.
- Patients with unsuccessful revascularization with minimal increase in lower limb blood flow still experience some improvement in pain, emotional reactions and family relationships in the first year.
- Significant, immediate and lasting benefit on HRQOL is seen after successful revascularization for critical limb ischemia although less pronounced than in claudicants. Despite long-term limb salvage and optimal graft functioning, patients successfully revascularized for CLI remain functionally disabled when compared to age-matched subjects, nevertheless they report similar well-being.
- Younger healthy amputees with successful prosthetic rehabilitation after below-knee amputation experience fairly good HRQOL while acceptable maintenance of HRQOL at the premorbid level is observed in older amputees though pain relief and ambulation with assistance devices.
- Further investigations are needed on the measurement of HRQOL before and after OVS and ET to best define the future role of patient-oriented outcome in the decision making process of vascular surgery in LEAD.

Appendix

Key facts of revascularization for lower extremity arterial disease

Level of disease	Type	Material	Mortality %	Indications	Expected 5-year patency %
Aorto- iliac	BPG[a]	Pro	3.3	Bilateral, Long aortic lesion	85–90
	biAxF	Pro	7		50–76
	ET	Stent	ND	<3 cm stenosis	77
Iliac arteries	ET	Stent	1	Focal stenosis	64–75
	Cxo	Pro	6	Unilateral occlusion	55–92
	AxF	Pro	6		44–79
CFA/ bifurcation	TEA	Patch	0–3	Focal stenosis	50
PFA	TEA	Pro or Ven			
SFA/ AK popliteal	BPG	Ven or Pro	1.3–6	Multiple lesions	66/50
	ET	Stent if failure	0.9	Focal lesion	33–62
BK popliteal	BPG	Ven (GSV)	1.3–6	Multiple lesions	66
	ET		ND	Focal stenosis	
Leg/pedal	BPG	Ven (GSV)	1.3–7	Multisegmental CLI only	74–80
	ET	Subintimal	ND		33–51

BPG bypass graft; *TEA* thromboendarterectomy; *ET*: endovascular therapy
[a]*BPG* aortobifemoral; *biAxF* axillo bifemoral; *AxF* axillofemoral; *Cxo* crossover BPG; *AK* above-knee; *BK* below-knee; *CFA* common femoral, *PFA* profunda femoris, *SFA* superficial femoral artery; *GSV* great saphenous vein, *Pro* prosthesis, *Ven* venous; *CLI* critical limb ischemia, *Nd* no data

References

ACC/AHA 2005 guidelines. (2006). J Am Coll Cardiol. 47: 1239–1312.

Aquarius AE, Denollet J, De Vries J, Hamming JF. (2007). J Vasc Surg. 46: 507–512.

Albers M, Fratezi AC, De Luccia N. (1992). J Vasc Surg. 16: 54–59.

BASIL trial participants. (2005). Lancet. 366: 1925–1934.

Bosch JL, van der Graaf Y, Hunink MGM. (1999). Circulation. 99: 3155–3160.

Breek JC, Hamming JF, De Vries M, van Berge Henegouwen DP, van Heck GL. (1992). J Vasc Surg. 36: 94–99.

Brothers TE, Robinson JG, Elliott BM. (2007). J Vasc Surg. 45: 701–708.

Cherr GS, Wang J, Zimmerman PM, Dosluoglu HH. (2007). J Vasc Surg. 45: 744–750.

Chetter IC, Spark JI, Scott JA, Kent PJ, Berridge DC, Kester RC. (1998). Br J Surg. 85: 951–955.

Chetter IC, Spark JI, Scott JA, Kester RC. (1999). Ann vac Surg. 13: 90–103.

Chong PF, Garratt AM, Golledge J, Greenhalgh RM, Davies AH. (2002). J Vasc Surg. 36: 764–771.

Currie IC, Wilson YG, Bairs RN, Lamont PM. (1995). Eur J Vasc Endovasc Surg. 10: 356–361.

Deneuville M, Perrouillet A. (2006). Ann Vasc Surg. 20: 753–760.

Deneuville M, Pierrot JM, N'Guyen R. (2008). Arch Cardiovasc Dis. 101: 23–29.

Deutschmann HA, Schoellnast H, Temmel W, Deutschmann M, Schwantzer G, Fritz GA, Brodmann M, Hausegger KA. (2007). AJR. 188: 169–175.

De Vries M, Ouwendijk R, Kessels AG, de Haan MW, Flobbe K, Hunink MGM, van Engelshoven JMA, Nelemans JP. (2005). J Vasc Surg. 41: 261–268.

Engelhardt M, Bruijnen H, Scharmer C, Jezdinsky N, Wölfle K. (2006). Eur J Vasc Endovasc Surg. 32: 182–187.

Feinglass J, McCarthy WJ, Slavensky R, Manheim LM, Martin GJ. (2000). J Vasc Surg. 31: 93–103.

Gallagher P, Desmon D. (2007). Prosthet Orthot Int. 31: 167–176.

Goshima KR, Mills JL Sr, Hughes JD. (2004). J Vasc Surg. 39: 330–335.

Guralnik JM, Ferrucci L, Simonsick EM, Salive ME, Wallace RB. (1995). N Engl J Med. 332: 556–561.

Gibbons GW, Burgess AM, Guadagnoli E, Pomposelli FB, Freeman DV, Campbell DR, Miller A, Marcaccio EJ, Nordberg P, LoGerfo FW. (1995). J Vasc Surg. 21: 35–45.

Hallin A, Bergqvist D, Fugl-Meyer K, Holmberg L. (1992). Eur J Vasc Endovasc Surg. 24: 255–263.

Hernandez-Osma E, Cairols MA, Marti X, Barjau E, Riera S. (2002). Eur J Vasc Endovasc Surg. 23: 91–94.

Holtzman J, Cadwell M, Walvatne C, Kane R. (1999). J Vasc Surg. 29: 395–402.

Johnson BF, Singh S, Evans L, Drury R, Datta D, Beard JD. (1997). Eur J Vasc Endovasc Surg. 13: 306–314.

Khaira HS, Hanger R, Shearman CP. (1996). Eur J Vasc Endovasc Surg. 11: 65–69.

Kalbaugh CA, Taylor SP, Blackhurst DW, Dellinger MB, Trent EA, Youkey JR. (2006). J Vasc Surg. 44: 296–303.

Klevsgård R, Risberg BO, Thomsen MB, Hallberg IR. (2001). J Vasc Surg. 33: 114–122.

Klevsgård R, Fröberg BL, Risberg BO, Hallberg IR. (2002). J Vasc Surg. 36: 310–317.

Mehta T, Venkata Subramaniam A, Chetter I, McCollum P. (2006). Eur J Vasc Endovasc Surg. 31: 46–52.

Morgan MBF, Crayford T, Murrin B, Fraser CA. (2001). J Vasc Surg. 33: 679–687.

Nehler MR, Coll JR, Hiatt WR, Regensteiner JG, Schnickel GT, Klenke WA, Strecker PK, Anderson MW, Jones DN, Whitchill TA, Moskowitz. (2003). J Vasc Surg. 38: 7–14.

Nguyen LL, Moneta GL, Conte MS, Bandyk DF, Clowes AW, Seely BL, for prevent III investigators. (2006). J Vasc Surg.44: 977–84.

Nicoloff AD, Taylor LM Jr, McLafferty RB, Moneta GL, Porter JM. (1998). J Vasc Surg. 27: 256–263.

Novgren L, Hiatt WR, Dormandy JA, Nehler MR, Harris KA, Fowkes FGR. (2007). J Vasc Surg. 45Suppl: 5A–65A.

Nylaende M, Abdelnoor M, Stranden E, Morken B, Sandbaek G, Risum O, Jorgensen JJ, Lindahl AK, Arnesen H, Seljeflot I, Kroese AJ. (2007). Eur J Vasc Endovasc Surg. 33: 3–12.

Paaske WP, Laustsen J. (1995). Eur J Vasc Endovasc Surg. 10: 226–230.

Peel JP, Donnan PT, Fowkes GR, Ruckley CV. (1993). Eur J Vasc Surg. 7: 448–451.

Pell JP on the behalf of the Scottish Vascular Audit Group. (1995). Eur J Vasc Endovasc Surg. 9: 469–472.

Rajagopalan S, Dellegrottaglie S, Furniss AL, Gillespie BW, Satayathum S, Lameire N, Saito A, Akiba T, Jadoul M, Ginsberg N, Keen M, Port FK, Mukherjee D, Saran R. (DOPPS) (2006). Circulation.114: 1914–1922.

Regensteiner JG, Hargarten ME, Rutherford RB, Hiatt WR. (1993). Angiology. 44: 1–10.

Rucker-Whitaker C, Greenland P, Liu K, Chan C, Guralnik JM, Criqui MH, Taylor L, Pearce WH, McGrae McDermott M. (2004). J Am Geriatr Soc. 52: 922–930.

Sabeti S, Czerwenka-Wenkstetten A, Dick P, Schlager O, Amighi J, Mlekusch I, Mlekusch W, Loewe C, Cejna M, Lammer J, Minar E, Schillinger M. (2007). J Endovasc Ther. 14: 431–437.

Seabrook GR, Cambria RA, Freischlag JA, Towne JB. (1999). Cardiovasc Surg. 7: 279–286.

Tangelder MJ, McDonnel J, Van Busschbach JJ, Buskens E, Algra A, Lawson JA, Eikelboom BC. (1999). J Vasc Surg. 29: 913–919.

Taylor SM, Kalbaugh CA, Blackhurst DW, Hamontree SE, Cull DL, Messich HS, Robertson RT, Lagan EM 3rd, York JW, Carsten CG 3rd, Snyder BA, Jackson MR, Youkey JR. (2005). J Vasc Surg. 42: 227–235.

Taylor SM, Kalbaugh CA, Blackhurst DW, Cass AL, Trent AE, Langan EMIII, Youkey JR. (2006). J Vasc Surg. 44: 747–756.

Thorsen H, McKenna S, Tennant A, Holstein P. (1992). Eur J Vasc Endovasc Surg. 23: 495–499.

Wann-Hansson C, Hallberg IR, Risberg B, Klevsgård R. (2004). Health Qual Life Outcomes. 17: 2–9.

Whyman MR, Fowkes FG, Kerracher EM, Gillespie IN, Lee AJ, Housley E, Ruckley CV. (1996). Eur J Vasc Endovasc Surg. 12: 167–172.

139 Quality of Life After Laser Surgery for Eye Disorders

K. Pesudovs · D. B. Elliott

1   Introduction 2380

2   Refractive Error 2381

3   Disease Burden of Refractive Error 2382

4   Treatments of Refractive Error 2383

5   Refractive Correction-Related Quality of Life 2383

6   Questionnaire Technology 2384

7   The Quality of Life Impact of Refractive Correction (QIRC) Questionnaire 2385

8   The Refractive Status Vision Profile (RSVP) 2388

9   The National Eye Institute Refractive Quality of Life (NEI-RQL) 2390

10 Other Instruments 2390

11 Comparing Quality of Life Questionnaire for Refractive Surgery Outcomes 2391

    Summary Points 2393

Abstract: Refractive error is common, and when uncorrected is a significant disease burden worldwide with 98 million people visually impaired and five million people blind from refractive error alone. Refractive error can be corrected by spectacles, contact lenses or laser refractive surgery, with the latter becoming an increasingly popular treatment. The outcome of laser refractive surgery is assessed by clinical measures and patient reported outcomes, most importantly quality of life (QOL). A number of questionnaires exist for the measurement of quality of life after refractive surgery but these vary in validity. A refractive error related quality of life instrument should include a breadth of content areas e.g., well being, convenience and concerns, not just functioning or satisfaction. ❷ Rasch analysis has been used in the development of The Quality of Life Impact of Refractive Correction (QIRC) questionnaire which facilitated optimization of question inclusion, unidimensionality and valid linear scoring. The QIRC questionnaire, and others, readily demonstrates the benefits of refractive surgery. However, QIRC is also sensitive to the negative impacts of surgical complications, providing a global assessment of QOL outcome. The Quality of Life Impact of Refractive Correction (QIRC) instrument is demonstrably superior to other instruments in terms of validity and reliability, so is the ideal outcome measure for laser refractive surgery.

List of Abbreviations: *ADVS,* Activities of Daily Vision Scale; *ICF,* International Classification of Functioning, Disability and Health; *LASEK,* Laser assisted sub-epithelial keratectomy; ❷ *LASIK,* Laser in situ keratomileusis; *NEI-RQL,* The National Eye Institute Refractive Quality of Life questionnaire; *PRK,* ❷ Photorefractive keratectomy; *PRO,* Patient reported outcome; *QIRC,* Quality of Life Impact of Refractive Correction questionnaire; *QOL,* Quality of Life; *RK,* Refractive keratectomy; *RSVP,* The Refractive Status Vision Profile; *WHO,* World Health Organization

1   Introduction

Refractive errors of the eye are common, and represent a significant burden in terms of disability arising from uncorrected refractive error and economically in the cost of the correction of refractive error. Refractive errors can be treated with spectacles, contact lenses or refractive surgery. Laser refractive surgery has become a highly refined and successful treatment increasingly performed worldwide. The success of laser refractive surgery is typically assessed using objective clinical measures such as postoperative uncorrected ❷ visual acuity and residual refractive error (Waring, 2000). However, these measures do not necessarily correlate well with patients' postoperative subjective impressions (McGhee et al., 2000). Ultimately, the patient's perspective is an important outcome of refractive surgery and a number of patient-reported outcomes (PROs) have been measured. The most important PRO domain is quality of life (QOL) as this includes all issues that impact a person undergoing laser refractive surgery. Several useful instruments exist including the Quality of Life Impact of Refractive Correction (QIRC) questionnaire (Pesudovs et al., 2004), the Refractive Status Vision Profile (RSVP) (Schein, 2000) and the National Eye Institute Refractive Quality of Life (NEI-RQL) (McDonnell et al., 2003b). These instruments, and other less formal questionnaires, have been used to show the improvement in QOL that occurs with laser refractive surgery, as well as the impact of complications that may arise (Ben-Sira et al., 1997; Garamendi et al., 2005; McDonnell et al., 2003b; McGhee et al., 2000; Schein et al., 2001). In this chapter we outline the important QOL instruments for measuring PRO of laser refractive surgery.

2   Refractive Error

Refractive error or ❷ ametropia is a very common disorder affecting millions of people and causes poor vision, headaches and eyestrain in addition to other less common symptoms. In a normal, emmetropic eye, the power of the refracting surfaces of the eye, the ❷ cornea and ❷ crystalline lens, are perfectly matched to the axial length of the eye so that light from a distant object is focussed onto the ❷ retina, the light sensitive lining of the eye, performing a function analogous to camera film (❷ *Figure 139-1*). Ametropia is caused by a mismatch of the refractive power of the eye and its axial length (❷ *Figure 139-2*). If the cornea and lens are too powerful and/or the eye is too long, then light from an object in the distance will be focused in front of the retina and distance vision will be blurred, although vision of close-up objects will be fine. This type of ametropia is called ❷ myopia or short or near sightedness. If the cornea and lens are too weak and/or the eye is too short, then light from an object in the distance will be focussed behind the retina. This type of ametropia is called ❷ hyperopia or long sighted-ness. Since the eye can increase its refracting power by adjusting the shape of the lens (this is called ❷ accommodation and describes how the eye is able to focus on near objects) the hyperopic eye tries to focus, the power of the lens and eye increases and the distant image can be made clear. The problem then becomes that there is less focusing power to bring close objects into focus as some of the focusing power has been used to see in the distance. Distance vision is typically fine, but near vision can be blurred. An individual with a lot of focusing

◨ Figure 139-1
The human eye shown in cross-section (courtesy of Dr. Karen Hampson). The human eye as though cut in half from front (cornea) to back, with the important structures named. The only parts of the eye that are visible are the white sclera surrounding the colored part of the eye, the iris. The iris has a central hole that allows light through, the pupil. The cornea and lens are transparent

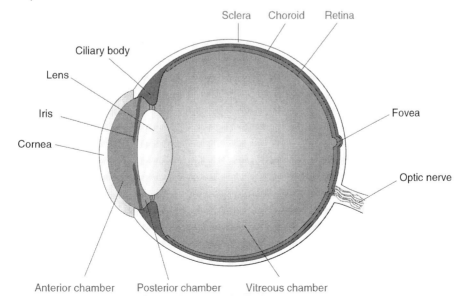

■ Figure 139-2

Refractive error as illustrated by the focus of parallel rays of light arising at infinity (courtesy of Dr. Karen Hampson). The focus of light from a far away object is shown to focus on the retina at the back of the eye in emmetropia, in front of the retina in myopia (short sightedness), and behind the retina in hyperopia (long sightedness)

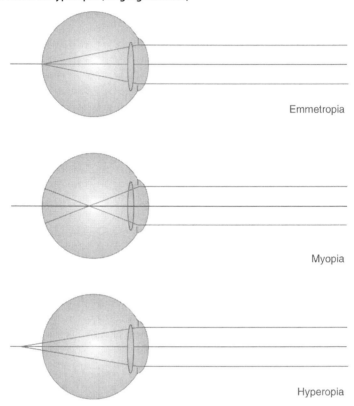

Emmetropia

Myopia

Hyperopia

power would be able to cope with a slight amount of hyperopia. Other people suffer from headaches due to exerting focusing effort for long periods. Unfortunately as we age, our focusing power decreases until we have relatively little at the age of 40–45 and none left at the age of about 55–60 (Charman, 1989), so that hyperopia becomes increasingly common after 40.

3   Disease Burden of Refractive Error

Estimates of the number of people worldwide with refractive error range from about 800 million to 2.3 billion. The accuracy of estimates is hampered by variation across gender and ethnicity and variation with the type of refractive error. Data from 29,281 people in the US, western Europe and Australia over 40 years of age showed a prevalence for hyperopia (3 ❷ diopters or greater) of 9.9%, 11.6%, and 5.8%, respectively, and for myopia (1 diopter or more) 25.4%, 26.6%, and 16.4% for these population samples (Kempen et al., 2004). Amongst Chinese in Singapore, the prevalence of myopia is twice as high (Wong et al., 2000), although in less developed Asian populations the prevalence of myopia is less than in Western populations (Wong et al., 2003). While refractive error is clearly a common problem, corrected refractive error really has only economic burden. However, uncorrected refractive error is a significant public health problem.

Worldwide, 259 million people are estimated to have ❷ visual impairment, and 42 million are estimated to be blind (Dandona and Dandona, 2006). Uncorrected refractive error is estimated to be responsible for 98 million cases of visual impairment and five million cases of blindness. Although Vision 2020 (the current WHO global initiative) imposes a mandate to correct refractive errors, little infrastructure and few resources are available to accomplish the task of correcting refractive errors. Access to general medical services is possible for about 25% of populations in developing countries, access to medical eye care, including refraction, could be obtained by only about 10%. It is likely that visual impairment and blindness due to uncorrected refractive error will remain a global public health problem.

In the developed world, uncorrected refractive error is also a burden. The economic burden of uncorrected refractive error is of the order of several billon dollars in the USA alone (Rein et al., 2006). However, the economic burden of correcting refractive error in the USA amounts to $5.5 billion per year in direct costs (Rein et al., 2006).

4   Treatments of Refractive Error

There are three main methods for the correction of refractive error; spectacles, contact lenses and refractive surgery. Spectacles dominate the refractive error correction market, in the USA approximately 12% of the adult population wears contact lenses and 6.1 million (2.2%) have had refractive surgery, including 1.2 million (~0.4%) in 2002 (Vision Watch, 2003). There are several different types of refractive surgery; incisional procedures such as radial keratotomy (RK) are now obsolete with excimer laser based procedures being the industry standard. Laser in Situ Keratomileusis (LASIK) is the most widely performed refractive surgery procedure in the USA today. Indeed, LASIK dominates the refractive surgery market with all other procedures way behind in terms of volume (Vision Watch, 2003). Photorefractive keratectomy (PRK), which has various synonyms (e.g., LASEK, epi-LASIK, surface ablation), is also a prevalent treatment. PRK and LASIK are fundamentally the same treatment, however, PRK us performed at the surface of the cornea (with only the epithelial cells removed) whereas LASIK is performed within the stroma of the cornea after a thin flap of tissue has been cut and rolled back. In both treatments, the shape of the cornea is altered to change its refractive power such that the ametropia is eliminated. Myopia is more commonly treated with laser refractive surgery than hyperopia, especially with PRK. However, treatment for hyperopia is performed at lower levels of refractive error and with LASIK.

5   Refractive Correction-Related Quality of Life

Quality of life (QOL) is a PRO in which all impacts on a person's enjoyment of life, ability to function, well being and all other life potentials are assessed. In Medicine, QOL is specifically modified to mean – health-related quality of life. That is, the measurement of health-related impacts on all aspects of life. For refractive surgery, the definition can be narrower still, in that the PRO need only tap all aspects of life impacted by the correction of refractive error. Many instruments (questionnaires are commonly called instruments in the QOL literature) purport to measure quality of life, but only measure a few dimensions; often vision-related activity limitation only (visual functioning or ❷ visual disability would be more appropriately called vision-related activity limitation to be in line with the World Health Organization (WHO) International Classification of Functioning, Disability and Health (ICF) (World Health Organization, 2001)). However, QOL has many other dimensions e.g., emotional, spiritual, vocational, economical attributes etc. So to purport to measure QOL but to only or principally measure activity limitation means that any inferences one may draw about QOL impacts will be incorrect unless they are confined to activity limitation only. This problem is called construct under representation (Downing and Haladyna, 2004), and is common in vision-related instruments including the popular National Eye Institute Visual Functioning Questionnaire (La Grow, 2007). So the name of an instrument is clearly very important in defining the concept that the instrument purports to measure. The title of the Visual Function Index 14 instrument and the research paper that introduced it quite clearly indicates that it measures activity limitation and does not claim to measure quality of life but it has often been misinterpreted as assessing QOL (Steinberg et al., 1994; Uusitalo et al., 1999; Valderas et al., 2004). For refractive surgery PROs, several QOL instruments do exist, and in the best examples they tap multiple domains of QOL including visual functioning, symptoms, convenience, health concerns, economic concerns and well being (Pesudovs et al., 2004).

6   Questionnaire Technology

Just as LASIK has improved continuously over 10 years due to improved technology, so too has the field of patient-reported measurement improved. Important improvements have occurred in the use of statistical methods for improving the validity and scoring of questionnaires. Considerations in selecting a QOL instrument should include its reliability and validity. Two of the major refractive surgery QOL instruments, the Refractive Status Vision Profile (RSVP) (Schein, 2000, Schein et al., 2001; Vitale et al., 1997, 2000) and National Eye Institute Refractive Quality of Life (NEI-RQL) (Berry et al., 2003; Hays et al., 2003; McDonnell et al., 2003a, 2003b) instruments use traditional Likert scoring (Likert, 1932) where patients' response scores for a selected set of items are summed to derive the overall score. Likert or summary scoring is based on the hypotheses that all questions (often called items in the QOL literature), have equal importance and equivalent response categories for each question have equal value, so that there are uniform increments from category to category for every question. For example, in a summary scaled visual activity limitation instrument, the Activities of Daily Vision Scale (ADVS), the response category of "a little difficulty" scores four, "extreme difficulty" is twice as bad and scores two, and "unable to perform the activity due to vision" is again twice as bad with a score of one. In cases where the items in an instrument do not have equal importance, the logic of averaging scores across all items becomes questionable. The ADVS ascribes the same response scale to a range of different items, such that "a little difficulty" "driving at night" receives the same numerical score as "a little difficulty" "driving during the day," despite the former being by far the more difficult and complex task. This rationale of "one size fits all" is flawed in this case, and Rasch analysis has been used to confirm that differently calibrated response categories can help to provide a valid and contextual scale that truly represents QOL (Pesudovs et al., 2003).

By resolving inequities in a scale arising from differential item difficulty, Rasch analysis provides a self-evident benefit in terms of accuracy of scoring. This process also removes noise from the measurement which in turn improves sensitivity to change and correlations with other variables (Garamendi et al., 2006; Norquist et al., 2004). For example, the standard scoring of the Refractive Status and Vision Profile (RSVP) failed to show any difference in QOL between a group of spectacle and contact lenses wearers in optometric practice and a group of spectacle and contact lenses wearers about to undergo refractive surgery. When Rasch analysis was used to differentially calibrate each item, significant differences between the groups were found, with the pre-refractive surgery group having a lower self-reported QOL than the control group, as might be expected (Garamendi et al., 2006). This occurs through the reduction of noise in the original measurement which chiefly arises from considering all items to be of the same value. Note that conventionally developed instruments can also be re-engineered using Rasch analysis (Garamendi et al., 2006; Massof and Fletcher, 2001; Pesudovs et al., 2003) and it is possible to use the Rasch calibrations from these studies to convert summary scaled data from these instruments (Lamoureux et al., 2006; Massof, 2005, 2007). However, this is second best to developing an instrument using Rasch analysis as this technique also gives unparalleled insight into the dimensionality of a questionnaire, so informs the content that should be included in the questionnaire.

The importance of Rasch analysis in the development and scoring of questionnaires has been recognized in standards proposed for the assessment of questionnaire quality (de Boer et al., 2004; Pesudovs et al., 2007; Terwee et al., 2007). Clearly, a Rasch-scaled questionnaire should be used wherever possible for the measurement of outcomes. Indeed, calls have been made for this to be the case when assessing refractive surgery outcomes (Weisinger, 2006). There is one Rasch scaled, highly validated instrument developed for measuring quality of life impact of refractive surgery: the Quality of Life Impact of Refractive Correction (QIRC) questionnaire (Pesudovs et al., 2004).

7 The Quality of Life Impact of Refractive Correction (QIRC) Questionnaire

This instrument was developed for the assessing the quality of life impacts of spectacles, contact lenses and refractive surgery (Pesudovs et al., 2004). Visual function, symptoms, convenience, cost, health concerns and well being are included in the content of this instrument which was rigorously developed using literature review, expert opinion, and focus groups. Content was determined using a pilot questionnaire with Rasch analysis for item reduction. A 90-item pilot instrument was implemented on over 300 participants across the United Kingdom. Analysis of these data led to the final 20 item questionnaire (❷ *Table 139-1*). QIRC has been ratified as a valid and reliable measure of refractive correction-related QOL by both Rasch analysis and standard psychometric techniques (Pesudovs et al., 2004). QIRC scores are reported on a 0–100 scale which is free of floor and ceiling effects with a higher score representing better QOL and the average score being close to 50 units (❷ *Figure 139-3*). The difficulty of the items is well matched to the ability of persons, so QIRC is well targeted to the patients. QIRC has been shown to be responsive to LASIK surgery, demonstrating significant improvements in QOL overall from a mean $\pm$ SD of 40.07 $\pm$ 4.30 to 53.09 $\pm$ 5.25 (Garamendi et al., 2005). Individual item analysis showed 15 of the 20 items demonstrated statistically significant improvement. Patients reported improved QOL on all five convenience items, both

◻ Table 139-1

The 20 items of QIRC

Item description
1	How much difficulty do you have driving in glare conditions?
2	During the past month, how often have you experienced your eyes feeling tired or strained?
3	How much trouble is not being able to use off-the-shelf (non prescription) sunglasses?
4	How much trouble is having to think about your spectacles or contact lenses or your eyes after refractive surgery before doing things; e.g., traveling, sport, going swimming?
5	How much trouble is not being able to see when you wake up; e.g., to go to the bathroom, look after a baby, see alarm clock?
6	How much trouble is not being able to see when you are on the beach or swimming in the sea or pool, because you do these activities without spectacles or contact lenses?
7	How much trouble is your spectacles or contact lenses when you wear them when using a gym/doing keep-fit classes/circuit training etc?
8	How concerned are you about the initial and ongoing cost to buy your current spectacles/contact lenses/refractive surgery?
9	How concerned are you about the cost of unscheduled maintenance of your spectacles/contact lenses/refractive surgery; e.g., breakage, loss, new eye problems?
10	How concerned are you about having to increasingly rely on your spectacles or contact lenses since you started to wear them?
11	How concerned are you about your vision not being as good as it could be?
12	How concerned are you about medical complications from your choice of optical correction (spectacles, contact lenses and/or refractive surgery)?
13	How concerned are you about eye protection from ultraviolet (UV) radiation?
14	During the past month, how much of the time have you felt that you have looked your best?
15	During the past month, how much of the time have you felt that you think others see you the way you would like them to (e.g., intelligent, sophisticated, successful, cool, etc)?
16	During the past month, how much of the time have you felt complimented/flattered?
17	During the past month, how much of the time have you felt confident?
18	During the past month, how much of the time have you felt happy?
19	During the past month, how much of the time have you felt able to do the things you want to do?
20	During the past month, how much of the time have you felt eager to try new things?

The 20 questions identified as the most useful to characterize aspects of quality of life influenced by refractive correction and used in the QIRC questionnaire. *QIRC* Quality of Life Impact of Refractive Correction
Reproduced from Complications in Refractive Surgery, 2008, Influence of refractive surgery complications in quality of life, Pesudovs K, *Table 139-1* with kind permission of Springer Science and Business Media

economic items, all four health concern items and on 4 of the 7 items in the well being domain (❯ *Figure 139-4*). QIRC is also sensitive to decreased QOL caused by complications of LASIK (Garamendi et al., 2005; Pesudovs et al., 2006). The major complications of LASIK include residual refractive error which can mean that the patient still needs to wear spectacles or

◻ **Figure 139-3**

Person/item map for the QIRC questionnaire. The figure plots the mean score for each item or question from the QIRC questionnaire on the right hand side against subjects on the left represented by # (# = 3 subjects). A higher score indicates a better QOL. The distribution of items is well matched to the distribution of persons (*M* mean; *S*1 standard deviation; *T* two standard deviations) and this question group exhibits excellent targeting of items to subjects. *QOL* Quality Of Life; *QIRC* Quality of life Impact of Refractive Correction questionnaire

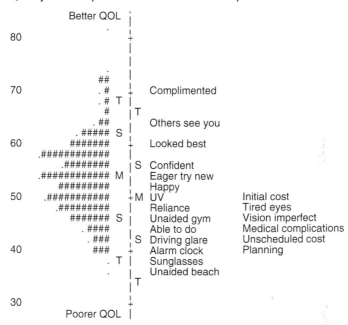

contact lenses after the surgery and chronic dry eye giving a gritty sensation that often requires regular eye drops to be administered and these lead to reduced quality of life. However, minor complications, like night vision disturbances, may not negatively impact QOL.

The QIRC questionnaire effectively differentiates between spectacle wearers, contact lens wearers and post-refractive surgery patients – with the refractive surgery group showing superior QOL (50.23 ± 6.31) than contact lens wearers (46.70 ± 5.49, $p < 0.01$) and spectacle wearers (44.13 ± 5.86, $p < 0.001$) (Pesudovs et al., 2006). There were significant differences between scores on 16 of the 20 questions; of the remaining four questions two health concerns and two well being questions did not detect differences between groups (❯ *Figure 139-5*). Our study also showed that those spectacle wearers with medium or high refractive error had worse QOL than those with low refractive error. We presume that this is partly due to the nature of spectacles for larger degrees of myopia and hyperopia and also due to the fact that these spectacles would have to be worn full-time as without them the person would have very poor vision. High powered spectacles are relatively heavy with thicker edges (myopic spectacles) or centers (hyperopic spectacles) and either greatly magnify (hyperopic spectacles) or minify (myopic spectacles) the patient's eyes behind their spectacles. In addition, these spectacles can affect QOL in terms of concerns over cost if patients attempt to improve the appearance and

◼ Figure 139-4

QIRC scores before and after LASIK surgery (Reproduced from Complications in Refractive Surgery, 2008, Influence of refractive surgery complications in quality of life, Pesudovs K, ❯ *Figure 139-1* with kind permission of Springer Science and Business Media). Mean ± 1SD scores for each question from the QIRC questionnaire for 66 people with myopia (short-sightedness) before and 3 months after refractive surgery by LASIK. A higher score after surgery indicates an improvement in quality of life related to refractive correction. *QIRC* Quality of life Impact of Refractive Correction questionnaire, LASIK – Laser in situ keratomileusis

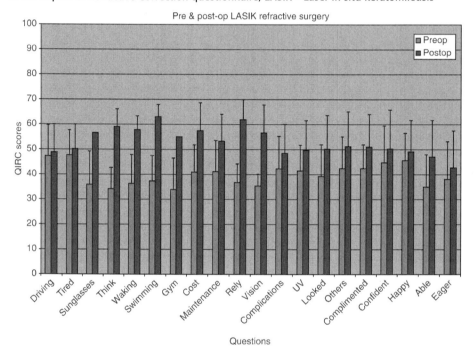

thickness of the lenses by obtaining thin (high refractive index and/or aspheric) lenses with special coatings. It should be noted that the superior QOL for refractive surgery patients comes with a risk in that patients may be one of the small number (approximately 5%) that have significant complications that can lead to reduced QOL (Pesudovs et al., 2006).

QIRC was developed to be as short as possible, so contains only 20 items and takes on average slightly under 5 min to complete (Pesudovs et al., 2004). The QIRC questionnaire, scoring spreadsheets and supporting material are available free from http://konrad.pesudovs.com/konrad/questionnaire.html.

8   The Refractive Status Vision Profile (RSVP)

The RSVP is a conventionally developed and Likert scaled instrument developed almost exclusively on a refractive surgery population (92% of subjects) (Schein, 2000), and is really

■ Figure 139-5

Mean ± 1SD responses on each QIRC question for spectacle, contact lens and refractive surgery groups. Average scores from each question on the QIRC questionnaire for a group of 104 spectacle wearers, 104 contact lens wearers and 104 people who had recently had refractive surgery. A higher score indicates a better quality of life related to refractive correction. *QIRC* Quality of life Impact of Refractive Correction questionnaire

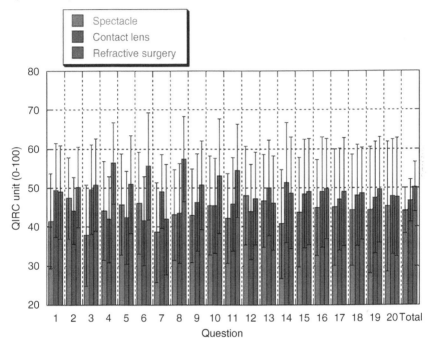

only valid for refractive surgery and not for spectacle or contact lens wearers. Indeed, the RSVP has been shown to be insensitive to QOL issues relevant to people wearing contact lenses (Nichols et al., 2001). Its 42 items fall into the domains of concern (6 items), expectations (2), physical/social functioning (11), driving (3), symptoms (5), glare (3), optical problems (5) and problems with corrective lenses (7 items) (Schein et al., 2001). The RSVP has been shown to be sensitive to QOL changes related to visual functioning and refractive error, and is responsive to refractive surgery (Schein et al., 2001). Improvements after refractive surgery occurred in the subscales: expectations, physical and social functioning and problems with corrective lenses.

The RSVP was developed using traditional techniques, but its psychometric properties were re-evaluated by Garamendi et al. using Rasch analysis (Garamendi et al., 2006). The original 42 item questionnaire showed poor targeting of item impact to patient QOL, items with a ceiling effect, underutilized response categories, a high level of redundancy and no valid subscales. Rasch analysis guided response scale restructuring and item reduction to a 20 item instrument with improved internal consistency and precision for discriminating between groups. It was shown that many of the 14 items relating to functioning and driving were redundant and could be reduced to five items without any loss of accuracy. In addition, many of the eight items related to symptoms and glare were shown to be redundant and this could be reduced to three. This is consistent with the content of the QIRC questionnaire, in which the use of Rasch analysis in the development of the original questionnaire identified that patients with corrected refractive error experienced few problems with visual function, and issues of convenience, cost, health concerns and well being were more influential on QOL (Pesudovs et al., 2004). Perhaps the reason why the original RSVP was so heavily weighted with functioning and symptoms questions was because the items were principally determined by clinicians (Schein, 2000), who tend to deal with patients' presenting complaints of symptoms or functional difficulties, instead of using more objective methodology to discover the important QOL issues for patients when their refractive error has been corrected and their functional vision is normal and they have no symptoms. Most of the time refractive corrections provide adequate functional vision without symptoms and it is only when patients are so motivated by a problem that they visit their clinicians that this is not the case.

9   The National Eye Institute Refractive Quality of Life (NEI-RQL)

The NEI-RQL is a conventionally developed and Likert scaled 42 item questionnaire that included subscales related to clarity of vision, expectations, near and far vision, diurnal fluctuations, activity limitations, glare, symptoms, dependence on correction, worry, suboptimal correction, appearance and satisfaction. The development and validation of the NEI-RQL was spread across three papers and despite rigorous work with focus groups, there is no report on how the final 42 items were selected (Berry et al., 2003; Hays et al., 2003; McDonnell et al., 2003b). The majority of the questions are again related to symptoms or functional difficulties and the content appears to be very clinician-led, similar to the RSVP. However, the NEI-RQL can discriminate between modes of refractive correction (Nichols et al., 2003, 2005) and is sensitive to QOL changes related to visual functioning and refractive error. (Schmidt et al., 2007) Two studies have used the NEI-RQL to demonstrate improved QOL after refractive surgery (McDonnell et al., 2003b; Nichols et al., 2005). The NEI-RQL has not been tested or scaled using Rasch analysis.

10   Other Instruments

The Vision Quality of Life Index is a simple six item questionnaire that does not compute an overall score but compares groups on the basis of agreement with each of six statements. People who had undergone refractive surgery had less concern about four of the six issues included in this questionnaire (Chen et al., 2007). The content of the questionnaire includes concern about injury, coping, friendships, ability to obtain assistance, fulfilling roles and confidence in joining in activities so therefore can be considered a quality of life instrument. This instrument can effectively inform of the rate of concerns within these content areas.

The Myopia Specific Quality of Life and the Canadian Refractive Surgery Research Group Questionnaires have been conventionally validated and shown to be responsive to refractive surgery (Brunette et al., 2000; Lee et al., 2005). Other studies that report QOL issues before and after refractive surgery have used informal, non-validated questionnaires (Bailey et al., 2003; Ben-Sira et al., 1997; McGhee et al., 2000; Rose et al., 2000).

11 Comparing Quality of Life Questionnaire for Refractive Surgery Outcomes

We recently compared several refractive surgery QOL PROs – QIRC, the NEI-RQL and the RSVP, across a comprehensive framework for assessing instrument validity and reliability. This study concluded that QIRC was superior in terms of methods used for item reduction, demonstration of unidimensionality, response scale construction, scoring system and aspects of reliability (Pesudovs et al., 2007). These findings are summarized in ❷ *Table 139-2*.

Disadvantages of the RSVP and NEI-RQL

- Likert or summary scoring (Likert, 1932). This scoring method assumes that categories of responses have specific values and that these values represents appropriate positions along a linear scale; this is invariably incorrect (Pesudovs et al., 2003). This method also assumes that all items have the same value; this is also invariably incorrect (Pesudovs et al., 2003). These two assumptions cause the scoring to be noisy and non-linear. This decreases both the accuracy and precision of measurement (Garamendi et al., 2006; Norquist et al., 2004) and leads to an increase in the required sample size for studies.
- Since neither were developed using Rasch analysis, neither have had the benefits of stringent assessment of internal consistency afforded by Rasch analysis. Rasch analysis gives greater insight into the dimensionality of a questionnaire than available with conventional methods, so items which do not fit the construct under measurement can be excluded. Importantly, redundant items can be identified by Rasch analysis and removed. If a Likert scored questionnaire contains redundant items this leads to overemphasis of that issue within the "score" and this is a serious problem of the RSVP (Garamendi et al., 2006). Conventionally developed questionnaires consistently require modification when assessed by Rasch analysis in that misfitting and redundant items need removal and often the response scale needs revision (Garamendi et al., 2006; Lamoureux et al., 2006; Massof Fletcher, 2001; Pesudovs et al., 2003).
- Despite four papers outlining the development and validation for the NEI-RQL, nowhere is the method for arriving at the final 42 items reported (Berry et al., 2003; Hays et al., 2003; McDonnell et al., 2003a, 2003b). This is a serious failing in content validity.
- The NEI-RQL does not allow for an overall score of quality of life, only subscale scores. The validity of these subscales has not been demonstrated and many contain too few items to validly form a subscale. The RSVP has the same problem with invalid subscales.

Advantages of QIRC over the RSVP or the NEI-RQL

- True linear scoring on an interval scale.
- More precise measurement of quality of life.
- More accurate measurement of quality of life.
- Smaller sample size required for outcome studies.
- All questions fit the construct of quality of life.
- Content of the questionnaire driven by patients, not by clinicians, which means that it is more relevant.

■ Table 139-2

Quality assessment of three refractive error-related quality of life instruments: the RSVP, NEI-RQL and QIRC

	Hypo-thesis	Intended popula-tion	Actual content area	Item identifi-cation	Item reduc-tion	Unidimen-sionality	Response scale	Scoring scale	Discrim-inant validity	Conver-gent validity	"Other" validity	Test-retest reli-ability	Inter-observer or inter-mode agree-ment	Rasch separa-tion reli-ability	Interpre-tation	Respons-iveness
RSVP[a]	✓✓	✓	✓✓	✓✓	✓	✗	✗	✗	0	✓	✓	✓	0	0	✓[b]	✓[b]
NEI-RQL	✓✓	✓✓	✓✓	✓✓	✗	✗	✗	✗	0	✓✓	✓✓	✓✓	0	0	✓✓	✓✓
QIRC	✓✓	✓✓	✓✓	✓✓	✓✓	✓✓	✓✓	✓✓	0	0	✓✓	✓✓	0	✓✓	✓✓	✓✓

[a]A Rasch-analyzed version of the RSVP (Garamendi et al., 2006) with a modified response scale and a reduced number of items has been shown to have greater responsiveness and test-retest reliability than the standard instrument. It also provides a unidimensional score, statistically justified response and scoring scales and good Rasch separation reliability

[b]Conflicting reports of normative data levels and responsiveness of the RSVP are provided by (Schein et al., 2001) and (Nichols et al., 2001)

An assessment of three questionnaires that attempt to assess aspects of quality of life influenced by refractive correction. The assessment rates aspects of their development, reliability and accuracy and scoring is either ✓✓ which is the top score and a positive rating; ✓ is a minimally acceptable or "just OK" score, ✗ which is a negative rating and 0 indicates that this aspect of quality has not been reported to date. More details of the quality assessment are provided in the paper listed in the title

RSVP Refractive Status Vision Profile; NEI-RQL National Eye Institute Refractive Quality of Life; QIRC Quality of Life Impact of Refractive Correction. Reproduced from Pesudovs et al. (2007)

- QIRC is less than half the length of the RSVP or the NEI-RQL, plus a consistent question and answer format ensures time of completion is less than half. Brevity encourages completion making QIRC more likely to supply a higher participation rate in a study and more complete data.

The need for Rasch scaled questionnaires is broadly recognized across ophthalmology (Massof, 2007; Pesudovs, 2006; Spaeth et al., 2006; Weisinger, 2006) There is no justification for using a non-Rasch analyzed questionnaire (both scored and developed using Rasch analysis) when one is available. To do so leaves the study open to criticism of its methodology and therefore its outcome. For refractive surgery outcomes research, QIRC is the preferred instrument.

Summary Points

- Refractive error is common.
- Uncorrected refractive error is a significant disease burden worldwide with 98 million people visually impaired and five million people blind from refractive error alone.
- Refractive error can be corrected by spectacles, contact lenses or laser refractive surgery.
- The outcome of laser refractive surgery is assessed by clinical measures of visual acuity and residual refractive error plus patient reported outcomes, especially quality of life.
- A number of questionnaires exist for the measurement of quality of life after refractive surgery but all questionnaires are not equal in validity.
- Rasch analysis is important in the development of questionnaires to optimize question inclusion, unidimensionality and to provide valid linear scoring.
- A refractive error related quality of life instrument should include a breadth of content areas e.g., well being, convenience and concerns, not just functioning or satisfaction.
- Quality of life instruments readily demonstrate the benefits of refractive surgery.
- A sound QOL instrument is also sensitive to the negative impacts of surgical complications, providing an insight into the real impact of the intervention on the person.
- The ideal QOL outcome measure for refractive surgery would contain broad content, be developed and validated with Rasch analysis and have valid linear scoring.
- The Quality of Life Impact of Refractive Correction (QIRC) instrument is superior to other instruments in terms of validity and reliability.

References

Bailey MD, Mitchell GL, Dhaliwal DK, Boxer Wachler BS, Zadnik K. (2003). Ophthalmology. 110: 1371–1378.

Ben-Sira A, Loewenstein A, Lipshitz I, Levanon D, Lazar M. (1997). J Refract Surg. 13: 129–134.

Berry S, Mangione CM, Lindblad AS, McDonnell PJ. (2003). Ophthalmology. 110: 2285–2291.

Brunette I, Gresset J, Boivin JF, Pop M, Thompson P, Lafond GP, Makni H. (2000). Ophthalmology. 107: 1790–1796.

Charman WN. (1989). Ophthalmic Physiol Opt. 9: 424–430.

Chen CY, Keeffe JE, Garoufalis P, Islam FM, Dirani M, Couper TA, Taylor HR, Baird PN. (2007). J Refract Surg. 23: 752–759.

Dandona L, Dandona R. (2006). BMC Med. 4: 6.

de Boer MR, Moll AC, de Vet HC, Terwee CB, Volker-Dieben HJ, van Rens GH. (2004). Ophthalmic Physiol Opt. 24: 257–273.

Downing SM, Haladyna TM. (2004). Med Educ. 38: 327–333.

Garamendi E, Pesudovs K, Elliott DB. (2005). J Cataract Refract Surg. 31: 1537–1543.

Garamendi E, Pesudovs K, Stevens MJ, Elliott DB. (2006). Vision Res. 46: 1375–1383.

Hays RD, Mangione CM, Ellwein L, Lindblad AS, Spritzer KL, McDonnell PJ. (2003). Ophthalmology. 110: 2292–2301.

Kempen JH, Mitchell P, Lee KE, Tielsch JM, Broman AT, Taylor HR, Ikram MK, Congdon NG, O'Colmain BJ. (2004). Arch Ophthalmol. 122: 495–505.

La Grow S. (2007). Optom Vis Sci. 84: 785–788.

Lamoureux EL, Pallant JF, Pesudovs K, Hassell JB, Keeffe JE. (2006). Invest Ophthalmol Vis Sci. 47: 4732–4741.

Lee J, Park K, Cho W, Kim JY, Kang HY. (2005). J Refract Surg. 21: 59–71.

Likert RA. (1932). Arch Psychol. 140: 1–55.

Massof RW. (2005). Ophthalmic Epidemiol. 12: 103–124.

Massof RW. (2007). Optom Vis Sci. 84: 689–704.

Massof RW, Fletcher DC. (2001). Vision Res. 41: 397–413.

McDonnell PJ, Lee P, Spritzer K, Lindblad AS, Hays RD. (2003a). Arch Ophthalmol. 121: 1577–1581.

McDonnell PJ, Mangione C, Lee P, Lindblad AS, Spritzer KL, Berry S, Hays RD. (2003b). Ophthalmology. 110: 2302–2309.

McGhee CN, Craig JP, Sachdev N, Weed KH, Brown AD. (2000). J Cataract Refract Surg. 26: 497–509.

Nichols JJ, Mitchell GL, Saracino M, Zadnik K. (2003). Arch Ophthalmol. 121: 1289–1296.

Nichols JJ, Mitchell GL, Zadnik K. (2001). Ophthalmology. 108: 1160–1166.

Nichols JJ, Twa MD, Mitchell GL. (2005). J Cataract Refract Surg. 31: 2313–2318.

Norquist JM, Fitzpatrick R, Dawson J, Jenkinson C. (2004). Med Care. 42: I25–136.

Pesudovs K. (2006). BMC Ophthalmol. 6: 25.

Pesudovs K, Burr JM, Harley C, Elliott DB. (2007). Optom Vis Sci. 84: 663–674.

Pesudovs K, Garamendi E, Elliott DB. (2004). Optom Vis Sci. 81: 769–777.

Pesudovs K, Garamendi E, Elliott DB. (2006). J Refract Surg. 22: 19–27.

Pesudovs K, Garamendi E, Keeves JP, Elliott DB. (2003). Invest Ophthalmol Vis Sci. 44: 2892–2899.

Rein DB, Zhang P, Wirth KE, Lee PP, Hoerger TJ, McCall N, Klein R, Tielsch JM, Vijan S, Saaddine J. (2006). Arch Ophthalmol. 124: 1754–1760.

Rose K, Harper R, Tromans C, Waterman C, Goldberg D, Haggerty C, Tullo A. (2000). Br J Ophthalmol. 84: 1031–1034.

Schein OD. (2000). Trans Am Ophthalmol Soc. 98: 439–469.

Schein OD, Vitale S, Cassard SD, Steinberg EP. (2001). J Cataract Refract Surg. 27: 665–673.

Schmidt GW, Yoon M, McGwin G, Lee PP, McLeod SD. (2007). Arch Ophthalmol. 125: 1037–1042.

Spaeth G, Walt J, Keener J. (2006). Am J Ophthalmol. 141: S3–S14.

Steinberg EP, Tielsch JM, Schein OD, Javitt JC, Sharkey P, Cassard SD, Legro MW, Diener-West M, Bass EB, Damiano AM, Steinwachs DM, Sommer A. (1994). Arch Ophthalmol. 112: 630–638.

Terwee CB, Bot SD, de Boer MR, van der Windt DA, Knol DL, Dekker J, Bouter LM, de Vet HC. (2007). J Clin Epidemiol. 60: 34–42.

Uusitalo RJ, Brans T, Pessi T, Tarkkanen A. (1999). J Cataract Refract Surg. 25: 989–994.

Valderas JM, Alonso J, Prieto L, Espallargues M, Castells X. (2004). Qual Life Res. 13: 35–44.

Vision Watch. (2003). Vision Correction Market Review. Jobson Publishing, New York.

Vitale S, Schein OD, Meinert CL, Steinberg EP. (2000). Ophthalmology. 107: 1529–1539.

Vitale S, Schein OD, Steinberg EP, Ware JE, Jr. (1997). Invest Ophthalmol Vis Sci. 38: S841.

Waring GO, 3rd. (2000). J Refract Surg. 16: 459–466.

Weisinger HS. (2006). J Refract Surg. 22: 14–15.

Wong TY, Foster PJ, Hee J, Ng TP, Tielsch JM, Chew SJ, Johnson GJ, Seah SK. (2000). Invest Ophthalmol Vis Sci. 41: 2486–2494.

Wong TY, Foster PJ, Johnson GJ, Seah SK. (2003). Invest Ophthalmol Vis Sci. 44: 1479–1485.

World Health Organization. (2001). The International Classification of Functioning, Disability and Health (ICF). World Health Organization, Geneva.

3 Quality of Life Measures and Indices

3.3 Early Life Stages and Aging

140 Intrauterine Growth Restriction and Later Quality of Life

D. Spence

1   *Introduction* *2398*
1.1 Definition 2398
1.2 Small for Gestational Age Versus Intrauterine Growth Restriction 2399
1.3 Overview of Intrauterine Growth Restriction 2399

2   *Etiological Determinants of IUGR* *2399*
2.1 Fetal Abnormality and Infections 2400
2.2 Maternal Disease 2400
2.3 Lifestyle Factors 2401

3   *Pediatric Implications* *2401*

4   *Long-term Implications for Adult Health* *2402*

5   *Original Research* *2402*
5.1 Quality of Life 2403
5.2 Short Form 36 Health Survey 2403
5.3 Definition and Measurement of Quality of Life 2404
5.4 1950's Cohort 2405
5.5 Health-Related Quality of Life 2405

6   *Conclusion* *2407*

     Summary Points *2408*

Abstract: ❷ Intrauterine growth restriction (IUGR) remains a major clinical problem in modern obstetrics. While technology has yet to aid significant prevention of IUGR, the past few decades has seen the introduction of some of the most innovative therapies in the history of ❷ neonatal intensive care. This has resulted in an increased survival rate of a heterogeneous group of babies, including those with intrauterine growth restriction. It is therefore important to assess if the associated problems with these babies, impact on health related ❷ quality of life long-term. Subtle psychological and social differences have been reported in childhood and early adult life and higher incidence of coronary heart disease, high blood pressure, and diabetes have also been reported in later life. However, it is unclear how this impacts on overall quality of life. Quality of life is considered an important outcome measure for healthcare interventions in adults and health status measures are key determinants of health service use. Despite the extensive cohort studies undertaken to date, there is a dearth of literature on the relationship between IUGR and quality of life, particularly in later life. A recent study addressed this gap in the literature, comparing subjects born with IUGR and a control group with normal birth weight for ❷ gestation. Quality of life in adulthood was assessed using the Short Form-36 health survey (SF-36). The two groups reported similar quality of life on each of the eight dimensions of the SF-36 and there were no significant differences between them. Adjusting for potential confounding variables did not alter this conclusion. This chapter summarizes the impact of IUGR on later quality of life.

List of Abbreviations: *AGA*, Appropriate for gestational age; *CI*, Confidence intervals; *CMV*, Cytomegalovirus; *g*, Grams; *GP*, General Practitioner; *IUGR*, Intrauterine growth restriction; *LMP*, Last menstrual period; *SD*, Standard deviation; *SF-36*, Short Form 36 health survey; *SGA*, Small for gestational age; *SPSS*, Statistical package for social sciences; *UK*, United Kingdom

1   Introduction

Intrauterine growth restriction (IUGR) continues to be a significant clinical problem in modern obstetrics. Whilst there has been substantial progress regarding IUGR, there is still some way to go as many difficulties and challenges still exist in improving clinical outcome and in understanding the scientific mechanism.

1.1   Definition

Growth is a basic fundamental of life and of particular importance is the intrauterine growth of the ❷ fetus. Normal fetal growth has been defined as "that which is neither significantly restricted nor promoted by extrinsic factors" (Robinson et al., 1997, p. 29). It may be assumed that the area of research surrounding growth disturbance is well established, yet definitions which are concise and rigorously laid out are not readily available. IUGR has been described as "a concept signifying that the fetus has not achieved its optimal growth" by Kingdom and Baker (2000, p. 1). Many factors affect fetal growth and inhibit it, yet although there is diversity in the causes of IUGR, the fact that the baby with IUGR would have been bigger were it not for suboptimal genetic and/or environmental factors, is common to all.

1.2   Small for Gestational Age Versus Intrauterine Growth Restriction

The International Committee at Geneva recommended a definition of prematurity in 1937 (Crosse, 1949). As a result, healthy full-term babies which often weigh less than 3,200 g, perhaps even as little as 2,300 g, were termed premature by definition if the birth weight was below 2,500 g. This meant babies born less than 2,500 g were regarded as premature, regardless of the period of gestation. This birth weight standard inevitably included some full-term but small for gestational age infants. Definitions have changed and since the abandonment of the concept that weight determines age, a variety of terms exist to describe babies who demonstrate altered growth. One such term is "small for gestational age" (SGA), with a synonym "small for dates." Henriksen (1999), indicates that SGA and IUGR are different concepts and views SGA as a size measurement which may or may not reflect restricted fetal growth. However, as they share core clinical problems, all infants with birth weight at or below the 10th percentile for gestational age are usually considered SGA (Fanaroff et al., 1989). By convention the 10th centile is the most commonly used cutoff (Bakketeig, 1996), however the 5th centile (Strauss, 2000) or even the 3rd centile (Paz et al., 1995) may be used. There are many reasons why a baby may be small and these are related to both maternal and fetal factors. Growth restriction, congenital infection, or congenital malformations are some examples which may lead to, or are associated with small for gestational age. The terms IUGR and SGA are frequently used in an interchangeable manner, however throughout this chapter the term IUGR will be used.

1.3   Overview of Intrauterine Growth Restriction

IUGR is a major cause of ❷ perinatal ❷ morbidity and ❷ mortality (Kilby and Hodgett, 2000). It is defined as less than 10% of predicted fetal weight for gestational age and can result in significant fetal morbidity and mortality if not properly diagnosed (Vandenbosche and Kirchner, 1998). IUGR is associated with increased risk of stillbirth, neonatal death, and other adverse outcomes (Clausson et al., 2001). Most cases of IUGR present during the third trimester, with most fetal deaths involving IUGR occurring after 36 weeks' gestation and before onset of labor. In accordance with the common definition of IUGR, the expected incidence of IUGR should be about 10%, however, the actual incidence is currently about 4–7%, increasing to around 15–25% in twins. On occasions, some infants thought to have IUGR, in retrospect can be found to be constitutionally small (Vandenbosche and Kirchner, 1998).

2   Etiological Determinants of IUGR

As outlined, IUGR refers to a biological process in which the fetus fails to achieve its genetically programed growth potential and contributing factors which interact, include the external environment, coexistent maternal disease, and the placental and fetal adaptive responses (Kingdom and Baker, 2000). Many different factors may lead to, or are associated with IUGR, including genetic, nutritional, uterine, and placental factors, fetal infection and maternal oxygen-carrying capacity may also be associated (Neerhof, 1995). ❷ Table 140-1 outlines attributable causes of IUGR for which etiological roles are well established.

◼ Table 140-1

Etiological determinants of intrauterine growth restriction in a developed country

Attributable causes of IUGR	
• Cigarette smoking	• Pregnancy induced hypertension
• Low weight gain	• Congenital anomalies
• Low body mass index	• Other genetics
• Primiparity	• Alcohol/drugs
• Short stature	• Unknown

These are attributable causes of intrauterine growth restriction (IUGR) for which etiological roles are well established. They refer to a developed country in which 25% of women smoke during pregnancy and a substantial minority are nonwhite

2.1   Fetal Abnormality and Infections

Fetal abnormality may be associated with IUGR (Vandenbosche and Kirchner, 1998) and trisomies likely to be associated are trisomy 18 (Edward syndrome) and 13 (Patau syndrome). Infection particularly viral can severely impair the growth potential of a fetus. The classic example is rubella, now uncommon in the United Kingdom (UK) due to widespread immunization, but which remains a problem worldwide. Rubella is an important embryopathic virus and if infection occurs in the first trimester, the fetus is at considerable risk of developing profound abnormalities such as blindness, cardiac malformations, and deafness. This virus appears to have the potential to interfere with the genomic drive to growth, which leads to a growth-restricted baby. There are other viral infections which are associated with growth restriction, including cytomegalovirus (CMV) and varicella (chickenpox), if they infect the fetus in the early weeks of pregnancy. Infections with agents such as *Treponema pallidum,* are uncommon in the UK, but globally are a significant cause of fetal growth failure (Gross, 1989).

2.2   Maternal Disease

A plethora of different coexistent maternal diseases has been linked to the development of IUGR. IUGR may ensue if any maternal disease is of sufficient severity. Maternal diseases such as hypertension, renal disease, autoimmune disorders, and microvascular disease associated with long-standing insulin dependent diabetes, can increase the risk of a fetus developing IUGR. Such conditions affect fetal growth, as they lead primarily to reduced blood supply via the uterine arteries. This arises from inadequate changes in the maternal spiral arteries at the time of placentation and in the subsequent weeks. Secondary changes known as acute atherosis also occur, a process which narrows the blood vessels still further. These changes combine to restrict blood supply and as a result, substrate delivery to the placental bed and thence to the fetus (Whittle, 1999). This situation is exacerbated if preexisting maternal vascular disease is present. The mother is at particular risk of developing pregnancy-induced hypertension or even preeclampsia and consequently the fetus fails to grow normally (Neerhof, 1995). Maternal illness can also indirectly create growth problems in the fetus, not necessarily from the illness itself, but from the drugs required to control it. A classic example is anticonvulsant therapy which is known to be associated with IUGR. It is assumed that these drugs affect cellular mechanisms, rather than the substrate supply previously described.

2.3   Lifestyle Factors

Toxins from smoking and excessive alcohol are also well recognized as being associated with IUGR, however maternal alcohol intake is not as consistent in affecting fetal growth as maternal smoking (Gross, 1989). The evidence linking smoking with IUGR is unequivocal and there is no doubt that fetotoxic effects result from high maternal alcohol intake. At its extreme form, this presents as fetal alcohol syndrome. It is thought that excessive alcohol taken in early pregnancy may act as a cellular poison, thus reducing the fetal potential for growth. The effect of smoking may be due to the vasoconstrictive effect of nicotine in the maternal circulation and also because of the displacement of oxygen from hemoglobin by carbon monoxide. Drugs such as cocaine and "crack" are potent vasoconstrictors which may have adequate influence on the uterine vasculature to be a potential cause of severe IUGR. Demographic studies have long linked inequalities in health to economic and social variables and many lifestyle factors may contribute to fetal growth restriction. Socioeconomic group is a factor which may be related to fetal growth, maternal height is another factor, and small women from certain ethnic groups are more likely to have small babies, but not necessarily babies with IUGR (Whittle, 1999). It is apparent that the impact of other factors which affect fetal size such as smoking and hypertension, is likely to be greatest amongst those women who have constitutional factors which also reduces fetal size. This presents the challenge in maternal-fetal medicine, to develop techniques which will successfully separate out these different factors and their relative contribution.

3   Pediatric Implications

IUGR babies can have a variety of problems, having an increased risk in various perinatal morbidities (Ergaz et al., 2005). Condition at birth is poorer compared with "appropriate for gestational age" (AGA) babies (Ariyuki et al., 1995). In the short-term they have difficulty with temperature control related to their small body mass to surface area, lack of glycogen stores, and low brown fat which reduces their nonshivering thermogenesis. Perinatal hypoxia is also associated with poor glycogen reserves. These babies are at increased risk of necrotizing enterocolitis due to the adaptation to prolonged intrauterine hypoxia associated with fetal gut ischemia. Babies born with IUGR can develop respiratory complications. However, lung maturity is not solely related to IUGR but is dependant on various factors including for example, gestational age. It has also long been recognized that these babies are at risk of neonatal hypoglycemia (Drossou et al., 1995). ❯ Table 140-2 outlines conditions specifically associated with IUGR. The care of these babies can be complex requiring advanced neonatal support. Subsequent development depends both on the extent and etiology of the IUGR and the gestational age at delivery. In infancy and early childhood IUGR infants are at risk for growth failure and neurodevelopmental sequelae, including cerebral palsy, cognitive deficit, and behavioral problems (Yanney and Marlow, 2004).

■ Table 140-2

Conditions specifically associated with intrauterine growth restriction

Neonatal condition
• Perinatal hypoxia
• Necrotizing enterocolitis
• Respiratory distress syndrome and respiratory complications
• Hypoglycemia
• Polycythemia
• Anemia, leucopenia, and low platelets
• Postnatal growth

Intrauterine growth restriction increases mortality and morbidity in the neonatal period

4   Long-term Implications for Adult Health

Epidemiological studies have influenced our thinking regarding IUGR. The work of Barker and his colleagues often referred to as the "fetal origins of adult disease" highlights the possibility that those babies born small for dates are more likely to develop hypertension and noninsulin dependent diabetes in adult life (Barker, 1992). It must be noted however, that it was the effect of low-birth weight rather than IUGR which formed the basis of Barker's studies (Whittle, 1999). These original UK findings have been replicated in different countries, leading to a wide acceptance that low rates of fetal growth is associated with ❷ cardiovascular disease in adult life (❷ Table 140-3).

5   Original Research

There are major gaps in the knowledge of long-term effects of IUGR. In our study the aim was to determine whether health problems reported in adult life, in particular health-related quality of life at age 50 years, are associated with IUGR at birth. We took account of gestational age and birth weight.

■ Table 140-3

Adult diseases associated with fetal growth restriction

Adult disease	
• Coronary heart disease	• Type 2 diabetes
• Stroke	• Hypertension
• Polycystic ovary syndrome	• Osteoporosis
• Hormone dependent cancers	

There is an inverse relationship between birth weight and the prevalence of chronic diseases in adulthood

5.1 Quality of Life

"Quality of life" is one of the fastest growing areas of research and policy. It has become an accepted endpoint in clinical research trials in recent years, particularly as interest in patients' experiences and preferences has grown. Health related quality of life is the primary outcome of this study and was measured at 48–50 years in two groups; those born with IUGR and those with normal birth weight. Despite the extensive cohort studies undertaken to date, there is a dearth of literature on the relationship between IUGR and quality of life. The past few decades has seen the introduction of some of the most innovative therapies in the history of neonatal intensive care (Saigal and Rosenbaum, 1996). This has resulted in a further decline in neonatal mortality of high-risk babies; however, improvements in morbidity have not been as significant. These major improvements in perinatal care have seen an increased survival rate of a heterogeneous group of babies, including those born preterm or low-birth weight and also those with intrauterine growth restriction (❯ Table 140-4). For some of these babies who survive there

❑ Table 140-4
Notes on intrauterine growth restriction

Birth weight is the most important determinant of perinatal outcome
IUGR is associated with many medical problems for the baby, before and after delivery
The mechanisms involved in fetal growth are not well understood
Various factors (maternal and fetal) may inhibit fetal growth
Diagnosis of IUGR is thus complex
Both stillbirths and neonatal deaths are strongly associated with IUGR
Effective monitoring of fetal growth is of major importance in antenatal care
Identification and management of the growth restricted baby are a major challenge for clinicians

Key points related to intrauterine growth restriction

may be adverse outcomes and such impairments may profoundly influence health and quality of life during childhood and adult life. These issues have received little attention to date, as focus has been on for example, physical handicap, academic difficulties, and behavioral problems experienced by these babies particularly in infancy, childhood, and adolescence (Hack et al., 1994; McCormick et al., 1992; Saigal et al., 1991), few extend to early adulthood. Concerns regarding the care of babies of borderline viability have resurfaced and the appropriateness of offering intensive care to all babies is being questioned. This creates ethical dilemmas and perhaps "bad publicity". It is therefore important to assess if the associated problems with these babies, impact on quality of life long-term. A quality of life approach is much broader than traditional measures of health outcome, including morbidity and mortality, which insufficiently capture the full spectrum of potential "health" problems. It is essential to promote a wider perspective on health and social wellbeing.

5.2 Short Form 36 Health Survey

The health status measure used to assess quality of life in this study was the Short Form 36 Health Survey (SF-36). This short 36-item questionnaire is used worldwide and covers a wide range of areas that may be adversely affected by illness. The SF-36 is a valuable tool in research which has undergone validity testing in the UK including assessment of the content, criterion, and construct validity of the instrument which is widely used particularly as it is appropriate for use with adults of working age (Jenkinson et al., 1993) and within the National Health Service (Garratt et al., 1993). It was chosen as the quality of life measurement in this study, as it is easy to administer and quick to complete and is a comprehensive tool applicable across social and demographic groups (Hayes et al., 1995). It has been used in a cohort of very low birth weight infants to determine if their birth weight had impacted on their lifestyle and quality of life at age 19–22 years. In this study, Cooke (2004) concluded that problems experienced by those born very preterm, were not perceived to influence quality of life in early adulthood. It covers a wide range of areas that may be adversely affected by illness. It measures eight multi-item dimensions (❯ *Table 140-5*). For each dimension item scores are coded, summed, and transformed onto a scale from 0 (worst possible health state measured by the questionnaire) to 100 (best possible health state).

◻ Table 140-5
Short Form-36 dimensions

Dimension	Label	No. of items
• Physical functioning	PF	10
• Role limitation due to physical problems	RP	4
• Pain	BP	2
• General health perception	GH	5
• Energy/vitality	EV	4
• Social functioning	SF	2
• Role limitation due to emotional problems	RE	3
• Mental health	MH	5

For each dimension item scores are coded, summed, and transformed onto a scale from 0 (worst possible health state measured by the questionnaire) to 100 (best possible health state)

5.3 Definition and Measurement of Quality of Life

The definition and measurement of quality of life has been an issue of considerable debate (Eiser and Morse, 2001). It is a term often used vaguely and without clear definition. This is due to the broad nature of a concept which incorporates physical functioning (can undertake activities of daily living including self-care and mobilizing), psychological functioning (emotional and mental wellbeing), social functioning (relationships with others and ability to take part in social activities), and perception of health status, pain, and general satisfaction with life (Sanders et al., 1998). Eiser and Morse (2001) outlined three key ideas which define the concept of quality of life. The first is the idea that individuals have their own distinct perspective on quality of life, depending on current lifestyle, past experience, hopes for the future, dreams, and goals. The second relates to a medical setting, where quality of life is usually viewed as a multidimensional construct incorporating numerous domains. The third idea is that quality of life can include both objective and subjective perspectives in each domain. The former perspective concentrates on what the individual can do and the latter includes what things mean to the individual.

More recently in all areas of medicine there is increasing recognition of the need to measure outcomes from the perspective of patients. To do so, it is essential to understand the personal experience and effect of disease and disabilities on individuals and their families (Saigal and Rosenbaum, 1996). The measurement of health-related quality of life provides useful descriptive and discriminative information about the various health problems of individuals. Attention to quality of life has emphasized the need to consider outcomes in terms of the individual as a whole, rather than focusing on a narrow range of clinical indicators. Mortality is no longer viewed as the only endpoint when considering the efficacy of medical intervention. Health related quality of life is now considered an important outcome measure for healthcare interventions in adults and health status measures are key determinants of health service use (Hofman et al., 2004).

5.4   1950's Cohort

The cohort in our study consisted of babies who were born in Royal Maternity Hospital, Belfast between 1954 and 1956 and who were traced and assessed in adulthood at the age of about 50 years. Information on each birth between 1954 and 1956 ($n = 6366$) was manually abstracted and entered on a database. Gestational age was calculated based on the first day of the last menstrual period (LMP) (Hypponen et al., 2003; Kiserud and Marsal, 2000; Strauss, 2000) and birth weight recorded in pounds and ounces was converted to grams.

The study group consisted of growth restricted babies (birth weight < 10th centile), born at term. The control group was term, normal birth weight babies ($\geq$10th centile). Exclusion criteria were multiple pregnancies, babies born with major congenital abnormalities, and surviving adults deemed inappropriate for the study by their General Practitioner (GP).

The study and control groups were selected from 4,667 births that met the inclusion criteria. Software from the Child Growth Foundation was used to adjust birth weight for gestation and gender and to convert these measures to standard deviation scores (SDS). SPSS (version 11) was used to identify the study group ($n = 491$). A random selection of the non-study group based on a one-to-one ratio formed the control group. Losses to follow up, dropouts, and nonparticipation were recorded at the various stages to enable the researcher to examine potential sample bias. The sample was traced with the assistance of the Central Services Agency in Northern Ireland and GPs.

For each dimension item scores were coded, summed, and transformed onto a scale from 0 to 100. Mean scores between groups were initially compared using t-tests. Multiple linear regression analysis was then undertaken to adjust for potential confounding variables.

5.5   Health-Related Quality of Life

Results from this study showed both groups reported similar health-related quality of life on each dimension of the SF-36 and there were no significant differences between them (Spence et al., 2007). Adjusting for potential confounding variables did not alter this conclusion (❯ *Tables 140-6–140-9*). The IUGR group did have a tendency to use Health Services more for example outpatient departments, accident and emergency, and reported having more GP consultations, illnesses, use of medication and admissions to hospital. This clearly has implications for Health Service resources.

◻ Table 140-6

Short Form 36 health survey sub-dimensions related to physical and social functioning before and after adjustment for confounding variables

SF-36	IUGR Group n = 111 Mean (Standard Deviation)	Control Group n = 124 Mean (Standard Deviation)	Mean Difference Unadjusted (95% Confidence Intervals)	P Value	Mean Difference Adjusted[a] (95% Confidence Intervals)	P Value
Physical function	86.3 (21.5)	82.9 (23.7)	3.4 (−2.5 to 9.2)	0.26	4.4 (−1.3 to 10.1)	0.13
Social functioning	85.8 (22.9)	86.0 (23.8)	−0.2 (−6.3 to 5.8)	0.94	1.1 (−4.7 to 6.8)	0.71

[a]Adjusted for gender, social class at birth, marital status, education, Townsend deprivation index, and age at time of study

The group with intrauterine growth restriction (IUGR) reported similar health-related quality of life on each of these dimensions of the Short Form 36 Health Survey (SF-36). Data are mean and standard deviation, with the scale from 0 (worst possible health state measured by the questionnaire) to 100 (best possible health state)

◻ Table 140-7

Short Form 36 health survey (SF-36) sub-dimensions related to role limitations before and after adjustment for confounding variables

SF-36	IUGR Group n = 111 Mean (Standard Deviation)	Control Group n = 124 Mean (Standard Deviation)	Mean Difference Unadjusted (95% Confidence Intervals)	P Value	Mean Difference Adjusted[a] (95% Confidence Intervals)	P Value
Role limitation due to emotional problems	79.9 (34.9)	81.7 (35.1)	−1.8 (−10.9 to 7.2)	0.69	0.2 (−8.3 to 8.7)	0.96
Role limitation due to physical problems	83.3 (32.7)	80.6 (35.9)	2.7 (−6.2 to 11.6)	0.55	4.8 (−3.8 to 13.3)	0.27

[a]Adjusted for gender, social class at birth, marital status, education, Townsend deprivation index, and age at time of study

The IUGR group reported similar health-related quality of life on each of these dimensions of the SF-36. Data are mean and standard deviation, with the scale from 0 (worst possible health state measured by the questionnaire) to 100 (best possible health state)

◘ Table 140-8

Short Form 36 health survey (SF-36) sub-dimensions related to mental health and energy level before and after adjustment for confounding variables

SF-36	IUGR Group n = 111 Mean (Standard Deviation)	Control Group n = 124 Mean (Standard Deviation)	Mean Difference Unadjusted (95% Confidence Intervals)	P Value	Mean Difference Adjusted[a] (95% Confidence Intervals)	P Value
Mental Health	72.3 (19.3)	73.4 (19.7)	−1.1 (−6.1 to 3.9)	0.67	0.4 (−4.4 to 5.1)	0.88
Energy/ Vitality	61.1 (21.7)	61.0 (21.1)	0.1 (−5.4 to 5.6)	0.98	1.5 (−3.8 to 6.8)	0.58

[a]Adjusted for gender, social class at birth, marital status, education, Townsend deprivation index, and age at time of study
The IUGR group reported similar health-related quality of life on each of these dimensions of the SF-36. Data are mean and standard deviation, with the scale from 0 (worst possible health state measured by the questionnaire) to 100 (best possible health state)

◘ Table 140-9

Short Form 36 health survey (SF-36) sub-dimensions related to bodily pain and general health before and after adjustment for confounding variables

SF-36	IUGR Group n = 111 Mean (Standard Deviation)	Control Group n = 124 Mean (Standard Deviation)	Mean Difference Unadjusted (95% Confidence Intervals)	P Value	Mean Difference Adjusted[a] (95% Confidence Intervals)	P Value
Pain	76.9 (25.6)	76.8 (24.1)	0.1 (−6.3 to 6.5)	0.98	1.3 (−4.9 to 7.6)	0.68
General health perception	70.1 (21.6)	71.0 (20.1)	−0.9 (−6.3 to 4.4)	0.74	0.3 (−5.0 to 5.6)	0.90

[a]Adjusted for gender, social class at birth, marital status, education, Townsend deprivation index, and age at time of study
The IUGR group reported similar health-related quality of life on each of these dimensions of the SF-36. Data are mean and standard deviation, with the scale from 0 (worst possible health state measured by the questionnaire) to 100 (best possible health state)

6 Conclusion

Most follow-up studies of those born preterm or very low-birth weight examine quality of life in childhood or adolescence, with only a few extending to early adulthood. Less is known about health-related quality of life in later adult life and there is little information on those born with IUGR. Health-related quality of life is regarded as an increasingly important outcome measure for healthcare interventions and health status measures are significant determinants of health care utilization (Hofman et al., 2004). The SF-36 is used worldwide to assess quality of life and general health and covers a wide-range of areas that may be adversely affected by illness. In our study the scores on each domain of the SF-36 were similar to published UK age-related norms for males and females aged 45–54 years (Ware et al., 1993). Similar findings have been reported in a study using the SF-36 to assess quality of life in 19–22 year olds who had been born very preterm (Cooke, 2004).

Our study indicates that adults who were born growth restricted do not perceive themselves to have worse health-related quality of life than their normally grown peers. It could be argued that participants in this study have survived the short-term effects of IUGR and although they see themselves as being healthy, this needs to be assessed by formal physical examination. The impact of being born with IUGR should not be underestimated in terms of later health and wellbeing and potential implications for Health Service resources.

Summary Points

- IUGR is a concept indicating a fetus has not reached its optimal growth.
- IUGR increases mortality and morbidity in the neonatal period but there is limited information on its effect on health-related quality of life in adulthood.
- The importance of measuring health-related quality of life is recognized by clinicians and policy makers to inform patient management and policy decisions.
- Our study indicates that adults who were born growth restricted do not perceive themselves to have worse health-related quality of life than their normally grown peers.
- Being born with IUGR has potential implications for Health Service resources.

References

Ariyuki Y, Hata T, Kitao M. (1995). Pediatrics. 96: 36–42.

Bakketeig LS. (1998). Eur J Clin Nutr. 52: Suppl 1.

Barker DJP (ed.). (1992). Fetal and Infant Origins of Adult Disease. BMJ Publishing Group, London.

Clausson B, Gardosi J, Francis A, Cnattingius S. (2001). Br J Obstet Gynaecol. 108: 830–834.

Cooke RWI. (2004). Arch Dis Child. 89: 201–206.

Crosse VM. (1949). The premature baby, 2nd ed. J & A Churchill Ltd, London.

Drossou V, Diamanti E, Noutsia H, Konstantinidis T, Katsougiannopoulos V. (1995). Acta Paediatr. 84: 1–5.

Eiser C, Morse R. (2001). Arch Dis Child. 84: 205–211.

Ergaz M, Avgil M, Ornoy A. (2005). Reprod Toxic. 20: 301–322.

Fanaroff AA, Hack M, Kliegman RM. (1989). In: Gross TL, Sokol RJ (eds.) Intrauterine Growth Restriction a Practical Approach. Year Book Medical Publishers Inc, London.

Garratt AM, Ruta DA, Abdalla MI, Buckingham JK, Russell IT. (1993). Br Med J. 306: 1440–1444.

Gross TL. (1989). In: Gross TL, Sokol RJ (eds.) Intrauterine Growth Restriction a Practical Approach. Year Book Medical Publishers Inc, London.

Hack M, Taylor G, Klein N, Eiben R, Schatschneider C, Mercuri-Minich N. (1994). N Engl J Med. 331: 753–759.

Hayes V, Morris J, Wolfe C, Morgan M. (1995). Age Ageing. 24: 120–125.

Henriksen T. (1999). Acta Paediatr Suppl. 88: 4–8.

Hofman A, Jaddoe VWV, MacKenbach JP, Moll HA, Snijders RFM, Steegers EAP, Verhulst FC, Witteman JCM, Buller HA. (2004). Paediatr Perinat Epidemiol. 18: 61–72.

Hyppönen E, Power C, Davey Smith G. (2003). Diabetes Care. 26: 2515–2517.

Jenkinson C, Coulter A, Wright L. (1993). Br Med J. 306: 1437–1440.

Kilby M, Hodgett S. (2000). In: Kingdom J, Baker P (eds.) Intrauterine Growth Restriction a Practical Approach. Year Book Medical Publishers Inc, London.

Kingdom J, Baker P (eds.). Intrauterine Growth Restriction Aetiology and Management. Springer-Verlag, London.

Kiserud T, Maršál K. (2000). In: Kingdom J, Baker P (eds.) Intrauterine Growth Restriction a Practical Approach. Year Book Medical Publishers Inc, London.

McCormick MC, Brooks-Gunn J, Workman-Daniels K, Turner J, Peckham GJ. (1992). JAMA. 267: 2204–2208.

Neerhof MG. (1995). Clin Perinatol. 22: 375–385.

Paz I, Gale R, Laor A, Danon YL, Stevenson DK, Seidman DS. (1995). Obstet Gynecol. 85: 452–456.

Robinson JS, Owens JA, McMillen IC, Erwich JJ, Owens PC. (1997). In: Cockburn F (ed.) Advances in Perinatal Medical. The Parthenon Publishing Group, London.

Saigal S, Rosenbaum P. (1996). Semin Neonatol. 1: 305–312.

Saigal S, Szatmari P, Rosenbaum P, King S, Campbell D. (1991). J Pediatr. 118: 751–760.

Sanders C, Egger M, Donovan J, Tallon D, Frankel S. (1998). Br Med J. 317: 1191–1194.

Spence D, Alderdice FA, Stewart MC, Halliday HL, Bell AH. (2007). Arch Dis Child. 92: 700–703.

Strauss RS. (2000). JAMA. 283: 625–632.

Vandenbosche RC, Kirchner DO. (1998). Am Fam Physician. 15: 1384–1393.

Ware JE, Snow KK, Kosinski M, Gandek B. (1993). The Health Institute, New England Medical Center, Boston, MA.

Whittle MJ. (1999). In: Rodeck CH, Whittle MJ (ed.) Fetal Medicine Basic Science and Clinical Practice. Churchill Livingstone, London.

Yanney M, Marlow N. (2004). Semin Fetal Neonatal Med. 9: 411–418.

141 Assessment of Quality of Life During Pregnancy and in the Postnatal Period

C. R. Martin · J. Jomeen

1   Introduction 2412

2   Quality of Life in Pregnancy 2412

3   Postnatal Quality of Life 2414

4   Measuring Perinatal Quality of Life 2416

5   SF-36 2416

6   The Mother Generated Index (MGI) 2416

7   Maternal Postpartum Quality of Life Tool 2418

8   Inventory of Functional Status after Childbirth 2420

9   Conclusion 2420

    Summary Points 2420

Abstract: Quality of life has become an area of increasing importance to the area of pregnancy and childbirth. Much has been written on specific clinical presentations that occur during the ❯ perinatal period that may deleteriously impact on perceived quality of life, for example ❯ postnatal depression, complications during labor or abnormalities in the baby. This chapter will explore the salient issues regarding assessment of quality of life during pregnancy and in the postnatal period.

List of Abbreviations: *EPDS*, Edinburgh Postnatal Depression Scale; *IFSAC*, The Inventory of Functional status after Childbirth; *MAPP-QOL*, The Maternal Postpartum Quality of Life Tool; *MGI*, Mother Generated Index; *SF-36*, Short-Form 36

1 Introduction

Pregnancy induces a unique physiological response, which stresses the body more than any other physiological event in a health women's life resulting in metabolic, hormonal, cardio-vascular, respiratory and musculo-skeletal adaptations (Sternfield, 1997). Many of theses changes manifest in many of the so called minor disorders of pregnancy such as nausea and vomiting, dizziness and fatigue (Gross and Pattison, 2007), some of which are transient some are more enduring. Following birth, the postnatal period is a time when a woman has to adjust to physical changes and new emotional demands and the impact of aspects such as perineal trauma and associated pain on women's general health (Albers and Borders, 2007), ability to fulfill daily activities (Lydon-Rochelle et al., 2001) and ability to adapt to mother-hood (Mason et al., 1999) has also been investigated and documented. The increasing literature, documenting the impact of pregnancy and childbirth on women's normal daily activities, identifies the concept of Quality of Life as an important psychological domain worthy of further debate, both as a concept but also in terms of its effective assessment in women across the perinatal period.

2 Quality of Life in Pregnancy

There is a general paucity of evidence exploring the relationship between perinatality and women's quality of life. Decreased physical functioning, as a dimension of quality of life, however has been demonstrated during normal pregnancy (Haas et al., 2005; Heuston and Kasik-Miller, 1998; Ochet et al., 1999). In pregnancy, nausea and vomiting, is experienced by more than 70% of pregnant women with 28% reporting the negative consequences of pregnancy on family, social and occupational functioning (Attard et al., 2002; O'Brien and Naber, 1992). However, broader quality of life limitations have also been identified by women themselves, including physical symptoms/aggravating factors; fatigue and emotions (Magee et al., 2002). In a study conducted at the end of pregnancy McKee et al. (2001) emphasized the impairment of pregnancy on the dimensions of life quality that require physical activity and in particular the detriment to "vitality" dimension of quality of life. More recently Forger et al. (2005) noted increased bodily pain and impaired physical functioning in a cohort of Austrian women during late pregnancy. There is very little work considering pregnant groups and physical activity in relation to clinical outcomes, indeed the association between quality of life decrements and pregnancy outcomes remains equivocal. Whilst poor physical functioning has been significantly associated with an increased risk of ❷ preterm labor (Haas et al., 1999), other studies conversely, have linked increased or strenuous domestic activity in ❷ multigravida women with higher rates of preterm labor (Launer et al., 1990) and small for dates babies (Woo, 1997). Some albeit rather scant evidence suggests that the restriction of physical activity is associated more with psychological rather than clinical outcomes, with implications for women's self-esteem and a sense of control associated with being active and the freedom to decide what activities to pursue (Gross and Pattison, 2007).

Clearly pregnancy related factors which impact on daily life are important to pregnant women. It is also feasible that a woman's perception of their pregnancy is important in assessments of life quality. Pesavento et al. (2005), investigating quality of life in pregnant Italian women, found that those with a normal pregnancy have a good perception of their quality of life, whilst women with a high risk pregnancy do not. This may link to the findings, which identify the unwelcome nature of the restrictions associated with a high risk pregnancy and suggest that any potential reduction in psychological wellbeing can be attributed more to the restrictions placed on activity than to the pregnancy risk itself (Mackey and Coster-Schultz, 1992; Monaham and De Joseph, 1991).

A further dimension to the debate around quality of life in pregnancy is explored by Kelly and colleagues (2001). They demonstrate the relationship between amplified physical symptoms in pregnancy and the existence of depression and anxiety. This concurs with findings from primary and secondary care settings, which have shown that unexplained medical symptoms are associated with psychopathology (Russo et al., 1994; Simon et al., 1999). Further, anxiety and depression amongst patients with a known medical disease are associated with an amplification of the disease specific and non-specific symptoms (Dwight et al., 2000). Physical symptoms are common in pregnancy, predominantly associated with the normal physiological changes that occur and expected by both clinicians and women themselves. However, an elevated incidence of somatic complaints or negative reports/perceptions of quality of life may rather be associated with psychological disturbance. This may also be true in reverse, and the amplification of somatic symptoms may contribute to the existence of anxiety and depression. The direction of this relationship is yet to be established but it seems legitimate, to suggest that quality of life detriment has often been perceived as a normative part of pregnancy and as such largely ignored.

Abundant evidence demonstrates a strong association between depression and decrements in self-reported functional status or quality of life (Simon, 2003) and also that effective treatment helps to restore function. Other studies have reported that outpatients with depressive disorders experienced functional impairment and decreased well-being comparable to or greater than that of people with chronic medical conditions (Hays et al., 1995; Wells et al., 1989). Other trials have demonstrated that improving depression leads to significant improvements in quality of life (Coulehan et al., 1997). Only a few studies to date have considered these relationships in pregnant women. An inverse relationship has been demonstrated between elevated levels of depressive symptomatology and lowered health-related functioning and perceived well-being in Black and Hispanic pregnant women (McKee et al., 2001) and in a more diverse group of pregnant American women (Nicholson et al., 2006). More recent study findings also identified that British women in early pregnancy classified as possibly anxious using the Anxiety subscale of the Hospital Anxiety and Depression Scale (Zigmond and Snaith, 1983) or suffering minor/major depression as measured by the Edinburgh Postnatal Depression Scale (Cox et al., 1987), experienced poorer quality of life compared with their non-anxious and non-depressed counterparts (Jomeen and Martin, 2005).

☐ Figure 141-1

Factors which may impact on antenatal quality of life. It shows the constellation of factors which may significantly impact on antenatal quality of life. This list is not exhaustive and the factors described may interact. Baby screen results in the figure explicitly means tests for the detection of fetal abnormality

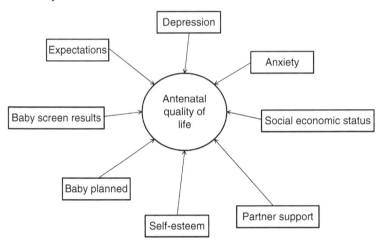

Once again, however, the direction of causality remains ambiguous but it seems clear that psychological detriment and quality of life are inherently linked. Factors which may impact on perceived antenatal quality of life are shown in ❯ *Figure 141-1.*

3   Postnatal Quality of Life

Women experience a broad spectrum of physical as well as emotional challenges following childbirth; some of these are persistent and clearly have the capacity to impact on a woman's quality of life. Recognition of the extent of maternal morbidity and its effect on quality of life has been on the increase in recent years (Symon et al., 2002) and as a result has become the focus of several studies. The impact of perineal trauma and associated perineal pain, a common complication of labor, is well documented. Perineal pain has been linked to both short term and long term perinatal morbidity including perineal pain, perineal healing, urinary incontinence, flatus incontinence, fecal incontinence, sexual morbidity and ❯ dyspareunia (Williams et al., 2007), as well as fatigue and depression (Brown and Lumley, 2000). Both the level of perineal trauma and the degree of suturing were significant in women's self-reports of poor general health (Eason et al., 2000). Women with an ❯ episiotomy, for example, demonstrated longer periods of disruption to their daily life including sleeplessness, difficulty bathing and resuming normal daily activities (Okubo et al., 2000). Quality of life in the postnatal period is a complex and personal area affected by many different aspects of health and well-being (Symon et al., 2002) and can determined by the physical experience of pregnancy and childbirth itself but also the emotional, social, sexual and spiritual dimensions of the transition to motherhood. From a physical perspective, women with significant obstetric morbidity in pregnancy and/or labor report lower general health (Waterstone et al., 2003). Important differences in fatigue have been observed with emergency and elective caesarean section women reporting more prolonged fatigue and lower physical quality of life. A study more specifically examining sleep quality, found positive relationships between good sleep quality and self-report health (Hyyppa et al., 1991) seeming to concur with Tulman and Fawcett (1990) that physical energy levels were overall the strongest correlate of functional status and highlights the dynamic of sleep and fatigue in terms of postnatal quality of life. Indeed in a study which assessed women's quality of life and sleep quantity/quality at 2 weeks and 6 months postnatal revealed profiles of improving quality of life concurrent with improved sleep patterns (Jomeen and Martin (in press)). Such findings seem intuitive and support the suggestion that functional status increases progressively to reflect the physical recovery and psychosocial adjustment to motherhood. Tulman and Fawcett (1990) reveal the significant relationships between mother's functional status and variables such as confidence in motherhood, family, relationship and demographic variables. Higher levels of physical energy, parity, confidence in mothering, and infants with predictable temperament were all associated with increased functional status in household, social, community and self-care activities.

A study which considered the role of quality of life and its relation to postnatal depressive symptomology in Mexican women, found antenatal family quality of life, and postnatal family quality of life to be significant predictors along with other risk factors to postnatal depression (Martinez-Schallmoser, 1992). As in the antenatal period, studies demonstrate a co-morbid relationship between postnatal depression and negative quality of life assessments (Small et al., 2000) yet once again the causality of the relationship is not firmly established. However a recent study exploring relationships between postnatal depression and quality of life implies that it is postnatal depression that negatively influences all dimensions of life quality explored using the SF-36 (De Tychey et al., 2007). An interesting dimension, which supports this assumption, appears to be the influence of baby gender on postnatal depression and postnatal quality of life, with the birth of a boy having negative consequences. Factors which may impact on perceived postnatal quality of life are shown in ❷ *Figure 141-2*.

◻ **Figure 141-2**
Factors which may impact on postnatal quality of life. It shows the myriad of factors which may significantly impact on postnatal quality of life. This list is not exhaustive and the factors described may interact

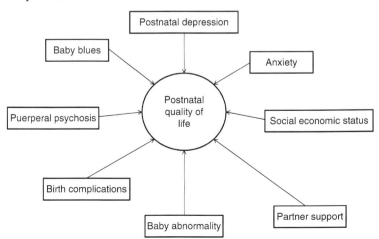

4   Measuring Perinatal Quality of Life

An increasing interest in quality of life as a psychological domain of interest and clinical significance requires a quality of life instrument that reliably measure both physical and psychological functioning. The concern around screening measures in pregnancy appears to focus around the unique and dynamic physiological nature of pregnancy. Several assessment and screening tools that have been demonstrated as reliable and valid in generic populations have been observed to be unstable in terms of factor structure, unreliable and inaccurate (Jomeen and Martin, 2004; Karimova and Martin, 2003; Martin and Jomeen, 2003).

5   SF-36

Quality of Life has been widely investigated in a number of clinical conditions utilizing the Medical Outcomes Survey Short Form 36 (SF-36: Ware and Sherbourne, 1992; Ware et al., 2000). This measure is a widely used generic, multipurpose self-report quality of life questionnaire. The SF-36 consists of 36 questions from which functional health and well-being sub-scale scores are calculated for eight sub-scale domains comprehensively describing quality of life attributes; these being physical functioning (1), role-physical (2), bodily pain (3), general health (4), vitality (5), social functioning (6), role-emotional (7) and mental health (8). Summary measures of physical health (scales 1–4) and mental health (scales 5–8) can also be calculated. An improved version of the SF-36 (version 2) has been introduced which incorporates instruction and item changes and a better layout for questions and answers. The psychometric properties of the SF-36 have been extensively evaluated with good support found for the taxonomy of eight scales and two higher order factors (physical health and mental health domains).

The SF-36 has been used in pregnancy (Heuston and Kasik-Miller, 1998) and in postnatal women (De Tychey et al., 2007; Small et al., 2000; Small et al., 2003). Its psychometric properties in early pregnancy have been recently explored by Jomeen and Martin (2005), utilizing Exploratory and Confirmatory Factor Analysis. The recommendations from this study are for the use of the SF-36 as an eight subscale measure. The merits of using the instrument as a two subscale measure of physical and mental health require further evaluation (Jomeen and Martin, 2005). The SF-36 has also demonstrated as a feasible and reliable tool ($\alpha > 0.7$) in postnatal women, able to discriminate between groups by mode of delivery and to detect moderate recovery in physical and small recovery in mental status over time, when combined with other health related quality of life measures (Jansen et al., 2007). There are a number of suggested measurement models of the SF-36 sub-scales (Jomeen and Martin, 2005) and these are described in ❷ *Figures 141-3–141-6.*

6   The Mother Generated Index (MGI)

The Mother Generated Index (MGI) is subjective tool designed specifically for use in postnatal women, in order to assess postnatal quality of life in new mothers. The MGI gives a primary index quality of life score and a secondary index that identifies those areas considered most important by the mother. The validity of the MGI was tested in a cohort of 103 postnatal women and was sought from concurrent use of the EPDS and the SF-12 which has both

◘ Figure 141-3

Diagrammatic representation of a uni-dimensional model of the SF-36. The figure shows the sub-scales of the SF-36 and their relationship to a single domain of quality of life. This presents a uni-dimensional measurement model of the SF-36

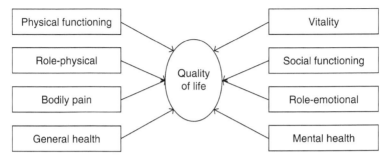

◘ Figure 141-4

Diagrammatic representation of a bi-dimensional model of the SF-36 specifying separable but correlated physical and mental quality of life domains. The figure shows the sub-scales of the SF-36 and their relationship to two higher order physical health and mental health domains. These higher order domains are often found to be significantly correlated in clinical groups. The Figure reveals one common measurement model of the SF-36, however a number of others have been proposed. Calculation of separate mental health and physical health component scores has been suggested and are often reported in the clinical research literature utilizing this commonly used quality of life assessment tool

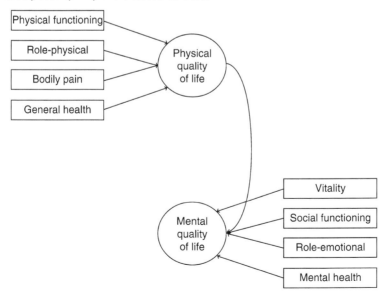

physical (PCS-12) and mental component (MCS-12) scores (Symon et al., 2002). The primary index correlated significantly with the EPDS and the MCS-12 yet not with the PCS-12 scores at both, the differences were more marked at the 8 month than 6–8 weeks observation point. The authors postulate that women do not consider physical problems as important

□ Figure 141-5

Diagrammatic representation of a bi-dimensional model of the SF-36 specifying uncorrelated physical and mental components within a higher order health quality of life domain. The figure shows the sub-scales of the SF-36 and their relationship to uncorrelated higher order physical health and mental health domains. These higher order domains may correlate significantly with the overall quality of life score but may not be correlated with each other. Though less established in the literature, this model may be relevant to certain clinical groups with specific symptom presentations, for example a group with very poor physical functioning but relatively normal levels of mental health functioning

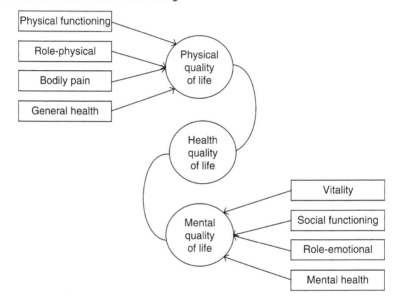

in terms of assessing quality of life, a conclusion not necessarily borne out by the other study findings, which have been previously explored in this chapter. Marked differences between high and low scores in terms of quality of life lead the authors to suggest that the measure might serve as a valuable screening tool and a cut-point score of six is also explored. The unique benefit of the MGI, which could also be considered its drawback for use in large scale research studies, is that it allows women to comment on any aspect of their own lives after childbirth and is individualized in its nature. Symon et al. (2002) study was not without limitations, including the small sample utilized and the MGI needs further testing in terms of its reliability and validity. Its use since its introduction appears to have been limited.

7   Maternal Postpartum Quality of Life Tool

A recent study developed and tested a 41 item self-report measure to assess postpartum experience and quality of life of new mothers in the early postnatal period (Hill et al., 2006). The Maternal Postpartum Quality of Life Tool (MAPP-QOL), adopted the definition, domains and conceptual model from the work of Ferrens (1990) and Ferrens and Powers (1992).

☐ Figure 141-6

Diagrammatic representation of a tri-dimensional model of the SF-36 specifying separable physical, mental and general well-being components within a higher order health quality of life domain. The figure shows the sub-scales of the SF-36 and their relationship to physical, mental and general well-being quality of life higher order domains. This represents a sophisticated conceptualization of a unique measurement model of the SF-36, informed by clinical research observations. These more sophisticated measurement models are of importance as they provide useful insights into the responding characteristics of distinct clinical groups on the instrument which may have unique responding "signatures" or profiles. This model also highlights the developing area of clinical interest in the measurement characteristics of commonly used quality of life assessment tools

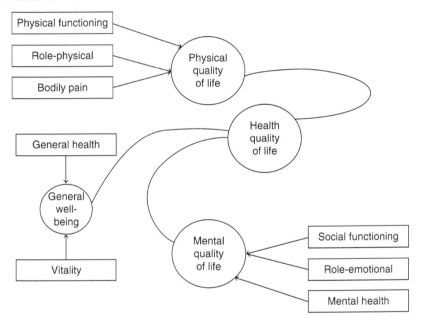

The Quality of Life Index (Ferrens, 1990) has core items and condition specific items and has demonstrated good internal consistency across various clinical groups. The bulk of the items in the MAPP-QOL replicate those of the QLI, with items modified or developed to fit specific aspects of quality of life domains for postpartum mothers. Component analysis revealed to scale to consist of five domains linked to postnatal quality of life including psychological/baby; socio-economic; relational/spouse-partner; relational/family-friends; health and functioning. The measure performed relatively well from a psychometric perspective, with alpha co-efficients across the domains ranging from 0.82–0.96, convergent validity was supported by a strong correlation (r = 0.69), whilst discriminate validity was supported by negative correlations with the four negative mood states of the Multiple Affect Adjective Check List Revised (anxiety; depression; hostility and dysphoria). Hill et al. (2006) study was not without limitations in terms of sample size and type and the utility of this scale clearly requires further evaluation. Despite it relatively good performance, this measure remains in its infancy.

8   Inventory of Functional Status after Childbirth

The Inventory of Functional status after Childbirth (IFSAC: Fawcett et al., 1988) was designed for assessment of the functional status in the specific situation of recovery from childbirth. With functional status in this context defined as the mother's readiness to assume infant care responsibilities and resume self-care, household, social, community and occupational activities. The model was conceptually derived from and an attempt to operationalized Roy's Adaptation model. The IFSAC is a 36 item measure arranged into five subscales, reflecting the definition above infant care responsibilities (six items); self care activities (eight items); household activities (12 items); social and community activities (six items) and occupational activities (four items). Items are scored on a four point scale ranging from "never" to "all the time," high mean scores for individual subscales and total scale indicated greater functional status. Initial psychometric testing revealed modest but acceptable levels of internal consistency, poor construct validity and correlations between subscales which suggested the need for further testing and refinement.

9   Conclusion

Pregnancy and childbirth are associated with intense physical changes and often a great deal of emotional upheaval, with the ability to perform usual roles affected (Attard et al., 2002). Even in an uneventful pregnancy women have subtle changes that may detract from their quality of life (Heuston and Kasik-Miller, 1998). It seems apparent that quality of life may have a significant role to play in the psychological well-being of pregnant and postnatal women, with a possible suggestion that recognition and validation by caregivers of the need for pregnant women to make changes in lifestyle will contribute to improved quality of life and less risk of psychological sequalae. However evidence regarding outcomes related to quality of life and maternity experience remains scant and merits further investigation before any clear associations can be made between quality of life issues and pregnant and postnatal women's psychological well-being. Further research must also concentrate on the utility of the measures available to measure quality of life and contribute to the debate on reliable instruments to identify and/or predict physical detriment and psychological sequelae.

Summary Points

- Pregnancy is associated with physiological and psychological changes which may impact in quality of life.
- The postnatal period is also associated with specific presentations such as postnatal depression which may impact negatively on quality of life.
- There is a relative vacuum in the research literature on the relationship of pregnancy and the postnatal period to quality of life.
- Depression can occur during pregnancy and have a negative impact on quality of life.
- The physical consequences of childbirth including birth trauma may impact negatively on perceived quality of life.
- The presence of a relatively low perceived quality of life during the antenatal period may predict later postnatal depression.

- Gender of the baby may be an important contributor to the mothers perceived quality of life, with a male baby having a more negative effect in this domain.
- Assessment of key psychological domains germain to quality of life is difficult during pregnancy and the postnatal period with evidence of a number of significant psychometric concerns related to measurement.
- The evidence base in relation to quality of life during pregnancy and in the postnatal period is developing rapidly but much further research is needed in this area.

References

Albers LL, Borders N. (2007). J Midwifery Womens Health. 52: 246–253.

Attard CL, Kohli MA, Coleman S, Bradley C, Hux M, Atanackovic G, Torrance GW. (2002). Am J Obstet Gynecol. 186: 222–227.

Brown S, Lumley J. (2000). Br J Obstet Gynaecol. 107: 1194–2001.

Coulehan J, Schulberg H, Block M, Madonia M, Rodriguez E. (1997). Arch Intern Med. 157: 1113–1120.

Cox JL, Holden J, Sagovsky R. (1987). Br J Psychiatry. 150: 782–786.

de Tychey C, Briancon S, Lighezzolo J, Spitz E, Kabuth B, de Luigi V, Messmebourg C, Girvan F, Rosati A, Thockler A, Vincent S. (2007). J Clin Nurs (Online Early Articles). Available from http://www.blackwell-synergy.com/doi/abs/10.1111/j.1365–2702.2006.01911.x.

Eason E, Labrecque M, Feldman P. (2000). Obstet Gynecol. 95: 464–471.

Dwight M, Kowdley K, Rus J, Ciechanowski P. (2000). J Psychosom Res 49: 311–317.

Fawcett J, Tulman L, Myers ST. (1988). J Nurse Midwifery. 33(6): 252–260.

Ferrens C. (1990). Oncol Nurs Forum. 17(3): 15–21.

Ferrens C, Powers M. (1992). Res Nurs Health. 15: 29–38.

Förger F, Østensen M, Schumacher A, Villiger PM. (2005). Ann Rheum Dis. 64: 1494–1499.

Gerard Jansen AJ, Essink-Bot M-L, Duvekot JJ, van Rhenen DJ. (2007). J Psychosom Res. 63: 275–281.

Gross H, Pattison H. (2007). Sanctioning Pregnancy. Routledge, Hove.

Haas JS, Jackson RA, Fuentes-Afflick E, Stewart AL, Dean ML, Brawarsky P, Escobar GJ. (2005). J Gen Intern Med. 20: 45–51.

Haas J, Meneses V, McCormick M. (1999). J Womens Health Gend Based Med. 8: 547–553.

Hays R, Wells K, Sherbourne C, Rogers W, Spritzer K. (1995). Arch Gen Psychiatry. 53: 899–904.

Heuston W, Kasik-Miller S. (1998). J Fam Pract. 47: 209–212.

Hill PD, Aldag JC. (2007). J Gynecol Neonatal Nurs. 36(4): 328–334.

Hill PD, Aldag JC, Hekel B, Riner G, Bloomfield P. (2006). J Nurs Meas. 14(3): 205–220.

Hyyppa MT, Kronholm E, Mattler CE. (1991). Br J Med Psychol. 64: 24–34.

Jansen G, Essink-Bot M-L, Duvekot JJ, van Rhenen DJ. (2007). J Psychosom Res. 63(3): 275–281.

Jomeen J, Martin CR. (2004). Psychol Health. 19: 787–800.

Jomeen J, Martin CR. (2005). J Psychosom Res. 59: 131–138.

Jomeen J, Martin CR. (in press). J Eval Clin Pract.

Karimova GK, Martin CR. (2003). Psychol Health Med. 8(1): 89–103.

Kelly RH, Russo J, Katon W. (2001). Gen Hosp Psychiatry. 23(3): 107–113.

Launer LJ, Villar J, Kestler E, de Onis M. (1990). Br J Obstet Gynaecol. 97: 62–70.

Lydon-Rochelle MT, Holt VL, Martin DP. (2001). Paediatr Perinat Epidemiol. 15(3): 232–240.

Magee LA, Chandra K, Mazzotta P, Stewart D, Koren G, Guyatt, G. (2002). Am J Obstet Gynecol. 186(5): 232–238.

Mackey MC, Coster-Schultz MA. (1992). Clin Nurs Res. 1: 366–284.

Martin CR, Jomeen J. (2003). J Reprod Infant Psychol. 21: 267–278.

Martinez-Schallmoser LD. (1992). Perinatal depressive symptoms, quality of life, social support and risk factors in Mexican-American women. PH.D., University of Illinois.

Mason L, Glenn S, Walton I, Appleton C. (1999). Birth. 26(3): 164–171.

McKee MD, Cunningham M, Janklowski MA, Zayas L. (2001). Obstet Gynecol. 97: 998–993.

Monaham PA, De Joseph JF. (1991). J Perinat Neonat Nurs. 4: 12–21.

Nicholson WK, Setse R, Hill-Briggs F, Cooper LA, Strobino D, Powe NR. (2006). Obstet Gynecol. 107: 798–806.

O'Brien B, Naber S. (1992). Birth. 19: 138–143.

Ochet F, Carey MA, Adam L. (1999). Obstet Gynecol. 94: 935–941.

Okubo N, Mitsuhashi Y, Saito K. (2000). 14: 35–44.

Pesavento F, Marconcini E, Drago D. (2005). Minerva Ginecol. 57: 451–460.

Russo J, Katon M, Sullivan M, Clark M, Buchwald D. (1994). Psychosomatics. 35: 546–556.

Simon GE. (2003). Biol Psychiatry. 54: 208–215.

Simon G, Von Korff M, Piccinelli C, Fullerton C, Ormel J. (1999). N Engl J Med. 341: 1329–1335.

Small R, Lumley J, Donohue L, Potter A, Waldenstrom U. (2000). Br Med J. 321: 1043–1047.

Small R, Lumley J, Yelland J. (2003). J Psychosom Obstet Gynaecol. 24: 45–52.

Sternfield B. (1997). Sports Med. 23: 33–47.

Symon A, MacDonald A, Ruta D. (2002). Birth. 29: 40–46.

Tulman L, Fawcett J. (1990). 22(3): 191–194.

Ware Jr JE, Sherbourne CD. (1992). Med Care. 30: 473–483.

Ware JE, Kosinski MA, Dewey JE. (2000). How to Score Version 2 of the SF-36 Health Survey. Quality Metric: Lincoln (RI)

Waterstone M, Wolfe C, Hooper R, Bewley S. (2003). Br J Obstet Gynaecol. 110: 128–133.

Wells K, Stewart R, Hays M, Burnam W, Rogers W, Daniels M, Berry S, Greenfield S, Ware J. (1989). JAMA. 283: 212–230.

Williams A, Herron-Marx S, Knibb R. (2007). J Clin Nurs. 16, 549–561.

Woo GM. (1997). Ann Behav Med. 19: 385–398.

Zigmond AR, Snaith RP. (1983). Acta Psychiatr Scand. 67: 361–370.

142 Generic Quality of Life Measures for Children and Adolescents

K. J. Zullig · M. R. Matthews · R. Gilman · R. F. Valois · E. S. Huebner

1	*Introduction*	*2424*
1.1	Relevance of Quality of Life Measurement to Health Care	2424
1.2	The Challenge of Quality of Life Measurement	2426
2	*Methodology*	*2426*
2.1	Generic Measures Including both Objective and Subjective Aspects of QOL	2427
2.1.1	Comprehensive Quality of Life Scale-School Version	2427
2.1.2	Quality of Life Profile: Adolescent Version	2428
2.2	Generic Subjective QOL Measures	2429
2.2.1	Youth Quality of Life-Research Version	2429
2.2.2	Multidimensional Students' Life Satisfaction Scale	2431
3	*Future Directions for Research*	*2433*
3.1	Quality of Life Measurement: How many Domains can and Should be Measured?	2434
4	*National Adolescent Indexes to Match Objective and Subjective QOL Data*	*2435*
4.1	Limitations of the CWI	2436
4.2	Conclusions	2436
	Summary Points	*2436*
	Appendix A	*2438*

Abstract: The purpose of this chapter was to review generic measures of child and adolescent (ages 18 or less) quality of life (QOL) that have been applied in at least two populations (e.g., age groups, nationalities, etc.) and have yielded strong psychometric properties. The chapter begins with a discussion regarding the relevance of quality of life measurement to health care. Next, we briefly review the challenges associated with QOL measurement in general followed by multidimensional measures that have been applied to various general (i.e., non-clinical) samples. Multidimensional measures were chosen for this review because they gather important information across a number of life domains. For example, understanding the contribution of environmental factors to an adolescent's behavioral, cognitive, and overall health functioning is critical to understanding human development In this regard, multidimensional QOL measures can help assess the potential influence of various proximal (e.g., quality of school experiences) and distal factors (e.g., quality of neighborhood environment) on life quality among youth.

The measures in this review are classified into two categories: (1) those that contain both objective and subjective QOL indicators, and (2) those comprised of subjective QOL measures only. Specifically, we review the Comprehensive Quality of Life Scale-School Version (Com-QOL-S5: Cummins, 1997), the Quality of Life Profile-Adolescent Version (QOLPAV: Raphael et al., 1996), the Youth Quality of Life (YQOL: Edwards et al., 2002; Patrick et al., 2002), and the Multidimensional Students' Life Satisfaction Scale (MSLSS: Huebner, 1994). Lastly, we recommend some suggestions for future research in youth QOL measurement, including promising efforts to use QOL as one overall index of well-being.

List of Abbreviations: *BASC 2*, behavior assessment system for children-second edition; *CWI*, child and youth well-being index; *CHIP-AE*, child health and illness profile; *CHQ-CF80*, child health questionnaire-child form; *CHQ-PF50*, child health questionnaire-parent form; *CDI*, children's depression inventory; *ComQOL-S5*, comprehensive quality of life scale-school version; *CADS-A*, conners' auxiliary adhd/dsm iv instrument; *FDI*, functional disability inventory; *GCQ*, generic children's quality of life measure; *KINDL*, German Munich quality of life questionnaire for children; *MSLSS*, multidimensional students' life satisfaction scale; *PedsQL*, pediatric quality of life inventory; *PWI-SC*, personal well-being index-school children; *QOL*, quality of life; *QOLPAV*, quality of life profile-adolescent version; *SF-36*, short form; *SF-12*, short form-12 health survey; *SIP*, sickness impact profile; *TedQL*, teddy quality of life; *C-QOL*, the quality of life measure for children; *YQOL*, youth quality of life

1   Introduction

1.1   Relevance of Quality of Life Measurement to Health Care

A number of recent studies consistently note how increasing levels of life quality appear to protect against factors that may potentially contribute to psychological and interpersonal distress. For example, Gilman and Huebner (2006) found that adolescents reporting exceedingly high overall QOL (i.e., scores in the top 20% of the distribution) were significantly less likely to report elevated levels of psychopathology (e.g., depression, anxiety), and to report significantly more positive interpersonal relationships and school attitudes than adolescents reporting exceedingly low QOL (i.e., scores in the bottom 20% of the distribution). Equally if not more important, adolescents in the high QOL group also reported greater adaptation than peers who reported "average" QOL (scores in the middle of the distribution), suggesting that optimal levels of QOL confer benefits that are not found among even among youth reporting typical levels (see Greenspoon and Saklofske, 2001 for further support). Similar findings have been reported in other studies-both with respect to self-reported overall QOL (Suldo and Huebner, 2006) and to specific QOL domains (e.g., school experiences; see Huebner and Gilman, 2006).

Given the findings that suggest that high QOL and various indices of positive behavioral, interpersonal, and educational adjustment are interrelated, the application of QOL measurement to healthcare professions is important for a number of reasons. First, the use of QOL ratings may provide important information above and beyond that what is traditionally measured in health care settings-typically symptom presence and severity (see Frisch, 1998). Nevertheless, anecdotal (Frisch et al., 1992) and empirical evidence (Keyes, 2007) finds that successful elimination of maladaptive behaviors does not necessarily lead to optimal life quality. That is, one cannot assume that individuals will behave or feel "good" simply because they no longer feel "bad". Although these findings and comments were specific to adults, similar statements have been made among adolescent researchers as well (Huebner et al., 2006).

Second, although most adolescents are healthy *and* report being in good health (Irwin et al., 2002), the assumption that physical health difficulties may go unrecognized among adolescents until an actual serious physical illness manifests itself is problematic. For example, Zullig et al. (2005) found that adolescents who reported just 1–2 poor physical health days during the past 30 were significantly more likely to report dissatisfaction with life. In this same study with dissatisfaction with life increasing linearly as number of reported poor days increased. Studies with adults have revealed associations between life satisfaction reports and a variety of health conditions (see Frisch et al., 2003 for a review). For instance, low life satisfaction reports are associated with physical health problems, including myocardial infarctions, chronic pain syndrome, respiratory tract infections, and colds. Low life satisfaction has been shown to predict mental health problems, such as depression, anxiety, and somatoform disorders as well as suicide. Individual differences in life satisfaction also significantly predict longevity (Frisch et al., 2003). Thus, youth reporting a greater number of poor physical health days during the past 30 days may be at greater risk for any of these conditions as they age.

Third, QOL ratings may help monitor how adolescents' in health care settings perceive the quality of their treatment, which is in turn a factor contributing to compliance. There is an axiom that what gets measured gets done (Moore et al., 2003). Yet often what is monitored is outcome data based solely on measures of psychopathology or objective indicators (e.g., frequency of disruptive behaviors observed). However, there is an association between intervention compliance and positive perceptions of the intervention itself. For example, among adults Carlson and Gabriel (2001) reported that patients in a drug treatment program who rated the quality of services as high were more likely to abstain from drugs even 1 year after receiving treatment. Among adolescents, QOL reports appear to show treatment sensitivity and compliance. For instance, longitudinal studies of adolescents first entering a residential treatment setting reported different (and consistently higher) QOL levels through the course of time, with the level of QOL related to treatment compliance (Gilman and Handwerk, 2001). These findings suggest that perceived life quality is an important and meaningful component of compliance and should be monitored throughout the course of treatment. Indeed, considering the aforementioned psychological, psychosocial, and psychoeducational benefits that are conferred to youth reporting optimal QOL, such monitoring may provide healthcare professionals with repeated opportunities to assess domain-specific life quality across treatment phases, in hopes that the reports change from "low" to "neutral" to "high."

Similarly, decrements in QOL reports across particular domains would suggest detrimental effects for youth receiving treatment.

1.2 The Challenge of Quality of Life Measurement

We must acknowledge at the outset that the definition of QOL and its subsequent measurement have been varied and diverse. Part of the challenge of QOL measurement stems from the fact that there has been little consensus as to what QOL "really is" (Schalock and Parameter, 2000), leading some QOL researchers to question the utility of the Term altogether (Rapley, 2003), mainly because it is not a directly measurable construct, nor is it a consistent entity across populations.

Historically, QOL measurement as a societal-level concern has been approached from two broad perspectives: objective and subjective. A traditional objective approach focused on external, quantifiable conditions of a particular culture or geographic area such as income levels, quality and available housing, crime rates, divorce rates, access to medical services, school attendance, life expectancy, and suicide rates. On the other hand, a traditional subjective approach disputed measuring QOL in an exclusively objective sense, and instead, suggested subjective indicators (e.g., sense of community, satisfaction with life, sense of safety, relationships with family, etc.) should take precedent and complement more traditional, objective QOL indicators.

Pragmatically speaking, the relationships between the two have been surprisingly modest, indicating that both approaches reveal unique information that is crucial to the understanding of overall life quality. As are result, some QOL instruments combine of self-reported subjective perceptions of life circumstances and objective circumstances (e.g., the number of physician visitations within a 3-month period, number of drugs or alcohol use events within the last 30 days, etc).

Our take on QOL measurement in general, but specifically for ❷ children and adolescents in this chapter, is the appropriateness of a measure for the research topic. For example, if a researcher is interested in measuring the QOL of adolescents' family life, then it is best to have a family domain measure of QOL in a chosen instrument. More importantly, that family measure should reliably and validly assess what it purports to assess. Thus, the purpose of this chapter is to review generic measures of child and adolescent (ages 18 or less) QOL that have been applied in at least two populations (e.g., age groups, nationalities, etc.) and have yielded strong psychometric properties. Given the relevance of quality of life measurement to health care, we have reviewed measures that fit our criteria for inclusion by offering credible ❷ reliability and ❷ validity evidence.

2 Methodology

In order for measures to be included in this chapter, instruments must have met the following criteria: they were developed for children and adolescents under the age of 18, applied in at least two populations (e.g., age groups, nationalities, etc.) and have yielded strong psychometric properties. When a particular measure was not reported directly from a child or adolescent respondent, or if a parent or guardian provided the response, these QOL measures were also included. Measures were considered to be generic if the measure demonstrated validity and applicability to non-clinical child or adolescent populations. Given these criteria, 15 generic quality of life measures for children and adolescents were identified through an extensive review of the literature.

In examining the 15 generic quality of life measures, four met our search criteria. These four are: (1) the Comprehensive Quality of Life Scale-School Version (ComQOL-S5; Cummins, 1997); (2) the Quality of Life Profile-Adolescent Version (QOLPAV; Raphael et al., 1996); (3) the Youth Quality of Life (YQOL; Edwards et al., 2002; Patrick et al., 2002); and (4) the Multidimensional Students' Life Satisfaction Scale (MSLSS; Huebner, 1994). Study sample demographics for each reviewed objective and subjective measure are provided in ❯ Table 142-1. Unless otherwise noted, additional tables and detailed scoring information of each reviewed scale are provided within the text.

The 11 others [The Quality of Life Measure for Children (C-QOL); Personal Well-Being Index-School Children (PWI-SC); Child Health and Illness Profile (CHIP-AE); Child Health Questionnaire-Child Form (CHQ-CF80); Child Health Questionnaire-Parent Form (CHQ-PF50); Pediatric Quality of Life Inventory (PedsQL); Generic Children's Quality of Life Measure (GCQ); Teddy Quality of Life (TedQL); Short Form-12 Health Survey (SF-12); Short Form (SF-36); Sickness Impact Profile (SIP)] were excluded because additional research is necessary or are they are not appropriate measures of QOL. All measures are completed by the child or adolescent with the exception of the CHQ-PF50, which is completed by the child's parent or guardian.

2.1 Generic Measures Including both Objective and Subjective Aspects of QOL

2.1.1 Comprehensive Quality of Life Scale-School Version

The ComQOL-S5 (Cummins, 1997) (see ❯ Table 142-1 for full study references) is self-administered and is comprised of seven domains (Material Well-Being, Health, Productivity, Intimacy, Safety, Place in Community, Emotional Well-Being). Scoring for each domain is computed by obtaining a satisfaction score for each domain and weighting that score by the perceived importance to the individual. Either component can be administered independently if so desired, and it has demonstrated validity and reliability with adolescents aged 12–18 years old (see Appendix for full scale complete with scoring instructions).

Being the fifth edition of the ComQOL-S, the ComQOL-S5 has similar validity and reliability measures as the ComQOL-S fourth edition (ComQOL-S4). The ComQOL-S4 was originally examined by Bearsley (1997) and included 524 adolescents aged 14–17 years old who were: (1) homeless or "at risk" for homelessness; (2) community school students (with a high frequency of behavioral, emotional, family, or learning problems); and (3) non-homeless secondary school students. For the subjective portion of the ComQOL-S4, Importance ($\alpha = 0.76$) and Satisfaction ($\alpha = 0.80$) yielded acceptable levels of internal consistency. For the objective portion of the scale, correlations for each of the individual items versus the domain score were found to be significant ($p < 0.01$). Criterion-related validity was determined through comparisons with the Life Attitude Profile-Revised Scale (Recker, 1992) and the ComQOL-S4's subjective portion. Results revealed the ComQOL-S4 was positively correlated with choice and responsibleness ($r = 0.45$), goal seeking ($r = 0.16$), and personal meaning ($r = 0.61$), and negatively with death acceptance ($r = -0.01$) and existential vacuum ($r = -0.48$).

◘ Table 142-1

Sampling characteristics of generic QOL measures for children and adolescents

Measure	Location	N	Mean Age	Gender	Race[a]
ComQOL-S5	Melbourne, Australia (Gullone and Cummins, 1998)	264	14.6	53% female	NA
	Australia (Bearsley, 1997)	524	15.8	57% female	NA
QOLPAV	Perth, Western Australia	363	13.8	67% female	NA
	(Meuleners et al., 2003, 2005)	167	17.4	62% female	NA
	Great Britain (Bradford et al., 2002)	899	14.0	46% female	94% C, 6% O
YQOL-R	Seattle, WA, USA (Patrick et al., 2002)	236	12–18	30% female	80% C, 5% AA, 1% H
	Seattle, WA, USA (Topolski et al., 2004)	214	14.8		80.5% C, 4.7% AA, 13.9% O
MSLSS	Columbia, SC USA (Huebner and Dew, 1993a, b)	222	15.5	52% female	50% C, 51% AA
	Columbia, SC USA (Huebner et al., 1998)	291	12.9	57% female	55% C, 41% AA, 4% O
	Columbia, SC USA (Gilman et al., 2000)	321	16.1	65% female	42% C, 56% AA, 2% H
	Midwest and Northeast, USA (Gilman et al., 2004)	159	13.0	44% female	84.3% C, 5% AA, 10.7% O
	South Korea and South Carolina, USA (Park et al., 2004)	1,657	12.8	49% female	50.4% K; 49.6% A
	Croatia and Southeast, USA (Gilman et al., 2005)	632	14.7	60% female	46% CRxO; 54% A
	Tokyo, Japan and Honolulu, USA (Ito and Smith, 2006)	995	NA	51% female	62% J; 38% A

NA not available

[a]*C* Caucasian; *AA* African American; *H* Hispanic; *O* other; *K* Korean; *CRO* Croatian; *J* Japanese; *A* American; *NA* not available

2.1.2 Quality of Life Profile: Adolescent Version

The Quality of Life Profile: Adolescent Version (QOLPAV) (Raphael et al., 1996) has also been applied to numerous populations (see ❷ *Table 142-1* for full study references). The QOLPAV began its development with six high school student focus groups (grades 9–13) to gather information regarding what the term "quality of life" means and to gain insight on specific concerns that adolescents have in their lives. Questions developed from these focus groups were then examined by different adolescents to verify content relevance, identify missing topics, and assess the wording of the QOLPAV. This information led to a 54-item questionnaire containing three broad domains (Being, Belonging, and Becoming), which were formed from nine subdomains (physical being, physical belonging, practical becoming, psychological being, social belonging, leisure becoming, spiritual being, community belonging, growth becoming). All items were responded to with a five-point Likert response scale ranging from 1 ("Not at all Important"/"No Satisfaction at All") to 5 ("Extremely Important"/"Extremely Satisfied").

Reliability for the QOLPAV was calculated using a Cronbach's alpha for each of the subdomains, the broad domains and for the overall score. For all of the broad domains, $\alpha \geq 0.80$ (Being items $\alpha = 0.85$, Belonging items $\alpha = 0.83$, Becoming items $\alpha = 0.87$). For the subdomains all coefficients approached or exceeded 0.70 (physical being $\alpha = 0.68$; physical belonging $\alpha = 0.67$; practical becoming $\alpha = 0.74$; psychological being $\alpha = 0.72$; social belonging $\alpha = 0.69$; leisure becoming $\alpha = 0.74$; spiritual being $\alpha = 0.71$; community belonging $\alpha = 0.68$; growth becoming $\alpha = 0.79$). The overall score demonstrated high internal consistency ($\alpha = 0.94$). To assess the validity of the QOLPAV, correlational analyses were performed on measures of self-esteem, life satisfaction, social support, and life chances taken from the Youth Transition Study (Bachman et al., 1967). The QOLPAV demonstrated significant ($p < 0.01$) correlations with all four measures (ranging from 0.45 to 0.56). The QOLPAV is a private domain scale and therefore the actual scale items are not provided. However, complete information regarding the QOLPAV, including ordering information can be located at http://www.utoronto.ca/qol/qolPublications.htm.

2.2 Generic Subjective QOL Measures

2.2.1 Youth Quality of Life-Research Version

The Youth Quality of Life-Research Version (YQOL-R: Edwards et al., 2002) has been administered to separate groups of youth aged 12–18 years with and without disabilities (see ❷ *Table 142-1* for full study references).

YQOL-R validity analyses included 210 adolescents (with and without disabilities) with a test battery of 49 items. Convergent validity was established by comparing the measure with the German Munich Quality of Life Questionnaire for Children (KINDL; Ravens-Sieberer and Bullinger, 1998) and the Children's Depression Inventory (CDI; Kovacs, 1992). Group/discriminant validity was assessed through the use of the Conners' Auxiliary ADHD/DSM IV Instrument (CADS-A; Conners, 1997), the Functional Disability Inventory (FDI; Walker and Greene, 1991), and the Youth Disability Screener (Patrick et al., 1998).

These analyses resulted in a 41-item measure consisting of five domains: Self, Relationship, Environment, and General Quality of Life. All of the domains in the YQOL-R correlated highly with all domains of the KINDL (average $r = 0.73$, $p < 0.05$). Additionally, findings indicate that the correlations between the YQOL-R and KINDL were significant and in the expected direction. These findings suggest that the YQOL-R is sensitive to adolescents' current symptom status (e.g., the YQOL-R perceptual scores were significantly lower for those adolescents who scored above the depression cut-point on the CDI, and above the ADHD cut-point on the CADS-A; Patrick et al., 2002). ❷ *Table 142-2* provides the YQOL-R items by domains. The QOL scores are summed and those are then transformed to a scale from 0 to 100 for ease of interpretation, where higher scores indicate higher QOL.

◼ Table 142-2

YQOL-R items by domain

Self
1. I keep trying even if at first I don't succeed
2. I can handle most difficulties that come my way
3. I am able to do most things as well as I want
4. I feel good about myself
5. I feel I am important to others
6. I feel comfortable with my sexual feelings and behaviors
7. I have enough energy to do the things I want to do
8. I am pleased with how I look
9. I feel comfortable with the amount of stress in my life
10. I feel it is okay if I make mistakes
11. I feel my life has meaning
12. My personal beliefs give me strength
13. I feel alone in my life
14. I feel left out because of who I am
Relationships
15. I feel most adults treat me fairly
16. I feel I am getting the right amount of attention from my family
17. I feel understood by my parents or guardians
18. I feel useful and important to my family
19. I feel my family cares about me
20. My family encourages me to do my best
21. I feel I am getting along with my parents or guardians
22. I feel my parents or guardians allow me to participate in important decisions which affect me
23. I try to be a role model for others
24. I can tell my friends how I really feel
25. I am happy with the friends I have
26. I am satisfied with my social life
27. I feel I can take part in the same activities as others my age
28. People my age treat me with respect
Environment
29. I feel my life is full of interesting things to do
30. I like trying new things
31. I like my neighborhood
32. I look forward to the future
33. My family has enough money to live a decent life
34. I feel safe when I am at home
35. I feel I am getting a good education
36. I know how to get the information that I need

◘ Table 142-2 (continued)

37. I enjoy learning new things
38. I feel safe when I am at school
General QOL
39. I enjoy life
40. I am satisfied with the way my life is now
41. I feel life is worthwhile

Items 2–4, 6–8, 9–11, 13–15, 19, 20, 23, 25, 26, 27, 33–36, 40, 41 use a 11-point rating scale with adjectival anchors "Not at All" to "Completely". Items 1, 5, 12, 16–18, 21, 22, 24, 28–32, 37, 39 use a 11-point rating scale with adjectival anchors "Not at All" to "A Great Deal"

2.2.2   Multidimensional Students' Life Satisfaction Scale

The Multidimensional Students' Life Satisfaction Scale (MSLSS) is a 40-item, subjective QOL instrument that assesses life satisfaction across five domains shown to important to the lives of youth (Family, Friends, School, Living Environment, and Self) in addition to an overall life satisfaction assessment (Huebner, 1994) (see ❷ *Table 142-1*).

The MSLSS is appropriate for use on children between the ages of 8 and 18 and has been administered to over 4,000 children and adolescents world-wide (see ❷ *Table 142-1*), making it one of the most frequently administered scales of its kind. The psychometric properties of the scale consistently yield robust values, with internal consistency estimates of each MSLSS domain ranging from 0.80 and higher. In addition, the Total score (which is an aggregate of all items and is akin to measure of general satisfaction) is 0.95 or higher in several studies (see Gilman and Huebner, 2000). Evidence for the construct validity has been found by comparing the domain scores with well-known behavior and self-concept scales, including the Behavior Assessment System for Children-Second Edition (BASC 2: Reynolds and Kamphaus, 2004) and the Self-Concept Scale (Marsh et al., 1984). Evidence for the construct validity has been consistently found using both exploratory (Huebner, 1994) and confirmatory factor analysis (Gilman et al., 1999). Finally, the factor structure of the scale is invariant with respect to nationality (Gilman et al., 2008). ❷ *Table 142-3* provides the MSLSS items by domains.

Scoring the MSLSS is straightforward. The four response options are assigned points as follows: (never = 1); (sometimes = 2); (often = 3); and (almost always = 4). Negatively-keyed items must be reverse scored (see ❷ *Table 142-3* for the list of negatively-keyed items). Hence, negatively-keyed items are scored so that almost always = 1, and so forth. Higher scores thus indicate higher levels of life satisfaction throughout the scale. It should be noted that a 6-point agreement format has been used with middle and high school students. In this case, response options are assigned points as follows: (1 = strongly disagree, 2 = moderately disagree, etc.). Because the domains consist of unequal number of items, the domain and total scores are made comparable by summing the item responses and dividing by the number of domain (or total) items.

An abbreviated version of the MSLSS is also available for research purposes or when resources are limited: the Brief Multidimensional Students' Life Satisfaction Scale (BMSLSS) (Seligson et al., 2003) (see ❷ *Table 142-4*). The BMSLSS contains one item for each domain of the MSLSS in addition to an overall item. Although space limits a detailed discussion of the BMSLSS, it has demonstrated acceptable psychometrics in several samples of youth ranging

◘ Table 142-3

Multidimensional students' life satisfaction (MSLSS) scale structure

Family
I enjoy being at home with my family
My family gets along well together
I like spending time with my parents
My parents and I doing fun things together
My family is better than most
Members of my family talk nicely to one another
My parents treat me fairly
Friends
My friends treat me well
My friends are nice to me
I wish I had different friends[a]
My friends are mean to me[a]
My friends are great
I have a bad time with my friends[a]
I have a lot of fun with my friends
I have enough friends
My friends will help me if I need it
School
I look forward to going to school
I like being in school
School is interesting
I wish I didn't have to go to school[a]
There are many things about school I don't like[a]
I enjoy school activities
I learn a lot at school
I feel bad at school[a]
Living environment
I like where I live
I wish there were different people in my neighborhood[a]
I wish I lived in a different house[a]
I wish I lived somewhere else[a]
I like my neighborhood
I like my neighbors
This town is filled with mean people[a]
My family's house is nice
There are lots of fun things to do where I live
Self
I think I am good looking

◻ Table 142-3 (continued)

I am fun to be around
I am a nice person
Most people like me
There are lots of things I can do well
I like to try new things
I like myself

[a]Reverse keyed items

◻ Table 142-4
Brief multidimensional students' life satisfaction scale (BMSLSS) items

I would describe my satisfaction with my family life as:
I would describe my satisfaction with my friendships as:
I would describe my satisfaction with my school experience as:
I would describe my satisfaction with myself as:
I would describe my satisfaction with where I live as:

Response options are a 7-point Likert-type scale based on anchors of terrible, unhappy, mostly dissatisfied, mixed (about equally satisfied and dissatisfied), mostly satisfied, pleased, and delighted

in age from elementary school to high school (Seligson et al., 2003, 2005). Furthermore, life satisfaction (via measurement with the BMSLSS) has been shown to be related to the six priority adolescent objective health behavior categories in the United States for premature morbidity and mortality as defined by the US Centers for Disease Control and Prevention. For instance, life dissatisfaction has been shown to be significantly associated with behaviors that lead to intentional and unintentional injuries (Valois et al., 2001, 2004a); increased use of tobacco, alcohol and other drugs (Zullig et al., 2001); increased risky sexual behavior (Valois et al., 2002); poor body image and dietary behavior (Valois et al., 2003); and physical inactivity (Valois et al., 2004b).

3   Future Directions for Research

In spite of the potential advantages of including multidimensional QOL measures in assessment strategies and prevention/intervention programs, several neglected areas remain. First, more theory-based research is needed. Although not necessarily problematic at the idiographic level, the selection of one QOL measure over another when examining QOL across groups and/or nations may only provide a partial explanation of the factors that contribute to QOL. Compounding this issue is the finding that not all QOL domains appear to have the same relevance across groups. For example, recent studies (Gilman et al., 2008; Park and Huebner, 2005) reported that mean scores were significantly different across QOL domains with the MSLSS, with these differences falling along the individualistic/collectivistic cultural continuum. Considering that many of the reviewed measures in this chapter have to date been administered to limited samples often representing only one cultural group, clearly additional studies are necessary to establish generalization of their findings. Such studies are necessary to expand the empirical understanding of what domains should be included when investigating QOL among adolescents.

Further, while the scales reviewed in this chapter have been administered to a variety of samples, many existing measures appear to be designed for a specific series of studies, or for a specific population. Few measures have attempted to expand their scope of focus to additional groups to address fundamental psychometric questions. For example, Gilman and Huebner (2000) recommended that existing child- or adolescent-focused QOL measures would benefit from rigorous studies of basic psychometric properties, including evaluations of normative samples, reliability, and validity. Additionally, research is needed to address limitations inherent in using self-reports, such as the potential effects of response distortions or social desirability. Although such strategies have been rarely used, other-raters (e.g., peers, teachers, parents) or the use of alternative methods of QOL assessment (such as using experiential time sampling) have been recommended as strategies to minimize response artifacts (see Huebner et al., 2007 for a comprehensive review of these strategies).

Moreover, research on QOL has been limited mostly to cross-sectional research. Studies of the correlates of QOL offer a useful initial step, but advancement of QOL research will require longitudinal and/or experimental studies to clarify the directionality of relationships. Although in their infancy, studies have shown that low QOL precedes the occurrence of psychological distress and poor health (e.g., Suldo and Huebner, 2004). Such findings provide unique and necessary information regarding the directionality of QOL effects as well as potential support for dual-factor models of mental health (Greenspoon and Saklofske, 2001).

3.1   Quality of Life Measurement: How many Domains can and Should be Measured?

Another area of future research is the consideration of what actually constitutes QOL in the terms of optimal number and types of domains to measure. Some research has been conducted that has attempted to name a specific number of QOL domains noteworthy across multiple QOL studies. Whereas Felce and Perry (1995) outline five domains of QOL (Material, Physical, Social, Emotional, and Productive Well-Being), Cummins' (1996) content analysis of 1,500 articles concerning the topic of QOL determined that at least seven domains compose subjective QOL: Material Well-Being, Health, Productivity, Intimacy, Safety, Community, and Emotional Well-Being. Of interest, Hagerty et al. (2001) suggest these domains should also be used to guide the use and selection of objective QOL assessments as well.

However, translating these domains to children and adolescents presents some challenges. For instance, Cummins' (1996) identified domains were based on studies of adults and support for the domains was primarily based on a content analysis procedures without following up with more psychometric analyses of particular scales (e.g., factor analyses, multitrait-multimethod tests of convergent and discriminant validity). The Multidimensional Students' Life Satisfaction Scale (MSLSS; Huebner, 1994) has offered empirical support, but contains five domains. Were we to strictly abide by Cummins' (1996) criteria, this would have precluded us from including the MSLSS in our review. What is more important to us is the appropriateness of the measure for the research topic. That is, if a researcher is interested in QOL among peers members, then the measure should contain a "peers" or "friends" domain; and each domain should be supported by research-based evidence of its validity.

Thus, continuing research is needed to empirically support the various multidimensional models available. There are also developmental issues we must acknowledge that challenge measurement in general, whether it is intelligence testing or QOL. If we borrow from Piaget's influential work, we understand that as youth age, they move through a series of stages with progressing cognitive abilities. Consequently, what is an appropriate QOL measure for youth in preoperational development (ages 2–7) where reasoning is limited owing to egocentrism, centering, and transductive reasoning may not be useful for youth in formal operational development (ages 11 and older) where youth are better equipped to think more abstractly, solve problems mentally, and engage in hypothetico-deductive reasoning. In other words, there is reason to believe that the nature and number of QOL domains that children and adolescents are able to differentiate may change across age groups. Younger children may be unable to distinguish domains to the same extent as older adolescents. Nevertheless, some preliminary research is emerging in the United States that attempts to maximize available data to assess child and adolescent QOL in the form of national index.

4 National Adolescent Indexes to Match Objective and Subjective QOL Data

Countries have long held the belief that monitoring QOL at the national-level is of great importance resulting in the creation of numerous indexes which were recently systematically reviewed (see Hagerty et al., 2001). Noteworthy conclusions from this comprehensive review (p. 86) include the need for: (1) the formulation of a domain structure common to all indexes; (2) additional predictive validity or sensitivity studies to establish causality; and (3) testing convergent validity against other QOL indexes. In this regard, there has been some progress, specifically pertaining to adolescent QOL measurement.

Promising efforts to match population objective and subjective QOL measurement into an overall index have been conducted by Land and colleagues (Land et al., 2001, 2007) using the Child and Youth Well-being Index (CWI). The CWI pulls from a variety of objective and subjective data sources (e.g., vital statistics and population-level survey data) and is based on 28 national-level indicators (see Land et al., 2001 for a full review and justification of these 28 indicators). Because 25 of the 28 indicators used in the CWI date back to 1975, while three (health insurance coverage, activity limitation reports, and subjective health assessments) were implemented in 1985, the CWI is calculated and indexed first by year: 1975 or 1985. According to Land et al. (2007, p. 112), "The base year value of the indicator is assigned a value of 100 and subsequent values of the indicator are taken as percentage changes in the index. The directions of the indicators are oriented so that a value greater (equal or lesser) than 100 in subsequent years means the social condition measured has improved (no change or deteriorated)," relative to its base year.

Land and colleagues (2007) have demonstrated the usefulness of the CWI by each of Cummins' (1996) QOL domains using 1975 as the referent year through 2003, indicating that from 1975 through 1993, overall adolescent QOL declined in the USA. However, from 1994 onward, the CWI indicated a sustained improvement in the QOL of American youth. When the CWI was computed by domain, Land et al. (2007) determined that much of the decline was in response to a decline in relationships and emotional/spiritual well-being. Even more interesting was an observed and persistent decrease in health from the mid-1980s through 2003. Land et al. (2007) attributes this decline to the increasing prevalence of obesity among youth in the United States and provides compelling sensitivity data showing that when the obesity indicator is included in the *Health* domain, it decreases by 24% from 1981 to 2001. When the obesity indicator is excluded, the health domain increases from 1975 to 1983 and has since remained relatively stable. Equally compelling comparisons are made by race, gender, and even overall life satisfaction levels of twelfth grade students. However, as with any developing index or measure, some limitations are extended to the CWI.

4.1 Limitations of the CWI

First, the CWI is highly reliant on objective indicators and restricted to currently available, national data resources. For example, only three of the 28 indicators are based on subjective assessments (e.g., self-perceived excellent/very good, good, fair, or poor health; activity limitation; and the importance of religion). Second, as observed by Land and colleagues (2007), the CWI domains of *Intimacy* and *Emotional and Spiritual Well-Being* are underdeveloped. In fact, a direct measure of *Emotional and Spiritual Well-Being* is not available and is instead measured via indicators of suicide, church attendance, and the importance of religion in one's life. As noted earlier, knowing the modest relationship between objective and subjective QOL indicators, despite the robust relationships identified between the CWI and several other adolescent health measures, additional adolescent QOL item development is recommended. Third, a comprehensive understanding of the relationship between mental "health" and mental illness needs to be made before such an index is realized. To date, quality of life studies have primarily focused on analyzing characteristics leading to positive outcomes, while the converse continues for those who research mental illness. There seems to be little discourse in the way of understanding the nexus between the two worlds. Although some efforts have been made in this area (e.g., Schwartz et al., 2007), much work remains in explaining adolescent psychosocial development.

4.2 Conclusions

Fortunately, there are quality measures already available that have yet to be incorporated into national-level youth surveys. For instance, all 15 identified generic adolescent QOL measures located for this chapter contain adequate measures of both intimacy and emotional well-being, elements which might be incorporated into national-level surveys to enhance the scope of measurement systems, such as the CWI. In conjunction with QOL researchers, local, regional, and national policy makers may wish to determine which particular QOL domains should be assessed to best serve their unique needs and interests, then select or develop various indices based on the research evidence available for the specific measures available, In short, they must address the question, "What should be measured for which specific purpose(s), with which particular population(s), under what specific conditions(s)?

Summary Points

- QOL appears to be a crucial psychological strength that is related to healthy adaptation in adolescents.

- The use of QOL ratings may provide important information above and beyond that what is traditionally measured in health care settings-typically symptom presence and severity.
- QOL measures can and should be used in conjunction with severity measures to monitor the effectiveness of a given intervention on enhanced life quality, in addition to symptom reduction.
- QOL reports can provide a multicontextual perspective because they gather important information across a number of life domains and may help monitor how adolescents' perceive the quality of interventions, which is in turn a factor contributing to treatment compliance.
- This chapter reviewed generic measures of child and adolescent (ages 18 or less) QOL that have been applied in at least two samples (e.g., age groups, nationalities, etc.) and have yielded strong psychometric properties.
- Four qualifying measures were identified and divided into two categories: (1) measures that assessed both objective and subjective ($n = 2$) and (2) measures that assessed subjective QOL only ($n = 2$).
- Acceptable objective and subjective QOL measures are: (1) the Comprehensive Quality of Life Scale-School Version (ComQOL-S5), and (2) the Quality of Life Profile-Adolescent Version (QOLPAV).
- Acceptable subjective QOL measures are: (1) the Youth Quality of Life (YQOL), and b) the Multidimensional Students' Life Satisfaction Scale (MSLSS).
- Eleven other measures [The Child Quality of life (C-QOL); Personal Wellbeing Index-School Children (PWI-SC); Child Health and Illness Profile (CHIP-AE); Child Health Questionnaire-Child Form (CHQ-CF80); Child Health Questionnaire-Parent Form (CHQ-PF50); Pediatric Quality of Life Inventory (PedsQL); Generic Children's Quality of Life Measure (GCQ); Teddy Quality of Life (TedQL); Short Form-12 Health Survey (SF-12); Short Form (SF-36); Sickness Impact Profile (SIP) were identified as, but are not being included.
- Although not necessarily problematic at the idiographic level, the selection of one QOL measure over another when examining QOL across groups and/or nations may only provide a partial explanation of the factors that contribute to perceived life quality.
- Few measures have attempted to expand their scope of focus to additional groups to address fundamental psychometric questions.
- Moreover, research on QOL has been limited mostly to cross-sectional research. Studies of the correlates of QOL offer a useful initial step, but advancement of QOL research will require longitudinal and/or experimental studies to clarify the directionality of relationships.
- Advocations for including well-being indicators as a national index of positive mental health have been made for adults and such an index would be salient for adolescents as well. Nevertheless, a comprehensive understanding of the relationship between mental "health" and mental illness needs to be made before such an index is realized.
- Efforts have been undertaken to address how many domains should QOL measure, but additional research is needed to empirically support a specific domain structure.
- The Child and Youth Well-being Index (CWI) currently being tested on youth in the United States is providing the first steps toward that empirical support.

Appendix A

ComQol-S5 Cummins, 1997

This scale has three sections. The first will ask you for some factual information. The next two will ask how you feel about various aspects of your life.

To answer each question put a (√) in the appropriate box. Please ask for assistance if there is anything you do not understand.

Please answer all the questions and do not spend too much time on any one item.

What is your date of birth?   _____/_____/_____

                                         day   month   year

What is your sex? (circle one)   Male   Female

Section 1

This section asks for information about various aspects of your life. Please tick the box that most accurately describes your situation.

*1(a)   Where do you live?

A house   ☐

A flat or apartment   ☐

A room (e.g. in a hostel) ☐
or caravan

Do your parents own the place where you live or do they pay rent?

Own   ☐

Rent   ☐

*b)   How many clothes and toys do you have compared with other people of your age?

More than almost anyone	More than most people	About average	Less than most people	Less than almost anyone
☐	☐	☐	☐	☐

*c)   **If either of your parents has paid work, please give the name of their job.**

Father   _____

Mother   _____

2a)   **How many times have you seen a doctor over the past 3 months?**

None	1–2	3–4 (about once a month)	5–7 (about every two weeks)	8 or more (about once a week or more)
☐	☐	☐	☐	☐

b)   **Do you have any on-going medical problems? (e.g. visual, hearing, physical, health, etc.).**

Yes ☐   No ☐

If **yes** please specify:

Name of medical condition	*Extent of medical condition*
e.g. Visual	Require glasses for reading
Diabetes	Require daily injections
Epilepsy	Requires daily medication

_____   _____

_____   _____

_____   _____

(c)   **What regular medication do you take *each day*?**

If none tick box   ☐

or

Name(s) of medication (don't worry if you get the spelling wrong)

_____

_____

_____

_____

3(a)   **How many hours do you spend on the following *each week*? (Average over past 3 months)**

Hours work for pay   0 ☐   1–10 ☐   11–20 ☐   21–30 ☐   31–40+ ☐
(not counting pocket
money)

Hours at school or college   0 ☐   1–10 ☐   11–20 ☐   21–30 ☐   31–40+ ☐

Hours unpaid child care   0 ☐   1–10 ☐   11–20 ☐   21–30 ☐   31–40+ ☐

(b)   **In your spare time, how often do you have <u>nothing</u> much to do?**

Almost always   Usually   Sometimes   Not Usually   Almost never
☐   ☐   ☐   ☐   ☐

(c)   **On *average*, how many hours TV do you watch each day?**

Hours per day

None   1–2   3–5   6–9   10 or more
☐   ☐   ☐   ☐   ☐

4(a)   **How often do you talk with a close friend?**

Daily	Several times a week	Once a week	Once a month	Less than once a month
☐	☐	☐	☐	☐

(b)   **If you are feeling sad or depressed, how often does someone show they care for you?**

(c)   **If you want to do something special, how often does someone else want to do it with you?**

(d)   **How often do you sleep well?**

(e)   **Are you safe at home?**

(f)   **How often are you worried or anxious during the day?**

Almost always	Usually	Sometimes	Not Usually	Almost never
☐	☐	☐	☐	☐

*6(a)   **Below is a list of leisure activities. Indicate how often in an *average_month* you attend or do each one for your enjoyment (not employment).**

Activity	Number of times per month
(1) Go to a club/group/society	_____
(2) Meet with friend(s)	_____
(3) Watch live sporting events (Not on TV)	_____
(4) Go to a place of worship	_____
(5) Chat with neighbours	_____
(6) Eat out	_____
(7) Go to a movie	_____
(8) Visit family	_____
(9) Play sport or go to a gym	_____
(10) Other (please describe)	_____

(b) **Do you hold an *unpaid* position of responsibility in relation to any team, club, group, or society?**

Yes ☐   No ☐   If no, go to question (c)

If '**yes**', please indicate the highest level of responsibility held:

☐ Committee Member

☐ Committee Chairperson/Convenor

☐ Secretary/Treasurer/Team Vice-captain

☐ Captain, Group President, Chairperson or Convenor

(c) **How often do people *outside your home* ask for your help or advice?**

Almost every day	Quite often	Sometimes	Not often	Almost never
☐	☐	☐	☐	☐

7(a) **How often can you do the things you *really* want to do?**

(b) **When you wake up in the morning, how often do you wish you could stay in bed *all day***

(c) **How often do you have wishes that *cannot* come true?**

Almost always	Usually	Sometimes	Not Usually	Almost never
☐	☐	☐	☐	☐

Section 2

How *Important* are each of the following life areas to you?

Please answer by placing a (√) in the appropriate box for each question.

There are no right or wrong answers. Please choose the box that best describes how **important each area is to you.** Do not spend too much time on any one question.

1. How *important to you* ARE THE THINGS YOU OWN?
2. How *important to you* is YOUR HEALTH?
3. How *important to you* is WHAT YOU ACHIEVE IN LIFE?
4. How *important to you* are CLOSE RELATIONSHIPS WITH YOUR FAMILY OR FRIENDS?
5. How *important to you* is HOW SAFE YOU FEEL?
6. How *important to you* is DOING THINGS WITH PEOPLE OUTSIDE YOUR HOME?
7. How *important to you* is YOUR OWN HAPPINESS?

Could not be more important	Very important	Somewhat important	Slightly important	Not important at all
☐	☐	☐	☐	☐

Section 3

How *satisfied* are you with each of the following life areas?

There are no right or wrong answers. Please (√) the box that best describes how **satisfied** you are with each area.

1. How *satisfied are you* with the THINGS YOU OWN?
2. How *satisfied are you* with your HEALTH?
3. How *satisfied are you* with what you ACHIEVE IN LIFE?
4. How *satisfied are you with* your CLOSE RELATIONSHIPS WITH FAMILY OR FRIENDS?
5. How *satisfied are you* with HOW SAFE YOU FEEL?
6. How *satisfied are you* with DOING THINGS WITH PEOPLE OUTSIDE YOUR HOME?
7. How *satisfied are you* with YOUR OWN HAPPINESS?

Delighted	Pleased	Mostly satisfied	Mixed	Mostly dissatisfied	Unhappy	Terrible
☐	☐	☐	☐	☐	☐	☐

Calculation of results for the ComQol-S5

1   Coding the objective data

The following information is relevant to the scoring procedures:

Missing values: Score as 9 (then get the computer to recognise ë9í as denoting a missing value).

Estimated income: The average adult Australian full-time wage in February 1997 was $38,063 per year. Users in other countries will need to modify the scoring of income on a pro rata basis.

MATERIAL WELL-BEING

1(a)   Accommodation:

house + own	= 5
flat/apartment + own	= 4
house + rent	= 3
flat/apartment + rent	= 2
Room + either	= 1

(b)   Possessions:

More than almost anyone	= 5	Less than most people	= 2
More than most people	= 4	Less than almost anyone	= 1
About average	= 3		

(c)   Estimated income:

More than $56,000	= 5	$11,000–$25,999	= 2
$41,000–$55,999	= 4	Below $10,999	= 1
$26,000–$40,999	= 3		

Below $10,999	**$11,000–$25,999**
Students	Laborers and related workers
People who are unemployed	

$26,000–$40,999

School teachers/Junior academics
Paraprofessionals
Clerks
Drivers
Personal service workers
Salespersons
Tradespersons

Farmers & farm managers
Managing supervisors
Artists & related professionals
Technical officers
Nurses
Police
Plant & machine operators/drivers

$41,000–$55,999

Legislators & government appoint officials
Managers and administrators
School principals
Professionals
Engineers & building professionals
Social professionals
Business professionals

56,000+

Managing directors/General managers
Medical doctors
Senior academics

HEALTH

2(a) **Doctor**   None = 5   5–7 = 2
                    1–2 = 4   8 or more visits = 1
                    3–4 = 3

b)   **Disability or medical condition**

5 =   No disability

4 =   Minor disability (e.g. eyeglasses) not likely to interfere with normal life activities or routines

3 =   Constant, chronic condition that interferes to some extent with daily life (e.g. diabetes, heart condition, Alzheimer's disease, migraines, infertility, asthma when nothing is recorded under medication, arthritis when nothing is recorded under medication)

2 =   Disability likely to restrict social activities (e.g. profound deafness, blindness, significant physical disability, depression, schizophrenia, arthritis, Parkinson's Disease, paraplegia, asthma needing regular medication, arthritis needing regular medication, limb missing)

1 =   Major disability likely to require daily assistance with personal care (e.g. severe psychiatric condition, advanced multiple sclerosis, severe cognitive or physical impairment, quadriplegia)

Note

It is sometimes difficult to choose between categories, eg. multiple sclerosis or Alzheimers in the early stages would probably score 3, but in the latter stages score 2. Put them into these categories unless there is some information that tells otherwise. Eg. Assume that a person who has Alzheimers, but is able to answer the questionnaire scores 3, because once social activities become markedly restricted they would probably not be capable of completing the questionnaire. If a person has mild deafness, score 3, but if they are completely deaf, score 2.

c)   **Medication**

No regular medication = 5
Single non-psychotropic medication = 4
Multiple non-psychotropic medication = 3
Psychotropic medication = 2
Psychotropic plus non psychotropic medication = 1

Note

Psychotropic medication indicates drugs for the control of epilepsy, psychoses, and other abnormal mental states. They include tranquilisers, sedatives, barbiturates and a host of others. Some of these drug names are provided in Appendix A.

PRODUCTIVITY

3a)   **Number of hours**

31–40+ work, education or child care = 5
21–30 hours combined work/education/child care = 4
11–20 hours combined work/education/child care = 3
1–10 hours combined work/education/child care = 2
Neither work nor education nor child care = 1

b)   **Spare time** (Note reverse score)

Almost always	= 1	Not usually	= 4
Usually	= 2	Almost never	= 5
Sometimes	= 3		

c)   **Hours TV each day**

None	= 5	6–9 hours	= 2
1–2 hours	= 4	10+ hours	= 1
3–5 hours	= 3		

INTIMACY

4a)   **Talk**

Daily	= 5	Once a month	= 2
Several	= 4	Less than once a month	= 1
Once a week	= 3		

b)   **Care**

Almost always	= 5	Not usually	= 2
Usually	= 4	Almost never	= 1
Sometimes	= 3		

c)   **Activity**

Almost always	= 5	Not usually	= 2
Usually	= 4	Almost never	= 1
Sometimes	= 3		

SAFETY

5a)   **Sleep**

Almost always	= 5	Not usually	= 2
Usually	= 4	Almost never	= 1
Sometimes	= 3		

b)   **Safe**

Almost always	= 5	Not usually	= 2
Usually	= 4	Almost never	= 1
Sometimes	= 3		

c)   **Anxiety**   (Note reverse score)

Almost always	= 1	Not usually	= 4
Usually	= 2	Almost never	= 5
Sometimes	= 3		

PLACE IN COMMUNITY

6a) **Activity**

(i)   For each separate activity calculate $0.2 + (0.2 \times \text{frequency})$ for each activity up to a maximum frequency of 4/month. i.e. Each activity is scored to a maximum of 1.0.

(ii) Aggregate the total scores across all activities up to a maximum of 5 activities. Round all fractions to the nearest integer, i.e. the maximum score possible is 5

Additional Comments

(6)	eat out	"take aways" - exclude
(7)	movies	"watched videos" - exclude
(8)	other	people sometimes write something that should come under one of the previous categories, [eg. tennis club or yacht club should come under (i)] put them under the category that seems most appropriate.

If rather than writing how many times in last month, people write:

occasionally	record	"1"
numerous		"4"
sometimes		"1"
seldom		"9" (i.e. missing value)
weekends		"4"

b) **Responsibility**

Chairperson/ President/ Convenor e.g: captain of basketball team, convenor of a social group = 5

Treasurer/ Secretary or other title denoting specific major area of responsibility eg: Immediate past-president, vice-captain = 4

Sub-committee chairperson or other indication of minor area of responsibility or active involvement eg: Responsible for catering arrangements = 3

Committee or team member = 2

If they say they hold a position but do not state what the position is = 1

None = 1

c)   **Advice**
Almost every day = 5   Not often   = 2
Quite often   = 4   Almost never = 1
Sometimes   = 3

EMOTIONAL WELL-BEING

7a)   **Can do**
Almost always = 5   Not usually   = 2
Usually   = 4   Almost never = 1
Sometimes   = 3

b)   **Bed** (reversed scored)
Almost always = 1   Not usually   = 4
Usually   = 2   Almost never = 5
Sometimes   = 3

c)   **Wishes** (reversed scored)
Almost always = 1   Not usually   = 4
Usually   = 2   Almost never = 5
Sometimes   = 3

4.2   Coding the subjective data

IMPORTANCE

Could not be more important	Very important	Somewhat important	Slightly important	Not at all important	Missing value
5	4	3	2	1	9

SATISFACTION

Delighted	Pleased	Mostly Satisfied	Mixed	Mostly Dissatisfied	Unhappy	Terrible	Missing value
7	6	5	4	3	2	1	9

Note

We use the score of 9 to allow computer identification of missing values. If this scheme is used, care needs to be taken that these '9' values are recognized as excluded values, and not included as data.

IMPORTANCE × SATISFACTION

In order to calculate a meaningful subjective QOL (SQOL) score (Importance x Satisfaction) for each domain, the satisfaction data need to be re-coded as follows:

Delighted	Pleased	Mostly Satisfied	Mixed	Mostly dissatisfied	Unhappy	Terrible
+4	+3	+2	+1	−2	−3	−4

Following this recoding procedure each SQOL domain score is calculated as $(I \times S)$, and the overall $SQOL = \Sigma (I \times S)$. As a result of this procedure the SQOL obtained for any domain ranges between −20 and +20.

References

Bachman JG, Kahn RL, Mednick MT, Davidson TN, Johnston LD. (1967). Youth in Transition: Volume 1: Blueprint For a Longitudinal Study of Adolescent Boys. Institute for Social Research, University of Michigan, Ann Arbor.

Bearsley C. (1997). No Place Called Home: Quality of Life and Meaning of Life of Homeless Youths. Honours Thesis, School of Psychology, Deakin University, Melbourne.

Bradford R, Rutherford DL, John A. (2002). J Adolesc. 25: 261–274.

Carlson MJ, Gabriel RM. (2001). Psychiatr Serv. 52: 1230–1236.

Conners CK. (1997) Conners' Auxillary ADHD/DSM-IV Adolescent Self-Report Scale (CADS-A). Multi-health systems, North Tonawanda, NY.

Cummins RA. (1996). Soc Indic Res. 38: 303–332.

Cummins RA. (1997). Comprehensive Quality of Life Scale-School Version (Grades 7–12), 5th (ed.). Deakin University.

Edwards TC, Huebner CE, Connell FA, Patrick DL. (2002). J Adolesc. 25: 275–28.

Felce D, Perry J. (1995). Res Devel Disabil. 16: 51–74.

Frisch MB. (1998). Clin Psychol: Sci Prac. 5: 19–40.

Frisch MB, Clark MP, Rouse SV, Rudd MD, Paweleck J, Greenstone A, et al. (2003). Predictive validity and sensitivity to change in quality of life assessment and life satisfaction: Further studies of the Quality of Life Inventory or QOLI in mental health settings. In: Sirgy MJ et al. (eds.) Advances in Quality of Life Theory and Research. Kluwer Academic Publishers, The Netherlands, pp. 191–210.

Frisch MB, Cornell J, Villanueva M, Retzlaff PJ. (1992). Psychol Assess. 4: 92–101.

Gilman R, Ashby J, Sverko D, Florell D, Varjas K. (2005). Pers Individ Dif. 39: 155–166.

Gilman R, Easterbrooks S, Frey M. (2004). Soc Indic Res. 66: 143–164.

Gilman R, Handwerk ML. (2001). Resid Treat Child Youth. 18: 47–65.

Gilman R, Huebner ES. (2000). Behav Change. 17: 178–183.

Gilman R, Huebner ES. (2004). Resid Treat Child Youth. 21: 7–17.

Gilman R, Huebner ES. (2006). J Youth Adolesc. 35: 311–319.

Gilman R, Huebner ES, Laughlin JE. (2000). Soc Indic Res. 52: 135–160.

Gilman R, Huebner ES, Park N, Tian L, O'Byrne J, Schiff M, et al. (2008). J Youth Adolesc. 2: 142–154.

Gilman R, Laughlin JE, Huebner ES. (1999). Sch Psychol Int. 20: 300–307.

Greenspoon PJ, Saklofske DH. (2001). Soc Indic Res. 54: 81–108.

Gullone E, Cummins RA. (1998). Behav Change. 16: 127–139.

Hagerty MR, Cummins RA, Ferriss AL, Land K, Michalos AC, Peterson M, Sharpe A, Sirgy J, Vogel J. (2001). Soc Indic Res. 55: 1–96.

Huebner ES. (1994). Psychol Assess. 6: 149–158.

Huebner ES, Dew T. (1993a). J Psychoeduc Assess. 11: 345–350.

Huebner ES, Dew T. (1993b). Sch Psychol Int. 14: 355–360.

Huebner ES, Laughlin JE, Ash C, Gilman R. (1998). 16: 118–134.

Huebner ES, Gilman R. (2006). Appl Res Qual Life. 1: 139–150.

Huebner ES, Gilman R, Suldo SM. (2007). Assessing perceived quality of life in children and adolescents. In: Handler L, Smith S (eds.) The Clinical Assessment of Children and Adolescents. A practitioner's handbook. Lawrence Erlbaum, Mahwah, NJ, pp. 347–363.

Huebner ES, Seligson JL, Valois RF, Suldo SM. (2006). Soc Indic Res. 79: 477–484.

Huebner ES, Valois RF, Suldo SM, Smith LC, McKnight CG, Seligson JL, Zullig KJ. (2004). J Adolesc Health. 34: 270–278.

Irwin CE, Burg SJ, Cart CU. (2002). J Adoles Health. 31: 91–121.

Ito A, Smith DC. (2006). The Comm Psychol. 38: 19–21.

Jirojanakul P, Skevington S. (2000). Br J Health Psychol. 5: 299–321.

Jirojanakul P, Skevington S, Hudson J. (2003). Soc Sci Med. 57: 1277–1288.

Keyes CLM. (2007). Am Psychol. 62: 95–108.

Kovacs M. (1992). Children's Depression Inventory (CDI). Multi-Health Systems, North Tonawanda, NY.

Land KC, Lamb VL, Meadows SO, Taylor A. (2007). Soc Indic Res. 80: 105–132.

Land KC, Lamb VL, Mustillo SK. (2001). Soc Indic Res. 56: 241–320.

Marsh HW, Barnes J, Cairns L, Tidman M. (1984). J Educ Psychol. 940–976.

Meuleners LB, Lee AH. (2005). Qual Life Res. 14: 1057–1063.

Meuleners LB, Lee AH, Binns CW, Lower A. (2003). Qual Life Res. 12: 283–290.

Moore KA, Brown BV, Scarupa MS. (2003). The uses (and misuses) of social indicators: Implications for public policy. Child Trends Research Brief, Publication #2003–01. Child Trends, Washington, DC.

Patrick DL, Connell FA, Edwards TC, Topolski TD, Huebner CE. (1998). Final report submitted to the Centers for Disease Control and Prevention: Special Interest Project #4 (96): Age Appropriate Measures of Quality of Life and Disability Outcomes among Children: Youth Quality of Life Study. Center for Disability Policy and Research, Seattle, WA.

Patrick DL, Edwards TC, Topolski TD. (2002). J Adolesc. 25: 287–300.

Park N, Huebner ES. (2005). J Cross-Cult Psychol. 36: 444–456.

Park N, Huebner ES, Laughlin JE, Valois RF, Gilman R. (2004). Soc Indic Res. 66: 61–79.

Raphael D, Rukholm E, Brown I, Hill-Bailey P, Donato E. (1996). J Adolesc Health. 19: 366–375.

Rapley M. (2003). Should we 'hang up quality of life as a hopeless term?. In: Rapley M (ed.) Quality of Life Research: A Critical Introduction. Sage Publications, Thousand Oaks, CA, pp. 212–226.

Ravens-Sieberer U, Bullinger M. (1998). Qual Life Res. 7: 399–407.

Recker GT. (1992). Life Attitude Profile-Revised. Trent University, Canada.

Reynolds CR, Kamphaus RW. (2004). Manual for the Behavioral Assessment System for Children, 2nd version. American Guidance Services, Circle Pines, MN.

Schalock RL, Parameter T. (2000). Preface. In: Quality of Life: Its Conceptualization, Measurement, and Application. IASSID, A Consensus Document. Washington. Schwartz SJ, Pantin H, Coatsworth JD, Szapocznik J. (2007). J Prim Prev. 28: 117–144

Selgison JL, Huebner ES, Valois RF. (2003). Soc Indic Res. 61: 121–145.

Seligson JL, Huebner ES, Valois RF. (2005). Soc Indic Res. 73: 355–374.

Suldo SM, Huebner ES. (2004). Sch Psychol Q. 19: 93–105.

Suldo SM, Huebner ES. (2006). Soc Indic Res. 78: 179–203.

Topolski TD, Edwards TC, Patrick DL, Varley P, Way ME, Buesching DP. (2004). J Atten Disord. 3: 163–173.

Valois RF, Zullig KJ, Drane JW, Huebner ES. (2001). Am J Health Behav. 25: 353–366.

Valois RF, Zullig KJ, Huebner ES, Drane JW. (2003). Eat Disord: J Treat Prev. 11: 271–288.

ValoisRF, Zullig KJ, Huebner ES, Drane JW. (2004a). J Sch Health. 74: 59–65.

Valois RF, Zullig KJ, Huebner ES, Drane JW. (2004b). Soc Indic Res. 66: 81–105.

Valois RF, Zullig KJ, Kammermann SK, Huebner ES, Drane JW. (2002). J Child Fam Stud. 11: 427–440.

Walker LS, Greene JW. (1991). J Pediatr Psychol. 16: 39–58.

Zullig KJ, Valois RF, Drane JW, Huebner ES. (2001). J Adolesc Health. 29: 279–288.

Zullig KJ, Valois RF, Huebner ES, Drane JW. (2005). Qual Life Res. 14: 1573–1584.

143 Quality of Life in Children with Cerebral Palsy

A. Aran

1	*Introduction*	2454
2	*Assessment Tools*	2456
2.1	Parental and Child Perceptions	2456
2.2	Measures	2456
3	*Generic Tools*	2457
4	*Specific Tools*	2458
4.1	Function and Participation	2461
5	*QOL in Children with CP*	2461
5.1	Parent's View	2461
5.2	Children's View	2461
5.3	Factors Affecting HRQL in Children with CP	2461
6	*Level of Motor Disability*	2462
7	*Cognitive Impairment*	2464
8	*Other Co-Morbidities*	2464
9	*Pain*	2465
10	*Socioeconomic Status*	2465
11	*Child Characteristics (Age, Gender)*	2465
12	*Parenting Style*	2465
13	*Summary and Recommendations*	2465
	Summary Points	2466

Abstract: ❷ Cerebral Palsy (CP) is a non-progressive disorder of movement and posture caused by a defect or injury to the immature brain and its impact is further exacerbated by disabilities other than the motor impairments, such as epilepsy, learning disabilities, behavioral and emotional problems. Traditionally, the treatment of children with chronic diseases, as Cerebral Palsy (CP) was focused on the physical aspects of the disease and the treatment efficacy was measured primarily by physical improvement. In the past two decades, quality of life (QOL), defined, as well-being across various broad domains, has become an important treatment goal, especially in chronic diseases like CP.

As studies on QOL, are highly subjective in nature and may have many inherent limitations, a combination of well valid, parent-based and child-based questionnaires as well as generic and disease specific tools is required.

Although several studies have found that parents report lower QOL for their children with CP (in every aspect of QOL measured), the children themselves, usually rate their quality of life in the emotional and social domains, equal to their typically developed peers. Further more, parents of children with severe impairment, often reported better quality of life in the psychosocial domains compared to the reports for children with mild impairment. These consistent findings suggest that children with cerebral palsy can adapt well to their activity limitations and may have satisfactory quality of life in spite of significant deficits. These results also mean that factors other than the impairment severity may have a major influence on QOL in disabled children.

The consensus that improving QOL is an important treatment goal in children with CP, mandates measures and treatments that enhance this goal.

List of Abbreviations: *CHQ*, ❷ Child Health Questionnaire; *CP*, Cerebral Palsy; *GMFCS*, ❷ Gross Motor Function Classification System; *PedsQL*, 4.0, Pediatric Quality of Life Inventory Version 4.0; *PODCI*, Pediatric Outcomes Data Collecting Instrument; *QOL*, Quality of Life

1 Introduction

Cerebral palsy (CP) is the most common cause of physical handicap in children, with an estimated rate of 2–2.5 per 1,000 live births (for Key Facts of cerebral palsy, please see ❷ *Table 143-1*). The term CP represents a group of conditions that are caused by a permanent static lesion of the motor areas in the developing brain. CP is caused by either inborn developmental problem or by acquired injury, like ischemic or hemorrhagic stroke, anoxia, traumatic injury or infection. The lesion occurred before the birth, during the birth, or within the first 2–3 years of life. Even though the lesion itself does not change, the clinical manifestations of the lesion change as the child grows and develops. The motor skills of most children with cerebral palsy improve as they grow, but the rate of improvement is slower in children with cerebral palsy compared to unaffected children. As a result of the lesion in the brain's motor areas, the child faces difficulties with stance and active motions. More than 50% of the patients are able to walk without arm assistance but cannot run or Jump; 20% can walk only with assistance and 25% cannot walk at all. If the lesion involves other brain areas in addition to the motor area, most commonly in large lesions that cause severe motor impairment, the physical disability is often associated with other problems such as epilepsy (35%) learning disabilities (50%), cerebral visual impairment (40%) and mental retardation (30%) (Koman et al., 2004).

For research and clinical purposes, CP is usually graded according to the Gross Motor Function Classification System (GMFCS). This scale measures severity of CP and rates

◘ **Table 143-1**

Key Facts of cerebral palsy

Definition	CP is an "umbrella term" for a group of physical disabilities (stance and movements) that are caused by a permanent static damage to the motor control centers of the developing brain
Causes	Common causes of CP are disturbances of the blood supply to the brain or infections that occur in most cases during pregnancy or in pre term infants and sometimes during infancy
Types	CP is commonly classified according to the anatomical distribution of the impairment: Diplegia – legs are involved much more than arms; Hemiplegia – involvement of arm and leg in the same side; Quadriplegia – all four limbs are involved. The dominant movement disorders are Spasticity (stiff muscles) and ataxia (lack of muscle coordination)

❯ *Table 143-1* summarizes briefly the definition, classification and the common causes of cerebral palsy. *CP* cerebral palsy

◘ **Table 143-2**

Overview of Gross Motor Function Classification System (Palisano et al., 1997)

Level I	Walks without restrictions; limitation in more advanced gross motor skills
Level II	Walks without assistive devices; limitation walking out doors and in community
Level III	Walks with assistive devices; limitation walking out doors and in community. (usually requiring wheelchair)
Level IV	Self mobility (usually with wheelchair) with limitations; children are transported or use power mobility out doors and in community
Level V	Self mobility (even with the use of power wheelchair) is very limited

❯ *Table 143-2* describes the Gross Motor Function Classification System – a common classification of the motor severity in Cerebral Palsy into five levels from the milder impairment (level I) to the most severe (level V)

outcome of motor function in a scale ranging from I to V (❯ *Table 143-2*). CP is usually described as mild if the child can walk independently (corresponds to levels I/II), moderate if the child is ambulant with assistive devices (level III) and severe if the child is wheelchair dependent (levels IV/V) (Oeffinger et al., 2004).

The impact of CP, the motor impairment and co-morbidities on most individuals and their families is usually substantial. The treatment is supportive (there is no cure for CP) and is often long term and complex. The exact treatment regimen depends on the specific type of CP and co-morbidities but usually includes physical and occupational therapy, special education, orthopedic surgery, and assistive devices. Frequently, further treatments are applied and the emotional and financial costs on the children, their parents, and the health services are substantial.

Whereas treatment modalities of CP have been documented in a multitude of studies, their subjective impact on children with CP and their families is an area that has been relatively neglected (Bjornson and McLaughlin, 2001; Majnemer and Mazer, 2004).

Considering the supportive rather than curative nature of the various treatment modalities, it is now well accepted that improving quality of life should be the main treatment goal for children with CP and specific assessment of QOL should be an integral part of any outcome measurement.

2   Assessment Tools

2.1   Parental and Child Perceptions

The challenge of assessing a highly subjective parameter like QOL in a quantitative tool led to the development of many different measurement instruments.

The first studies of QOL in children, were based on the parent's perspective in most cases (Bullinger and Ravens-Sieberer, 1995). With time, data based on children self-reports began to accumulate, driven by a strong recommendation of the World Health Organization and the International Association for Child Psychology and Psychiatry, that measures of QOL in children will use self-reports whenever possible (World Health Organization, 1993). The accumulating data demonstrated good psychometric properties even in young children and gradually, child based, self reported QOL measurements, became standard of care (Connolly and Johnson, 1999; Harding, 2001; Landgraf and Abetz, 1996). However, QOL assessment in children, especially those with developmental problems, cannot be based only on self-report tools. For many children, parent's report, is the only option due to a young age, severe motor disability, or cognitive impairment. Even if the child is capable of self-reporting, some studies have found children's reports to be less reliable (Goodwin et al., 1994).

Several studies compared the parents'–proxy report on the QOL of their children to the children's self-report. Interestingly, the correlation between the parents and the children reports, is depended considerably on the children's health status. While parents generally perceive the QOL of their healthy children as higher than the children themselves (Cremeens et al., 2006; Theunissen et al., 1998; Waters et al., 2003), They score the QOL of their disabled children, lower than the self-reports of the disabled children (Bastiaansen et al., 2004; Havermans et al., 2006; Majnemer et al., 2007; Ronen et al., 2003; Russell et al., 2006; Shelly et al., 2008; Varni et al., 2005; White-Koning et al., 2007).

While many factors can influence this discrepancy between parental and child's views, a recent large study, found that parental stress and child's pain are important contributors. When parents experience difficulties in their own lives they tend to report lower QOL for their children and conversely, when a child reports a severe pain, his self QOL report is lower compared to his parent's report, suggesting that parents may underestimate the extent to which pain affect their child's life (White-Koning et al., 2007).

Considering the subjective nature of Quality of life, the question whose perspective reflects the child's QOL more "reliably" (the child's perspective or the parental), is somewhat irrelevant. Today, it is usually accepted that each type of instrument, highlights different aspects of the child QOL and both are important. Together they create a complementary picture of the child's health status that helps us to define the child's needs for better QOL (De Civita et al., 2005; Eiser and Morse, 2001a, b; Shelly et al., 2008; White-Koning et al., 2007).

2.2   Measures

QOL measurements are based on the use of standardized and validated questionnaires.

For the assessment of❷ health-related quality of life (HRQL) in people with CP, two major types of questionnaires are available: Generic and disease specific.

❷ Generic questionnaires were developed to measure the HRQL of the general population regardless of health condition. These tools are generally being used for discrimination studies: the comparison of different aspects of QOL between patients and the healthy population or between different groups of patients, separated by severity of the disease or any other physical or psychosocial parameter. The advantage of these questionnaires is the general nature of their items, that allows them to be relevant for wide spectrum of health conditions. This general nature is also a disadvantage when it comes to detection of minor changes in HRQL following a disease specific intervention. To answer this need, ❯ disease specific questionnaires have been developed. These questionnaires contain many items that are more relevant to patients with a certain type of disease, which enable them to be sensitive to changes across time and interventions.

As mentioned above, when we deal with children, each type of questionnaire is further subdivided according to whether it is supposed to be answered by the children themselves or by a proxy of the children, usually a parent. Some generic questionnaires has both child and parent versions for the same items.

While currently, most of the assessment instruments for QOL in children with CP, are generic questionnaires that approach the parents, more specific and child based questionnaires, appears recently.

In the last two decades, studies of QOL in children with CP have used many different tools. A recent metanalysis identified 17 instruments, which have been used in more than 100 studies (Viehweger et al., 2008).

It is beyond the scope of this article to describe all those different tools and only questionnaires used in numerous and/or large studies, will be discussed.

3   Generic Tools

Various aspects of some of the more common generic questionnaires used for assessment of QOL in children with CP, are summarized in ❯ Table 143-3.

Child Health Questionnaire (CHQ) is a generic questionnaire that taps physical and psychosocial aspects of QOL as well as impact on family (❯ Table 143-4). A score of zero represents the worst health state and 100 the best. Each scale has its own score and additionally there are two summary scores: physical and psychosocial. The CHQ has demonstrated very good reliability and validity in population and clinical studies all over the world (Landgraf and Abetz, 1996). As other generic questionnaires, the CHQ is less sensitive to changes over time or following interventions, and may fail to detect meaningful improvements in functioning (Vargus-Adams, 2006). Nevertheless, the CHQ appears to be a reliable, valid, and acceptable tool for children with CP across a range of severities (Vargus-Adams, 2005; Wake et al., 2003). It can reliably reflect how parents perceive the health and well-being of their children and is extensively used in both the research and clinical fields. A common clinical use is as a screening tool for lower QOL (especially in the psychosocial aspects of QOL) of the child with CP or for a higher burden of care carried by the family, than would be anticipated by the clinical assessment. The CHQ has three parent's forms that contain 28, 50, or 87 items (CHQ PF – 28, CHQ PF – 50 and CHQ PF – 87 respectively) as well as a child's form with 87 questions (CHQ CF – 87).

❯ *KIDSCREEN* – KIDSCREEN is a relatively new, generic questionnaire that has child and adolescent (ages 8–18 years) as well as parent/proxy versions. Three KIDSCREEN instruments are available: KIDSCREEN-52 (long version) covering ten HRQOL dimensions, KIDSCREEN-27 (short version) covering five HRQOL dimensions and the KIDSCREEN-10 Index as a global HRQOL score. The questionnaire has been psychometrically validated recently on 22,110

■ Table 143-3

Common generic questionnaires, for QOL assessment in children with CP

Instrument	Versions	Age	Scales and number of items
CHQ	Child	10–18	Physical functioning; General health; Pain, Social limitations due to Physical disability and due to Emotional difficulties; Behavior; Mental health; Self esteem; Impact on family activities, on Parent's emotions and on Parent's free time; Family cohesion. 28/50 or 87 items
	Parent	5–18	
Kidscreen	Child	8–18	Physical well-being; Psychological well-being; Moods and emotions; Self-perception; Autonomy; Relationships with parents; Social support and peers; School environment; Social acceptance; Financial resources. 27/52 or 10 questions
	Parent	8–18	
PedsQL	Child	5–18	Physical functioning; Moods and emotions; Social functioning, School functioning
	Parent	5–18	23 items

❯ *Table 143-3* expresses important features of the three most common quality of life questionnaires, designed for the general population and used to assess quality of life in children with cerebral palsy. The ages approached by each version (the child and the parent versions), the scales covered by each tool and the total items in the various questionnaires are listed above. *CHQ* Child Health Questionnaire; *QOL* Quality of Life; *PedsQL* Pediatric Quality of Life Inventory; *CP* Cerebral Palsy

European children (Ravens-Sieberer, 2005).The version that has been used for disabled children, the KIDSCREEN-52 covers the following 10 dimensions: physical well-being, psychological well-being, moods and emotions, self-perception, autonomy, relationships with parents, social support and peers, school environment, social acceptance and financial resources. For each domain, item responses are summed and a score out of 100 is computed with higher scores indicating better QOL. The time required for administration is 15–20 min. This questionnaire have been used in the largest study so far, on QOL of children with CP (818 parents have answered the parent's version and 500 children have answered the child's version).

❯ *Pediatric Quality of Life Inventory* (PedsQL) – The PedsQL is a 23 items generic questionnaire, which was designed to enable integration of disease-specific modules (its PedsQL-CP Module is described in the next paragraph). It has parent's form and three versions of child's form (5–7 years, 8–11, 12–18) with good psychometric properties both in healthy children and children with chronic conditions (Varni et al., 2007, 2006).

The PedsQL covers four domains: Physical functioning (eight items), Emotional functioning (five items), Social functioning (five items) and School functioning (five items) and the mean of the last three domains creates the Psychosocial summary score (the sum of the items divided by the number of items answered).

4   Specific Tools

Various aspects of disease specific questionnaires for assessment of QOL in children with CP, are summarized in ❯ *Table 143-5.*

◘ Table 143-4

Description of the CHQ scales – Adapted from the US CHQ manual (Landgraf and Abetz, 1996)

Domain	Scale	Description
Physical	Physical Functioning	The extent of limitations in physical activities, including self-care, due to health problems
	General Health Perceptions and Global health	Parent subjective assessment of overall child's health; past, present, and future
	Role/Social Limitations-Physical	Limitations on school work and activities with friends as a result of physical health problems
	Bodily Pain	Intensity and frequency of general pain and discomfort
Psychosocial	Role/Social Limitations-Emotional/Behavioral	Limitations on school work and activities with friends due to emotional or behavioral difficulties
	Behavior and Global Behavior	Frequency of behavior problems: improper, aggressive or delinquent behavior
	Mental Health	Frequency of depressive or anxiety versus happy states
	Self-esteem	Satisfaction with school and athletic abilities, looks, relationships, and life overall
Family	Family Activities	Frequency of interruption of child's general health to family activities
	Family Cohesion	How well the family gets along with one another
	Parent Impact-Emotional	Level of distress experienced by parent due to child's health and well-being
	Parent Impact-Time	Limitation on parental time for personal needs due to child's health and well-being

❯ *Table 143-4* explains each of the 12 scales of the child health questionnaire, covering three domains of quality of life: Physical, Psychosocial and impact on family. *CHQ* Child Health questionnaire

❯ *Pediatric Outcomes Data Collection Instrument (PODCI)* is a 55 questions, disease specific questionnaire that is available as self- or proxy report forms for Adolescents (11–18 years) and as parent's form for children 2–10 years old. The American Academy of Orthopedic Surgeons (AAOS) developed the PODCI to measure general health and problems related to bone and muscle conditions in children (AAOS, 1997). The questionnaire contains six domains: Upper extremity and physical function, transfers and basic mobility, sports and physical function, pain/comfort, expectations from treatment and happiness with physical condition (Daltroy et al., 1998). Zero is the poorest score and 100 reflects best health status. A general function and symptom score is computed as a composite of the first four domains (the three physical function domains and the pain and comfort domain). This instrument allows orthopedic surgeons to assess the functional health and efficacy of treatment of their patients at baseline and follow-up, but provides less information on the impact of the condition on the family and the individual's self-esteem.

PedsQL-CP Module – The PedsQL CP Module was designed to measure HRQOL dimensions specific to CP. The module is applicable for both child self-report and parent proxy-report. Child self-report versions include ages 5–7 years, 8–12 years, and 13–18 years. Parent proxy

◼ Table 143-5

Specific instruments for QOL assessment in children with CP

Instrument	Versions	Age	Scales and number of items
PODCI	Child	11–18	Upper Extremity and physical function; Transfers and basic mobility; Sports; Pain; Expectations from treatment; Happiness with physical condition. (55 items)
	Parent	2–18	
DISABKIDS	Child	4–16	Autonomy; Moods and emotions; Social integration and Social exclusion; Physical limitations; Treatment. (37 or 12 items)
	Parent	4–16	
CP-QOL	Child	9–12	Friends and family; Participation; Communication; General health; Equipment; Pain. (53 items). The parents form includes also access to treatment and parental health. (66 items)
	Parent	4–12	
PedsQL-CP	Child	5–18	Daily activities; School activities; Movement and balance; Pain and hurt; Fatigue; Eating activities; Speech and communication. (35 items, the toddler's form – less items)
	Parent	2–18	

❯ *Table 143-5* describes four common questionnaires, which were designed specifically to tap health related quality of life in Children with cerebral palsy. All four instruments have both a child version, for self-report and a parent version. The ages approached by each version and the scales covered by each tool are listed above. *PODCI* Pediatric Outcomes Data Collecting Instrument; *QOL* Quality of Life; *PedsQL* Pediatric Quality of Life Inventory; *CP* Cerebral Palsy

report versions includes ages 2–4 years (toddler), 5–7 years (young child), 8–12 years (child), and 13–18 years (adolescent).

This 35-item's questionnaire encompasses seven scales: Daily activities (nine items), School activities (four items), Movement and balance (five items), Pain and Hurt (four items), Fatigue (four items), Eating Activities (five items); and Speech and communication (four items) (Toddlers' questionnaire contains fewer items). Higher scores indicate better HRQOL. The PedsQL 3.0 CP Module, demonstrated good psychometric properties in children with CP (Varni et al., 2006).

❯ *CP-QOL* – This disease specific questionnaire was developed based on views of children with CP and their parents regarding what the child needs in order to have a good QOL. The parent/proxy version assesses seven domains of QOL including social well-being and acceptance, feelings about functioning, participation and physical health, emotional well-being, access to services, pain and feeling about disability, and family health. The child self-report version assesses all of the above domains except access to services and family health. The parent proxy form (parents of children aged 4–12 year) comprises 66 items and the child self-report form (9–12 year) comprises 52 items. Both the child's and the parent-proxy's forms has demonstrated good psychometric properties (Waters et al., 2007).

❯ *DISABKIDS* – DISABKIDS is a new family of instruments, developed in Europe for the assessment of HRQOL in Children and adolescents with various chronic conditions. The instruments are available as self- or proxy report forms for three age groups: 4–7, 8–12 and 13–16, in three versions: long form (37 items), short form (12 items) and Smiley Measure.

These questionnaires can be used to assess HRQOL in patients with any type of chronic medical condition and have specific modules for some common childhood chronic conditions, including cerebral palsy. After completing the validation process (Simeoni et al., 2007) theses instruments will probably have a major role in QOL assessment of children with CP.

4.1 Function and Participation

Over the years, various instruments have been developed for the assessment of different aspects of function in children with CP; their description is beyond the scope of this chapter.

Likewise, Participation is another emerging model for the evaluation of children with CP, although related to quality of life this is a different concept that will not be discussed in this chapter.

5 QOL in Children with CP

5.1 Parent's View

Several studies have found that parent's perceive the QOL of their children with CP to be lower than the QOL of their healthy siblings or other typically developed kids, regardless of CP severity (❯ Table 143-6). These findings are consistent across various populations and measurement tools and apply to almost any aspect of QOL (Aran et al., 2007; Arnaud et al., 2008; Shelly et al., 2008; Vargus-Adams, 2006; Wake et al., 2003).

Siblings of children with CP had normal QOL regardless of disease severity (Aran et al., 2007).

5.2 Children's View

In spite of their parents view, and the common assumption that disabled children have a lower quality of life, the opinion of the disabled children themselves as reflected in two recent large studies (Dickinson et al., 2007; Shelly et al., 2008) as well as several smaller studies before (Grue, 2003; Varni et al., 2005; Watson and Keith, 2002), seems to be quite different (❯ Table 143-7). In the largest study ever, to tap self reported QOL in children with CP (Dickinson et al., 2007), 500 children aged 8–12 years, from six European countries, reported their QOL using KIDSCREEN. Over all, children with cerebral palsy had similar scores to children in the general population in all the KIDSCREEN's domains except schooling, in which evidence was equivocal, and physical wellbeing, in which comparison was not possible. It should be noticed though, that pain was more common then expected based on the proxy reports and it was associated with lower QOL on all domains.

5.3 Factors Affecting HRQL in Children with CP

Various factors have been found to affect quality of life in children with CP (see ❯ Table 143-8 for details) but most of them are child's characteristics (like disease severity) that are less treatable.

◨ Table 143-6

QOL in children with CP, as perceived by their parents

Study	Participants	Instruments	Major outcome
Arnaud et al., 2008 (SPARCLE)	Parents of 818 European children, age 8–12 year, mild to severe CP	Kidscreen	Parents reported lower scores in most domains, compared to the general population. The scores in the physical, but not the psychosocial domains, were lower in more disabled children (see ❯ Table 143-8 for more details)
Vargus-Adams et al., 2005	Parents of 177 children age 5–18; mild to severe CP	CHQ-PF50	Parents reported lower scores in all domains, compared to the general population. The scores in the physical, but not the psychosocial domains correlated with level of disability
Kennes et al., 2002	Parents of 408 children age 5–13; mild to severe CP	HUI-3	Rates of functional limitations were lower for more disabled children but scores in emotion and pain were not correlated with disability
Wake et al., 2003	Parents of 80 children, mild to moderate CP, age 5–18	CHQ-PF 50	Parents reported lower scores compared to the general population in all domains. The scores in the physical, but not the psychosocial domains, correlated with the level of disability

❯ *Table 143-6* summarizes the results of recent four large studies, which assessed the quality of life in children with Cerebral Palsy, by asking their parents to complete the Kidscreen, CHQ or HUI-3 questionnaires. All four studies found that children with CP have lower QOL scores (that reflect poorer quality of life), compared to the general population in every aspect of quality of life. In the physical domains, children with mild motor disability had higher scores but in the psychosocial domains, the scores were low regardless of motor impairment. *SPARCLE* Study of Participation of Children with Cerebral Palsy Living in Europe; *QOL* Quality of Life; *CHQ-PF 50* Child Health Questionnaire Parent Form 50 (items); *CP* Cerebral Palsy; *HUI-3* Health Utilities Index – Mark 3

Furthermore, those factors primarily influence the physical aspects of QOL, which usually simply reflect the physical functioning rather than the more variable psychosocial aspects.

6   Level of Motor Disability

Level of motor disability is a proven determinant of QOL in children with CP (Arnaud et al., 2008; Kennes et al., 2002; Liptak et al., 2001; Livingston et al., 2007; Majnemer et al., 2007; Shelly et al., 2008; Vargus-Adams, 2005; Varni et al., 2005; Wake et al., 2003).

In all of these studies, the physical scales scores were significantly lower in children with severe motor disability compared to those with mild or moderate disability. However, in most of the studies the degree of motor disability did not affect the social or emotional functioning in a similar manner. In fact, the scores on the psychosocial scales were often lower for children with mild CP than for those with moderate CP. A possible explanation is that children with mild CP measure themselves and are compared by their parents to the healthy population while children with moderate to severe CP are less likely to attend mainstream classes.

◘ Table 143-7

QOL in children with CP, as reported by the children themselves (with comparison to their parents view when applicable)

Study	Participants	Instruments	Major outcome
Dickinson, 2007 (SPARCLE)	500 European children, age: 8–12, mild to severe CP	KIDSCREEN	Children with CP reported similar QOL scores compared to children in the general population in most domains of the Kidscreen, regardless of physical impairment.
Oeffinger, 2007	Parents of 562 children age 4–18; 495 children age 5–18 (PedsQL); 247 children age 11–18 (PODCI); mild to moderate CP	PODCI PedsQL 4.0	Children with varying levels of disability have similar Quality of Life scores. Children rate themselves higher, for most of the PODCI and PedsQL scales, than their parents do and the difference increases with the level of disability.
Shelly et al., 2008	Parents of 205 children age 4–12; 53 children age 8–12; mild to severe CP	CP-QOL	Parents reported all domains of the CP-QOL to be lower in more disabled children. The children themselves reported high psychosocial QOL scores regardless of disability.
Varni et al., 2006	Parents of 235 children age 2–18; 77 children age 5–18. mild to severe CP	PedsQL PedsQL-CP	Parents and disabled children reported lower QOL scores, in all the PedsQL domains, compared to typically developed children, with correlation to disease severity. Children reported higher scores than their parents in both tools.
Bjornson, 2008	81 youth with mild to moderate CP age 10–13y and 30 typically developing youth age 10–13y	CHQ-CF87	Disabled youth reported lower QOL scores in the physical domains of the CHQ and equal scores in the psychosocial domains, compared to the typically developing youth.
Majnemer, 2007	Parents of 95 children age 6–12; 55 children age 6–12; mild to severe CP	CHQ-PF50 PedsQL 4.0	Parents and children reported lower QOL in physical domains, compared to healthy kids, but half reported equal scores in the psychosocial domains, regardless of disease severity. Children scores correlated with the parents' scores but they were higher.
Varni et al., 2005	Parents of 148 children age 5–18; 69 children age 6–18; mild to severe CP	PedsQL 4.0	Parents and children reported lower QOL in all domains, compared to healthy kids with correlation to disease severity. Children reported higher scores than their parents.

◗ Table 143-7 summarizes recent studies of quality of life in children with Cerebral Palsy, that used both child's self-reports and parent's reports. In all seven studies, the children rated their quality of life higher (better QOL) compared to their parents and in most of them the QOL scores in the psychosocial domains of the children self reports were equal to those of the general population. SPARCLE Study of Participation of Children with Cerebral Palsy Living in Europe; QOL Quality of Life; PODCI Pediatric Outcomes Data Collecting Instrument; CP Cerebral Palsy; PedsQL 4.0 Pediatric Quality of Life Inventory Version 4.0; CHQ-PF 50 Child Health Questionnaire Parent Form 50 (items); CHQ-CF 87 Child Health Questionnaire Child Form 87 (items)

◻ Table 143-8

Elements affecting QOL in children with CP in a recent large, population based study with 818 participants, using the Kidscreen (Arnaud et al., 2008)

Element	Effect	Domains affected
Severity of motor impairment	Negative	Physical well being, autonomy
	Positive	Social acceptance, school environment
Cognitive impairment	Negative	Social support
	Positive	Moods and emotions, self perception
Pain	Negative	Physical well being, psychological well being, Self perception
Epilepsy	Negative	Social support
High parental education	Negative	Parent relations/home life
Single parent household	Negative	Moods and emotions
Speech difficulties	Negative	Physical well being
Visual impairment	Negative	Physical well being
Hearing impairment, age, gender, parental occupation	No effect	Any domain of kidscreen

❯ *Table 143-8* describes the impact of different aspects of CP (right column) on various domains of the QOL (left column), as reflected in this large European study. Positive effect (middle column) means that children with higher disability have higher scores (which reflect better QOL) and Negative effect means that children with higher disability had lower QOL scores. *QOL* quality of life; *CP* cerebral palsy

7   Cognitive Impairment

As children with cognitive impairment are usually unable to reliably answer the QOL questionnaires, data regarding the impact of cognitive impairment on QOL is based on parental perception. In children with CP, this data is inconclusive. In an Australian study with 80 participants, CHQ scores were similar for children with and without cognitive delay (Wake et al., 2003) and this was also the finding in the study of McCarthy et al. (2002). Another large study, which used the KIDSCREEN, found that children with CP and cognitive impairment have lower QOL scores in the Social support domain but higher scores in the Moods and emotions and Self-perception domains, compared to children with CP and normal cognition (Arnaud et al., 2008).

8   Other Co-Morbidities

Parents of children with CP and epilepsy reported lower QOL on the Self-esteem and Family Cohesion scales of the CHQ (Wake et al., 2003) compared to parents of children with CP per se, the same pattern was found in the much larger study of Arnaud et al. (2008), for the social support domain of the Kidscreen.

Other co-morbidities of CP including Learning, behavioral, vision, hearing and communication difficulties were occasionally reported to affect a single, related aspect of QOL in these children (Arnaud et al., 2008; Majnemer et al., 2007).

9 Pain

Chronic pain correlates with reduced social contacts and activities with peers (Houlihan et al., 2004; Kennes et al., 2002) and with lower scores in the Physical well being, Psychological well being and Self perception (Arnaud et al., 2008) in the parent's reports. In the child's reports, pain was the most consistent influencing factor on QOL (Dickinson et al., 2007; Shelly et al., 2008).

10 Socioeconomic Status

As oppose to typically developed children and children with other chronic conditions, there is no evidence that disabled children from lower socioeconomic background have lower QOL scores compared to disabled children from higher socioeconomic background (Arnaud et al., 2008; Majnemer et al., 2007).

11 Child Characteristics (Age, Gender)

Many studies demonstrated that age and gender are not correlated with QOL in children with CP (Arnaud et al., 2008; Majnemer et al., 2007), However, such a correlation was found in some smaller studies (Bottos et al., 2001) and for other chronic conditions.

12 Parenting Style

In a recent study, the QOL of children with CP and their siblings were measured along with the parenting style of their mother (Aran et al., 2007). For the children with CP, autonomy allowing parenting style was found to correlate with higher CHQ scores in both the physical and the psychosocial domains. Accepting parenting style also positively correlated with the psychosocial domain. The impact of parenting style was greater than factors, such as severity of illness, IQ, SES and anxiety level. For the siblings there was no such a correlation.

As studies suggest that both the physical and psychosocial well being of children with CP deteriorate with the transition from youth to adulthood (Bottos et al., 2001), autonomy allowing parenting style during childhood may prepare children with CP for more independent lives as adults.

13 Summary and Recommendations

Good quality of life is the main goal for all children: disabled or typically developed. The World Health Organization defined QOL as "an individual's perception of their position in life in the context of the culture and value systems in which they live, and in relation to their goals, expectations, standards and concerns" (WHO, 1995) and naturally, this should be reported by the individual himself. However, when dealing with children, the parent's opinion must be considered as well, especially for young or mentally impaired children.

Several studies on QOL in children with CP revealed the dismal fact that parents perceive the QOL of their children with CP (even mild CP), to be lower in almost any aspect, compared to their healthy siblings and the general population. QOL scores in the physical domains correlate well with the level of disability, but the scores in the psychosocial scales are low regardless of the impairment severity. This finding emphasizes the importance of factors, other than the level of disability that may affect QOL in these kids.

In two recent studies, family variables as Parenting style and Family functioning were found to be important factors affecting the psychosocial aspects of QOL of children with CP (Aran et al., 2007; Majnemer et al., 2007). Autonomy allowing and accepting parenting styles, in contrast to controlling and rejecting parenting styles, were reflected in improved mental health, higher self-esteem, better behavior and less social and emotional limitations.

These findings can and should be translated to implementation of family interventions, particularly those focusing on parenting style, early in the disease course.

As other potentially treatable factors probably affect the psychosocial aspects of QOL in children with CP, any effort should be made to identify and treat those factors.

Summary Points

- Cerebral Palsy (CP) is a term that describes various motor problems that their cause is a permanent and stable brain damage that happened in early life. CP is the most common cause of motor disability in childhood.
- The treatment of CP is supportive (there is no cure for CP) and is often long term and complex. The exact treatment regimen depends on the specific type of CP and usually includes physical and occupational therapy, special education, orthopedic surgery, and assistive devices.
- Considering the supportive rather than curative nature of the various treatment modalities, it is now well accepted that improving quality of life should be the main treatment goal for children with CP and specific assessment of QOL should be an integral part of any outcome measurement.
- As studies on QOL, are highly subjective in nature and as such have many inherent limitations, a combination of well valid, parent-based and child-based questionnaires as well as generic and disease specific tools is required.
- Parents of children with CP usually report lower quality of life scores, for their disabled children, in every aspect of the quality of life and regardless of disease severity (even parents of children with mild CP reports lower scores).
- Parents of children with severe impairment often reported better quality of life in the psychosocial domains compared to the reports for children with mild impairment.
- As oppose to typically developed children, disabled children usually report higher quality of life scores compared to their parents.
- Children with CP, usually rate their quality of life in the emotional and social domains, equal to their typically developed peers.
- The findings listed above, suggest that children with cerebral palsy can adapt well to their activity limitations and may have satisfactory quality of life despite of significant deficits.
- These findings also mean that factors other than the impairment severity may have a major influence on QOL in disabled children.

- The consensus that improving QOL is an important treatment goal in children with CP mandates measures and treatments that enhance this goal.
- For example: the recent findings that family variables as Parenting style and Family functioning have major impact on the psychosocial aspects of QOL of children with CP, can and should be translated to implementation of family interventions, early in the disease course.

References

American Academy of Orthopedic Surgeons. (1997). Pediatric Outcomes Data Collection Instrument version 2.0. In: American Academy of Orthopedic Surgeons. Boston, Massachusetts.

Aran A, Shalev RS, Biran G, Gross-Tsur V. (2007). J Pediatr. 151(1): 56–60, e1.

Arnaud C, White-Koning M, Michelsen SI, Parkes J, Parkinson K, Thyen U. (2008). Pediatrics. 121(1): 54–64.

Bastiaansen D, Koot HM, Ferdinand RF, Verhulst FC. (2004). J Am Acad Child Adolesc Psychiatry. 43: 221–230.

Bjornson KF, Belza B, Kartin D, Logsdon RG, McLaughlin J. (2008). Arch Phys Med Rehabil. 89 (1): 121–127.

Bjornson KF, McLaughlin JF. (2001). Eur J Neurol. 8(Suppl 5): 183.

Bottos M, Feliciangeli A, Sciuto L, Gericke C, Vianello A. (2001). Dev Med Child Neurol. 43: 516–528.

Bullinger M, Ravens-Sieberer U. (1995). Revue Europeenne de Psychologie Appliquee. 45: 245–254.

Connolly MA, Johnson JA. (1999). Pharmacoeconomics. 16: 605–625.

Cremeens J, Eiser C, Blades M. (2006). Health Qual Life Outcomes. 4: 58.

Daltroy LH, Liang MH, Fossel AH, Goldberg MJ. (1998). J Pediatr Orthop. 18: 561–571.

De Civita M, Regier D, Alamgir AH, Anis AH, Fitzgerald MJ, Marra CA. (2005). Pharmacoeconomics. 23: 659–685.

Dickinson HO, Parkinson KN, Ravens-Sieberer U, Schirripa G, Thyen U, Arnaud C, et al. (2007). Lancet. 369(9580): 2171–2178.

Eiser C, Morse R. (2001a). Qual Life Res. 10: 347–357.

Eiser C, Morse R. (2001b). Health Technol Assess. 5: 1–157.

Grue L. (2003). Dev Med Child Neurol. 45(October Suppl): 8 (abstr).

Goodwin DA, Boggs SR, Graham-Pole J. (1994). Psychol Assess. 6: 321–328.

Harding L. (2001). Clin Psychol Psychother. 8: 79–96.

Havermans T, Vreys M, Proesmans M, De Boeck C. (2006). Child Care Health Dev. 32: 1.

Houlihan CM, O'Donnell M, Conaway M, Stevenson RD. (2004). Dev Med Child Neurol. 46: 305–310.

Kennes J, Rosenbaum P, Hanna SE, Walter S, Russell S, Raina P, Bartlett D, Galuppi B. (2002). Dev Med Child Neurol. 44: 240–257.

Koman LA, Smith BP, Shilt JS. (2004). Lancet. 363: 1619–1631.

Landgraf J, Abetz LN. (1996). In: Spilker B. (ed.) Quality of Life and Pharmacoeconomics in Clinical Trials. Lippincott-Raven, Philadelphia, PA, pp. 793–802.

Liptak GS, O'Donnell M, Conaway M, Chumlea WC, Wolrey G, Henderson RC. (2001). Dev Med Child Neurol. 43: 364–370.

Livingston MH, Rosenbaum PL, Russell DJ, Palisano RJ. (2007). Dev Med Child Neurol. 49(3): 225–231.

Majnemer A, Mazer B. (2004). Semin Pediatr Neurol. 11: 11–17.

Majnemer A, Shevell M, Rosenbaum P, Law M, Poulin C. (2007). J Pediatr. 151(5): 470–475, 5 e1–3.

McCarthy ML, Silberstein CE, Atkins EA, Harryman SE, Sponseller PD, Hadley-Miller NA. (2002). Dev Med Child Neurol. 44(7): 468–476.

Oeffinger D, Gorton G, Bagley A, Nicholson D, Barnes D, Calmes J. (2007). Dev Med Child Neurol. 49(3): 172–180.

Oeffinger DJ, Tylkowski CM, Rayens MK, Davis RF, Gorton GE, 3rd, D'Astous J. (2004). Dev Med Child Neurol. 46: 311–319.

Palisano R, Rosenbaum P, Walter S, Russell D, Wood E, Galuppi B. (1997). Dev Med Child Neurol. 39: 214–223.

Ravens-Sieberer U, Gosch A, Rajmil L. (2005). Expert Rev Pharmacoeconomics Outcomes Res. 5: 353–364.

Ronen GM, Streiner DL, Rosenbaum P. (2003). Epilepsia. 44: 598–612.

Russell KM, Hudson M, Long A, Phipps S. (2006). Cancer. 106: 2267–2274.

Shelly A, Davis E, Waters E, Mackinnon A, Reddihough D, Boyd R. (2008). Dev Med Child Neurol. 50(3): 199–203.

Simeoni MC, Schmidt S, Muehlan H, Debensason D, Bullinger M, Group tD. (2007). Qual Life Res. 16 (5): 881–893.

Theunissen NC, Vogels TG, Koopman HM. (1998). Qual Life Res. 7: 387–397.

Vargus-Adams J. (2005). Arch Phys Med Rehabil. 86: 940–945.

Vargus-Adams J. (2006). Dev Med Child Neurol. 48(5): 343–347.

Varni JW, Burwinkle TM, Berrin SJ, Sherman SA, Artavia K, Malcarne VL. (2006). Dev Med Child Neurol. 48(6): 442–449.

Varni JW, Burwinkle TM, Sherman SA. (2005). Dev Med Child Neurol. 47: 592–597.

Varni JM, Limbers CA, Burwinkle TM. (2007). Health Qual Life Outcomes. 3: 1.

Viehweger E, Robitail S, Rohon MA, Jacquemier M, Jouve JL, Bollini G. (2008). Ann Readapt Med Phys. 51(2): 129–137.

Wake M, Salmon L, Reddihough D. (2003). Dev Med Child Neurol. 45: 194–199.

Waters E, Davis E, Boyd R. (2007). Dev Med Child Neurol. 49: 49–55.

Waters E, Stewart-Brown S, Fitzpatrick R. (2003). Child Care Health Dev. 29: 501–509.

Watson SMR, Keith KD. (2002). Ment Retard. 40: 304–312.

White-Koning M, Arnaud C, Dickinson HO, Thyen U, Beckung E, Fauconnier J. (2007). Pediatrics. 120(4): e804–e814.

World Health Organization. (1993). Geneva, Switzerland: Division of Mental Health, World Health Organization, Geneva, Switzerland.

World Health Organization. (1995). Soc Sci Med. 41: 1403–1409.

144 Quality of Life Measures in Children with Cancer

C. H. Yeh · Y.-P. Kung · Y.-C. Chiang

1	Introduction	2470
2	The Criteria for Selection	2471
2.1	Conceptual Definitions of HRQL	2471
2.2	Disease Specific and Generic Instruments to Measure HRQL	2474
2.3	Respondent	2477
3	Discussion	2477
3.1	Problems with the Conceptual Definition of HRQL	2477
3.2	Proxy Agreement	2478
3.3	Developmental Concerns of HRQL	2479
4	Conclusion	2479
	Summary Points	2480

Abstract: Health related quality of life (HRQL) in pediatric oncology patients has gained much attention in the past three decades due to the advances in medical technology which has dramatically increased survival rates. The purpose of this review is to identify, describe and critique HRQL measures developed or applied in pediatric oncology patients. Considerable progress has been made in the development of HRQL for pediatric oncology patients in the past two decades. Measures reviewed in this chapter have been examined for many factors: multidimensional constructs, patient's subjective assessment, as well as supplemental information provided by parents or healthcare providers. Evidence of strong psychometric qualities has also been provided for the studies reviewed here. Still, there are problems regarding HRQL measures for pediatric oncology patients which need to be solved, including additional consensus of conceptual and operation definitions of HRQL. Issues related to concordances of proxy agreement remain. Few HRQL measures have taken developmental issues into account, especially for younger children. Interpretation of quantitative HRQL may ignore the qualitative meaning to children's perception of HRQL.

List of Abbreviations: *ARM*, adolescent resilience model; *CHI*, child health and illness; *CHQ*, child health questionnaire; *CHRIs*, child health rating inventories; *FS-II*, functional status II; *HCP*, health care professionals; *HRQL*, health related quality of life; *HUI*, health utilities index; *PCQL-32*, pediatric cancer quality of life inventory; *PEDQOL*, quality of life in children and adolescents with cancer; *PedsQL™*, pediatric quality of life inventory™; *POQOLS*, pediatric oncology quality of life scale; *PPSC*, play performance scale for children; *QOLCC*, quality of life for children with cancer; *QWB*, quality of well being; *WHO*, World Health Organization

1 Introduction

The survival rate for pediatric oncology patients has dramatically increased due to the advances in medical technology over the past two decades. The overall 5 year survival rate for all forms of pediatric cancer has improved, and is now up to 80% for some types of cancer (Adamson et al., 2005). Along with the improved outcomes for pediatric oncology, much attention has been directed toward health related quality of life (HRQL) issues for both cancer patients and long term cancer survivors. The co-morbidity of cancer treatment continues to be a major factor in providing care for oncology patients further increasing the need for Health Care Professionals (HCP) to attend to quality of life issues. The purpose of this chapter is to review and critique the research that has been published in the area of assessing and measuring HRQL for pediatric oncology patients and their families. HRQL has become an important outcome indicator for assessing the effectiveness of these recent advances in cancer treatment (Hinds et al., 2006; Pickard et al., 2004). Consensus in the field of HRQL has been achieved for both the subjective and objective perspectives of the conceptual and theoretical underpinnings (Cella, 1994; Eiser, 2004; Hinds et al., 2006; Pickard et al., 2004).

In the past three decades, a significant amount of literature has been published in the area of HRQL associated with pediatric oncology patients. The objective of this review is to identify, describe and critique HRQL measures developed or applied in pediatric oncology patients. Measures related to HRQL for pediatric oncology patients, have especially burgeoned over the past 20 years. The organization of this chapter is as follows: after a brief historical overview of HRQL, the current consensus of conceptual definitions for HRQL will be presented, the remaining sections of the chapter will describe the methods used to select and review the most rigorous research studies that have developed and tested measures for assessing HRQL in pediatric oncology patients and their families. Generic and disease specific HRQL instruments used for pediatric oncology patients will be described, issues associated with self-report and proxy measurements will be addressed as will concerns regarding reliability and validity of measures. The chapter will end with conclusions for further research.

2 The Criteria for Selection

The following section describes the process used for selecting the specific research studies that will be reviewed and critiqued in this chapter. An initial computer search (MEDLINE) was conducted using the headings "quality of life," "children," and "cancer." The bibliographies of other related review articles (Eiser and Morse, 2001; Hinds et al., 2006; Nathan et al., 2004; Pickard et al., 2004; Varni et al., 2007) were also reviewed and each selected article provided a partial cross-check on the completeness of the library-based search. Only articles published in the English-language, and in nationally circulated publications were included in the review.

When the titles were appropriate, the articles were retrieved and examined to determine if they met the selection criteria for this review. First, the article had to qualify as a research report. To qualify as a research report, the manuscript had to reflect the five major research elements recommended by Duffy (1985), which include: evidence of problem formation, data collection, evaluation of data points, analysis and interpretation, and presentation of results. The scientific merit of each study was reviewed according to criteria elaborated by Duffy (1985), according to title, abstract, problem, literature review, methodology, data analysis and discussion. The following is based on the searches and criteria just described.

The introduction of the concept of quality of life in medical research begin in the definition delineated by the World Health Organization (WHO) (1947) as "the complete state of physical, mental and social well being and not merely the physical, mental, and social dimensions (p.29)." Since that time, over 53,836 publications have appeared related to quality of life. Not surprising, only 0.5% (n = 285) of the publications identified are related to children (with cancer). Using a weighting for the search terms "quality of life," "children," and "cancer" resulted, only 156 publications that specifically focused on quality of life in children. In the 156 articles examined, the majority referred to theoretical or conceptual work (n = 95, 60%), empirical quality of life research in children with specific chronic conditions (n = 48, 30%), while the testing of assessment instruments (quality of life in children) or empirical quality of life research in general was less prominent.

2.1 Conceptual Definitions of HRQL

Until recently there was no consensus on the conceptual definitions associated with HROL. That has now changed and the accepted definitions are presented in ❷ Table 144-1 for conceptual definition and ❷ Table 144-2 for theoretical definition. In their article Hinds and Haase (1998), highlight function-based and meaning-based models, as well as Substantive models for quality of life in pediatric oncology patients. Each of these has contributed to the development of different scientific knowledge. Function-based models focus primary on objective assessment of one's functioning while subjective based models examine the meaning of the illness and the meaning of quality of life to the individual. A typical definition of

◼ Table 144-1

Conceptual definition of quality of life for pediatric oncology patients

References	Conceptual definition	Dimensions
Hinds et al. (2004)	An overall sense of well-being based on being able to participate in usual activities; to interact with others and feel cared about; to cope with uncomfortable physical, emotional, and cognitive reactions; and to find meaning in the illness experience	Symptoms, usual activities, social and family interactions, health status, mood, meaning of being ill
Woodgate and Degner, (2003)	Patient's changing perceptions of themselves across the trajectory of treatment were a major influence on their QOL or well-being. An inductively identified process labeled by the researchers as "keeping the spirit alive" represented the patients' efforts to live with cancer. Cancer-related symptoms precipitated changes in self-perceptions; the same symptoms were viewed as part of the entire cancer experiences, in part, represented by a process labeled "getting through all the rough spots." Cancer was described as profoundly affecting adolescents' sense of self, particularly with physical changes	
Yeh et al. (2004a)	QOL is defined as the impact of disease and treatment on the child's appraisal and satisfaction of functioning as measured in the following scales: (1) *physical function*, defined as functional status in the activities of daily living; (2) *psychological dysfunction*, defined as the degree of emotional distress; (3) *social function*, defined as interpersonal functioning in peer/school relationships; (4) *treatment/disease-related symptoms*, defined as anxiety and worry about the illness and treatments; and (5) *cognitive function*, defined as cognitive performance in problem solving	Physical function, psychological dysfunction, social function, treatment/disease-related function and cognitive function

function-based quality of life is "a multidimensional construct" that includes but is not limited to social, physical, and emotional functioning (Varni et al., 1998). Most of the measures represented in ❷ *Table 144-2* are based on a function-based model. Hinds and Haase (1998) believe the function-based definition may not detect patients' experiences which are meaningful to them. For example, adolescents may choose to answer an item asking if he or she is able to see friends at school with a "no" when in fact they could see friends but choose not to because they have lost their hair and choose to stay home due to their

□ Table 144-2

Theoretical definition of health related quality of life for pediatric oncology patients

References	Models	Theoretical definition
Haase et al. (1999)	Adolescent resilience model	Illness-related risk (i.e., symptom distress and uncertainty), social integration (i.e., relationships with peers and healthcare providers), and spiritual perspective meaning, positive coping, defensive coping, and family atmosphere, resilience and self-transcendence. The process of identifying or developing resources and strengths to flexibly manage stressors to gain a positive outcome, a sense of confidence, mastery and self-esteem
Hinds and Martin, (1988)	Self-sustaining model for adolescent	It is defined as a natural progression adolescents experiencing serious health threats move through to comfort themselves and to achieve competence in resolving health threats
Woodgate (1999)	Resiliency model	This model includes stressors or risk situations (i.e., cancer diagnosis, hair lose), vulnerability factors or protective factors, and outcomes (adaptation and maladaptation as a continuum)
Taieb et al. (2003)	Post-traumatic stress disorder	The symptoms of PTSD are grouped into three categories: reexperiencing (recurrent distressful memories or dreams), avoiding or numbing (shunning talking or thinking about the event), and increased arousal (behavioral or cognitive problems, sleep disturbances)
Hinds et al. (2005)	Pediatric QOL at end-of_life model	This model depicts the transition from curative to end-of-life care and reflects a dual focus on the QOL of the terminally ill child or adolescent and that of the family
Nuss et al. (2005)	Relational decision making at end of life in pediatric oncology	It depicts the centrality of three interdependent perspectives in end-of-life decision making: those of the child or adolescent, the parent or guardian, and the healthcare provider. Relational decision making is depicted as being influenced by communication skills, competence, emotions, faith, and hope

Table 144-2 was adapted from Hinds and Haase (1998) and updated

appearance and this alters their attendance at school, rather than the severity of their illness. Thus their quality of life score may be misinterpreted.

Hinds (1990) proposed a model of environmental influence on quality of life: that the internal environment (i.e., the child's feelings about him or herself), the immediate environment (i.e., significant others such as family or health care providers) and the institutional environment (i.e., financial support) all influence quality of life. The Adolescent Resilience Model (ARM) also indicates that the individual, family, and societal characteristics directly influence quality of life (Haase et al., 1999).

The different definitions of health-related quality of life in the current literature have resulted in an international consensus about the components of quality of life. An operational definition of the term has evolved. Varni et al. have recently identified this consensus definition as: health-related quality of life is viewed as a psychological construct which describes the physical, mental, social, psychological and functional aspects of well-being and function from the patient perspective (Varni et al., 2007). This operational definition stresses the multidimensionality of the quality of life concept as well as the relevance of patients' self-report.

2.2 Disease Specific and Generic Instruments to Measure HRQL

Two categories of instruments have been used to measure HRQL (❷ *Table 144-3*). This table is adapted from Pickard et al. (2004) and updated. Those developed specifically for children with cancer and generic instruments designed to measure quality of life in other chronic illnesses. These are separated and identified in ❷ *Table 144-2*. Generic measures refer to instruments used to assess functional status or quality of life across disease groups which are not designed specifically for the assessment of cancer patients, but they have been used in some of the reports that will be presented here, such as Child Health and Illness (CHI), Child Health Questionnaire (CHQ), Functional status II (FS-II), Quality of Well Being (QWB), Health Utilities Index (HUI) Mark 2 (HUI2) and Mark 3 (HUI3), Play Performance Scale for Children (PPSC).

The PPSC and FS-II were designed to measure physical functioning for pediatric oncology patients. The Health Utilities Index (HUI) Systems (HUI 2and HUI 3) (Feeny et al., 1996, 1999) have been used extensively to examine health status in pediatric cancer patients. The HUI is a multi-attribute instrument, with objective scoring criteria and brevity (Feeny et al., 1996, 1999). The Child Health Questionnaire (CHQ) (Landgraf et al., 1998) is designed to reveal a multidimensional profile of OQL for children, which measures various concepts not normally included in adult assessment tools, such as self-esteem, behavior and, the impact of the children's QOL on the family and parents.

Measurements developed to assess cancer-specific HRQL include the Pediatric Cancer Quality of life Inventory (PCQL-32) (this measure has also been expanded to the Pediatric Quality of life Inventory™, PedsQL™), Miami Pediatric Quality of Life Questionnaire, the Pediatric Oncology Quality of Life Scale (POQOLS), the Child Health Rating Inventories (CHRIs), the Quality of Life in Children and Adolescents with Cancer (PEDQOL), the Royal Marsden Hospital Pediatric quality of life questionnaire, and the Quality of Life for Children with Cancer (QOLCC). Psychometric testing with establish reliability and validity of these measures are well documented.

Disease-specific HRQL instruments are believed to enhance sensitivity for health (physical and disease) domains specifically for cancer. Cancer-specific HRQL measures described above allow us to evaluate psychological factors in addition to physical functioning and have sound psychometric qualities. Both the Child Health Rating Inventories (CHRIs) (Parsons et al., 1999) and the Pediatric Cancer Quality of Life Inventory-32 (PCQL-32) (Varni et al., 1998a) employ parent/child proxy to assess QOL and report variability in different domains of QOL. While these studies represent the significant advancement in QOL research on children with

◘ Table 144-3
Health-related quality of life measures in pediatric oncology patients

Instrument	Domains/items	Respondent	Items	Age
Generic				
Child Health and Illness Profile – Adolescent Edition (CHIP-AE) (Starfield et al., 1995)	Activity, disorders, discomfort, satisfaction with health, achievement of social roles, resilience	Child	153	11–17
Child Health Questionnaire (CHQ-PF50) (Landgraf et al., 1998)	Physical functioning, role/social physical/ emotional behavior, general health, parental time/emotional impact, self-esteem, mental health, general behaviors, family activities, family cohesion	Parent and child	50	5–16
Functional status II (R) (Stein and Jessop, 1990)	Physical, psychological, social	Parent	Long: 43	0–16
			Short: 14	
KINDL (Ravens-Sieberer and Bullinger, 1998)	Psychological well-being, social relationships, physical function, everyday life activities	Child	40	10–16
		Parent proxy		
		Parent (interview) (4–7 years)		
Sixteen-dimensional health-related measures (16-D, 17-D) (Apajasalo et al., 1996a,b)	Mobility, vision, hearing, breathing, sleeping, eating, elimination, speech, mental function, discomfort and symptoms, school and hobbies, friends, physical appearance, depression, distress, vitality (may varies due to different items included)	Child	16	12–15
Health Utilities Index (HUI)-Mark 2 and 3 (Barr et al., 1994; Feeny et al., 1996)	Mark 2: sensation, mobility, emotion, pain, fertility, cognition and self-care	Parent, child, physician	Interviewer:40;	≥6
	Mark 3: vision, hearing, speech, ambulation, dexterity, emotion, cognition and pain		Self-complete: 15	

◨ Table 144-3 (continued)

Instrument	Domains/items	Respondent	Items	Age
Child Health Rating Inventories (CHRIs) (Parsons et al., 1999)	Physical function, role function, mental health, overall quality of life, social/personal resources, cognitive function and energy	Child Parent Doctor	30	5–18
Quality of well-being scale (QWB) (Bradlyn et al., 1993)	Mobility, physical functioning, social activity, current symptomatology	Parent Child Adolescent	40	0–18
Behavioral, affective, and somatic experiences scale (BASES) (Phipps et al., 1994)	Somatic distress, compliance, mood/ behavior, interactions, activity	Nurse (BASE-N) Parent (BASE-P) Child (BASE-C)	38	2–20
Perceived illness experience (PIE) (Eiser et al., 1995)	Physical functioning (symptoms, functional disability, and restrictions), psychological functioning (symptoms)	Child	34	Adolescent
Play performance Scale for children (Lansky et al., 1987)	Level of activity	Parent	1–16	1
Cancer specific measures				
Pediatric cancer quality of life inventory (PCQL), PCQL-32, PedsQL™ (Varni et al., 1998a, 1999)	Disease/treatment related symptoms, physical, psychological, social, and cognitive functioning	Child, adolescent Parent	8–12 (child) 13–18 (adolescent)	Child: 84 Adolescent: 87
PEDQOL: quality of life in children and adolescents with cancer (Calaminus et al., 2000)	Physical functioning, autonomy, emotional functioning, cognition, social functioning/friends, social functioning/family, body image	Child Parent	8–18	34
Miami Pediatric Quality of life questionnaire (Armstrong et al., 1999)	Social competence, emotional stability, self-competence	Parent	1–18	40
Pediatric oncology quality of life scale (POQOLS) (Goodwin et al., 1994)	Physical functions and role restriction, emotional distress, reaction to current medical treatment	Parent	Not stated	21

◘ Table 144-3 (continued)

Instrument	Domains/items	Respondent	Items	Age
Royal Marsden Hospital Pediatric quality of life (Watson et al., 1999)	Functional status, global quality of life, physical symptoms, emotional status, social functioning, cognitive functioning, behavioral problems, school/educational progress	Parent	Not stated	78
Quality of life for children with cancer (QOLCC) (Yeh et al., 2004a)	Physical, social, cognitive disease/treatment, and psychological functioning	Child	7–18	34
		Adolescent		
		Parent		

Table 144-3 was adapted from Pickard et al. (2004) and updated

cancer, most have been conducted in western countries. Only one measure (Quality of Life in Children with Cancer, QOLCC) originated in Taiwan, is published in English, and was developed using a qualitative approach to explore life experiences of Taiwanese children with cancer. Based on the items from PCQL-32, QOLCC is a multidimensional measure to assess HROL (Yeh et al., 2004a,b).

2.3   Respondent

Information collected regarding HRQL includes patient, parent or healthcare providers. Among generic measures (n = 11), 4 includes respondent from patient and parent assessment, 3 from child only, 4 from parent only, and 1 from healthcare provider as well. Among cancer-specific measures (n = 6), 3 include responses from patient and parent assessment, and 3 from parent only.

3   Discussion

Considerable progress has been made in the development of HRQL for pediatric oncology patients in the past two decades. Measures reviewed in this article have considered many factors: multidimensional constructs, patient's subjective assessment, as well as supplemental information provided by parents or healthcare providers. Evidence of strong psychometric qualities has also been provided for the studies reviewed here. Still, there are problems regarding HRQL measures for pediatric oncology patients which need to be solved.

3.1   Problems with the Conceptual Definition of HRQL

Several conceptual definitions and models of HRQL for pediatric oncology patients have been developed or proposed. The development of a valid measure of a theoretical construct is the cornerstone of QOL research, which ensures that the construct under investigation is measurable in an applied setting (Hendrick and Hendrick, 1986). The importance of accuracy in measurement has been emphasized in the discipline of nursing. However, this may not be true in other disciplines. For example, many HRQL measures used in the literature are not supported by conceptual definitions, but only include the domains assessed in the measures. The lack of theoretical development for QOL concepts in pediatric cancer patient research may result in false conclusions, and subsequently, improper clinical interventions (Hinds and Haase, 1998). Some conceptual definitions are proposed, but limited HRQL measures are grounded under their conceptual definitions. For example, the meaning-based model of HRQL is very important because HRQL is a subjective construct (Hinds and Haase, 1998). However, few HRQL measures have considered the meanings from patients' perspective. Indeed, assessment of qualitative HRQL in addition quantitative measures has its challenge of how to collect both qualitative and quantitative data simultaneously. Triangulated data collection and data analysis are sometimes employed in nursing research in order to capture the meaning for the whole individual. Nursing focuses on caring and sensitivity for the individual and the holistic nature of that care to the point of also including the family and understanding the meaning of an event to all of them. Such methodological challenge of triangulation of data collection and analysis still limits many empirical studies.

3.2   Proxy Agreement

One of the challenges of a valid and reliable measure for children with cancer is that the cognitive capacity for self-evaluation changes with the normal process of maturation. One of the overall definitions of HRQL assessment as a subjective construct should be from patients themselves. Assessing the QOL of children is complex due to developmental differences in understanding the content being measured (Landgraf and Abetz, 1996). A few HRQL measures have been developed considering the perspective of children. Different versions of the same measures have been developed especially for children of different ages; child and adolescent self-report versions are available for both the PCQL-32 (Varni et al., 1998a,b) and the QOLCC (Yeh et al., 2004a,b). Proxy reports may be the only available source of data when children are too young to understand the content of self-report measures or too sick to answer a questionnaire. However, inconsistencies between children's self-reports and parent-proxy reports have been reported frequently in the literature (Chang and Yeh, 2005; Cotterill et al., 2000; Feeny et al., 1999; Varni et al., 1998a). Proxy reports tend to be more valid on objective assessments (such as hyperactivity, acting out) than on subjective assessments (depression and anxiety) (Varni et al., 1999). Differences between the degree of concordance between parents and young children and parents and adolescents have been established (Cotterill et al., 2000). Parents may have limited knowledge regarding children's HRQL, however, parents can still provide useful information (Jokovic et al., 2004). The understanding of differences between patients and parent proxy report may also be limited by cross-sectional study design. Agreement of HRQL among patient and parent may change during a course of cancer treatment. In a study examining the agreement on quality of life measures between children's self-reports and parent-proxy reports at different points in time, parent proxy consistently overestimated QOL. They tended to report better QOL (lower score of QOLCC) than did children (in both the on- and off-treatment groups) on baseline and

6-month follow-up assessments, with the one exception being the cognitive subscale at 6-month follow-up (Yeh et al., 2005). In a review study of proxy agreement in research conducted between 1980 and 1999 on QOL in pediatric populations, the authors concluded that before implementing QOL measures, the relationship between child and proxy rating must be clarified (Eiser and Morse, 2001).

3.3 Developmental Concerns of HRQL

HRQL for pediatric oncology patients include a broad range of age and developmental concerns up to age 18. It has been emphasized that HRQL should be able to detect the issues related to growth and development for children and adolescents. However, few measures have been designed to address developmental concerns. Some measures have been developed and tested using separate version of HRQL for children and adolescents (i.e., PCQL-32, QOLCC) (Varni et al., 1998a; Yeh et al., 2004a,b). The items included in these two versions are only different in wording levels regarding different cognitive maturity, but there are no differences in actual item content for children and adolescents. Issues regarding HRQL for children and adolescent may be different. For example, adolescents may focus on their peer relationships and career development but children are more concerned about their limited ability to actively play with others (Yeh, 2001). How the HRQL measures consider developmental changes across childhood is a very important issues in assessing children. In addition, another important issue is whether the same HRQL measure used to collect data when a patient is newly diagnosed is appropriate for patients during follow up courses of cancer treatment or even for survivors.

4 Conclusion

It is evident that the development and testing of HRQL measures for pediatric oncology patients have made considerable progress over the past 20 years. Measures of HRQL specific for pediatric oncology patients have been developed and tested with established reliability and validity. Agreements of proxy report are also examined. Nevertheless, there are still issues in measures of HRQL that need to be solved. First, the development of conceptual definitions for children and adolescents' perspectives of HRQL need to clearly defined according to cognitive differences. The perceptions of HRQL across the cancer treatment trajectory for survivors need to be addressed. Rigorous qualitative studies can be employed to explore children and adolescent's perception of HRQL. Second, the conceptual and operational definition of HRQL should be explicitly stated and matched with underlying conceptual assumptions. Measures of HROL should be tested in cross-sectional studies as well to examine their appropriateness for longitudinal follow up studies. Third, a measure of HRQL for young children (younger than 6 years) needs to be developed. Due to the limited cognitive development of young children, few empirical studies report the HRQL in younger children. In addition patient self-report data, parent proxy assessment should be used as complementary information to increase understanding of HRQL. Finally, HRQL measures need to consider the meaning of HRQL measures to children and adolescents. How we can interpret HRQL correctly is important for health care providers.

Summary Points

- The need for accurate measurement of Health related quality of life (HRQL) for assessment and evaluation of pediatric cancer treatment is essential due to the dramatic increase in the survival rate. Several conceptual definitions associated with HRQL have been proposed but many HRQL measures still lack explicit conceptual definitions.
- The meaning of HRQL measures may be misinterpreted and more work remains to solve how the interpretation of quantitative of HRQL can capture the meaning of HRQL to pediatric oncology patients.
- Differences between the degree of concordance between parents and young children and parents and adolescents have been established but are still limited by the use of cross sectional study designs.
- Developmental issue of HRQL measures have been addressed, but few measures have been designed to consider developmental concerns.
- Due to the limited cognitive development of young children, few empirical studies report the HRQL in younger children.

Acknowledgments

This review was supported by a grant to Dr. Yeh from National Health Research Institutes, Taiwan (Grant number: NHRI-EX95–9302PI) and National Science Council (NSC94–2314-B-182–014). Special thanks to Dr. Susan Jay for the manuscript editing.

References

Adamson P, Law G, Roman E. (2005). Lancet. 365: 753.

Apajasalo M, Rautonen J, Holmberg C, Sinkkonen J, Aalberg V, Pihko H, Siimes MA, Kaitila I, Makela A, Erkkila K, Sintonen H. (1996a). Qual Life Res. 5: 532–538.

Apajasalo M, Sintonen H, Holmberg C, Sinkkonen J, Aalberg V, Pihko H, Siimes MA, Kaitila I, Makela A, Rantakari K, Anttila R, Rautonen J. (1996b). Qual Life Res. 5: 205–211.

Armstrong FD, Toledano SR, Miloslavich K, Lackman-Zeman L, Levy JD, Gay CL, Schuman WB, Fishkin PE. (1999). Int J Cancer Suppl. 12: 11–17.

Barr RD, Pai MK, Weitzman S, Feeny D, Furlong W, Rosenbaum P. (1994). Int Oncol. 4: 639–648.

Bradlyn AS, Harris CV, Warner JE, Ritchey AK, Zaboy K. (1993). Health Psychol. 12: 246–250.

Calaminus G, Weinspach S, Teske C, Gobel U. (2000). Klin Padiatr. 212: 211–215.

Cella DF. (1994). J Pain Symptom Manag. 9: 186–192.

Chang PC, Yeh CH. (2005). Psychooncology. 14: 125–134.

Cotterill SJ, Parker L, Malcolm AJ, Reid M, More L, Craft AW. (2000). Brit J Cancer. 83: 397–403.

Duffy ME. (1985). Nurs Health Care. 6: 538–547.

Eiser C. (2004). Children with Cancer: The quality of life. Lawrence Erlbaum Associates, Mahwah.

Eiser C, Havermans T, Craft A, Kernahan J. (1995). Arch Dis Child. 72: 302–307.

Eiser C, Morse R. (2001). Arch Dis Child. 84: 205–211.

Feeny D, Furlong W, Mulhern RK, Barr RD, Hudson M. (1999). Int J Cancer Suppl. 12: 2–9.

Feeny DH, Torrance GW, Furlong WJ. (1996). In: Spilker B (ed.) Quality of Life and Pharmacoeconomics in Clinical Trials. Lippincott-Raven Publishers, Philadelphia, PA, pp. 239–252.

Goodwin DAJ, Boggs SR, Graham-Pole J. (1994). Psychol Assess. 6: 321–328.

Haase JE, Heiney SP, Ruccione KS, Stutzer C. (1999). Int J Cancer Suppl. 12: 125–131.

Hendrick C, Hendrick S. (1986). J Pers Soc Psychol. 50: 392–402.

Hinds PS. (1990). Semin Oncol Nurs. 6: 285–291.

Hinds PS, Gattuso JS, Fletcher A, Baker E, Coleman B, Jackson T, Jacobs-Levine A, June D, Rai SN, Lensing S, Pui CH. (2004). 13: 761–772.

Hinds PS, Burghen EA, Haase JE, Phillips CR. (2006). Oncol Nurs Forumm. 33: 23–29.

Hinds PS, Haase JE. (1998). In: King CR, Hinds PS (eds.) Quality of Life: from Nursing and Patient Perspective: Theory, Research, Practice. Jones and Bartlett Publishers International, London, pp. 54–63.

Hinds PS, Martin J. (1988). Nurs Res. 37: 336–340.

Hinds PS, Oakes LL, Hicks J, Anghelescu DL. (2005). Semin Oncol Nurs. 21: 53–62.

Jokovic A, Locker D, Guyatt G. (2004). Qual Life Res. 13: 1297–1307.

Landgraf JM, Abetz LN. (1996). In: Spilker B (ed.) Quality of Life and Pharmacoeconomics in Clinical Trials. Lippincott-Raven Publishers, Philadelphia, PA, pp. 793–802.

Landgraf JM, Maunsell E, Speechley KN, Bullinger M, Campbell S, Abetz L, Ware JE. (1998). Qual Life Res. 7: 433–445.

Lansky SB, List MA, Lansky LL, Ritter-Sterr C, Miller DR. (1987). Cancer. 60: 1651–1656.

Nathan PC, Furlong W, Barr RD. (2004). Pediatr Blood Cancer. 43: 215–223.

Nuss SL, Hinds PS, LaFond DA. (2005). Semin Oncol Nurs. 21: 125–134.

Parsons SK, Barlow SE, Levy SL, Supran SE, Kaplan SH. (1999). Int J Cancer Suppl. 12: 46–51.

Phipps S, Hinds PS, Channell S, Bell GL. (1994). J Pediatr Oncol Nurs. 11: 109–117.

Pickard AS, Topfer LA, Feeny DH. (2004). J Natl Cancer Inst Monographs. 33: 102–125.

Ravens-Sieberer U, Bullinger M. (1998). Qual Life Res. 7: 399–407.

Starfield B, Riley AW, Green BF, Ensminger ME, Ryan SA, Kelleher K, Kim-Harris S, Johnston D, Vogel K. (1995). Med Care. 33: 553–566.

Stein RE, Jessop DJ. (1990). Med Care. 28: 1041–1055.

Taieb O, Moro MR, Baubet T, Revah-Levy A, Flament MF. (2003). Eur Child Adolesc Psychiatry. 12: 255–264.

Varni JW, Katz ER, Seid M, Quiggins DJ, Friedman-Bender A. (1998a). Cancer. 82: 1184–1196.

Varni JW, Katz ER, Seid M, Quiggins DJ, Friedman-Bender A, Castro CM. (1998b). J Behav Med. 21: 179–204.

Varni JW, Limbers CA, Burwinkle TM. (2007). Health Qual Life Outcomes. 5: 43.

Varni JW, Seid M, Rode CA. (1999). Med Care. 37: 126–139.

Watson M, Edwards L, Von EL, Davidson J, Day R, Pinkerton R. (1999). Int J Cancer Suppl. 12: 65–70.

Woodgate RL. (1999). J Pediatr Oncol Nurs. 16: 35–43.

Woodgate RL, Degner LF. (2003). J Pediatr Oncol Nurs. 20: 103–119.

World Health Organization. (1947). The constitution of the World Health Organization. WHO Chron 1: 29.

Yeh CH. (2001). Nurs Sci Q. 14: 141–148.

Yeh CH, Chang CW, Chang PC. (2005). Nurs Res. 54: 354–362.

Yeh CH, Chao KY, Hung LC. (2004a). Psychooncology. 13: 161–170.

Yeh CH, Hung LC, Chao KY. (2004b). Psychooncology. 13: 171–176.

145 Quality of Life in Healthy and Chronically Ill Icelandic Children: Agreement Between Child's Self-Report and Parents' Proxy-Report

E. K. Svavarsdottir

1	*Introduction*	*2484*
1.1	HRQOL from the Child's, the Adolescent's and the Parent's Perspective	2485
1.2	Level of Agreement Between Child's Self-Report and the Parents' Report on HRQOL	2486
2	*Methodological Considerations*	*2487*
2.1	Procedure	2487
2.2	Subjects/Sample	2488
2.3	Instruments	2490
2.4	Data Analysis	2490
3	*An Analysis of the Agreement Between Pre-Teenagers' Self Report and Parents' Proxy Report*	*2491*
3.1	Mean Differences between Pre-Teenagers' Self-Report and Mothers' and Fathers' Proxy-Report	2491
3.2	Level of Agreement Between Pre-Teenagers' Self-Report and Parents' Proxy-Report	2493
3.3	Mean Differences and Agreements Between Pre-Teenagers' Self-Report and Single Parents' and Dual Parents' Proxy-Reports	2495
3.4	Mean Differences and Agreement Between Pre-Teenagers' Self-Report and Parents' Proxy-Report Based on the Gender of the Child and the Gender of the Parent	2496
3.5	Discussion	2498
4	*Conclusion*	*2500*
	Summary Points	*2501*

Abstract: The purpose of this chapter is to report on findings on level of agreement between 10 and 12-year-old healthy and chronically ill Icelandic pre-teenagers' reports and their mothers' and fathers' proxy-reports on the children's ❷ health related quality of life (HRQOL) and to view the findings in the light of the international literature. The research is cross-sectional and was introduced to 1,079 children in 5th and 6th grade and their parents. Out of those, 480 children (209 boys and 271 girls) and 912 parents (510 mothers and 402 fathers) gave their written consent and participated in the study. Data were collected from March to early June 2004 in 12 randomly selected public elementary schools in Reykjavik, Iceland. Descriptive statistics and dependent *t*-test were used to answer the research questions and to test the hypotheses. The main findings were that Icelandic pre-teenagers' ❷ self-report differed significantly from their mothers' and fathers' proxy-report on the social and school functioning subscales of the HRQOL measure, as well as on the overall HRQOL score. Further findings were that mothers of healthy children and both parents of chronically ill children differed significantly from their children in their perception of the physical functioning of the child. These findings emphasize that ❷ parents' proxy-report cannot be substituted for the pre-teenagers' report on their own HRQOL. However, within the subscale of emotional functioning, the children and their parents were found to agree. Agreement was also found between fathers and their healthy children on the physical functioning subscale. This suggests that Icelandic parents can provide valid information on their children's physical and emotional functioning, which can be used as a substitute for the children's own response. Although parents' proxy-report can only substitute a child's self-report within the emotional and physical functioning subscale, a proxy-report can add needed and valid information regarding parents' perspective on their pre-teenagers' HRQOL.

List of Abbreviations: *HRQOL,* health related quality of life; *QOL,* quality of life

1   Introduction

Parents of healthy as well as chronically ill pre-teenagers play a crucial role in their children's life. In their pre-teenage years, children who receive support and encouragement from their parents, other close family members, and school personnel are developing an identity, independency, and a sense of accomplishment when achieving normal growth and development. Parents are expected to encourage, support and stimulate children's development towards adulthood by providing a safe environment and by guiding and strengthening the development of educational, emotional, relational and behavioral skills as the children progress through the adolescent years. Early information on health related quality of life (HRQOL) among school children can help identify health related problems and give school nurses an opportunity to develop interventions, but one factor that greatly influences developmental outcomes and quality of life in children is their health status.

Quality of life (QOL) has been defined broadly as life satisfaction (Vila et al., 2003). Further, Varni et al. (2004) have emphasized the importance that HRQOL instruments are sensitive to cognitive development and include both the child's self-report and parents' proxy-report to reflect both perspectives. However, lack of agreement between self- and proxy-report has been documented in the literature (Annett et al., 2003; Guyatt et al., 1997; le Coq et al., 2000; Varni et al., 2004). No correlation was found between asthma control as viewed by clinician and the quality of life scores of the children (Williams and Williams, 2003). In addition, low correlation was found between the children's and the parents' rating of HRQOL.

Self-report is considered the standard for measuring perceived HRQOL among adolescents (Janse et al., 2005). HRQOL measures include both physical and psychological functioning but, in order to evaluate the impact of illness on day-to-day functioning, investigators have, in a range of clinical studies, included both disease specific and generic HRQOL questionnaires. Nevertheless, it is typically the parents' perceptions of their children's HRQOL that influence health care utilization. Therefore, it is important to determine whether proxy-reports are valid and whether they can be used to assess children's QOL for example, when children's self-report data is not possible to obtain.

Little is known about quality of life of pre-teenagers and about parental perception of HRQOL when a child in the general population is diagnosed with a chronic health condition or illness. The purpose of this study is to evaluate agreement between pre-teenagers' self-reports on HRQOL and their parents' proxy-report (both the mothers' and the fathers' perspective) among 10- to 12-year-old healthy and chronically ill Icelandic children.

1.1 HRQOL from the Child's, the Adolescent's and the Parent's Perspective

Health related quality of life has been studied among children and adolescents with variety of chronic illnesses, both from the child's or the adolescent's own perspective (Charron-Prochownik, 2002; Faulkner, 2003; Faulkner and Chang, 2007; Fiese et al., 2005; Mednick et al., 2004; Varni et al., 2003) as well as from the parents' or caregivers' perspective (Bothwell et al., 2002; Hays et al., 2006; Knowles et al., 2007; Landolt et al., 2002; Markham and Dean, 2006; Sheppard et al., 2005; Whitney, 2005). In a recent study on quality of life among children with asthma, the children's perception of their own quality of life was found to be associated with the parents' report of routine burden (Fiese et al., 2005). The authors emphasized that pediatric asthma management is a multifaceted activity and that in family environments where parents are overwhelmed or burdened by care there is a cost to the child as well. However, when families are able to create predictable routines around daily care, their children may be better equipped to follow doctor's orders, less likely to have anxiety-related symptoms, and have a better overall quality of life (Fiese et al., 2005). Ungar et al. (2006) pointed out in a study on analysis of a dyad approach to health related quality of life measurement in children with asthma that by bringing parent and child together, the dyad provides a forum for discussion and elaboration of perceptions of HRQOL. The authors highlighted that through skilled interviewer facilitation, parent and child may learn from each other's judgments and the child may be enabled to provide more reliable responses to structured HRQOL questionnaire items.

International literature on quality of life among families of children with asthma has among other things focused on life satisfaction. In a sample of Swedish families, Rydström et al. (2004) found that a desire to be like other families and hope and longing for a better life was the families' strategy to handle uncertainty regarding the disease. However, Dalheim-Englund et al. (2004) found in a sample of 371 Swedish parents of children with asthma that most of the parents evaluated their own quality of life as being close to the positive end of the scale, and there was close agreement in the scoring between parents within the same family. In that study, children with asthma were not found to influence the parents' QOL to a great degree.

Further, in a US sample of children with diabetes, the parents of 10- to 12-year-old school age children were found to experience greater life satisfaction (within the health related quality of life subscale) than parents of adolescents (13–18 years) (Faulkner and Clark, 1998). In another study on 99 African-American families of school age children and adolescents with type 1 diabetes, Faulkner and Chang (2007) found that emphasizing open family communication and providing emotional support for diabetic management would benefit the families regarding developmentally appropriate levels of self-care and quality of life. For families of children with cancer, the number of days from central venous catheter placement in the child and the child's coping was found to significantly predict the children's quality of life, which in turn predicted parental trust in the medical care (Tremolada et al., 2005). Further, a difference in perception of quality of life has been found between parents of chronically ill children and pediatricians (Janse et al., 2005) not only at diagnosis but also within 6 months follow-up measures.

Few researches have focused on quality of life among healthy school age children. Chen et al. (2005) conducted a study on the association of lifestyle factors with quality of life in 7,794 Japanese children aged 9–10 years and found unfavorable lifestyles in childhood, like almost never participating in exercise or having seldom breakfast, to be associated with poor quality of life in early adolescence. However, comparing quality of life among healthy as well as chronically ill children has received some attention in the literature. Meuleners et al. (2002) conducted a Delphi study regarding teachers', parents' and health care professionals' perception of the relative importance of different aspects of quality of life for adolescents with chronic illnesses. Half of the panels of parents and health professionals, and 68% of teachers, perceived the chronically ill adolescents to have worse QOL than their healthy counterparts. Reasons cited by the panels included: a poorer attitude as result of the chronic illness, the adolescent can be limited by what he or she can do, poor physical health, lack of independence, having greater obstacles to overcome than a healthy adolescent, the illness makes the chronically ill children different to everyone else and that the health condition prevents chronically ill children from making long term plans.

1.2   Level of Agreement Between Child's Self-Report and the Parents' Report on HRQOL

Little research has been published on the agreement between children's and parents' proxy-report on quality of life, neither in the literature on chronic illnesses nor in the general population literature. Upton et al. (2005) conducted a study on 69 children (aged 8–18 years) in public care and their carers (requited through routine pediatric assessments) and 662 children not in public care (recruited from local schools). The results indicated significant correlation with generic module scores between proxy and self-report scores. However, in a study on health related quality of life among 1,760 French adolescents and their parents (Simeoni et al., 2001), the parents' score was found to be significantly higher than the corresponding scores from the adolescents; this was true for the total index and for each dimension score except for the subscales of inaction and relationships with friends. In addition, in a study on families of children with cystic fibrosis (Epker and Maddrey, 1998), the parents were found to perceive the QOL of their children to experience greater impairment in the domains of behavior, self-esteem and general health perception than the children themselves reported. Further, Noyes (2007) found, in a study on health related quality of life among seventeen 4- to 18-year-old children that were dependent on ventilator, that the children and their parents reported the children's overall health-related quality of life the same, but parents reported significantly lower scores for their child's relationships with friends and their disease. The author emphasizes the need for both child and parent perspectives in order to understand the impact of ventilator-dependency on the child's life.

The level of agreement between children's perception and their parents' perception on quality of life has, over the last few years, received increased attention, both among health care professionals and researchers. Contradictory findings have nevertheless been reported regarding the child's perception and the parents' proxy-report. Chang and Yeh (2005) conducted a study on the agreement between children's self-reports and their parents' proxy-reports to evaluate quality of life in 141 Taiwanese children and adolescents with cancer (age 7–18 years) and their parents. Different statistical approaches were employed to evaluate convergence of self-reports and proxy-reports, such as product-moment correlation coefficient and the comparison of group means on the seven subscales (physical, psychological, social, disease symptom, cognitive, understanding and communication) as well as on the total score of the Quality of Life for Children with Cancer scale (QOLCC) (Yeh and Hung, 2003; Yeh et al., 2004a,b). The results indicated that children and parents had the largest discrepancy on the understanding subscale. For the adolescents (children age 12 and older), the mean differences were largest for the subscales of psychological factors and understanding, which indicates less agreement for these subscales than for the other subscales. The results suggested that for children who were younger and not able to evaluate QOL assessment due to their developmental limitation or severity of illness, the parents can provide valid information about the children's QOL. However, parent-proxy of QOL for adolescents provided significantly different information than the adolescents' self-report. The authors concluded that proxy-data of QOL for adolescents should be used with caution. However, Varni et al. (2003) conducted a study among 10,241 families of healthy as well as chronically ill children, age 2–16 years, and found a trend toward higher inter-correlations among parents proxy-report and increasing age of the children.

Little is known about agreement on HRQOL between healthy and chronically ill pre-teenagers (10–12 years old children) and their parents' proxy-report. Further, no study was found that evaluated agreement between pre-teenagers' perception on their own HRQOL and their parents' perception based on the children's family type (single parent families or dual parent families) or on the gender of the child and the gender of the parent.

Based on the review of the literature, it was hypothesized that there would be no significant difference on the total HRQOL scale nor on any of the subscales of the HRQOL measure between: (1) ❷ healthy pre-teenagers and their parents; (2) chronically ill pre-teenagers and their parents; (3) children and their mothers' proxy-report not matter what type of families the children lived in (single parent families or dual parent families); and (4) there would be no significant difference on the total HRQOL scale nor on any of the subscales of the HRQOL scale based on the gender of the pre-teenager nor on the gender of the parent. The following research questions were asked: (1) Is there a difference between healthy and chronically ill pre-teenagers' levels of agreement on HRQOL (both the total score and within all subscales) and their parents' proxy-report? (2) What is the association between pre-teenagers' self-reports and parents' proxy-reports on the total HRQOL scale as well as on all the subscales of the HRQOL measure?

2 Methodological Considerations

2.1 Procedure

This is a cross sectional study that is based on a larger study on generic health related quality of life (HRQOL) (from the children's and the parents' perspective) among 10- to 12-year-old

Icelandic school children, which included both healthy and chronically ill pre-teenagers (Svavarsdottir and Orlygsdottir, 2006a,b). Data were collected from March to early June 2004 in 12 randomly selected public elementary schools in Reykjavík, Iceland. The study was introduced to 1,079 children in 5th and 6th grade and their parents. Out of those, 480 children (209 boys and 271 girls) and 912 parents (510 mothers and 402 fathers) gave their written consent (both the child and its parents signed the consent) and participated in the study (45% participation of parent(s)-child pairs). The inclusion criteria for the study were: (1) the children needed to be in 5th or 6th grade, and (2) needed to read and write Icelandic. The parents had to be able to read and write Icelandic.

The research was approved by the Institutional Review Board of the Reykjavik Health Care Services, the Reykjavik Council of Education, the principals in the 12 elementary schools, the National Bioethics Committee, and the study was reported to the Data Protection Committee. All children in 5th and 6th grade of the participating schools were informed about the study by the data collection personnel and the school nurse in each school, who gave the children a package of documents to bring home to their parents. The package included an introduction letter, a form for informed consent, two questionnaire booklets (one for the mother and one for the father), and empty envelopes to bring back to the school nurse with a signed consent form (from both parents (if applicable) and the child) and completed questionnaires from the parents. The data collection personnel and the school nurse met with the children who had brought back a signed consent form from their parents. The children who participated were taken out of the classroom to answer the questionnaires. The data collection personnel and the school nurse gave verbal instructions and answered questions from the children. If the children had reading difficulties, either the data collection personnel or the school nurse read the questions out loud for the students.

2.2   Subjects/Sample

A majority of the families were dual parent families (n = 414; 72.71%) and 18.9% (n = 99) one parent families. Parents' mean age was 40.27 years (SD = 5.45), ranging from 24 to 63 years. The mean age of the children was 10.95 years (SD = 0.645) (range 10–12 years), 56.5% were girls and the remainder boys. As reported by the parents, 24.6% (n = 118) of the children had a chronic health condition (chronic illnesses). Of the children, 94 were diagnosed with one health condition (disease), 20 children had two diseases, and 4 children had three diseases. The chronic health condition varied among the 118 children, from being a physical illness (79 health conditions, 54.11%; e.g., allergy/eczema, n = 23 (15.8%); migraine, n = 19 (13%); asthma, n = 15 (10.3%)) to mental and learning disabilities (67 health conditions, 45.89%; e.g., learning disabilities, n = 23 (15.8%); hyperactivity/attention deficit disorder, n = 23 (15.8%); dyslexia, n = 6 (4.1%) (see ❷ *Table 145-1*). Range in the children's visits to the school nurse varied from being "every day" (n = 2; 3%), up to "once that week" (n = 20; 27%). The children who indicated that they were bullied in school last week reported being bullied from "often a day" (n = 3; 9%) to "once that week" (n = 8; 23%). Further, sample information regarding the mean score of the total HRQOL scale as well as all the subscales of HRQOL (physical, emotional social and school functioning) are listed in the Figure, for the parents and the pre-teenagers (see ❷ *Figure 145-1*).

◻ Table 145-1

Demographics of Icelandic school age children and their parents

Variables	Children (N = 480)		Parents (N = 911)		
	(n) Mean	% SD	(n) mean	% SD	Range
Gender of the children					
Female	(271)	(56.5)			
Male	(209)	(43.5)			
Age	10.5	0.665			
Gender of the parents					
Female			(510)	(59.8)	
Male			(401)	(44.02)	
Age			41.11	5.77	24–63
Martial status					
Single parent families			(99)	(18.9)	
Dual parent families			(424)	(81.2)	
Child with chronic health condition					
Yes			(142)	(29.58)	
No			(338)	(70.42)	

Gender of the pre-teenagers' and their parents' gender, age and marital status. The parents' perception of their children's chronic illnesses

◻ Figure 145-1

Mean scores of healthy (N = 117) and chronically ill pre-teenagers' report (N = 360) and their parents' proxy-report

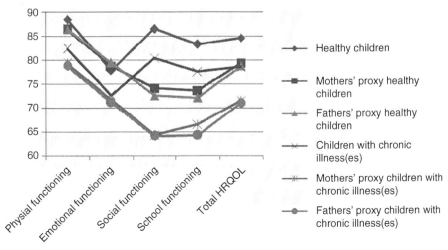

- Healthy children
- Mothers' proxy healthy children
- Fathers' proxy healthy children
- Children with chronic illness(es)
- Mothers' proxy children with chronic illness(es)
- Fathers' proxy children with chronic illness(es)

2.3   Instruments

The questionnaires were translated and culturally adapted to Icelandic from English. Two Icelandic health care providers independently translated the questionnaires into Icelandic (forward translation), and, after discussion and consultation with specialists, came to an agreement on a reconciled version. A professional bilingual translator, who is a native speaker of English and an Icelandic linguistic scholar, performed a back translation. Together, the back and forward translators decided on a new conceptually equivalent Icelandic version, which was pilot tested and validated on seven school children and their families. The instruments were finally proofread by an Icelandic professional. Validity of all the instruments that were used in the study was established by translating the instruments into Icelandic according to the steps described above.

Demographic and background information. Demographic information such as age, gender, grade, after school activities, visits to school nurse and experience of bullying victimization was reported by the children themselves. In addition, the parents answered questions regarding their own background and about their child's chronic health condition/illness(es).

Children's quality of life. The children's health related quality of life (HRQOL) was measured by the 23-item instrument "Pediatric Quality of Life Inventory" (PedsQL), the Generic Core Scale for 8- to 12-year-old children (children's self-report scale), which is to be administered to healthy school children, community population, or children with acute or chronic illnesses. The instrument has four subscales, physical functioning (eight items), emotional functioning (five items), social functioning (five items), and school functioning (five items). The children are asked how much of a problem each item has been for them for the past 1 month, ranging from "never" to "almost always a problem." The items are scored reversely and put on a 0–100 scale, where higher scores point to a higher HRQOL (0 = 100, 1 = 75, 2 = 50, 3 = 25, 4 = 0) (Varni et al., 2002). The internal consistency of the total scale is 0.88 for US children. For the Icelandic children, the alpha reliability was 0.90 for boys and 0.86 for girls. The internal consistency scores for the subscales ranged from 0.68 to 0.80 for the US sample (Varni et al., 2001), 0.70–0.79 for the Icelandic boys and 0.66–0.77 for the Icelandic girls.

Children's quality of life as perceived by their parents. The children's HRQOL as perceived by parents was measured by the 23-item instrument Pediatric Quality of Life Inventory (PedsQL), the Generic Core Scale for 8- to 12-year-old children (parent proxy-report; Varni et al., 1999, 2001). The instrument is a multidimensional parent proxy-report scale that is to be administered to parents of healthy school children or children with acute or chronic illness. The questionnaire is identical to the PedsQL (children's self-report) except that it is phrased in the third person. As described above the instrument has four subscales: physical functioning (eight items), emotional functioning (five items), social functioning (five items) and school functioning (five items). The parents were asked to rate how much of a problem each item had been for their child in the past month, ranging from "never a problem" to "almost always a problem." The items are scored reversely on a 0–100 scale (Varni et al., 2002). The internal consistency of the total scale is 0.90 for US parents. For the Icelandic parents, the alpha reliability for the total scale was 0.86 for mothers and 0.87 for fathers.

2.4   Data Analysis

The data on major study variables (average score for each participant on the total HRQOL score as well as for all the subscales) were normally distributed according to Stem and Leaf plots and histograms. Descriptive statistics, such as means and standard deviations or frequency distributions, were calculated for the major study variables on HRQOL, both the total score and the subscales, as well as for the demographic variables. Descriptive statistics and dependent t-tests were used to answer the research questions and to test the hypotheses of no significant difference in agreement between pre-teenagers' reports on HRQOL (both for the total score and subscales) and their parents' proxy-report. Alpha level of significance was set at 0.05 to reduce the likelihood of committing a Type I error.

In order to compare the differences between the child's self-report and parent's proxy-report, the mean scores and standard deviations were summarized separately. Further, the means of the differences (mean bias) (the children's group – parents' group) and the standard deviation of difference were computed (Chang and Yeh, 2005). A mean difference of less than zero indicates that the parents tend to overestimate their children's HRQOL and a mean difference greater than zero indicates that parents tend to underestimate it. The ❷ effect size d was used to examine the magnitude of this difference, which was found by dividing the mean difference by the SD of the mean score (Chang and Yeh, 2005). The value of the d was judged by the guideline provided by Cohen (1992) and as presented in a research by Chang and Yeh (2005), where $d = 0.2$ was categorized as a small effect size, $d = 0.5$ a medium effect size and $d = 0.8$ a large effect size. In addition, the agreement between the children and parents was further quantified using Person correlation coefficients. The Person product correlation coefficient's effective size was categorized further. When the correlation coefficient was smaller than 0.3 the effective size was labeled as small, when the correlation coefficient was between 0.3 and 0.5 it was evaluated to be medium, and when the correlation coefficient was equal or larger than 0.5 the effective size was considered to be large (Chang and Yeh, 2005; Cohen, 1992).

3   An Analysis of the Agreement Between Pre-Teenagers' Self Report and Parents' Proxy Report

3.1   Mean Differences between Pre-Teenagers' Self-Report and Mothers' and Fathers' Proxy-Report

For healthy pre-teenagers, a significant difference was found between the children's self-report and the mothers' proxy-report on the subscale of physical functioning. The mothers were found to report significantly lower physical functioning of their children than the children themselves. A significant difference was also found between healthy pre-teenagers' self-report and their mothers' proxy-report and between the children and their fathers perception on social functioning and school functioning. Thus, the mothers and the fathers were found to report significantly lower social functioning and significantly lower school functioning than the pre-teenagers. Further, a significant difference was found between the children's total health related quality of life score and the mothers' and the fathers' response; both the mothers and the fathers reported significantly lower health related quality of life (total score) than their healthy pre-teenagers. Interestingly, however, no difference was found between the children's self-report and their fathers' proxy-report on the physical functioning subscale, or between the parents' and the children's subscale of emotional functioning (see ❷ Table 145-2).

For children with chronic illness(es) (both physical illnesses and psychological illnesses), a significant difference was found between the pre-teenagers' self-report and their parents' proxy-report (both the mothers' and the fathers' proxy); the parents reported significantly

■ Table 145-2

Icelandic schoolage children's (N = 480) mean differences in self-report and parents'(N = 524) proxy report regarding HRQOL (subscales and total score)

Variables	Mean	SD	t-value[a]	df	p-value
Healthy children (n = 362)					
Physical functioning					
Self-report (n = 330)	88.41	9.48			
Mothers'-proxy report (n = 330)	86.40	14.66	−2.308	329	0.02
Self-report (n = 251)	87.98	9.36			
Fathers'-proxy report (n = 251)	86.42	14.46	−1.568	250	0.12
Emotional functioning					
Self-report (n = 325)	77.89	14.92			
Mothers'-proxy report (n = 325)	78.92	13.46	1.142	324	0.25
Self-report (n = 248)	77.54	14.95			
Fathers'-proxy report (n = 248)	79.64	12.88	1.869	247	1.63
Social functioning					
Self-report (n = 324)	86.50	14.84			
Mothers'-proxy report (n = 324)	74.25	22.94	−9.194	323	0.00
Self-report (n = 249)	85.64	15.18			
Fathers'-proxy report (n = 249)	72.76	22.91	−8.293	248	0.00
School functioning					
Self-report (n = 324)	83.66	12.84			
Mothers'-proxy report (n = 324)	73.60	19.00	−8.508	323	0.00
Self-report (n = 248)	83.28	13.21			
Fathers'-proxy report (n = 248)	72.05	20.19	−7.696	247	0.00
Total HRQOL score					
Self-report (n = 327)	84.77	9.96			
Mothers'-proxy report (n = 327)	79.45	79.45	79.45	326	0.00
Self-report (n = 250)	84.36	10.19			
Fathers'-proxy report (n = 250)	78.87	12.87	5.999	249	0.00
Children with chronic illness(es) (n = 118)					
Physical functioning					
Self-report (n = 114)	82.60	13.52			
Mothers'-proxy report (n = 114)	79.27	16.08	−2.074	113	0.04
Self-report (n = 88)	82.72	14.03			
Fathers'-proxy report (n = 88)	78.61	18.03	−2.114	87	0.04
Emotional functioning					
Self-report (n = 112)	72.83	17.28			
Mothers'-proxy report (n = 112)	71.70	14.44	0.724	111	0.47
Self-report (n = 87)	73.35	16.65			
Fathers'-proxy report (n = 87)	71.14	14.48	−1.26	86	0.21

◼ Table 145-2 (continued)

Variables	Mean	SD	t-value[a]	df	p-value
Social functioning					
Self-report (n = 110)	80.74	16.92			
Mothers'-proxy report (n = 110)	64.26	20.89	−7.560	109	0.00
Self-report (n = 86)	81.86	16.19			
Fathers'-proxy report (n = 86)	64.00	19.69	−7.371	85	0.00
School functioning					
Self-report (n = 112)	77.51	15.94			
Mothers'-proxy report (n = 112)	66.62	17.35	−5.403	111	0.00
Self-report (n=85)	79.03	14.22			
Fathers'-proxy report (n=85)	64.58	18.13	−6.162	84	0.00
Total HRQOL score					
Self-report (n = 113)	78.73	12.86			
Mothers'-proxy report (n = 113)	71.53	12.14	−5.697	112	0.00
Self-report (n = 87)	79.56	12.33			
Fathers'-proxy report (n = 87)	71.00	12.71	−5.84	85	0.00

Difference between pre-teenagers own report and their parents'report regarding health related quality of life.
n = varies due to missing data
[a]Paired t-tests

lower physical functioning than the ❯ pre-teenagers with chronic illnesses. Further, significant difference was found between the self-report of the children with chronic illness(es) and their parents' proxy on the subscales of social functioning, school functioning and on the total health related quality of life score. Parents of children with a chronic health condition reported lower social functioning, school functioning and lower total health related quality of life score than the children themselves. Nevertheless, no differences were found between the children's report and their parents' proxy-report on the subscale of emotional functioning. Hypotheses (1) and (2) were therefore only partly supported (see ❯ Table 145-2).

3.2   Level of Agreement Between Pre-Teenagers' Self-Report and Parents' Proxy-Report

When the ❯ level of agreement between the children's and their parents' proxy-report was further evaluated (to answer the research questions), healthy children and their parents' proxy differed the most on the social and the school functioning subscales. The mean differences on these two subscales varied from 10.06 to 12.88 (see ❯ Table 145-3). Similarly, for the children with chronic illness(es), their self-report and their parents' proxy-report differed the most on the subscales of social and school functioning, where the mean difference varied from 10.89 to 17.86 (see ❯ Table 145-3). As introduced by Chang and Yeh (2005), a mean difference below zero between self- and proxy-report equals ❯ overestimation, whereas a mean difference greater than zero equals ❯ underestimation. For these Icelandic pre-teenagers, both healthy children and children dealing with chronic illness(es), mean difference on all the subscales as well as on the total HRQOL score was greater than 0 for both the mothers' (varied from 1.03 to

◘ Table 145-3

Level of agreement between children's self report (N = 480), and the parents' proxy report (mothers N = 510; fathers N = 401) of HRQOL (subscales and total score)

Variables	Mean difference	Pearson's correlation	SD of difference	Effect size d
Healthy children				
Mothers versus children				
Physical functioning (n = 330)	2.01	0.20*	15.80	0.13
Emotional functioning (n = 325)	1.03	0.35*	16.27	0.06
Social functioning (n = 324)	12.25	0.25*	23.98	0.51
School functioning (n = 324)	10.06	0.15*	21.29	0.47
Total HRQOL score (n = 327)	5.32	0.24*	14.14	0.38
Fathers versus Children				
Physical functioning (n = 251)	1.56	0.18*	15.77	0.10
Emotional functioning (n = 248)	2.09	0.20*	17.64	0.12
Social functioning (n = 249)	12.88	0.22*	24.50	0.53
School functioning (n = 248)	11.23	0.10	22.99	0.49
Total HRQOL score (n = 250)	5.49	0.23*	14.46	0.38
Children with chronic illness(es)				
Mothers versus Children				
Physical Functioning (n = 114)	3.33	0.34*	17.13	0.19
Emotional Functioning (n = 112)	1.14	0.46*	16.64	0.07
Social Functioning (n = 110)	16.48	0.28*	22.86	0.72
School Functioning (n = 112)	10.89	0.18	21.32	0.51
Total HRQOL score (n = 113)	7.20	0.42*	13.43	0.54
Fathers versus Children				
Physical Functioning (n = 88)	4.11	0.38*	18.23	0.23
Emotional Functioning (n = 87)	2.21	0.45*	16.38	0.14
Social Functioning (n = 86)	17.86	0.23**	22.47	0.79
School Functioning (n = 85)	14.45	0.12	21.61	0.67
Total HRQOL score (n = 87)	8.56	0.40*	13.67	0.63

Agreement between children's report and their parents report on health related quality of life
*p < 0.01
**p < 0.05

12.25 for healthy children; and from 1.14 to 16.48 for children with chronic illness(es)) and the fathers' proxy-report (varied from 1.56 to 12.88 for healthy children; and from 2.21 to 17.86 for children with chronic illness(es)) (see ❷ *Table 145-3*). These results indicate that the Icelandic pre-teenagers and their parents had the largest discrepancy on the subscales of social and school functioning, which shows less agreement on these two subscales than the subscales of physical and emotional functioning. Further, these findings indicate that the parents of both health and chronically ill pre-teenagers had a tendency to underestimate their children's HRQOL when compared to the report of the children's themselves.

In order to evaluate further the level of difference between the children's self-report and the parents' proxy-report, the magnitude of the difference was found by dividing the mean difference with the SD of the mean score (Chang and Yeh, 2005; Cohen, 1992). For the healthy pre-teenagers, the effect size d was small for the physical and the emotional functioning subscales as well as the total HRQOL score, but medium for the social and the school functioning subscales. However, for the pre-teenagers with physical and psychological chronic illness(es), the effect size was small for the physical and emotional subscales, but medium or high for the total HRQOL score and the subscales of social and school functioning (see ❯ *Table 145-3*).

The association between the children's self-report and their parents' proxy-report was further evaluated by Pearson r correlation. As indicated by Chang and Yeh (2005) and Cohen (1992), Pearson product correlation coefficient smaller than 0.3 equals small effect size, correlation coefficient between 0.3 and 0.5 equal medium effect size, and correlation coefficient equal to or larger than 0.5 equals large effect size. For the families of the healthy children, Pearson product correlation between the children and their parents' proxy-report, ranged from 0.15 (school functioning, small correlation) to 0.35 (emotional functioning, medium correlation) (p < 0.01), indicating a small to medium degree of association (see ❯ *Table 145-3*). Similarly, Pearson product correlation between children with chronic illness(es) and their parents' proxy-report, ranged from 0.23 (social functioning, small correlation) to 0.46 (emotional functioning, median correlation) (p < 0.01), indicating small to medium association (see ❯ *Table 145-3*).

3.3 Mean Differences and Agreements Between Pre-Teenagers' Self-Report and Single Parents' and Dual Parents' Proxy-Reports

A significant difference was found between single mothers' proxy-report and their pre-teenagers on the social and school functioning subscales and on the total HRQOL scale. The single mothers were found to report significantly lower total HRQOL score as well as significantly lower social and school functioning score than the pre-teenagers themselves. For mothers and children living in dual parent families, a significant difference was also found on the mothers' proxy-report and their children's self-report on the total HRQOL scale as well as on the physical, social and school functioning subscales. Thus, mothers' proxy-report in dual parent families was significantly lower on the subscales of physical, social and school functioning as well as on the total HRQOL score than the pre-teenagers' self-report scores. Hypothesis (3) was therefore only partly supported (see ❯ *Table 145-4*).

For all the children who were living with a single parent or living in dual parent families, mean difference on the subscales as well as on the total HRQOL score was greater than 0. Difference scores between children and their single parent varied from 1.98 to 15.38 (see ❯ *Table 145-4*). Difference scores between children and their mothers in dual parent families varied from 1.02 to 12.71, indicating that Icelandic school age children, no matter what family type they were living in, had the largest discrepancy with their mother's proxy-report on the subscales of social and school functioning of the HRQOL scale (see ❯ *Table 145-4*). Interestingly, the magnitude (effect size) of the difference was small for the subscales of physical and emotional functioning, both for children in single and dual parent families, but medium for the social an school functioning in both family types. However, for children living in single parent families, the magnitude (effect size) of the difference between the child and their single mothers was medium for the total HRQOL score but small for children living in dual parent families. The association between the children's self-report and their parents' proxy-report

☐ Table 145-4

Mean differences and level of agreement between Icelandic school age children (N = 480), single parent families' (n = 99) and dual parent families' proxy report (n = 424) on HRQOL (both subscales and total score)

Variables	Mean diff.	Pearsons correlation	SD of diff.	t-value[a]	Effect size d
Schoolage children (N = 480)					
Single mothers versus children					
Physical functioning (n = 82)	3.95	0.25[*]	19.21	−1,848	0.21
Emotional functioning (n = 81)	1.98	0.44**	15.39	−1,155	0.13
Social functioning (n = 79)	15.38	0.35**	22.30	−6,130***	0.69
School functioning (n = 80)	12.59	0.22*	19.90	−5,622***	0.63
Total HRQOL score (n = 81)	7.99	0.35**	13.79	−5,216***	0.58
Dual parent families versus Children					
Physical functioning (n = 361)	1.98	0.29**	15.41	−2,445*	0.13
Emotional functioning (n = 354)	1.02	0.39**	16.61	1,160	0.06
Social functioning (n = 353)	12.71	0.27**	23.97	−9,961***	0.53
School functioning (n = 315)	9.67	0.18**	21.58	−8,427***	0.45
Total HRQOL score (n = 354)	5.29	0.34**	13.95	−7,164***	0.38

Difference in agreement between pre-teenagers and their single parent families and their dual parents families on their health related quality of life
*paired t-tests; $p < 0.05$
**$p < 0.01$
***$p < 0.001$

ranged from 0.18 (school functioning, small correlation) to 0.44 (emotional functioning, medium correlation) ($p < 0.01$), indicating a small to medium degree of association for both family types (see ❯ *Table 145-4*).

3.4   Mean Differences and Agreement Between Pre-Teenagers' Self-Report and Parents' Proxy-Report Based on the Gender of the Child and the Gender of the Parent

A significant difference was found between the mothers' proxy-report and their daughters' self-report on the physical, social and school functioning subscales and on the total HRQOL scale. The mothers were found to report significantly lower total HRQOL score as well as significantly lower physical, social and school functioning score than the pre-teenagers themselves. Further, a significant difference was found between the fathers' proxy-report and their daughters' self-report on the physical, social and school functioning subscales and on the total HRQOL scale. The fathers reported significantly lower total HRQOL score as well as significantly lower physical, social and school functioning score compared to the pre-teenagers themselves. Hypothesis (4) was therefore partly supported (see ❯ *Table 145-5*).

◻ Table 145-5

Mean difference and the level of aggrement between parents proxy report (N = 524) of HRQOL and the child's self report (N = 580) based on the gender of the school age child

Variables	Mean diff.	Pearson's correlation	SD of diff.	t-value[a]	Effect size d
School age children (n = 524)					
Mothers versus daughters					
Physical functioning (n = 250)	3.03	0.27[*]	16.02	−2,987[*]	0.19
Emotional functioning (n = 247)	0.30	0.45[*]	15.30	0,305	0.02
Social functioning (n = 245)	15.68	0.30[*]	22.82	−10,756[**]	0.69
School functioning (n = 247)	13.08	0.14[***]	21.78	−9,436[**]	0.60
Total HRQOL score (n = 249)	7.19	0.35[*]	13.25	−8,568[**]	0.54
Fathers versus Daughters					
Physical functioning (n = 196)	2.44	0.32[*]	14.90	−2,294[***]	0.16
Emotional functioning (n = 195)	1.63	0.33[*]	16.74	1,362	0.10
Social functioning (n = 195)	14.29	0.25[*]	23.46	−8,504[**]	0.61
School Functioning (n = 195)	13.28	0.09	23.28	7,964[**]	0.57
Total HRQOL score (n = 197)	6.70	0.33[*]	13.60	−6,920[**]	0.49
Mothers versus Sons					
Physical functioning (n = 194)	1.47	0.30[*]	16.30	−1,255	0.09
Emotional functioning (n = 190)	0.71	0.34[*]	17.72	0.549	0.04
Social functioning (n = 189)	10.26	0.28[*]	24.62	−5,729[**]	0.42
School functioning (n = 189)	6.61	0.25[*]	20.07	−4,529[**]	0.33
Total HRQOL score (n = 191)	3.98	0.34[*]	14.70	−3,749[**]	0.27
Fathers versus sons					
Physical functioning (n = 143)	1.92	0.25[*]	18.43	−1,247	0.10
Emotional functioning (n = 140)	0.06	0.27[*]	18.43	0,38	0.00
Social functioning (n = 140)	13.97	0.20[***]	18.30	−6,624[**]	0.56
School functioning (n = 138)	10.32	0.15	24.96	−5,587[**]	0.48
Total HRQOL score (n = 140)	5.69	0.29[*]	21.71	−4,403[**]	0.37

Agreement between parents and the pre-teenagers on health related quality of life based on the gender of the child

[a]$p < 0.01$
[b]$p < 0.001$
[c]$p < 0.05$

When the parent-son dyads were evaluated, a significant difference was also found between the mothers' proxy-report and their sons' self-report on the social and school functioning subscales and on the total HRQOL scale. The mothers were found to report significantly lower total HRQOL score as well as significantly lower social and school functioning score than their sons' themselves. In addition, a significant difference was also found between the fathers' proxy-report and their sons' self-report on the social and school functioning subscales and on the total HRQOL score, indicating that fathers reported significantly lower total HRQOL score as well as significantly lower social and school functioning score than their sons' in their self-report. Hypothesis (4) was therefore partly supported (see ❯ *Table 145-5*).

When all the school age children were put together in one group (healthy as well as chronically ill children), mean difference based on the gender of the parents as well as on the gender of the child was greater than 0 for both the total score of HRQOL as well as all the subscales of HRQOL (see ❯ *Table 145-5*). Difference score between mothers and their daughters varied from 0.30 to 15.68; difference score between fathers and their sons varied from 0.06 to 13.97; difference scores between fathers and daughters varied from 1.63 to 14.29 and difference scores between mothers and sons varied from 0.71 to 10.26; indicating that the parents and their pre-teenagers disagreed the most on the social and school functioning subscales of the HRQOL scale, no matter what gender combination of the "parent-child dyad" was evaluated, which shows less agreement on these two subscales than the subscales of physical and emotional functioning (see ❯ *Table 145-5*). Further, these findings indicate that the parents had a tendency to underestimate their children's HRQOL no matter what parent-child gender pair was evaluated (see ❯ *Table 145-5*).

The magnitude (effect size) of the difference was small for the physical and emotional functioning subscales both for the mother-daughter pairs and the father-daughter pairs, but medium for these same gender pairs regarding social and school functioning as well as for the total HRQOL scale. However, for the mother-son pairs and the father-son pairs, the magnitude of the difference was none or small on the physical and emotional functioning, but small for the school functioning subscale as well as for the total HRQOL score (see ❯ *Table 145-5*). For the father-son pairs, the magnitude of difference was medium regarding the social functioning subscale but small for the mother-son pairs. The association between the mother-daughter pairs ranged from 0.14 (school functioning, small correlation) to 0.45 (emotional functioning, medium correlation) ($p < 0.01$), indicating small to medium degree of association. For the father-daughter pairs, the association ranged from 0.25 (social functioning, small correlation) to 0.33 (emotional functioning; total HRQOL score, medium correlation) ($p < 0.01$); indicating small to medium degree of association. The association between the mother-son pairs ranged from 0.25 (school functioning, small correlation) to 0.34 (emotional functioning, total HRQOL score, small correlation) ($p < 0.01$), indicating small to medium correlation. For the father-son pairs, the association ranged from 0.20 (social functioning, small correlation) to 0.29 (total HRQOL score, small correlation) ($p < 0.01$), indicating a small degree of association (see ❯ *Table 145-5*).

3.5   Discussion

Key findings from the hypotheses testing add to our understanding of health related quality of life among healthy as well as chronically ill Icelandic pre-teenagers. Knowing that both healthy and chronically ill Icelandic pre-teenagers' perspective differs significantly from their mothers' and their fathers' perspective on their social and school functioning as well as on the overall HRQOL measure, and that the mothers of healthy children and both parents of chronically ill children differed significantly from their children in their perception of physical functioning, is important information for health care professionals and school personnel. These findings emphasize that parents' proxy-report cannot be substituted for the pre-teenagers' perspective on their own HRQOL. In all of these cases the parents reported significantly lower mean scores of social, school and physical functioning than their healthy or chronically ill pre-teenagers; thus, Icelandic parents underestimated their pre-teenagers on these subscales of HRQOL. These findings on 10- to 12-year-old Icelandic school age children and their parents are contradictory to the findings of Chang and Yeh (2005), who reported that parents could provide valid information of QOL for their children under 12 years of age and that parents' response could be used as substitute for the children's response. In this Icelandic study, it was only within the subscale of emotional functioning that the children and their parents were found to agree. A good agreement was also found between the fathers and their healthy children on the physical functioning subscale. This finding has not been previously reported in the literature, but indicates that Icelandic parents can provide valid information on their children's emotional functioning, and that that information can be used as a substitute for the healthy children's or the chronically ill children's own response. Interestingly, however, a gender difference was found between the parents. Icelandic fathers were found to be in agreement with their healthy pre-teenagers regarding their children's physical functioning. Fathers in Iceland might therefore be a good source of information for school personnel such as school nurses regarding physical functioning of their healthy children and could be used as a valid source or as a supplement for the children's own response.

Nevertheless, the magnitude of the mean bias for healthy children and their parents on the physical and the emotional functioning scales was found to be small, but medium on the social and school functioning subscales. However, for the pre-teenagers with chronic illnesses and their parents, the magnitude of the mean bias was small for the physical and emotional functioning subscales, but medium to high for the social and school functioning subscales. For the total HRQOL scale, the magnitude of the difference between the pre-teenagers' report and their parents' proxy-report was found to be small for the healthy children and their parents but medium for the pre-teenagers with chronic illness and their parents' proxy-report. In this sample of pre-teenagers and their mothers and fathers, there was a consistent bias for parental proxies to underestimate physical, social and school functioning as well as the total HRQOL scale score for both the healthy as well as chronically ill pre-teenagers. This finding emphasizes the need for school personnel and health care professionals to gather both parents' and the pre-teenagers' perspectives on children's HRQOL. Knowing both the children's and their parents' perception is important in order to gain a more holistic information from family members regarding both healthy as well as chronically ill children's HRQOL. Parents' proxy-report needs to be used with caution as a substitute information regarding 10- to 12-year-old children's HRQOL. However, the parents' perception of their pre-teenagers' HRQOL is valid additional information for health care professionals and school personnel. At the same time, this information needs to be used as such, that is, as additional information and not as substitute information for the pre-teenagers' own response.

According to Varni et al. (2003) and Chang and Yeh (2005), it is useful to evaluate the level of agreement between children's self-report and their parents' proxy-reports by examining the Pearson product correlation coefficient. In this study, all subscales of the HRQOL scale as well as the total scale score were found to be low or moderately correlated between mothers and their healthy children. Correlation was also low for the fathers and their healthy children except on the school functioning subscale, where no correlation was found. Similarly, for both parents and their chronically ill children, a moderate or low correlation was found on all subscales of the HRQOL scale as well as on the total scale score except for the school functioning subscale, where no correlation was found between the parents and their chronically ill pre-teenagers. According to Chang and Yeh (2005), Pearson correlation has been the most used approach to examine the proxy-validity and has been referred to as the level of agreement. However, according to these authors, this method has been criticized and they point out that Pearson correlation coefficient only measures the strength of a relation between two variables, rather than agreement. These authors emphasize that, since the Pearson correlation coefficient is insufficient to evaluate agreement between children's self-report and parents' proxy-report, group differences should be used to further supplement information provided by correlation coefficients.

In this Icelandic study, significantly lower mean differences were found between single mothers' proxy-report and the pre-teenagers' self-report on the social and school functioning subscales and on the total HRQOL. Similarly, for mothers and children living in dual parent families, a significantly lower mean difference was also found on the mothers' proxy-report and their pre-teenagers self-report and the total HRQOL scale as well as on the physical, social and school functioning subscales. This finding is new and has not been reported previously in the literature. Interestingly, however, for the subscales of emotional functioning, there was an absence of between-group difference for the pre-teenagers and their mothers' proxy-response, indicating that the children and their mothers had a high level of agreement on the emotional functioning subscale no matter what family type the children lived in (single or dual parent families). Similarly, no difference was found between the children and their single mothers on the physical functioning subscale, indicating good agreement between the single mothers and their pre-teenagers regarding the child's physical functioning. This was however not the case for children living in dual parent families.

When gender difference was evaluated, it was interesting to notice how alike the mothers' and the fathers' proxy responses were. A possible explanation of this similarity in the parents' responses regarding their perception of their pre-teenagers' HRQOL is the age of the parents; the mothers mean age was 40.07 and the fathers' mean age was 42.15, which indicates that the parents were experienced individuals. Nevertheless, and contrary to expectations, a significant difference was found between mothers and their daughters and the fathers and their daughters on the subscales of physical, social and school functioning as well as on the total HRQOL scale score. Interestingly, however, for the mothers and the fathers and their sons, a significant difference was only found on the subscale of social and school functioning and the total HRQOL scale score. These findings emphasize a gender difference between the pre-teenagers and their parents regarding the level of agreement on HRQOL. The Icelandic parents, both the mothers and the fathers, showed a higher level of agreement with their sons than their daughters on the pre-teenagers' HRQOL.

4   Conclusion

International researchers have reported contradictory findings on agreement between parents' proxy-reports and children's own response on HRQOL. Most of these researchers have focused on a variety of different chronic illnesses in different cultures and on how developmentally capable children are, based on their age, to report themselves on their HRQOL and whether their parents' report can serve as substitute report for the children. In order to achieve normal growth and development, healthy and chronically ill children need support from families, school personnel and health care professionals. Children's health status has been found to influence developmental outcomes and QOL in children. Therefore, information regarding children's HRQOL early on can help identify health related problems and give school nurses and other professionals opportunity to intervene appropriately. However, contrary to expectation, in this study on Icelandic pre-teenagers and their parents, lack of agreement was found between the pre-teenagers and their parents' proxy-report on the children's HRQOL. This finding emphasizes that for 10- to 12-year-old Icelandic healthy as well as chronically ill children, parents can only provide valid substitute report regarding their children's emotional functioning and the Icelandic fathers can provide valid substitute report for their healthy children's physical functioning. Nevertheless, parents' proxy-report can add valid information regarding both the mothers' and the fathers' perspective on their pre-teenagers' HRQOL and need therefore to be treated as such. Interestingly, in this study, single mothers were found to have a higher level of agreement with their pre-teenagers than mothers in dual parent families; and both mothers and fathers were found to have a higher level of agreement with their male pre-teenager than with their female pre-teenager. These findings indicate that within the Icelandic culture, family type and gender of the child influence the level of agreement between the pre-teenagers' self-report and the parents' proxy-report.

Summary Points

- Children's health status influences developmental outcome and quality of life. Therefore, early information regarding health related quality of life (HRQOL) can help identify health related problems.
- Lack of agreement between pre-teenagers' self report and parents' proxy report has been documented in the international literature.
- The instrument used in this study, "Pediatric Quality of Life Inventory" (PedsQL) developed by Varni et al. (2001, 2002), is a self-report intended for 8- to 12-year-old children has four subscales: physical functioning, emotional functioning, social functioning, and school functioning. Parents' perspective on their children's HRQOL was measured by a questionnaire identical to the children's self-report (but addressed to the parents).
- The pre-teenagers were in their self-report found to differ significantly from their mothers' and fathers' proxies on the social and school functioning subscales of the HRQOL measure as well as on the overall HRQOL score. These findings emphasize that parents' proxy report cannot be totally substituted for the pre-teenagers' report on their own HRQOL.
- Children and their parents showed a high level of agreement on the subscale of emotional functioning within the HRQOL scale. Agreement was also found between fathers and their healthy children on the physical functioning subscale.
- Even though parents' proxy report can only be substituted within the emotional and physical functioning subscale it can add needed and valid information regarding parents' perspective on their pre-teenagers HRQOL.

References

Annett RD, Bender BG, DuHamel TR, Lapidus J. (2003). J Asthma. 40: 577–587.

Bothwell JE, Dooley JM, Gordon KE, MacAuley A, Camfield PR, MacSween J. (2002). Clin Pediatr. 41: 105–109.

Chang PC, Yeh CH. (2005). Psychooncology. 14: 125–134.

Charron-Prochowinik D. (2002). J Pediatr Nurs. 17: 407–413.

Chen X, Sekine M, Hamanishi S, Yamagami T, Kagamimori S. (2005). Child Care Health Dev. 31: 433–439.

Cohen J. (1992). Psychol Bull. 112: 155–159.

Dalheim-Englund AC, Rydström I, Rasmussen BH, Möller C, Sandman PO. (2004). J Clin Nurs. 13: 386–395.

Epker J, Maddrey AM. (1998). Int J Rehabil Health. 4: 215–222.

Faulkner MS. (2003). Pediatr Nurs. 29: 362–368.

Faulkner MS, Chang LI. (2007). J Pediatr Nurs. 22: 59–68.

Faulkner MS, Clark FS. (1998). Diabetes Educ. 24: 721–727.

Fiese BH, Wamboldt FS, Anbar RD. (2005). J Pediatr. 146: 171–176.

Guyatt GH, Juniper EF, Griffith LE, Feeny DH, Ferrie PJ. (1997). Pediatrics. 99: 165–168.

Hays RM, Valentine J, Haynes G, Geyer JR, Villareale N, Mckinstry B, Varni JW, Churchill, SS. (2006). J Palliat Med. 9: 716–728.

Janse AJ, Sinnema G, Uiterwaal CSPM, Kimpen JLL, Gemke RJBJ. (2005). Arch Dis Child. 90: 486–491.

Knowles RL, Griebsch I, Bull C, Brown J, Wren C, Dezateux C. (2007). Arch Dis Child. 92: 388–393.

Landolt MA, Grubenmann S, Meuli M. (2002). J Trauma. 53: 1146–1151.

Le Coq EM, Boeke AJ, Bezemer PD, Colland VT, van Eijk JT. (2000). Qual Life Res. 9: 625–636.

Markham C, Dean T. (2006). Int J Lang Commun Disord. 41: 189–212.

Mednick L, Cogen FR, Streisand R. (2004). Child Health Care. 33: 169–183.

Meuleners LB, Binns CW, Lee AH, Lower A. (2002). Child Care Health Dev. 28: 341–349.

Noyes J. (2007). J Adv Nurs. 58: 1–10.

Rydström I, Dalheim-Englund AC, Segesten K, Rasmussen BH. (2004). J Pediatr Nurs. 19: 85–94.

Sheppard L, Eiser C, Kingston J. (2005). Child Care Health Dev. 31: 137–142.

Simeoni MC, Sapin C, Antoniotti S, Auquier P. (2001). J Adolesc Health. 28: 288–294.

Svavarsdottir EK, Orlygsdottir B. (2006a). J Sch Nurs. 22: 178–185.

Svavarsdottir EK, Orlygsdottir B. (2006b). Scand J Caring Sci. 20: 209–215.

Tremolada M, Axia V, Pillon M, Scrimin S, Capello F, Zanesco L. (2005). J Pain Symptom Manage. 30: 544–552.

Ungar WJ, Mirabelli C, Cousins M, Boydell KM. (2006). Soc Sci Med. 63: 2354–2366.

Upton P, Maddocks A, Eiser C, Barnes PM, Williams J. (2005). Child Care Health Dev. 31: 409–415.

Varni JW, Burwinkle TM, Rapoff MA, Kamps JL, Olson N. (2004). J Behav Med. 27: 297–318.

Varni JW, Burwinkle TM, Seid M, Skarr D. (2003). Ambul Pediatr. 3: 329–341.

Varni JW, Seid M, Kurtin PS. (2001). Med Care. 39: 800–812.

Varni JW, Seid M, Knight TS, Uzark K, Szer IS. (2002). J Behav Med. 25: 175–193.

Varni JW, Seid M, Rode CA. (1999). Med Care. 37: 126–139.

Vila G, Hayder R, Bertrand C, Falissard B, de Blinc J, Mouren-Simeoni MC, Scheinmann P. (2003). Psychosomatics. 44: 319–328.

Whitney B. (2005). Fam Community Health. 28: 176–183.

Williams J, Williams K. (2003). Pediatr Pulmonol. 35: 114–118.

Yeh CH, Chao, Hung LC. (2004a). Psychooncology. 13: 161–170.

Yeh CH, Hung LC. (2003). Psychooncology. 12: 345–356.

Yeh CH, Hung LC, Chao, KY. (2004b). Psychooncology. 13: 171–176.

146 Health-Related Quality of Life in Obese Children and Adolescents

M. de Beer · R. J. B. J. Gemke

1   Introduction 2504

2   Concepts and Definitions of HRQOL Instruments for Children and
    Adolescents 2505
2.1 Generic HRQOL Measures 2505
2.2 (Disease) Specific Instruments 2507

3   Obesity and HRQOL in Children and Adolescents 2508
3.1 Summary of Effect of Interventions on HRQOL of
    Obese Children and Adolescents 2510

4   Directions for Further Research 2513

    Summary Points 2514

Abstract: Prosperity is accompanied by a rapidly increasing prevalence of overweight and obesity, especially among children and adolescents. This has major implications for the occurrence of cardiovascular (e.g., hypertension, stroke) and metabolic (e.g., insulin resistance and dyslipidemia) diseases in adulthood, not only regarding their prevalence but also as they increasingly occur at a relatively younger (adult of even adolescent) age. Obesity is not only responsible for these slowly and sub clinically presenting somatic conditions but is also closely associated with development of adverse psychological and social conditions. This burden of obesity has both short and long term effects while children and adolescents are particularly vulnerable for adverse psychosocial consequences. Health related quality of life is a concept that enables to assess overall well-being in large groups of healthy subjects and those with a (acute or chronic) condition. In this chapter the concepts of measuring health related quality of life in children and adolescents will be reviewed followed by the introduction and discussion of generic and condition (obesity) specific measures for assessment of health related quality of life. Subsequently the relation of obesity with (impairment of) health related quality of life will be reviewed by a number of relevant studies. Rather than to provide an exhaustive review we sought to provide a representative sample of studies that (1) were methodologically sound; (2) comprised an adequate sample size; (3) comprised individuals across a broad range of relative body weight (body mass index, ❷ BMI [kg/m^2];) and (4) used generally well-validated measures of HRQL. Thereafter the effects of interventions on health related quality of life in obese children and adolescents will be discussed and finally a perspective for future research on this topic is proposed.

List of Abbreviations: *BMI*, body mass index; *CHQ*, child health questionnaire; *CHQ-CF*, child health questionnaire child form; *CHQ-PF*, child health questionnaire parent form; *HRQOL*, health related quality of life; *HUI*, health utilities index; *IWQOL*, impact of weight on quality of life; *KINDL*, kinderlebensqualität fragenbogen; *MHS*, municipal health service; *PedsQL*, pediatric quality of life inventory; *QOL*, quality of life; *SF-36*, short form 36; *SG*, standard gamble; *TACQOL*, TNO-AZL children quality of life; *TAPQOL*, TNO-AZL preschool children quality of life; *TTO*, time trade-off; *VAS*, visual analogue scales

1   Introduction

In the past decade the increasing prevalence of children and adolescents with overweight or obesity has reached alarming proportions (Hedley et al., 2004; Van den Hurk et al., 2007). Although currently this is primarily a problem in the Western world, a huge expansion in the developing countries, especially in those with a rapidly emerging market economy is expected. There is growing awareness of the long term health consequences of this condition, not only in adults, but also in children (Ten and Maclaren, 2004; Weiss et al., 2004). Particularly type 2 diabetes and cardiovascular diseases, developing at an early age are among the most important obesity associated comorbid conditions (Weiss et al., 2004). It has increasingly become clear that the problems associated with obesity are not restricted simply to causing or exacerbating medical conditions. Obesity also appears to have a substantial impact on a person's functional capacity and quality of life. It is important to know more about quality of life in obesity in order to understand which impairments of function and well-being are associated with this condition and what kind of needs for medical and/or psychosocial care may emerge. Also, assessment of changes in quality of life can be used as an outcome measure to evaluate the effects of interventions.

❯ Health-related quality of life (HRQOL) is a multidimensional construct of an individual's subjective evaluation of his/her health, encompassing physical (e.g., sensory and locomotor function), psychological (e.g., emotional functioning) and social domains (e.g., occupational or, in children and adolescents, school functioning) (Schipper et al., 1996). HRQOL is commonly measured using instruments including several domains and/or (sub)scales and/or items. In these instruments usually an item is a single question, a scale contains the available categories for expressing the response to the question, a domain (also called dimension or attribute) identifies a particular focus of attention and may comprise the response to a single item or to several related items, and an instrument is the aggregated collection of all items.

In this chapter, we will review the current knowledge on the impact of obesity on HRQOL and briefly address the effect of interventions (e.g., weight reduction) on the HRQOL of obese adolescents.[1] We will also discuss issues regarding the assessment of HRQOL in obese youngsters, and highlight potential directions for future research.

2   Concepts and Definitions of HRQOL Instruments for Children and Adolescents

Assessment of HRQOL in children and adolescents poses unique problems. Especially at younger age, rapid changes in physical and mental performance occur as part of the normal development in children. In contrast to adolescents, whose ability to respond to questionnaires is similar to adults, assessment of HRQOL in younger children needs special attention and requires separate instruments that (also) allow for proxies (parents) as respondents. The ability of younger children to use rating scales, understand the language, and generally complete lengthy questionnaires of the type used in adult work, is largely affected by age and cognitive development. Children are often regarded as unreliable respondents, and for this reason, early attempts to rate children's QOL were solely based on data provided by mothers. However, children and parents do not necessarily share similar views about the impact of illness, and therefore there are appropriate calls to involve children more directly in decisions about their own care and treatment (Schipper et al., 1996). As a consequence, any evaluation of current approaches to measuring children's QOL needs to consider the provision made for children to rate their own QOL (Eiser and Jenney, 1996; Eiser and Kopel, 1997). There are two ways in which HRQOL can be assessed, namely with generic and with disease specific instruments.

2.1   Generic HRQOL Measures

Generic instruments are measures that attempt to assess all important aspects of HRQOL. They can be applied to a variety of populations allowing for broad comparisons of the relative impact of health and disease. They are classified into health profiles and health indexes (or utilities).

Health profiles consist of multiple items that are grouped together into specific domains of health and functioning, providing patients, clinicians and researchers with information on the

---

[1] Refer to chapter by Jonda et al. Implementing interventions to enhance QOL in overweight children and adolescents

impact of diseases or treatments on different aspects of QOL. In addition, summary scores may been derived for some health profile instruments by averaging across domains. For adults several robust generic instruments are available in numerous languages. The Medical Outcomes Study 36-Item Short Form (SF36, developed in 1992) is today probably the most widely used generic health status questionnaire around the world for adults (Ware, 1996).

Although in adolescents generic health status measures for adults may (also) be used, for younger children health status and HRQOL measures are still in a developmental stage (Eiser and Morse, 2001). At present the following questionnaires are available for younger children. The Child Health and Illness Profile-adolescent edition,(Starfield et al., 1993) Child Health Questionnaire,(Landgraf et al., 1996) Functional Status II-R,(Stein and Jessop, 1990) KINDL, (Ravens Sieberer and Bullinger, 1998) TACQOL,(Vogels et al., 1998) TAPQOL,(Fekkes et al., 2000) the Warwick Child Health and Morbidity Profile,(Spencer and Coe, 1996) Health Utilities Index (HUI) mark 2 and 3 (Boyle et al., 1995). The Child Health Questionnaire (CHQ) is a frequently used instrument which has the same structure as the SF-36 does, but has been developed specifically for children and adolescents (Landgraf et al., 1996).

Preference-based measures of HRQOL particularly the HUI2 and HUI3 that have been developed especially for children provide a single overall score representing the net aggregate impact of physical, emotional and social functioning on QOL. Traditionally the preference or utility scale in health extends from 1 (perfect health) to 0 (death) (Boyle et al., 1995). Preference scores are advantageous in the application of economic evaluations of the cost-utility of alternative programs. Two main types of preferences exist: values and utilities. Values are preferences measured under certainty (meaning that there is no risk or uncertainty in the preference measurement question). The time trade-off (TTO) and the visual analogue scales (VAS) are preference measurement instruments that produce values. Utilities are preferences measured under uncertainty (there is risk or probability involved in the preference based measure). The standard gamble (SG) is a measurement that produces utilities. The SG resembles a kind of structured lottery in which the respondent is presented two alternatives, one of which is uncertain. The probability p is varied systematically until the respondent is indifferent between the two alternatives i.e., based on the probability p, the utility for the health state in each alternative can be calculated (Bennett and Torrance, 1996; Boyle et al., 1995; Apajasalo et al., 1996a,b) (❷ *Table 146-1*).

◘ Table 146-1

Commonly used generic HRQOL measures

Child health and illness profile-adolescent edition
Child health questionnaire
Functional status II-R
KINDL kinderlebensqualität fragenbogen
TACQOL TNO-AZL children quality of life,
TAPQOL TNO-AZL pre-school children quality of life
The warwick child health and morbidity profile
Health utilities index (HUI) mark 2 and 3
Pediatric quality of life inventory

Perhaps the best known and validated (Eiser and Morse, 2001) generic HRQOL instruments for children and adolescents are the Child Health Questionnaire (CHQ) (Landgraf et al., 1996) and the Pediatric Quality of Life Inventory (PedsQL) (Varni et al., 1999). These measures are applicable for both children (including proxy versions for young children) and adolescents in a wide variety of populations and allow for comparisons across a diversity of medical conditions. The CHQ Child Form 87 (CHQ-CF87) questionnaire encompasses 12 domains of which each item contains 4, 5 or 6 response alternatives. Per scale the items are summed up (some recoded/recalibrated) and transformed to a 0 (worst possible score) to 100 (best possible score) scale (Landgraf et al., 1996). Also parental (proxy) versions of the CHQ are available (CHQ-PF50 and CHQ-PF28, respectively) for application in younger children. The 23-item PedsQL 4.0 questionnaire encompasses physical functioning (8 items), emotional functioning (5 items), social functioning (5 items) and school functioning (5 items). A 5-point Likert scale is used for response (0 = never a problem; 4 = almost always a problem). Items are reversely scored and, if appropriate, linearly transformed to a 0–100 scale, so that higher scores indicate better HRQOL. A total scale score, a physical summary score and a psychosocial health summary score may be calculated (Varni et al., 1999). Commonly used generic HRQOL measures are listed in ❷ *Table 146-1*.

2.2   (Disease) Specific Instruments

(Disease) specific HRQOL measures focus on aspects of health status that are specific to the area of primary interest. The instruments may be specific to a condition or disease (e.g., obesity, asthma, heart failure), to a population, to a certain function or to a problem. The major advantage of (disease) specific measures is that they are frequently more responsive to changes after treatment than generic instruments (Guyatt et al., 1993, 2007). Another feature is that specific measures have the advantage of relating closely to areas routinely analyzed by physicians. Until recently there was no disease-specific HRQOL measurement available for obese children or adolescents. In 2006 Kolotkin et al. (2006) developed a measure of weight-related quality of life for adolescents, the Impact of Weight on Quality of Life (IWQOL)-Kids. This questionnaire consists of 27 items which were modeled after weight-related quality of life measures in adults, namely the IWQOL-Lite (Kolotkin and Crosby, 2002) and the original (adult) IWQOL (Kolotkin et al., 1997). Four factors were identified: physical comfort (6 items), body esteem (9 items), social life (6 items), and family relations (6 items). Response options range from always true (1) to never true (5). Preliminary analyses provide support for the measures strong psychometric properties, discrimination among BMI groups and between clinical and community samples, and responsiveness to a weight loss/social support interaction (Kolotkin et al., 2006) (❷ *Table 146-2*).

◻ Table 146-2
Commonly used condition (obesity) specific HRQOL measures

| Impact of weight on quality of life (IWQOL)-adults |
| Impact of weight on quality of life (IWQOL)-kids |
| Impact of weight on quality of life (IWQOL)-lite |

3   Obesity and HRQOL in Children and Adolescents

So far, a limited number of studies assessing HRQOL in juvenile obesity have been performed. Probably due to a relation between the severity (and obviousness) of obesity and physical and social problems, a negative association between HRQOL and BMI has been described in adults, which may also apply to adolescents and to a lesser extend to children (Kortt and Clarke, 2005; Lee et al., 2005). In clinical studies on chronic health problems, including juvenile obesity, HRQOL is an important indicator of outcome complementary to clinical (e.g., biometric) and laboratory (e.g., biochemical) markers.

The published studies concerning this issue are briefly discussed below and also summarized in ❷ *Table 146-1*. We did not intend to provide an exhaustive review of all published studies that have estimated the effect of obesity on HRQOL in children and adolescents. Rather, we sought to provide a representative sample of studies that (1) were methodologically sound; (2) comprised an adequate sample size; (3) comprised individuals across a broad range of relative body weight (body mass index, BMI $[kg/m^2]$;) and (4) used generally well-validated measures of HRQOL.

Studies which exclusively address younger children will not be discussed here.

A longitudinal study published in 2001 put forward that obese children and adolescents (n = 584, mean age 12 years) experience more restriction in quality of life compared to children and adolescents with asthma and atopic dermatitis (Ravens-Sieberer et al., 2001). Of the total score, 37% of the variance was explained by stress level, coping, lack of emotional support and poor global health. However, it was unclear which criteria were used for the assessment of obesity and whether possible co-morbid diseases were accounted for. Furthermore a comparison with a normal weight control group is lacking. Therefore the generalizability of these findings is limited.

Nine studies have used the Pediatric Quality of Life inventory (PedsQL) or a derived measure to assess self-report and/or parent–proxy report of HRQOL in obese youth.

In 2003, Schwimmer et al. reported a decrease in all domains of PedsQL (physical, emotional, social and school), in a group of 106 severely obese children and adolescents aged 5–18 years (Schwimmer et al., 2003). In this study, obese children and adolescents appeared to have a similar reduction in HRQOL as those with cancer. The confounding factors that were adjusted for (age, gender, socio-economic status and ethnicity) were not accountable for these findings. BMI z-score among obese children and adolescents was inversely associated with physical functioning. Furthermore obesity-related comorbid conditions were not responsible for differences in HRQOL (Schwimmer et al., 2003).

Comparable impairments in all domains of functioning were found by Zeller et al. (Zeller and Modi, 2006). In a clinical study among 166 children and adolescents aging 8–18 years they specifically addressed possible racial differences between obese African Americans and Caucasians. No differences between these groups were found. Furthermore, similar to findings from Schwimmer et al. (2003) they found discrepancies between parents and children in reported HRQOL; parents reported significantly worse HRQOL than their children across many dimensions, especially on emotional and social domains. The authors put forward that maternal distress, which is often reported by mothers of treatment-seeking obese youth, can be a possible explanation for this finding. Furthermore, previous research suggests that parents and youth tend to show greater agreement for observable ("objective") behavior than internal ("subjective") states reflected in reported emotional and social domains (Matza et al., 2004). Again BMI z-score was inversely related with physical and social HRQOL. Furthermore, the study elucidated robust relations among impaired HRQOL, depressive symptoms, lower perceived social support, and degree of overweight. The strongest predictors of HRQOL for obese youth were depressive symptoms and perceived social support from class mates. Thus, obese youth who feel supported by their school-based peer group and who are less depressed may have better HRQOL (Zeller and Modi, 2006).

In 2007 Janicke et al. (2007) demonstrated an association between increased parent distress, and peer victimization with lower HRQOL in overweight youth, aged 8–17 years. Depressive symptoms mediated the relationships between these (potential) external risk factors and child-reported HRQOL. Hence, the authors emphasize the important impact of those elements. Incorporating peer support in treatment for example, may improve weight loss in overweight youth and moreover interventions which address parents' personal coping and distress will likely be beneficial in the treatment of their overweight children (Jelalian et al., 2006). In contrast with the studies mentioned earlier, BMI z-score was not related to HRQOL, indicating that the degree of overweight made no difference in perceived HRQOL. Similar to findings of Zeller et al. (2006), there was no relationship between weight status and HRQOL within different racial groups (Janicke et al., 2007).

Another study (Ingerski et al., 2007), with partially the same patient population as that in the previously mentioned study, (Janicke et al., 2007) extends the findings of Zeller et al. (Zeller and Modi, 2006) and Janicke et al. (Janicke et al., 2007). Taken together, these studies suggest that social support is especially important to obese youth's HRQOL. Again no relation between the degree of overweight (as measured by BMI z-score) with HRQOL was found in this study (Ingerski et al., 2007).

By the same token Stern et al. (2007) found that both teasing (partially mediated by self esteem) and low self esteem were associated with obesity in a clinical population. The main focus of this study was to investigate the influence of gender and race on psychosocial factors and dietary habits associated with pediatric overweight. Few gender or ethnic differences on psychosocial variables were found (Stern et al., 2007).

Results from a study from Doyle et al. suggest that overweight adolescents at high risk for the development of eating disorders also experience elevated levels of negative affect, impairment in HRQOL (physical, emotional and social aspects), and eating disturbances. (Doyle et al., 2007).

In a group of 33 extremely obese adolescents who presented for evaluation of bariatric surgery marked decreases in HRQOL across all domains were found (Zeller et al., 2006). The level of impairment characterizing this population was worse than that in less extreme obese subjects (Schwimmer et al., 2003). The authors speculate that the severity of HRQOL impairment in these extremely obese adolescent was due to of the visible nature of extreme obesity, the social stigma attached to it, and the cumulative impact of medical comorbidities. Furthermore, their analysis revealed gender differences in HRQOL indicating that obese adolescent girls may be at particular risk in the social domain (Zeller et al., 2006). This gender difference was confirmed in several studies (Ingerski et al., 2007; Janicke et al., 2007; Jelalian et al., 2006; Matza et al., 2004; Schwimmer et al., 2003; Stern et al., 2007; Zeller and Modi, 2006) although others failed to demonstrate these differences (Zeller and Modi, 2006).

A cross-sectional study of children and adolescents from community pediatrics clinics (39 obese and 94 normal weight controls) and a hospital-based obesity clinic (49 children), showed significant differences in physical and social domain scores even in moderate obesity (Pinhas-Hamiel et al., 2006). Both physical and social domain scores decreased progressively with increased BMI z-scores. The perceived HRQOL of obese children treated in a hospital setting was similar to that of obese children in the community (Pinhas-Hamiel et al., 2006).

In a series by the authors of this chapter, HRQOL was measured by the PedsQL and CHQ, among 31 obese adolescents (Mean BMI = 34.9 kg/m^2) in weight-loss program in a tertiary centre (De Beer et al., 2007). For every patient, two age and sex matched controls, with normal weight for height, were enrolled. These controls were randomly selected from adolescents at their regular visit to the preventive school physician from the regional Municipal Health Service (MHS). Substantial differences in HRQOL were found between obese and control adolescents, mainly in the physical and social domains (De Beer et al., 2007). Furthermore we found an inverse relation between BMI z-score and HRQOL. Obesity-related comorbidity appeared to be an important explanatory variable in the impairments found in physical and social domains, experienced by obese adolescents. This is in contrasts with findings by Schwimmer et al. (2003) and Zeller et al. (2006).

Based on cross-sectional data from a sample of 110 treatment seeking extremely over-weight adolescents and 34 normal weight controls, Fallon and al. found a decreased reported HRQOL regarding Social/Interpersonal, Self-esteem, and Daily living HRQOL similar to adults seeking weight loss treatment (Fallon et al., 2005). Interestingly, overweight had a greater impact among heavier whites, compared with blacks, with regard to social and psychological well-being, aspects of daily living, health efficacy, and physical appearance. This is the first study among overweight adolescents which used the disease specific instrument IWQOL-A, and therefore may have been more sensitive to distinctive impairments experienced by obese youth (Fallon et al., 2005).

The only population based study among adolescents was published in 2005 by Swallen et al. (Swallen et al., 2005). Using a US nationally representative sample of 4,743 adolescents, they demonstrated that obesity in ❷ adolescence is linked with poor physical HRQOL. In the general population, adolescents with above normal body mass did not report poorer emotional, school, or social functioning (Swallen et al., 2005).

In summary, studies attempting to estimate the effect of obesity on HRQOL in children and adolescents indicate that: (1) obese children and adolescents report significantly impaired HRQOL; (2) obesity appears to have a greater impact upon physical and social functioning than on mental health domains; (3) there appears to be a relevant association between BMI and the degree of HRQOL impairment; (4) race may have a modulating effect that needs to be further examined; (5) social support is especially important to HRQOL in children and adolescents; and (6) obesity-related comorbid conditions may have a contribution to the negative effect obesity seems to have on HRQOL (❷ *Table 146-3*).

3.1   Summary of Effect of Interventions on HRQOL of Obese Children and Adolescents

Until now, most studies which evaluate the effect of obesity treatment focus on the effect of interventions on children's and adolescent self esteem. Only few studies used HRQOL as an outcome measure, these studies are briefly reviewed here.

A multidisciplinary behavioral program, published in 1990, produced significant weight losses in black female adolescents, which were associated with improvement in psychological status (Wadden et al., 1990). End-of-treatment scores of participating subjects on standardized tests indicated increased self-esteem and decreased feelings of depression (Wadden et al., 1990).

◼ Table 146-3

Summary of relevant studies assessing HRQOL in children overweight or obesity

References	Study and sample	HRQOL measure	General finding
Ravens-Sieberer et al. (2001)	Longitudinal study of 584 obese children and adolescents (mean age: 12 years)	German KINDL[R]	Decreased HRQOL in all domains (except physical functioning)
Schwimmer et al. (2003)	Cross-sectional data from clinically severe obese children and adolescents (5–18 yrs, n = 106)	PedsQL 4.0	Decreased HRQOL in all domains (physical, emotional, social and school domains)
Swallen et al. (2005)	Community based, cross-sectional study of 4,743 adolescents	Derivative measure of PedsQL 4.0	Decreased HRQOL in physical domain
Fallon et al. (2005)	Cross-sectional study of 110 overweight adolescents and 34 nonoverweight controls	IWQOL-A HRQOL CHQ-PF50	Overweight is associated with poorer HRQOL, regardless of race
Zeller et al. (2006)	Cross-sectional data of 33 extremely obese adolescents, presenting for evaluation at a bariatric surgery program	PedsQL 4.0	Marked impairments in HRQOL across all domains
Pinhas-Hamiel et al. (2006)	Cross-sectional study of 182 children and adolescents from community pediatrics clinics and a hospital-based obesity clinic	PedsQL 4.0	Obese children had lower HRQOL scores in the physical, social and school domains. Severity of obesity affected the pattern of the HRQOL scores. No difference between community and clinical obese children
Zeller et al. (2006)	Cross-sectional study, children and adolescents of 8–18 yrs (n = 166)	PedsQL 4.0	Depressive symptoms, perceived social support from classmates, degree of overweight, and socioeconomic status seem tot be strong predictors of HRQOL
Janicke et al. (2007)	Cross-sectional data, 96 at-risk-for-overweight and overweight youth, 8–17 years of age	PedsQL 4.0	Increased parent distress, child depressive symptoms, and peer victimization were associated with lower HRQOL
Ingerski et al. (2007)	Cross-sectional study of 107 clinically overweight youth, ages 12–17 years	PedsQL 4.0	HRQOL obese adolescents lower than in healthy children. Degree of overweight was not related to HRQOL
Stern et al. (2007)	Cross-sectional study of 100 treatment seeking overweight adolescents	PedsQL 4.0	HRQOL among overweight adolescents is associated with both teasing and low self-esteem. The relation between teasing and HRQOL is partially mediated by self-esteem

☐ Table 146-3 (continued)

References	Study and sample	HRQOL measure	General finding
Doyle et al. (2007)	Cross-sectional study of 81 treatment seeking adolescents	PedsQL 4.0	Overweight adolescents at high risk for the development of eating disorders also experience impairment in physical, emotional and social aspects of HRQOL
De Beer et al. (2007)	Cross-sectional study of 31 treatment seeking adolescents, compared to 62 matched normal-weight controls	PedsQL 4.0, CHQ CF-87	Substantial differences between obese and normal weight adolescents in physical and social domains, partially explained by obesity-related comorbidity

CHQ-CF child health questionnaire child form; *CHQ-PF* child health questionnaire parent form; *HRQOL* health-related quality-of-life; *IWQOL* impact of weight on quality of life; *KINDL* kinderlebensqualität fragenbogen); *PedsQL* pediatric quality of life inventory

Another treatment protocol which incorporated peer social support proved to be beneficial for weight loss and its maintenance in adolescents (Jelalian and Mehlenbeck, 2002). Group activities included both mental and physical challenges that fostered development of trust, social skills and self-confidence. Measures of height and weight, as well as questionnaires assessing self-concept, physical self-worth, and social functioning, were obtained prior to treatment, immediately following the 16-week intervention, and 6 months after completion of active treatment. They observed significant decreases in percent overweight during the course of the intervention. Furthermore, decreases in weight were accompanied by improvements in self-confidence related to physical appearance and physical self-worth. These findings provided some preliminary support for the application of a peer-based program as an adjunctive treatment for adolescent weight management intervention (Jelalian and Mehlenbeck, 2002).

In a large systematic review a comprehensive assessment of pediatric weight management programs was conducted to evaluate the impact of these programs on child and adolescent self-esteem (Walker Lowry et al., 2007). The results of this review suggest overall positive effects on self esteem by pediatric weight management programs across a variety of settings and common treatment components, although the authors question the methodological soundness of the studies. They assume that components related to self-esteem improvements include weight status change, consistent parent involvement, the use of a peer group format to target self-esteem and develop positive peer interactions. The authors put forward that studies indicate that certain components of self-esteem may be affected first (such as body image) and subsequently lead to global self-esteem improvements (Walker Lowry et al., 2007).

According to Ravens-Sieberer et al. in-patient rehabilitative treatment for obesity in children is associated with an increase in HRQOL. After a rehabilitation program, psychosocial factors explained 28% of the variance compared to 37% before treatment (Ravens-Sieberer et al., 2001).

In a 6-month, randomized, double-bind, placebo-controlled trial, the use of sibutramine in 40 obese Mexican adolescents was evaluated (García-Morales et al., 2006). HRQOL was assessed at the study start and end using the 36-item Short-Form Health Survey (SF-36) questionnaire. Interestingly, no differences were found between the sibutramine and the placebo group; both groups showed significant increases in total HRQOL scores (García-Morales et al., 2006).

As seen in the majority of studies in adult populations, weight reduction induced surgically, produced dramatic improvements in the majority of HRQOL indices (Fontaine and Barofsky, 2001). However, it is unclear whether weight reduction would have beneficial effects on HRQOL among persons who have lower degrees of obesity and participate in less invasive forms of weight-loss treatment. Inge et al. performed early observations in a sample of 16 extremely obese adolescents (mean BMI 59.9 kg/m^2) presenting for bariatric surgery, which revealed that at 12-months post surgery adolescents experience significant improvement in HRQOL and depressive symptomatology despite continued obesity (mean BMI 36.9 kg/m^2) (Inge et al., 2007). The authors suggest that these psychosocial changes may substantively alter the psychological health and socioeconomic trajectory of the adolescent to a greater extent than if surgery is performed later in adulthood (Inge et al., 2007).

In summary, studies attempting to estimate the effect of intervention in obese children and adolescents indicate on HRQOL that: (1) obese adolescents report significantly improved self esteem and less feelings of depression after obesity treatment; (2) peer social support appears to be additionally advantageous; (3) HRQOL significantly improves after various types of obesity treatment (e.g., mediation or placebo based, surgery); (4) obesity treatment should commence early, preferably well before adulthood, because the negative impact on psychological health and the socioeconomic prospects can then still be modified.

4 Directions for Further Research

In most studies, groups of children and adolescents seeking treatment were assessed. It should be realized that these are selective samples of adolescents that usually are highly motivated to achieve weight loss through therapy, which may have been driven by their level of psychosocial distress. Whether these psychosocial difficulties also characterize children and adolescents with obesity who are not currently in treatment or seeking methods to lose weight remains unknown. Studies which assessed children in an unselected population setting suggest a lesser degree of impairments in the various HRQOL domains (Wake et al., 2002; Williams et al., 2005).

The cross-sectional nature of all studies performed up till now precludes conclusions regarding causality, and therefore, their generalizability is limited. Prospective longitudinal studies examining the impact of overweight status on children and adolescents may help to further clarify the relationship between weight, BMI and HRQOL.

Furthermore, so far only few studies have used the overweight-specific HRQOL measures, particularly the recently developed IWQOL. We would recommend future research to use this or similar condition specific measures, complementary to generic measures. While generic measures of HRQOL allow for comparison with other chronic conditions, they usually lack the sensitivity to detect differences in HRQOL in cross sectional or longitudinal analysis of an exclusively overweight sample. Using both measures, they can complement each other.

Comparison of the relation of obesity with HRQOL among different countries and cross-cultural validation of condition (i.e., obesity) specific HRQOL measures are also important topics for future research.

☐ Table 146-4
Summary of directions for future research on obesity and HRQOL

Focus on longitudinal instead of cross-sectional studies
Usage of condition (obesity) specific HRQOL measures
Cross cultural comparison of impact of obesity on HRQOL
Attention for (long term) efficacy and cost-effectiveness of interventions on HRQOL

Finally, a lot of attention is directed at various available treatment options, such as cognitive behavioral therapy (with or without peer-based support), drug treatment, and (bariatric) surgical treatment. Well-designed, prospective studies, which evaluate the efficacy, (cost)effectiveness and safety of these weight loss interventions are mandatory, particularly to assess which therapy is most appropriate for an individual obese child or adolescent (❷ Table 146-4).

Summary Points

- Obese children and adolescents report significantly impaired HRQOL.
- Obesity appears to have a greater impact upon physical and social functioning than on mental health domains.
- A relevant association between BMI and the degree of HRQOL impairment has been described.
- Race may have a modulating effect on the relation between BMI and HRQOL.
- Social support is especially important to HRQOL in children and adolescents.
- Obesity-related comorbid conditions may aggravate the negative effects of obesity on HRQOL.

References

Apajasalo M, Rautonen J, Homberg C. (1996a). Qual Life Res. 5: 532–538.

Apajasalo M, Sintonen H, Holmberg C, et al. (1996b). Qual Life Res. 5: 205–211.

Bennett K, Torrance GW. (1996). Measuring health state preferences and utilities: rating scale, time trade-off, and standard gamble techniques. Spilker B (ed.) Quality of Life and Pharmacoeconomics in Clinical Trials. Lippincott-Raven, Philadelphia, PA, pp. 253–265.

Boyle MH, Furlong W, Feeny D, et al. (1995). Qual Life Res. 4: 249–257.

De Beer M, Hofsteenge GH, Koot HM, HiraSing RA, Delemarre-van de Waal HA, Gemke RJBJ. (2007). Acta Paediatr. 96: 710–714.

Doyle AC, Le Grange D, Goldschmidt A, Wilfley DE. (2007). Obesity (Silver Spring). 15: 145–154.

Eiser C, Jenney MEM. (1996). BR J Cancer. 73: 1313–1316.

Eiser C, Kopel SJ. (1997). Children's perception of health ad illness. In: Petrie KJ, Weinman JA, (ed.) Perceptions of Health and Illness: Current Research and Applications. Harwood Academic Publishers, Singapore.

Eiser C, Morse R. (2001). Arch Dis Child. 84: 205–211.

Fallon EM, Tanofsky-Kraff M, Norman AC, McDuffie JR, Taylor ED, Cohen ML et al. (2005). J Pediatr. 147: 443–450.

Fekkes M, Theunissen NC, Brugman E, Veen S, Verrips EG, Koopman HM, Vogels T, Wit JM, ad Verloove-Vanhorick SP. (2000). Qual Life Res. 9: 961–972.

Fontaine KR, Barofsky I. (2001). Obes Rev. 2: 173–182.

García-Morales LM, Berber A, Macias-Lara CC, Lucio-Ortiz C, Del-Rio-Navarro BE, Dorantes-Alvárez LM. (2006). Clin Ther. 28: 770–782.

Guyatt GH, Feeny DH, Patrick DL. (1993). Ann Int Med. 118: 622–629.

Guyatt GH, Ferras CE, Halyard MY, Revicki DA, Symonds TL, Varricchio CG et al. (2007). Mayo Clin Proc. 82: 1229–1239.

Hedley AA, Ogden CL, Johnson CL, Carroll MD, Curtin LR, Flegal KM. (2004). JAMA. 291: 2847–2850.

Inge TH, Xanthakos SA, Zeller MH. (2007). Int J Obes. 31: 1–14.

Ingerski LM, Janicke DM, Silverstein JH. (2007). J Pediatr Psychol. 32: 869–874.

Janicke DM, Marciel KK, Ingerski LM, Novoa W, Lowry KW, Sallinen BJ et al. (2007). Obesity (Silver Spring). 15: 1799–1807.

Jelalian E, Mehlenbeck R. (2002). J Clin Psychol Med Settings. 9: 15–23.

Jelalian E, Mehlenbeck R, Lloyd-Richardson EE, Birmaher V, Wing RR. (2006). Int J Obes (Lond). 30: 31–39.

Kolotkin RL, Crosby RD. (2002). Qual Life Res. 11: 157–171.

Kolotkin RL, Head S, Brookhart A. (1997). Obes Res. 5: 434–441.

Kolotkin RL, Zeller MH, Modi AC, Samsa GP, Quinlan NP, Yanovski JA et al. (2006). Obesity (Silver Spring).14: 448–457.

Kortt MA, Clarke PM. (2005). Qual Life Res. 14: 2177–2185.

Landgraf JMJM, Abetz L, Ware JE. (1996). The CHQ User's Manual. The Health Institute, New England Medical Center, Boston, MA.

Lee AJ, Morgan CL, Morrissey M, Wittrup-Jensen KU, Kenedy-Martin T, Currie CJ. (2005). Diabet Med. 22: 1482–1486.

Matza LS, Swensen AR, Flood EM, Secnik K, Leidy NK. (2004). Value Health. 7: 79–92.

Pinhas-Hamiel O, Singer S, Pilpel Fradkin A, Moda D, Reihman B. (2006). Int J Obes (Lond). 30: 267–272.

Ravens Sieberer U, Bullinger M. (1998). Qual Life Res. 7: 399–407.

Ravens-Sieberer U, Redegeld M, Bullinger M. (2001). Int J Obes Relat Metab Disor. 25 (Suppl 1): S63–S65.

Schipper H, Clich JJ, Olweny CL. (1996). Quality of life studies: definitions and conceptual issues. In:

Spilker B (ed.) Quality of Life and Pharmacoeconomics in Clinical Trials, 2nd ed. Lippincott-Raven, Philadelphia, PA, pp. 11–23.

Schwimmer JB, Burwinkle TM, Varni JW. (2003). JAMA. 289: 1813–1819.

Spencer NJ, Coe C. (1996). Child Care Health Dev. 22: 367–379.

Starfield B, Bergner M, Ensminger M, et al. (1993). Pediatrics. 91: 430–435.

Stei RE, Jessop DJ. (1990). Med Care. 28: 1041–1055.

Stern M, Mazzeo SE, Gerke CK, Porter JS, Bean MK, Laver JH. (2007). J Pediatr Psychol. 32: 90–94.

Swallen KC, Reither EN, Haas SA, Meier AM. (2005). Pediatrics. 115: 340–347.

Ten S, Maclaren N. (2004). J Clin Endocrinol Metab. 89: 2526–2539.

Van den Hurk K, van Dommelen P, van Buuren S, Verkerk PH, Hirasing RA. (2007). Arch Dis Child. 92: 992–995.

Varni JW, Seid M, Rode CA. (1999). Med Care. 37: 126–139.

Vogels T, Verrips GH, Verloove-Vanhorick SP, et al. (1998). Qual Life Res. 7: 457–465.

Wadden TA, Stunkard AJ, Rich L, Rubin CJ, Sweidel G, McKinney S. (1990). Pediatrics. 85: 345–352.

Wake M, Salmon L, Waters E, Wright M, Hesketh K. (2002). Int J Obes Relat Metab Disord. 26: 717–724.

Walker Lowry K, Sallinen BJ, Janicke DM. (2007). J Pediatr Psychol. 32: 1179–1195.

Ware JEJ. (1996). The SF-36 health survey. In: Spilker B (ed.) Quality of Life ad Pharmacoeconomics in Clinical Trials. Lippincott-Raven, Philadelphia PA, pp. 337–345.

Weiss R, Dziura J, Burgert TS, Tamborlane WV, Taksali SE, Yeckel CW et al. (2004). N Engl J Med. 350: 2362–2374.

Williams J, Wake M, Hesketh K, Maher E, Waters E. (2005). JAMA. 293: 70–76.

Zeller MH, Modi AC. (2006). Obesity (Silver Spring). 14: 122–130.

Zeller MH, Roehrig HR, Modi AC, Daniels SR, Inge TH. (2006). Pediatrics. 117: 1155–1561.

147 Implementing Interventions to Enhance Quality of Life in Overweight Children and Adolescents

J. Lamanna · N. Kelly · M. Stern · S. E. Mazzeo

1	Introduction	2518
2	Quality of Life	2518
3	Specific QOL Improvements Associated with POI	2519
3.1	Physical QOL	2519
3.1.1	Weight Management	2519
3.1.2	Physiological Functioning	2520
3.1.3	Physical Fitness Improvements	2521
3.2	Psychological QOL	2521
3.2.1	Depression	2521
3.2.2	Self-Esteem	2521
3.2.3	Eating Behavior	2522
3.2.4	Body Perceptions	2523
3.3	Social QOL	2523
3.3.1	Peer Relationships	2523
3.3.2	Teasing	2524
3.3.3	Family Relationships	2524
4	Components of Programs	2524
4.1	Physical Activity	2524
4.2	Nutrition Counseling	2525
4.3	Behavioral Modification	2526
4.4	Parent Involvement	2526
5	Multidisciplinary POI Programs	2527
5.1	Outpatient Intervention	2527
5.2	Inpatient Intervention	2527
6	Conclusion	2531
	Summary Points	2534

Abstract: The rates of pediatric overweight in the United States and in other industrialized countries have risen dramatically in recent years. Pediatric overweight is associated with poor physical, psychological, and social Quality of Life (QOL). Overweight children and adolescents are at greater risk for weight-related health problems, emotional and psychological problems, and social stigmatization than their normal-weight peers. To address the pediatric overweight crisis and to improve QOL in this population, a number of interventions have been developed. Rather than focusing on weight loss, interventions tend to encourage the development of healthy lifestyle behaviors such as regular physical activity and a nutritious diet. Interventions have been found to yield promising enhancements in QOL. These programs offer one or more treatment components, including physical activity, nutritional counseling, behavioral modification, and parent involvement. Inpatient and outpatient facilities are the primary outlets for these services. This chapter focuses primarily on the impact of pediatric overweight interventions on QOL, and also describes the modalities through which they enhance QOL.

List of Abbreviations: *BM*, Behavior Modification; *BMI*, Body Mass Index; *CBT*, Cognitive Behavioral Therapy; *NC*, Nutritional Counseling; *PA*, Physical Activity; *PI*, Parent Involvement; *POI*, Pediatric Overweight Intervention; *QOL*, Quality of Life; *TEENS*, Teaching, Education, Exercise, Nutrition, and Support

1 Introduction

The prevalence of overweight among children and adolescents is increasing at alarming rates in both the United States (Ogden et al., 2006) and in other industrialized countries (Kiess et al., 2001; Rudolf et al., 2001). In response to this crisis, a number of pediatric overweight interventions (POIs) have been developed. These interventions are administered primarily through inpatient and outpatient treatment facilities and include components addressing physical activity, nutritional counseling, behavioral management, and parental involvement (Barlow and Expert Committee, 2007, Haddock et al., 1994). In addition to the research available on interventions, there is evidence to support the efficacy of these components individually.

In addition to promoting weight management and healthy lifestyle habits, POIs have been found to enhance quality of life (QOL). In this chapter, we first highlight some specific QOL improvements related to participation in POI. Next, we discuss types of interventions and intervention program components, focusing on the mechanisms through which they improve QOL. Finally, we provide readers with special considerations for POI.

2 Quality of Life

In the literature, little consensus has been reached regarding an exact definition of QOL. Definitions vary widely. For example, QOL has been described as the degree to which human physical, spiritual, social, economic, and psychological needs are met (Dempster and Donnelly, 2000) and as a multidimensional construct subjectively based on the individual's perception of his or her well-being or objectively based on societal standards of well-being (Felce and Perry, 1995). According to Schipper et al. (1996), physical QOL refers to strength, energy, and the ability to carry on normal daily activities in addition to normal physical functioning. Psychological QOL refers to mental well-being with regard to psychological processes, such as anxiety and depression. Also according to Schipper and colleagues, social QOL refers to the quality of an individual's relationships with peers, family, and the general community. For the purposes of this chapter, we use Schipper's conceptualization of QOL in our discussions of the enhancements in QOL associated with POI.

When compared to their normal weight peers, overweight children and adolescents have been found to have lower QOL in the physical (Friedlander et al., 2003; Schwimmer et al., 2003; Pinhas-Hamiel et al., 2006), psychological (Friedlander et al., 2003; Schwimmer et al., 2003), and social domains (Pinhas-Hamiel et al., 2006; Schwimmer et al., 2003). It is beyond the scope of this chapter to discuss the impact of pediatric overweight on QOL. However, it is clear that the detrimental effects of pediatric overweight on QOL provide a strong rationale for POI.

3   Specific QOL Improvements Associated with POI

Because of the negative effects of pediatric overweight on QOL, overweight children and adolescents should seek some type of intervention to improve their QOL (Barlow and Expert Committee, 2007). While unstructured attempts to reduce overweight may be successful for some children and adolescents, Barlow and Expert Committee (2007) recommend that when primary care efforts to treat pediatric overweight fail, overweight children and adolescents should enroll in a multidisciplinary POI. Multidisciplinary POIs that promote healthy eating and physical activity can decrease the degree of overweight in children and adolescents (Wilfley et al., 2007) and have the greatest capacity for long-term efficacy (Jelalian and Saelens, 1999).

Many POIs encourage participants to emphasize increasing their frequency of healthy lifestyle habits and focus very little, if at all, on weight loss (Stern et al., 2006; Stern et al., 2007). POIs that promote healthy lifestyle changes, as opposed to weight-focused diets, have been suggested to have the greatest potential for success (Wilfley et al., 2007). Because healthy lifestyle habits are associated with long-term weight management, and QOL improvements have been found to be associated with successful weight management (Dreimane et al., 2007; Fullerton et al., 2007), it seems plausible to infer that positive healthy lifestyle changes are vital to improving QOL. These enhancements have been observed in the physical, psychological, and social domains of QOL (see ❷ *Figure 147-1*).

3.1   Physical QOL

A number of physical QOL enhancements have been associated with POI. Some of these enhancements include weight management, improvements in anthropometric measurements, improved physiological functioning, and enhanced physical fitness.

3.1.1   Weight Management

The goal of most POIs is to promote weight management via the implementation of healthy lifestyle habits, such as eating low-fat, nutrient dense foods and engaging in regular physical

■ Figure 147-1

Quality of Life components addressed by pediatric overweight intervention programs

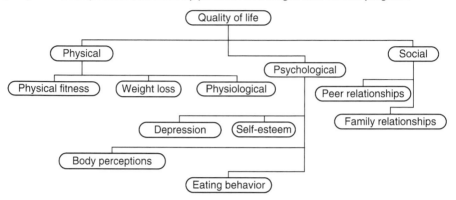

activity (Barlow and Expert Committee, 2007). Weight management is necessary for reducing the risk of future weight-related health problems (Spear et al., 2007). In addition, weight loss is associated with improved well-being (Dreimane et al., 2007) and physical QOL (Fullerton et al., 2007).

Changes in body composition subsequent to POI are measured in terms of a variety of anthropometric measurements. Because the degree of overweight in children and adolescents is measured using the BMI percentile rank, most outcome studies report changes in BMI percentile. Many studies have yielded significant decreases in BMI (e.g., Myers et al., 1998; DeStefano et al., 2000; Braet et al., 2004; Gately et al., 2005; Jiang et al., 2005; Kirk et al., 2005; Edwards et al., 2006); however others have not (Cameron, 1999; Yin et al., 2005; Daley et al., 2006). Nonetheless, studies often find decreases in anthropometric measurements such as percentage of body fat (Gately et al., 2005; Kirk et al., 2005; Nemet et al., 2005; Yin et al., 2005; Savoye et al., 2007), fat mass (DeStefano et al., 2000; Gately et al., 2005), waist circumference (Gately et al., 2005), and hip circumference (Gately et al., 2005) as well as increases in lean body mass (Kirk et al., 2005; Yu et al., 2008).

3.1.2   Physiological Functioning

Another primary goal of POIs is to improve physiological functioning. There is evidence to suggest that POI can improve physiological processes that have been negatively impacted by overweight (Barlow and Expert Committee, 2007). Specifically, decreases in blood pressure (Gately et al., 2005; Jiang et al., 2005; Kirk et al., 2005; Reinehr et al., 2006a; Reinehr et al., 2006b), cholesterol (Jiang et al., 2005; Kirk et al., 2005; Reinehr et al., 2006a; Reinehr et al., 2006b; Savoye et al., 2007), insulin levels (Kirk et al., 2005; Reinehr et al., 2006a; Savoye et al., 2007), triglyceride levels (Reinehr et al., 2006b) and increases in bone mineral density (Yin et al., 2005) have been observed in children and adolescents who have participated in POIs. Further, a decrease in BMI has been linked to the reduction of sleep disorders in children, specifically sleep apnea (Chan et al., 2004).

3.1.3   Physical Fitness Improvements

Physical fitness improvements are also associated with POI. Specifically, increases in physical activity (Nemet et al., 2005; Piko and Keresztes, 2006), endurance (Nemet et al., 2005), and physical fitness (Nemet et al., 2005; Yu et al., 2008) have been observed. In a 12-week exercise program for overweight boys, aerobic and resistance training led to increases in peak volume of oxygen uptake and resting energy expenditure (DeStefano et al., 2000). QOL enhancements resulting from physical fitness improvements include increased cardiovascular (Carrel et al., 2005; Yin et al., 2005) and aerobic fitness (Gately et al., 2005; Kirk et al., 2005) and psychosocial enhancement (Piko and Keresztes, 2006; Yu et al., 2008). Overall, these positive findings on physical fitness provide evidence of direct improvements in QOL as a result of POI.

3.2   Psychological QOL

There is evidence to suggest that POI can enhance psychological QOL, especially with regard to depression, self-esteem, eating behaviors, and body perceptions.

3.2.1   Depression

Overweight children and adolescents report higher rates of depression than their normal weight peers (Pinhas-Hamiel et al., 2006). Despite the potential benefit of enhanced mood in response to POI, relatively few studies report changes in depression scores. However, some have yielded promising results (Myers et al., 1998; Edwards et al., 2006). Edwards and colleagues suggest that socialization with children with similar problems along with increased self-efficacy for weight control may contribute to decreased depression.

The exercise components of intervention programs, in particular, appear to have a positive effect on depression. Stella et al. (2005) suggest that aerobic exercise is associated with reduced depression because it causes biochemical changes in the brain that increase serotonin levels which elevate mood. However, not all studies manipulating exercise in overweight children and adolescents have yielded reductions in depression scores. Daley et al. (2006) found no changes in depression, positive affect, or negative affect in response to an exercise intervention.

3.2.2   Self-Esteem

Overweight children and adolescents tend to have lower self-esteem than their normal weight peers (Erermis et al., 2004). In a review of the impact of pediatric overweight programs on self-esteem, Lowry et al. (2007) reported that the majority of studies examining self-esteem change as a result of intervention reported significant increases in either global self-esteem or a related construct, such as self-worth, self-concept, perceived competence, and physical appearance. The mechanisms through which interventions affect self-esteem are not entirely clear. However, Lowry and colleagues proposed some plausible hypotheses. First, decreases in weight status may be associated with increases in self-esteem. It may be that children who lose weight experience increased self-esteem as a result of the satisfaction associated with their success. Second, Lowry and colleagues suggest that the parental involvement often encouraged by POIs can be associated with increased self-esteem. Parents can provide a supportive environment that promotes a healthy lifestyle, reinforces healthy behaviors, and institutes family lifestyle changes. Third, Lowry and colleagues suggest that group interventions enhance self-esteem because they provide peer social support.

Other studies have also documented changes in overall self-esteem (Braet et al., 2004; Savoye et al., 2005; Daley et al., 2006; Jelalian et al., 2006), and in a number of self-esteem domains. Improvements in perceived physical appearance (Braet et al., 2003; Braet et al., 2004; Jelalian et al., 2006) and athletic competence (Braet et al., 2003; Braet et al., 2004) perhaps develop subsequent to improvements in physical activity. Increased perceived social acceptance (Braet et al., 2003; Braet et al., 2004) may be attributed to the peer support provided by intervention programs or from decreased peer stigmatization.

Despite these promising findings, some studies have not found significant improvements in self-esteem following participation in POI. For example, one study reported no change in self-esteem (Dremaine et al., 2007) and one found changes due only to weight loss (Huang et al., 2007). Further, one study found that self-esteem actually *decreased* after intervention, perhaps because those in the intervention felt "singled out" for treatment (Cameron, 1999).

Although high self-esteem is generally thought to promote positive adaptation, it can also be associated with negative healthy lifestyle perceptions and behaviors. Stern and colleagues (2006) found that overweight treatment-seeking adolescents with higher self-esteem were less likely to believe that their weight was a problem, less likely to believe that their appearance would improve if they lost weight, and were less likely to exercise regularly than those with lower self-esteem. These maladaptive perceptions and behaviors about weight are potential barriers to successful POI.

Despite the potential barriers high self-esteem poses to overweight intervention, many studies have documented increases in self-esteem in response to POIs (Lowry et al., 2007). Not only has self-esteem been shown to increase after participation, but self-esteem appears to affect other components of QOL. For example, Stern and colleagues (2007) found that in an adolescent treatment seeking-sample, self-esteem partially mediated the relationship between teasing and QOL, thereby serving as a protective factor against the adverse effects often associated with teasing.

3.2.3   Eating Behavior

Eating behavior modification is a healthy lifestyle change encouraged by many POIs. The consumption of food high in fat and calories and low in nutrients contributes to overweight. Therefore, most POIs promote healthy modification of eating behavior. However, relatively few studies report changes in eating-related behavior and attitudes. Results are mixed among the studies that have yielded changes in eating behaviors. One study (Edwards et al., 2006) found no differences in food preoccupation, dieting patterns, and eating attitudes among 8- to 13-year-olds who participated in a family-based POI. Studies have found that intervention has no impact on emotional eating (Braet et al., 2003; Braet et al., 2004), but may be effective in decreasing dietary restraint (Braet et al., 2004). Changes in actual eating behavior, however, are difficult to measure as they are based largely on self-report of behaviors that occur outside of the intervention setting.

Disordered eating behaviors such as binge eating have been observed in POI seeking populations (Decaluwe et al., 2003). Binge eating poses a specific challenge for POI programs because it is often associated with other underlying psychological issues (Stice et al., 2002) such as depression (Ross and Ivis, 1999) and low self-esteem (Decaluwe et al., 2003), and because it requires specific behavior modification to treat (Glasofer et al., 2007). This evidence illustrates the need for POI programs to specifically address binge eating. One possible intervention technique, cognitive behavioral therapy (CBT), has been found to be effective in treating binge eating in the pediatric overweight population (Braet et al., 2004).

3.2.4   Body Perceptions

Overweight children and adolescents are susceptible to sensitivity about their weight, poor body image, and low body satisfaction (Huang et al., 2007). Therefore, POI programs have begun to investigate changes in body perceptions as a result of intervention. Some specific changes that have been observed are decreased drive for thinness (Braet et al., 2003; Braet et al., 2004), body dissatisfaction, weight concern, and shape concern (Braet et al., 2004).

However, other evidence suggests that participation in POI alone does not yield changes in body perceptions. Some studies indicate that only adolescents who participate in a POI *and* either lose or maintain weight experience positive changes in body perceptions such as body image (Huang et al., 2007), body satisfaction, and physical appearance esteem (Walker et al., 2003). In these studies, weight loss appeared to make the difference, as those who lost or maintained weight experienced the greatest changes in body perceptions.

It is important to monitor how changes in body perceptions relate to weight loss. That is, beneficial improvements in body perceptions contribute to improvements in QOL. However, some children and adolescents may interpret improvements in body perceptions as indicators that their weight is no longer a health issue, perhaps contributing to reduced motivation to continue engaging in healthy lifestyle behaviors. Another concern is that too much emphasis on weight and associated health risks in POIs could contribute to poor body perceptions (Huang et al., 2007). To prevent the development of maladaptive body perceptions, it has been recommended that intervention programs maintain a supportive, non-critical environment (Barlow and Dietz, 1998).

3.3   Social QOL

Overweight, treatment-seeking children and adolescents have been described by their mothers as being socially withdrawn and isolated (Zeller et al., 2004b). However, POI programs have been found to have the capacity to enhance social QOL, particularly regarding peer and family relationships. These enhancements include increased social competence (Myers et al., 1998), improved social well-being (Braet et al., 2004), and decreased social problems (Epstein et al., 1998; Myers et al., 1998). Consideration of social functioning in intervention programs is vital, given the isolating and stigmatizing effects of pediatric overweight (Strauss and Pollack, 2003). Improvements in social functioning and social QOL are therefore key potential benefits of POIs.

3.3.1   Peer Relationships

Youth who have participated in POIs report increased peer support (Resnicow et al., 2000). Peer support has been linked to several positive treatment outcomes, including increased participation in physical activity (Andersen and Wold, 1992) and enhanced QOL (Zeller and Modi, 2006). Myers and colleagues propose that these programs work because as children lose weight, they become less socially stigmatized and develop improved peer relationships. The improved peer relationships, in turn, increase the availability of peer-related physical activity while decreasing opportunities for overeating, thereby helping children maintain these healthy lifestyle behaviors.

3.3.2 Teasing

Overweight children and adolescents are often subjected to teasing by peers (Robinson, 2006). Although some studies have shown that POI contributes to improvements in social functioning (Epstein et al., 1998; Myers et al., 1998; Braet et al., 2004) to our knowledge, there has been no documented evidence of reduced frequency of teasing subsequent to POI. Teasing should certainly be addressed by POIs. Its reduction is an important target for future clinical research.

3.3.3 Family Relationships

Improved family functioning has been found to be a result of POI programs, especially those that provide family or parent involvement components. Prior to treatment, families of overweight children and adolescents are characterized by high maternal psychological distress, high family conflict, and negative meal-time interaction (Zeller et al., 2007). Although only a limited amount of research has examined the effects of POIs on family functioning, preliminary findings have been encouraging. For example, some families experienced increased cohesion (Kirschenbaum et al., 1984; Dreimane et al., 2007), increased mutual support (Kirschenbaum et al., 1984), reductions in parental distress (Epstein et al., 2000; Epstein et al., 2001), and reductions in maternal psychopathology (Myers et al., 1998).

4   Components of Programs

Many POIs are comprised of a combination of four components: physical activity, nutritional counseling, behavioral modification, and parent involvement. The purpose of this section is to describe the mechanisms through which POIs seem to enhance QOL. ❷ *Figure 147-2* provides a representation of these components.

4.1   Physical Activity

Exercise is a necessary and vital component of effective POI (Barlow and Expert Committee, 2007) and a wide variety of approaches have been implemented to increase physical activity (Snethen et al., 2006). While increasing physical activity is an important component of weight management, it does not appear to be sufficient if implemented alone (Spear et al., 2007).

POIs encourage participants to engage in physical activity outside of the intervention facility using such techniques as self-monitoring energy expenditure (e.g., Epstein et al., 2000) and tracking physical activity using devices such as accelerometers or pedometers (Resnicow et al., 2000; Salmon et al., 2005). Some programs encourage the reduction of sedentary

□ Figure 147-2

Common components of outpatient pediatric overweight intervention programs

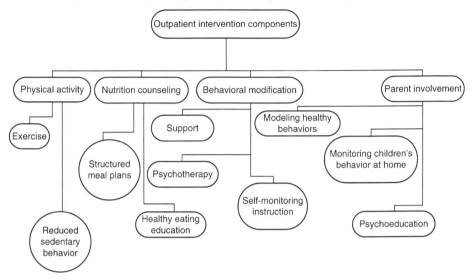

behaviors such as television viewing (Robinson, 1999; Epstein et al., 2000; Epstein et al., 2004). Other programs take a more active approach by providing exercise facilities (Sothern et al., 2002; Savoye et al., 2007) or teaching participants athletic skills (Resnicow et al., 2000; Salmon et al., 2005; Yin et al., 2005). Studies have noted several improvements in pediatric QOL outcomes resulting from increased physical activity including increased self-esteem (Calfas and Taylor, 1994; Weiss et al., 1990), decreased depression (Shepard, 1995; Stella et al., 2005), increased self-image (Kirkcaldy et al., 2002), and improved self-efficacy (Sallis et al., 2000; Neumark-Sztainer et al., 2003).

4.2 Nutrition Counseling

Adopting nutritious eating habits is also a central component of a healthy lifestyle. It has therefore been one of the main areas of focus in multidisciplinary POI. Often, participants are given information regarding nutrition and healthy eating via individual or group nutrition counseling sessions (Valverde et al., 1998; Savoye et al., 2005; Savoye et al., 2007).

POIs that include a nutrition component are more effective in producing positive outcomes when compared to those without a nutrition component (Collins et al., 2006). Although it appears that having a nutrition component is vital to successful POI, it is not clear which of the many different nutrition components is most effective (Collins et al., 2006). However, a review of the extant studies suggests that a few conclusions can be drawn. First, research suggests that the long-term maintenance of weight loss is better achieved through educational-based activities and diet modifications (Murphree, 1994), rather than through severe diet restriction (Valverde et al., 1998) or structured meal plans (Savoye et al., 2005). Second, the inclusion of a nutrition component in which participants are taught to make better food choices is preferable to those that focus on prohibiting certain foods (Savoye et al., 2007). Further, although it is difficult to identify the specific effects of a nutritional component of POI on QOL, it is clear that in order to maximize long-term improvements in QOL, it is necessary to target and change maladaptive eating styles in addition to promoting physical activity.

4.3   Behavioral Modification

Specific behavioral modification techniques may be necessary to change the unhealthy lifestyle habits that contribute to overweight, as education alone is often inadequate in effective weight management (Spear et al., 2007). To facilitate behavioral change, many POIs provide some type of behavioral modification or behavioral support component. Behavioral modification modalities include self-monitoring of eating behavior and physical activity, stimulus control strategies, and contingency management (Jelalian and Saelens, 1999).

In addition to behavioral modification, the efficacy of cognitive behavioral therapy (Duffy and Spence 1993; Braet et al., 2004; Herrera et al., 2004; van den Akker et al., 2007) has also been examined. With cognitive behavioral therapy (CBT) for POI, children and adolescents learn to monitor and understand how their thoughts are associated with weight-related behaviors. In a review of POI behavioral modification components, Spear and colleagues (2007) suggest that when compared to cognitive techniques, behavioral techniques are more effective in improving healthy lifestyle behaviors such as diet and physical activity.

Like physical activity and nutritional components, it is difficult to evaluate the specific effects of behavioral modification within multidisciplinary POIs. However, because these comprehensive programs that include behavioral modification have yielded some successes overall, we can argue here that the behavioral component may be an important element, although further study is needed to determine how much of a relative effect this component has on outcomes.

4.4   Parent Involvement

Many POIs encourage or require parental participation and there is evidence to support the effectiveness of parental involvement (e.g., Golan, 2006). Young et al. (2007) suggest that those interventions that promote active parental involvement yield larger effect sizes than those that do not. Parents' capacity to role model healthy eating and physical activity is the primary rationale for involving them in their children's overweight intervention (Jelalian and Saelens, 1999; St Jeor et al., 2002). In addition, parental involvement is needed in POI, as children most often depend on parents to provide food and opportunities to engage in physical activity.

Unfortunately, children do not always agree with their parents on weight and healthy lifestyle-related issues. For example, parents may perceive their overweight children as having poorer QOL than the overweight children perceive themselves as having (Hughes et al., 2007). Parents and children may also have discrepant views on weight status issues. Stern and colleagues (2006) found that although daughters are more likely than mothers to be currently trying to lose weight, daughters are less likely to understand genetic influences on weight and more likely to believe that if one is active, weight status is not important.

One reason parents may refer their children to POI is that they tend to view their offspring's overweight as more detrimental than does the child (Zeller et al., 2004b; Hughes et al., 2007). Thus, differences in child and parent perceptions of the magnitude of QOL impairments resulting from overweight may be one barrier to child motivation to change. Despite the potential for differences in parent and child perceptions on the impact of overweight, parents and children should be encouraged to work together to achieve a healthier lifestyle.

Although many parents of children who are involved in POIs have accurate perceptions of their children's problems, some parents have distorted views of their children's overweight. They may see their children as 'big-boned' or 'solid' rather than overweight (Young-Hyman et al., 2000; Stern et al., 2006). These distorted perceptions are another possible barrier to beneficial parental involvement in POI.

5 Multidisciplinary POI Programs

There is evidence for the effectiveness of the four major component areas of POI (i.e., physical activity, nutritional counseling, behavioral modification, and parent involvement) in both community and clinical pediatric overweight populations. Multidisciplinary POIs that provide all four of these components include primarily inpatient and outpatient clinics, but also smaller interventions conducted in school (Cole et al., 2006) or weight-management camp settings (e.g., Walker et al., 2003; Gately et al., 2005). Successes observed in POIs conducted in schools and camps suggest that healthy behavior modifications can be effectively promoted and implemented in a number of youth-friendly environments. Although findings ascertained from POIs conducted in schools and camps are important, there is a relative paucity of evidence for their effectiveness. Therefore, our focus in this section will be exclusively on formal inpatient and outpatient POIs that include physical activity, nutritional counseling, behavioral modification, and parent involvement.

5.1 Outpatient Intervention

The majority of literature on POI evaluates outpatient programs. Many of these programs are university-based and are comprised of physical activity, nutritional counseling, behavioral modification, and parental involvement components (see ❯ Table 147-1). ❯ Table 147-2 provides a detailed description of the Teaching, Education, Exercise, Nutrition, and Support (TEENS) program, the outpatient multidisciplinary POI program with which we are affiliated. We provide this description as a prototype for outpatient POI. ❯ Figure 147-3 illustrates the TEENS timeline.

5.2 Inpatient Intervention

Inpatient POIs offer the most intensive intervention available for pediatric overweight. For severely overweight children and adolescents, inpatient care may be necessary, as outpatient treatment programs are not very successful in treating the severely overweight population

■ Table 147-1
Outpatient POI programs

Program Name	Sample	Method	Intervention	QoL Outcomes	Reference
Bright Bodies	209 overweight 8- to 16-year olds; (105 treatment; 69 control)	Treatment: Family based program included exercise, nutrition, and behavioral modification Control: Weight counseling every 6 months	**Behavior modification:** 1x/wk during first 6 months; included self-awareness, goal setting, stimulus control, coping skills, cognitive behavior strategies, contingency management **Exercise:** 2x/wk during first 6 months; 50 minutes of warm-up, aerobic exercise, cool-down **Nutrition:** Promoted low-fat, nutritious foods and portion control **Parent involvement:** Parents attended nutrition counseling sessions	6- and 12-month follow-up intervention vs. control group: Significant decreases in weight, BMI, body fat %, kg of estimated body fat mass, total cholesterol, fasting insulin, insulin resistance	Savoye et al., 2007
Committed to Kids	93, 13- to 17-year-olds (BMI ≥ 85th% percentile)	1-year medical, psychosocial, nutrition, & exercise intervention; family involvement encouraged	**Behavior modification:** Weekly sessions to discuss accomplishments; positive reinforcement of healthy eating & physical activity; self-monitoring, commitment, setting goals, relapse prevention also discussed **Exercise:** Frequency and intensity based on overweight severity; increases over the course of the program **Nutrition:** Recommendations based on overweight severity, but includes calorie monitoring, portion control; increased protein consumption, reduced carbohydrate & fat consumption **Family involvement:** Group nutrition education sessions attended by patient and family; focus on identifying food groups, cooking activities, tips on reading labels and grocery shopping, tips for dining out	Participants reduced BMI from 32.3 (SD=1.3) at baseline to 28.2 (SD=1.2) at 1-year.	Sothern et al., 2002

Program	N	Description	Intervention	Outcomes	Citation
Kids N Fitness	264, 7- to 17-year-olds, (BMI ≥ 85th%ile) (180 enrolled in an 8 wk program; 84 enrolled in a 12 wk program)	8- or 12-week program; participants attended once per week; exercise, nutrition education, behavior modification, family involvement combined into one, 90-minute per week, session	**Behavior modification:** Instruction on healthy lifestyle habits **Exercise:** Included exercise intervals, exercise videos, walking, dancing, and modified sports (participants were kept continually active) **Nutrition:** Included instruction on food guide pyramid, reading food labels, and monitoring portion sizes; tips for dining out, reducing sugar and cholesterol consumption, and understanding food nutrients and additives **Parent involvement:** Parents were informed of the risks of overweight, and the importance of healthy lifestyle habits	**8 week program:** Improved parent perception of child's general health, physical functioning, bodily pain, behavior, and mental health. **12 week program:** Improved parent perception of child's physical limitations, bodily pain, behavior, health, and family cohesion.	Dreimane et al., 2007
Obeldicks	240, 6-to 14-year-olds (203 treatment, 37 control)	1 year intervention program; reduction in intensity every 3 months; follow-up 2 years after starting intervention	**Behavior modification:** Behavior therapy 2x/week during first 3 months; individual family psychotherapy from months 3 to 9 **Exercise:** 1x/week throughout program **Nutrition:** 6 group sessions of a nutritional course during the first 3 months; "Optimized Mixed Diet" was taught – dietary recommendations based on German dietary guidelines **Parent involvement:** Parent groups met 2x/month during the first three months, 1x/month from months 3 to 9	Intervention group over 2 year period: decreased BMI, systolic blood pressure, insulin level, and cholesterol concentration	Reinehr et al., 2006a

Listed above are the results of studies conducted on several multidisciplinary outpatient pediatric overweight intervention programs. Their sample sizes, research methodologies, intervention strategies, and QoL outcomes are provided.

BMI - Body Mass Index

SD - Standard Deviation

◼ Table 147-2

TEENS program description

Component	Description
Behavioral treatment	1. At enrollment, behavioral specialists (counseling psychology doctoral students) conduct a detailed intake session to evaluate each participant's developmental history, past or current methods for controlling weight, dietary intake, level of physical activity, family functioning, and goals for participation in the program. 2. After the participant has received medical clearance to enroll in the program, the participant and behavior specialist meet biweekly for 30 minutes. The purpose of these sessions is to make and maintain goals, monitor program adherence, and to address personal or family issues that may be impacting treatment. 3. After approximately 2 to 3 sessions, the behavior specialist refers the participant to group behavioral support sessions. During the behavioral group support sessions, each participant has the opportunity to discuss with his or her same sex-peers issues related to their treatment.
Physical Activity	1. The TEENS program facility has a gym complete with cardiovascular equipment, resistance machines, and free weights. 2. The goal for each exercise session is to reach a maximum heart rate at or above 150 beats per minute, or 70-80% of the participant's maximum heart rate. 3. Typical sessions include: a. 10 minutes warm-up b. 20-30 minutes cardiovascular activity c. 20-30 minutes strength training d. 10 minute cool down
Nutritional counseling	1. Registered dieticians provide individual nutrition lessons to the participants and their parents.
Parent Involvement	1. TEENS is a family-based program and participants' parents are expected to be involved in their child's treatment. 2. Parents are required to attend enrollment and intake sessions, as well as progress meetings with staff members at various points throughout the program. They are encouraged, and may be required, to attend their child's individual behavioral support and nutrition sessions. 3. There is a 12-week, psychoeducational group for parents only. Topics such as family meal planning, environmental and genetic precursors of overweight, promoting healthy body image, and dealing with teasing are discussed.

Listed above is a description of TEENS, a multidisciplinary outpatient pediatric overweight intervention program. TEENS - Teaching, Education, Exercise, Nutrition, Support

(Braet et al., 2003). Inpatient programs are especially valuable for overweight children who come from families who are less supportive of their efforts by offering a live-in environment in which they can learn healthy eating behaviors and engage in physical activity (Braet et al., 2004). A sample of inpatient POIs, their descriptions, and outcomes are listed in ❯ *Table 147-3*.

☐ Figure 147-3

Virginia Commonwealth University TEENS program timeline. *TEENS* Teaching, Education, Exercise, Nutrition, and Support; *PA* Physical Activity; *BM* Behavior Modification; *NC* Nutritional Counseling; *PI* Parent Involvement

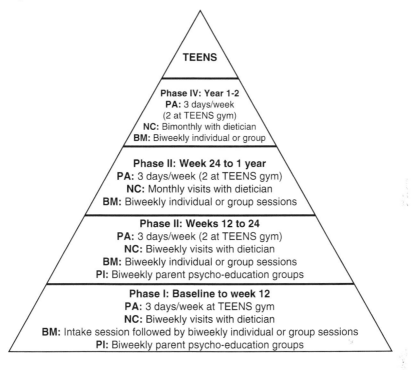

TEENS

Phase IV: Year 1-2
PA: 3 days/week
(2 at TEENS gym)
NC: Bimonthly with dietician
BM: Biweekly individual or group

Phase II: Week 24 to 1 year
PA: 3 days/week (2 at TEENS gym)
NC: Monthly visits with dietician
BM: Biweekly individual or group sessions

Phase II: Weeks 12 to 24
PA: 3 days/week (2 at TEENS gym)
NC: Biweekly visits with dietician
BM: Biweekly individual or group sessions
PI: Biweekly parent psycho-education groups

Phase I: Baseline to week 12
PA: 3 days/week at TEENS gym
NC: Biweekly visits with dietician
BM: Intake session followed by biweekly individual or group sessions
PI: Biweekly parent psycho-education groups

6   Conclusion

The prevalence of pediatric overweight is rising at alarming rates. Overweight is associated with poor physical, psychological, and social QOL. In response to the high rates of pediatric overweight and its detrimental effects on QOL, POIs have been established in a number of countries worldwide. These interventions offer physical activity, nutritional counseling, behavioral modification, and parent involvement components. In this chapter, we have discussed the specific QOL improvements associated with POI and have described the ways in which these programs enhance QOL.

One challenge of evaluating multidisciplinary POIs is that it is difficult to determine which components are most effective (Braet et al., 2003) in producing QOL enhancements. However, the successes that multidisciplinary POIs yield suggest that this approach may be most effective.

There are a number of demographic, economic, psychological, and cultural factors that need to be more successfully integrated into POIs. For example, economic factors (Cote et al., 2004), minority status, depression, and poor self-concept (Zeller et al., 2004a) have been found to predict attrition. There is a need for intervention programs that are sensitive to African Americans, as they are at increased risk of overweight (Ogden et al., 2006). Treatment

■ Table 147-3
Inpatient POI programs

Program Name	Sample	Method	Intervention	QoL Outcomes	Reference
Zeepreventorium	76 obese 10- to 17-year olds (38 treatment; 38 control)	10-month inpatient treatment program; Compared treated children to wait-list controls	**Nutrition:** 1500-1800 kcal/day; 3 meals, 2 snacks per day **Physical activity:** 10 + hr/week **Psychological intervention:** cognitive behavioral modification **Parent involvement:** Received information on healthy food preparation and physical activity	**Intervention group: 48%** decrease in median adjusted BMI; decreased drive for thinness & external eating; increased self-perceived physical appearance, athletic competence, & social acceptance	Braet et al., 2003
Zeepreventorium	122 inpatient overweight 7- to 17-year olds	10-month inpatient treatment program	**Nutrition:** 100-1600 cal/day; 3 meals, 2 snacks per day **Physical activity:** 14+ hr/week **Psychological intervention:** cognitive behavioral modification; food cue resistance training; random assignment to extended coping program or to standard treatment program	**Pre- vs. post intervention;** *Decreased* percentage overweight, body mass index, & weight; parent-reported overall behavioral & internalizing problems; external eating, eating concern, frequency of binge eating, and bulimic symptomatology; drive for thinness, body dissatisfaction, weight concern, and shape concern. *Increased* global sense of self-worth, and perceived athletic & physical competence; dietary restraint *All changes were maintained at a 14-month follow-up; also increased perceived academic competence and social acceptance at follow-up	Braet et al., 2004

| Overweight Intervention Program at the Medical Psychiatric Unit of Schneider Children's Medical Center of Israel | BMI $\geq$ 95th percentile with presence of severe, overweight-related health issue | 3 phases: 1.) Pre-admission phase 2.) Weight loss and maintenance establishment 3.) Cognitive-behavioral treatment for addressing obstacles | **Nutrition:** Moderate caloric restriction **Physical activity:** Individualized plans based on physiological functioning **Psychological intervention:** cognitive behavioral psychotherapy **Parent involvement:** 1x/week individual training sessions with dietician and behavioral specialist; taught ways to enhance healthy habits for the whole family | None reported | Fennig & Fennig, 2006 |

Listed above are the results of studies conducted on several multidisciplinary outpatient pediatric overweight intervention programs. Their sample sizes, research methodologies, intervention strategies, and QoL outcomes are provided.

BMI - Body Mass Index
SD - Standard Deviation

programs specifically for African American girls have been somewhat successful, perhaps because they are more culturally relevant (Resnicow et al. 2000, 2005). The available literature suggests those who are financially disadvantaged, of diverse racial backgrounds, or who have psychological or emotional issues are at particularly high risk for attrition from POIs. A greater understanding of strategies that can be used to decrease attrition among these populations is clearly necessary.

Despite some promising results, many POIs have failed to yield significant QOL enhancements. Some proposed reasons for these failures include the difficulty involved in adhering to intense intervention protocols (Epstein et al., 1996; Yanovski and Yanovski, 2003), the costs associated with intervention (Jelalian and Saelens, 1999), and a lack of research evidence for effective intervention (Wilson et al., 2003). In addition, what differentiates successful pediatric overweight participants from unsuccessful pediatric overweight participants is largely unknown (Reinehr et al., 2003). Clearly, more research is needed to help increase our understanding of why some POIs show success overall whereas others do not. Such information should help us make real changes to our multidisciplinary POIs and thereby improve our intervention strategies.

Summary Points

- The rates of pediatric overweight are high in the United States and in many other industrialized countries.
- Intervention programs have been developed to address the pediatric overweight epidemic.
- Intervention programs have the capacity to enhance QOL in all domains.
- To promote long-term weight management, intervention programs encourage healthy lifestyle behaviors, not weight loss.
- POIs typically include physical activity, nutritional counseling, behavioral modification, and parent involvement components.
- Multidisciplinary programs, primarily housed in outpatient or inpatient clinics, have the greatest capacity for success because they address multiple issues related to pediatric overweight.

References

Andersen N, Wold B. (1992). Res Q Exerc Sport. 63(4): 341–348.

Barlow SE, Dietz WH. (1998). Pediatrics. 102: e29.

Barlow SE. (2007). Expert Committee Pediatrics. 120: S164–S192.

Braet C, Tanghe A, De Bode P, Franckx H, Van Winckel M. (2003). Eur J Pediatr. 162: 391–396.

Braet C, Tanghe A, Decaluwe V, Moens E, Rosseel Y. (2004). J Pediatr Psychol. 29(7): 519–529.

Calfas KJ, Taylor WC. (1994). Pediatr Exerc Sci. 6: 406–423.

Cameron JW. (1999). Issues Compr Pediatr Nurs. 22: 75–85.

Chan J, Edman JC, Koltai PJ. (2004). Am Fam Physician. 69(5): 1147–1154.

Cole K, D'Auria J, Garner H. (2006). J Spec Pediatr Nurs. 11(3): 166–177.

Collins CE, Warren J, Neve M, McCoy P, Strokes BJ. (2006). Archives of Pediatr Adolesc Med. 160: 906–922.

Cote MP, Byczkowski T, Kotagal U, Kirk S, Zeller M, Daniels S. (2004). Int J Qual Health Care. 16(2): 165–173.

Daley AJ, Copeland RJ, Wright NP, Roalfe A, Wales JKH. (2006). Pediatrics. 118(5): 2126–2134.

Decaluwe V, Braet C, Fairburn CG. (2003). Int J Eat Disord. 33: 78–84.

Dempster M, Donnelly M. (2000). Soc Work Health Care. 32(1): 45–56.

DeStefano RA, Caprio S, Fahey JT, Tamborlane WV, Goldberg B. (2000). Pediatr Diabetes. 1: 61–65.

Dreimane D, Safani D, MacKenzie M, Halvorson M, Braun S, Conrad B, Kaufman F. (2007). Diabetes Res Clin Pract. 75: 159–168.

Duffy G, Spence SH. (1993). J Child Psychol Psychiat. 34 (6): 1043–1050.

Edwards C, Nicholls D, Croker H, Van Zyl S, Viner R, Wardle J. (2006). Eur J Clin Nutr. 60: 587–592.

Epstein LH, Coleman KJ, Myers MD. (1996). Med Sci Sports Exerc. 28(4): 428–435.

Epstein LH, Goldfield GS. (1999). Med Sci Sports Exerc. 31, (11), Suppl 1, S553.

Epstein LH, Myers MD, Raynor HA, Saelens BE. (1998). Pediatrics. 101:554–570.

Epstein LH, Paluch RA, Gordy CC, Dorn J. (2000). Archives of Pediatr Adolesc Med. 154: 220–226.

Epstein LH, Paluch RA, Kilanowski CK, Raynor HA. (2004). Health Psychol. 23(4): 371–380.

Epstein LH, Paluch RA, Saelens BE, Ernst M, Wilfley DE. (2001). J Pediatr. 139: 58–65.

Erermis S, Cetin N, Tamar M, Bukusoglu N, Akdeniz F, Goksen D. (2004). Pediatr Int. 46: 296–301.

Felce D, Perry J. (1995). Res Dev Disabil. 16(1): 51–74.

Friedlander SL, Larkin EK, Rosen CL, Palermo TM, Redline S. (2003). Arch Pediatr Adolesc Med. 157: 1206–1211.

Fullerton G, Tyler C, Johnston CA, Vincent JP, Harris GE, Foreyt JP. (2007). Obesity. 15(11): 2553–2556.

Gately PJ, Cooke CB, Barth JH, Bewick BM, Radley D, Hill AJ. (2005). Pediatrics. 116(1): 73–77.

Glasofer DR, Tanofsky-Kraff M, Eddy KT, Yanovski SZ, Theim KR, Mirch MC, Ghorbani S, Ranzenhofer LM, Haaga D, Yanovski JA. (2007). J Pediatr Psychol. 32(1): 95–105.

Golan M. (2006). Int J Pediatr Obes. 1(2): 66–76.

Haddock CK, Shadish WR, Klesges RC, Stein RJ. (1994). Ann Behav Med. 16(3): 235–244.

Herrera EA, Johnston CA, Steele RG. (2004). Children's Health Care. 33(2): 151–167.

Huang JS, Norman GJ, Zabinski MF, Calfas K, Patrick K. (2007). J Adolesc Health. 40: 245–251.

Hughes AR, Farewell K, Harris D, Reilly JJ. (2007). Int J Obes. 31: 39–44.

Jelalian E, Mehlenbeck R, Lloyd-Richardson EE, Birmaher V, Wing RR. (2006). Int J Obes. 30: 31–39.

Jelalian E, Saelens BE. (1999). J Pediatr Psychol. 24 (3): 223–248.

Jiang JX, Lia XL, Greiner T, Lian GL, Rosenqvist U. (2005). Arch Dis Child. 90: 1235–1238.

Kiess W, Galler A, Reich A, Muller G, Kapellen T, Deutscher J, Raile K, Kratzsch J. (2001). Obesity Rev. 2: 29–36.

Kirk S, Zeller M, Claytor R, Santangelo M, Khoury PR, Daniels SR. (2005). Obes Res. 13(5): 876–882.

Kirkcaldy BD, Shephard RJ, Siefen RG. (2002). Social Psychiatry and Psychiatr Epidemiol. 37: 544–550.

Kirschenbaum DS, Harris ES, Tomarken AJ. (1984). Behav Ther. 15: 485–500.

Lowry KW, Sallinen BJ, Janicke DM. (2007). J Pediatr Psychol. 32(10): 1179–1195.

Murphree D. (1994). J Fam Pract. 38: 45–48.

Myers MD, Raynor HA, Epstein LH. (1998). Arch Pediatr Adolesc Med. 152: 855–861.

Nemet D, Barkan S, Epstein Y, Friedland O, Kowen G, Eliakim A. (2005). Pediatrics 115: e443--e449.

Neumark-Sztainer D, Story M, Hannan PJ, Tharp T, Rex J. (2003). Arch Pediatr Adolesc Med 157(8): 803–810.

Ogden CL, Carroll MD, Curtin LR, McDowell MA, Tabak CJ, Flegal KM. (2006). JAMA. 295(13): 1549–1555.

Piko BF, Keresztes N. (2006). J Community Health. 31(2): 136–145.

Pinhas-Hamiel O, Singer S, Pilpel N, Fradkin A, Modan D, Reichman B. (2006). Int J Obes 30: 267–272.

Reinehr T, Brylak K, Alexy U, Kersting M, Andler W. (2003). Int J Obes. 27: 1087–1092.

Reinehr T, de Sousa G, Toschke AM, Andler W. (2006a). Am J Clin Nutr. 84: 490–496.

Reinehr T, de Sousa G, Wabitsch M. (2006b). J Pediatr Gastroenterol Nutr. 43(4): 506–511.

Resnicow K, Taylor R, Baskin M, McCarty F. (2005). Obes Res 13(10): 1739–1748.

Resnicow K, Yaroch AL, Davis A, Wang DT, Carter S, Slaughter L, Coleman D, Baranowski T. (2000). Health Educ Behav. 27(5): 616–631.

Robinson S. (2006). J Sch Nurs. 22(4): 201–206.

Robinson TN. (1999). JAMA 282(16): 1561–1567.

Ross HE, Ivis F. (1999). Int J Eat Disord. 26(3): 245–260.

Rudolf MCJ, Sahota P, Barth JH, Walker J. (2001). BMJ. 322:1094–1095.

Sallis JF, Prochaska JJ, Taylor WC. (2000). Med Sci Sports Exerc. 32: 963–975.

Salmon J, Ball K, Crawford D, Booth M, Telford A, Hume C, Jolley D, Worsley A. (2005). Health Promot Int. 20: 7–17.

Savoye M, Berry D, Dziura J, Shaw M, Serrecchia JB, Barbetta G, Rose P, Lavietes S, Caprio S. (2005). J Am Diet Assoc. 105: 364–370.

Savoye M, Shaw M, Dziura J, Tamborlane WV, Rose P, Guandalini C, Goldberg-Gell R, Burgert TS, Cali AMG, Weiss R, Caprio S. (2007). JAMA. 297: 2697–2704.

Schipper H, Clinch JJ, Olweny CLM. (1996). In: Spilker B (ed) Quality of Life and Pharmacoeconomics in Clinical Trials 2nd ed. Lippencott-Raven, Philadelphia, pp. 11–23.

Schwimmer JB, Burwinkle TM, Varni JW. (2003). JAMA. 289(14): 1813–1819.

Shepard RJ. (1995). Res Q Exerc Sport. 66(4): 298–302.

Snethen JA, Broome ME, Cashin SE. (2006). J Pediatr Nurs. 21: 45–56.

Sothern MS, Schumacher H, von Almen TK, Carlisle LK, Udall JN. (2002). J Am Diet Assoc. 102(3): S81–S85.

Spear BA, Barlow SE, Ervin C, Ludwig DS, Saelens BE, Schetzina KE, Taveras EM. (2007). Pediatrics. 120 (Supp 4): S254--S288.

Stella SG, Vilar AP, Lacroix C, Fisberg M, Santos RF, Mello MT, Tufik S. (2005). Braz J Med Biol Res 38(11): 1683–1689

Stern M, Mazzeo SE, Gerke CK, Porter JS, Bean MK, Laver JH. (2007). J Pediatr Psychol. 32(1): 90–94.

Stern M, Mazzeo SE, Porter J, Gerke C, Bryan D, Laver J. (2006). J Clin Psychol Med Settings. 13(3): 217–228.

Stice E, Presnell K, Spangler D. (2002). Health Psychol. 21(2): 131–138.

St Jeor ST, Perumean-Chaney S, Sigman-Grant M, Williams C, Foreyt J. (2002). J Am Diet Assoc. 102(5): 640–644.

Strauss RS, Pollack HA. (2003). Arch Pediatr Adolesc Med. 157:746–752.

Valverde MA, Patin RV, Oliveira FLC, Lopez FA, Vitolo MR. (1998). Int J Obes. 22: 513–519.

van den Akker ELT, Puiman PJ, Groen M, Timman R, Jongejan MTM, Trijsburg W. (2007). J Pediatr. 151: 280–283.

Walker LLM, Gately PJ, Bewick BM, Hill AJ. (2003). Int J Obes. 27: 748–754.

Weiss MR, McAuley E, Ebbeck V, Wiese DM. (1990). J Sport Exerc Psychol. 12: 21–36.

Wilfley DE, Tibbs TL, Van Buren DJ, Reach KP, Walker MS, Epstein LH. (2007). Health Psychol. 26 (5): 521–532.

Wilson P, O'Meara S, Summerball C, Kelly S. (2003). Qual Saf Health Care. 12: 65–74.

Yanovski JA, Yanovski SZ. (2003). JAMA. 289(14): 1851–1853.

Yin Z, Gutin B, Johnson MH, MooreJ. Hanes JB, Cavnar M, Thornburg J, Moore D, Barbeau P. (2005). Obes Res. 13(12): 2153–2161.

Young KM, Northern JJ, Lister KM, Drummond JA, O'Brien WH. (2007). Clin Psychol Rev. 27: 240–249.

Young-Hyman D, Herman LJ, Scott DL, Schlundt DG. (2000). Obes Res. 8: 241–248.

Yu CC, Sung RY, Hau KT, Lam PK, Nelson EA, So RC. (2008). J Sports Med Phys Fitness. 48: 76–82.

Zeller M, Kirk S, Claytor R, Khoury P, Grieme J, Santangelo M, Daniels S. (2004a). J Pediatr. 114: 466–470.

Zeller MH, Modi AC. (2006). Obesity. 14(1): 122–130.

Zeller MH, Reiter-Purtill J, Modi AC, Gutzwiller J, Vannatta K, Davies WH. (2007). Obesity. 15(1):126–36.

Zeller MH, Saelens BE, Roehrig H, Kirk S, Daniels SR. (2004b). Obes Res. 12(10): 1576–1586.

148 Adolescent Quality of Life in Australia

A. H. Lee · L. B. Meuleners · M. L. Fraser

1	Introduction	2538
2	Health and Well-Being of Australian Adolescents	2539
3	Importance of Measuring QOL in the Adolescent Population	2539
4	Challenges for Measuring Adolescent QOL	2540
5	Dimensions of Adolescent QOL: Existing Evidence	2541
6	Generic Measures for Assessing Adolescent QOL	2541
7	Western Australian Study of Adolescent QOL	2545
7.1	Study Overview	2545
7.2	Research Design	2545
7.3	The Measuring Instrument	2545
7.4	Statistical Analyses and Results	2546
7.4.1	QOL and Its Determinants	2546
7.4.2	Assessing Measurement Properties Using Structural Equation Modeling	2546
7.4.3	Variations in QOL over a Six Month Period	2547
7.5	Contribution to Adolescent QOL Research	2549
7.6	Limitations	2551
8	Conclusions and Future Research	2552
	Summary Points	2552

Abstract: Although the majority of adolescent ❷ quality of life (QOL) research has focused on chronic diseases, the QOL measure can be highly useful in providing a broader understanding of the health and well-being of the general adolescent population. Adolescent QOL is a relatively new field so researchers face several challenges. Adolescents are a unique group and the unique dimensions that make up their QOL are only just emerging. Several generic assessments of adolescent QOL are being produced but predominantly in Europe and North America. One particular Australian based longitudinal study has contributed to the understanding of adolescent QOL. Encouragingly, it reported that Australian adolescents, both with and without a chronic disease, describe their QOL positively. It also provided initial validation for adolescent QOL in Australia to comprise of five dimensions, namely, "physical health," "environment," "social," "psychological" and "opportunities for growth and development," and showed that these dimensions are interdependent. The longitudinal nature of the study also revealed the dynamic nature of QOL and that potentially modifiable variables of adolescent "control" and "opportunities" could have a significant positive impact on QOL. Research would be enhanced by the development of pertinent adolescent QOL measures based on the most recent modification and validation of internationally developed instruments. Aboriginal and Torres Strait Islanders and rural or remote adolescents are at particular risk of poor QOL and these groups should be targeted for improvement. It is recommended that QOL research be used for developing policy, health intervention programs, monitoring the QOL status of the general adolescent population and identifying those at risk of low QOL.

List of Abbreviations: *AIHW,* Australian Institute of Health and Welfare; *CFA,* ❷ confirmatory factor analysis; *CHQ,* child health questionnaire; *ComQOL-S,* comprehensive quality of life scale – school version; *EFA,* ❷ exploratory factor analysis; *HRQOL,* ❷ health-related quality of life; *QOL,* quality of life; *QOLPAV,* quality of life profile- adolescent version; *SEM,* structural equation modeling; *WA,* Western Australia; *WHO,* World Health Organization

1   Introduction

Adolescent quality of life (QOL) is a relatively new field in Australia. While the majority of research has focused on adolescents with a ❷ chronic illness, QOL can also be an extremely useful measure for the general, healthy adolescent population. It is a complex concept and there is a lack of agreement regarding precisely what is meant by this term (Wallander et al., 2001). One definition is "the degree to which the person enjoys the important possibilities of his/her life" (Raphael et al., 1996). This holistic approach draws attention to the determinants of health at a range of levels and dimensions. Health-related quality of life (HRQOL) is a measure developed specifically to examine the impact of illness, injury or medical treatment on an individual's QOL. Previously it included dimensions related to illness or treatment only but is now evolving to incorporate broader factors, blurring the boundary with QOL (Ravens-Sieberer et al., 2006).

Adolescents are a unique group with a unique set of dimensions and factors that make up their QOL. A particular challenge is to determine the dimensions of adolescent QOL (Wallander et al., 2001). In addition, few QOL instruments have been developed or validated specifically for use with Australian adolescents. A longitudinal study of adolescent QOL in Western Australia (WA) included healthy adolescents in their sample and has provided valuable information on their QOL, potential dimensions to measure QOL and the interrelationships between these dimensions (Meuleners et al., 2003).

This chapter discusses the current health and well-being of Australian adolescents, the challenges for measuring QOL and evidence for the inclusion of dimensions to measure adolescent QOL. In addition, existing measures of adolescent QOL are reviewed and the WA adolescent QOL study is discussed in detail. Finally, future directions in the field will be explored.

2 Health and Well-Being of Australian Adolescents

It is not easy to gauge or measure how adolescents in Australian society are faring (Eckersley et al., 2006). A recent report compiled by the Australian Institute of Health and Welfare (AIHW) on young Australians aged 12–24 years compared different data sources and highlighted the contradictory information on their health and well being (AIHW, 2007).

Several traditional statistical measures of health and well-being have indicated a positive picture of young people in Australia. For example, life expectancy and mortality continues to improve, largely due to decreases in death due to transport injury, suicide and drug dependence disorder (AIHW, 2007). Australian youths are generally highly educated and in 2004–2005, 94% rated their own health as either "good," "very good" or "excellent" (AIHW, 2007).

However, other sources showed that adolescents in Australia are not faring well physically or psychologically. For example, approximately 25% were overweight or obese and less than half met recommended physical activity guidelines in 2004–2005 (AIHW, 2007). The 2004 National Drug Strategy Household Survey reported almost one third of young people drank alcohol at levels that placed them at risk of alcohol-related harm in the short term, 23% had used an illicit drug in the 12 months prior to the survey and around 17% were smokers (AIHW, 2005a). In addition, mental disorders were the leading contributor to the burden of disease and injury in young people with depression, anxiety and substance use accounting for the majority (AIHW, 2007). The rate of completed suicide for young Australians was also among the highest in the world (AIHW, 2000).

These statistics thus portray a considerably blurred picture of the overall QOL of Australian adolescents. Research that can provide information over a broad range of aspects of adolescent life is lacking in Australia, meaning conclusions about QOL have to be based on the accumulation of studies examining a single issue or a few key areas (Smart and Sanson, 2005). A recent overview noted that young people commonly self-report optimism and well-being in qualitative studies but their lives appear fairly negative with respect to objective criteria (Eckersley et al., 2006). Several explanations for this contradiction have been proposed. Young people are resilient and adaptable. Moreover, what may be considered a health risk, such as drug use, may be regarded as a life enjoying experience by young people (Eckersley et al., 2006).

3 Importance of Measuring QOL in the Adolescent Population

❷ Adolescence is a period of rapid emotional, physical and intellectual transition. Stressors can put this group at risk of various health and behavioral problems (Hurrelmann and Richter, 2006). There is ample evidence that adolescents' decisions and behaviors can impact on their health and QOL. Physical health, mental health, education and employment outcomes can be affected immediately and into the future (AIHW, 2005b; Eckersley et al., 2006). Therefore, adolescence is a key period for preventive health intervention.

Past research on adolescent QOL has focused on individuals with chronic disease. Disease and treatment have shifted to areas of chronic disease over the years with Attention Deficit Hyperactivity Disorder, conduct disorders and mental disorders becoming highly prevalent in Australian adolescents (AIHW, 2007). This shift has made the development of QOL measures extremely important for planning prevention and care programs (Eiser and Morse, 2001).

In terms of healthy adolescents, QOL research allows the monitoring of population health status over time, detection of sub-groups who may be at risk of poor QOL, as well as assessment of the impact of public health interventions (Ravens-Sieberer et al., 2001). While mortality, morbidity and behavioral risk measures are important in tracking health trends, they do not capture the perspective of adolescents themselves (Patrick et al., 2002). A recent review has suggested the need for a more holistic approach to health and well-being research for young Australians (Eckersley et al., 2006). QOL measures gather data over a broad range of aspects of adolescent life that are essential for the development of effective policies and interventions.

4   Challenges for Measuring Adolescent QOL

It is clear that measuring and monitoring the QOL of healthy Australian adolescents have many benefits. However, there are several challenges.

Firstly, QOL research in general is a relatively new field. While it is widely agreed that QOL is multidimensional (Rajmil et al., 2004; Raphael et al., 1996; Ravens-Sieberer et al., 2006), precisely which dimensions make up this construct is still under investigation. This issue is important as measuring too few dimensions can lead to ignoring meaningful information whereas measuring too many will result in non-interpretable and unreliable measurement dimensions (Coste et al., 2005). Furthermore, the concept of HRQOL which was once considered a sub-domain of QOL (Schipper et al., 1996), is now evolving to become broader, blurring the boundary between the two concepts (Zullig et al., 2005).

Secondly, the majority of research and instrument development in the field has focused on adult QOL. Adolescents operate within different frames of reference and their life experience and daily activities differ markedly from the adult population (Bullinger et al., 2006; Ravens-Sieberer et al., 2006). Consequently, there are fundamental differences in the way they understand and assess their own QOL.

Additionally, research that has targeted adolescents has focused mostly on the chronically ill (Ravens-Sieberer et al., 2006). While disease-specific research is useful, the measuring instruments cannot be applied generically and do not enable comparisons across conditions and healthy populations. These instruments also place emphasis on presence of symptoms and functional abilities (Eiser and Morse, 2001) that are not of high importance to the QOL of a healthy population.

Finally, information on the QOL of healthy adolescents and how it should be measured is only just emerging in Australia. While international research is informative, the adolescent experience, their priorities and perception of QOL could be influenced by their culture and values (Bullinger et al., 2006). For example, one study identified academic achievement as the most pressing concern for adolescents in Hong Kong (Hui, 2000), which may not be the case in Australia.

5   Dimensions of Adolescent QOL: Existing Evidence

The concept of adolescent QOL has emerged from frameworks initially developed with the adult population (Schipper, 1990). However, one qualitative study has provided evidence that the major components usually measured for adults are meaningful for adolescents but that the importance, spread and distribution of these components change throughout age groups (Rajmil et al., 2004). While dimensions of adult QOL are still controversial, measurement instruments consist at a minimum of physical, psychological and social dimensions (Bullinger, 2002; Ware, 2003). Previous research also indicates that personal characteristics such as age, gender and socioeconomic status could be associated with QOL and should be assessed (Ravens-Sieberer et al., 2007; Vingilis et al., 2002).

Adolescents face experiences that are unique to their specific age group. Past research has highlighted the dimensions of family, school and friendships as being particularly important for adolescent QOL (AIHW, 2007; Matza et al., 2004; Raphael et al., 1996). These groups provide their main form of social support and their health and wellbeing has been shown to be associated with a sense of connectedness to family, school and the community (AIHW, 2003). Most Australian adolescents live with their parents, siblings and other family members who provide them with physical, emotional and economic support (AIHW, 2007) and have a direct influence on their QOL. In addition, dimensions commonly assessed for adult QOL including the performance of basic functional tasks and economic or vocational status (Fayers and Machin, 2000), are much less relevant for adolescents.

A recent review of the major components of HRQOL instruments for children and adolescents cited physical well-being, psychological well-being, energy and vitality, self perception, cognitive functioning, social functioning and support including friends, sexual life and family, autonomy and independence, psychosocial relations to the material environment and general health perception/life quality as the major components (Ravens-Sieberer et al., 2006).

Other possible but less commonly assessed dimensions are also emerging from Australian and international adolescent studies. These include environmental factors such as neighborhood socioeconomic disadvantage, ❯ social capital and neighborhood safety (Drukker et al., 2006; Meyers and Miller, 2004). A role for less tangible, more difficult to measure factors such as beliefs, values and spirituality has also been suggested (Eckersley et al., 2006; WHOQOL SRPB Group, 2006).

An Australian study of adolescents in rural Queensland identified loneliness and neighborhood and school belongingness as being significantly associated with adolescents' subjective QOL (Chipuer et al., 2003). Another study of Western Australian adolescents indicated that improved control and opportunities in the adolescent's life had a positive impact on adolescent QOL (Meuleners and Lee, 2003).

Although an extensive list of possible dimensions is emerging, it is unsure whether they comprehensively encompass adolescent QOL and whether some dimensions should be weighted more heavily than others.

6   Generic Measures for Assessing Adolescent QOL

An increasing number of generic assessments of QOL suitable for the general adolescent population are being produced, predominantly in Europe and North America. The majority of these questionnaires measure HRQOL but considering the overlap with QOL, all of these measures are included in the discussion.

Reviews of QOL questionnaires for adolescents have revealed a reasonably coherent understanding of QOL, but the distribution of items among dimensions varies considerably (Rajmil et al., 2004; Ravens-Sieberer et al., 2006). The features of ten such questionnaires are listed in ❷ *Table 148-1*. All of them cover physical, psychological, social and school dimensions (Cummins, 1997; Landgraf et al., 1998; Patrick et al., 2002; Raphael et al., 1996; Ravens-Sieberer and Bullinger, 1998; Ravens-Sieberer et al., 2005; Sapin et al., 2005; Starfield et al., 1993; Varni et al., 1999; Vogels et al., 1998). Some also address personal care (Landgraf et al., 1998; Raphael et al., 1996; Ravens-Sieberer et al., 2005; Varni et al., 1999; Vogels et al., 1998) while others extend to environmental dimensions (Raphael et al., 1996; Ravens-Sieberer et al., 2005; Sapin et al., 2005; Varni et al., 1999; Vogels et al., 1998).

All instruments were self-report and the majority included parent or teacher-report questionnaires to cater for younger children. It is appropriate to collect information by self report as long as the age, maturity and cognitive development of the respondents are accounted for during instrument development (Ravens-Sieberer et al., 2006).

A limitation of existing instruments is the lack of international comparability. Moreover, since adolescents vary in their age and developmental stage, a single questionnaire may not be suitable for both younger and older adolescents (Ravens-Sieberer et al., 2006). Some instruments were also validated on small or non-representative samples (e.g., Starfield et al., 1993) or target small age ranges (e.g., Patrick et al., 2002; Sapin et al., 2005; Vogels et al., 1998). Finally, not all the instruments generated items with input from the target group (e.g., Starfield et al., 1993) while others were originally created for the chronically ill (e.g., Varni et al., 1999; Vogels et al., 1998).

The KIDSCREEN Quality of Life Questionnaire (Ravens-Sieberer et al., 2005), developed for 8- to 18-year-olds, is the first generic instrument to comprehensively fulfil the standards promoted by the World Health Organization (WHO) for measuring child and adolescent HRQOL (WHO, 1994). It was developed in seven European countries with consultation from the target group and was tested through random sampling of over 15,000 children and adolescents (Ravens-Sieberer et al., 2005). The questionnaire was valid and reliable and could be applicable in Australia after validation.

The Comprehensive Quality of Life Scale – School Version (ComQOL–S) was the only instrument that was developed for an Australian population although it was originally designed and evaluated for adults (Cummins, 1997). Few modifications were made for the adolescent population. While it addresses psychological and social dimensions in depth, very few school or neighborhood factors are included.

Both the child/adolescent and parent versions of the Child Health Questionnaire (CHQ), developed in the US (Landgraf et al., 1998), have been validated and modified in Australia. It performed well at an item and scale level. Although the physical and psychosocial dimension scores were not supported for population level analyses, the CHQ may be of value for adolescents with health problems (Waters et al., 2000). The Quality of Life Profile- Adolescent Version (QOLPAV), developed in Canada (Raphael et al., 2006), was validated for a study of Western Australian adolescents (Meuleners et al., 2001). This questionnaire was developed with direct input from adolescents and covered a broad range of dimensions including control and opportunities for improvement and change.

■ Table 148-1

Generic QOL instruments for adolescents

Name	Country of origin	Dimensions included[a]	Age (years)	Method of response	Number of items[b]	Reference
Child Health and Illness Profile (CHIP)	US	Satisfaction Complaints Resilience Health conditions Attainments of social goals Risk behaviors	12–17[c] 6–11 6–11	Self report Self report Parent report	188 45 45–188	Starfield et al. (1993)
Quality of Life Profile – Adolescent Version (QOLPAV)	Canada	Being Belonging Becoming	14–20	Self-report	54	Raphael et al. (1996)
Comprehensive Quality of Life Scale – School Version (ComQOL – S)	Australia	Material well-being Health Productivity Intimacy Safety Community Emotional well-being	11–18	Self report	35	Cummins (1997)
Child Health Questionnaire (CHQ)	US	General health Physical functioning Limitations in schoolwork and activities with friends Behavior Mental health Emotional or time impact on the parent Family cohesion Change in health Bodily pain or discomfort Self esteem Limitations in family activities	10–18 5–18	Self report Parent report (three versions)	87 28, 50, 98	Landgraf et al. (1998)
Revidierter KINDer Lebensqualitatsfragebogan (KINDL–R)	Germany	Physiological well-being Psychological well-being Self-esteem Family Friends School	4–7[d] 8–12 13–16 4–16	Self report Self report Self report Parent report	12 24 24 24	Ravens-Sieberer and Bullinger (1998)
The Netherlands Organization for Applied Scientific Research – Academic Medical Centre Child QOL Questionnaire (TACQOL)	The Netherlands	Physical complaints Mobility Independence Cognitive function Social function Positive emotions Negative emotions	8–15 5–15	Self report Parent report	56	Vogels et al. (1998)

◼ Table 148-1 (continued)

Name	Country of origin	Dimensions included[a]	Age (years)	Method of response	Number of items[b]	Reference
The Pediatric Quality of Life Inventory Generic Scores Scale (Peds QL 4.0)	US	Physical Emotional Social School	5–18 2–18	Self report Parent report	23	Varni et al. (1999)
Youth Quality of Life Instrument-Research Version (YQOL-R)	US	Self Relationships Surroundings General quality of life	12–18	Self report	57	Patrick et al. (2002)
KIDSCREEN Quality of Life Questionnaire	Austria Switzerland Germany Spain France The Netherlands UK	Physical well-being Psychological well being Moods and emotions Self-perception Autonomy Parents relations and home life Peers and social support relations School environment Bullying Financial resources	8–18	Self report Parent report	52/27[e]	Ravens-Sieberer et al. (2005)
Vecu de Sante Percue Adolescent (VSP-A)	France	Physical well being Body image Vitality Psychological well being Relationship with friends Relationship with parents Relationship with teachers Relationship with medical staff School performance Leisure activities	11–17	Self report Parent report Teacher report	40	Sapin et al. (2005)

This table summarizes the features of ten generic measures for assessing adolescent QOL

[a]Dimensions refer to the broader areas addressed in each instrument. Each dimension consists of several items

[b]Items refer to the total number questions making up the dimensions

[c]The CHIP has two different forms for two different age groups

[d]The KINDL-R has three different forms for three different age groups

[e]The KIDSCREEN has a full version consisting of 52 items and an abbreviated version consisting of 27 items

7 Western Australian Study of Adolescent QOL

7.1 Study Overview

This study aimed to provide a better understanding of adolescent QOL in WA (Meuleners et al., 2001). Although the study included adolescents with and without a chronic illness, the questionnaire and conceptual framework emphasized a ❷ wellness approach rather than illness approach (Raphael et al., 1996). The QOLPAV questionnaire was administered to investigate adolescent QOL (Meuleners et al., 2001). Five dimensions possibly underlying adolescent QOL, the interdependent relations between them (Meuleners et al., 2003), and the effects of covariates on QOL were also investigated (Meuleners and Lee, 2005). Finally, the dynamic changes in adolescent QOL over a 6 month period were documented and modeled (Meuleners and Lee, 2003).

7.2 Research Design

Study participants were recruited through the public and private secondary school system in the Perth metropolitan area of WA during 1999–2000. Stratified sampling with replacement was employed and a total of 30 schools, reflecting diversity in socio-economic status were approached. Of these, 20 schools agreed to participate and questionnaires were sent to the home of each student aged between 10 and 19 years after consent was granted from parents. Of the 500 consented adolescents who initially agreed to participate, 112 with a chronic condition and 251 without returned the questionnaire, giving an overall response rate of 72.6% (Meuleners et al., 2001).

7.3 The Measuring Instrument

The instrument QOLPAV (Raphael et al., 1996) was suitable for this study of healthy adolescents and those with a chronic illness. It was found to be reliable and correlated with measures of adolescent personality, self-reported health status and tobacco and alcohol use (Raphael et al., 1996). The framework underlying this instrument focused on possibilities for adolescents in three areas of life, "being," "belonging" and "becoming." As shown in ❷ Figure 148-1, these domains were further divided into nine sub-domains. The domains encompassed a multidimensional approach and emphasized the holistic nature of adolescent QOL. The QOLPAV consisted of 54 items and was a self-administered questionnaire. Each of the 54 items was scored using a five-point ❷ Likert scale. Adolescents rated the importance of each item and their satisfaction with the item. Scores were computed for the three domains, each of the nine sub-domains as well as the overall QOL. It also included items concerning control over the nine sub-domains and nine more items referring to opportunities for improvement and change (Meuleners and Lee, 2003).

Additional demographic variables, information related to gender, age, school, grade, family living situation, socio-economic status, presence of a chronic condition, its type and duration and sick time was also collected using the structured questionnaire. Two questions regarding the adolescent's perception of his/her overall physical health and QOL were also included in the questionnaire as a means of validating the overall QOL score (Meuleners et al., 2001). After review

□ **Figure 148-1**

Essential dimensions and sub-dimensions making up the QOLPAV. This figure summarizes the domains and sub-domains of adolescent QOL underlying the instrument QOLPAV

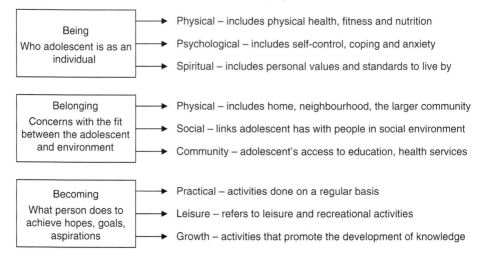

Being Who adolescent is as an individual	→ Physical – includes physical health, fitness and nutrition → Psychological – includes self-control, coping and anxiety → Spiritual – includes personal values and standards to live by
Belonging Concerns with the fit between the adolescent and environment	→ Physical – includes home, neighbourhood, the larger community → Social – links adolescent has with people in social environment → Community – adolescent's access to education, health services
Becoming What person does to achieve hopes, goals, aspirations	→ Practical – activities done on a regular basis → Leisure – refers to leisure and recreational activities → Growth – activities that promote the development of knowledge

by two adolescent health experts, the questionnaire incorporating QOLPAV and demographic section was pilot tested on a sample of 20 Australian adolescents, which led to minor modifications. Assessment of reliability and content validity was also undertaken (Meuleners et al., 2001).

7.4   Statistical Analyses and Results

7.4.1   QOL and Its Determinants

After administration of the baseline questionnaire, the results indicated that overall QOL scores for chronically ill and healthy adolescents were positive with both groups reporting an acceptable to very good QOL (Meuleners et al., 2001). There was no significant difference between the two groups. Stepwise regression was undertaken on the combined sample of participants to explore the latent factor determinants of QOL. Age, perceptions of health and control and opportunity were found to be significant determinants of QOL. No significant differences were observed between males and females (Meuleners et al., 2001).

7.4.2   Assessing Measurement Properties Using Structural Equation Modeling

Next, confirmatory factor analysis (CFA) was applied to determine the measurement properties of the latent factors or dimensions underlying adolescent QOL. Recursive structural equation modeling (SEM) was then undertaken to determine the direction and magnitude of the interdependent effects (Meuleners et al., 2003).

Exploratory factor analysis (EFA) was conducted as a preliminary to CFA. Weak items, accounting for a low percentage of the variance, were deleted from further analysis. The EFA results together with a literature review provided guidelines for selecting items to be included in the CFA. Five dimensions consisting of 18 items in total were retained. These domains were "social," "environment," "psychological," "physical health" and "opportunities for growth and development" (Meuleners et al., 2003).

A second-order CFA was conducted to address the factor structure of the five dimensions and 18 items. The completely standardized solution to the second-order CFA is shown in ❷ *Figure 148-2*. Results showed that the 18 items were reliable measures of their respective dimensions with associations ranging from 0.45 to 0.80. The direct effect of the five dimensions on QOL was strong (ranging from 0.68 to 0.90), thus convergent validity was achieved (Meuleners et al., 2003).

A recursive SEM was next fitted to estimate the direction and magnitude of the effects among the five identified dimensions of QOL. ❷ *Figure 148-3* illustrates the best fitting solution, with standardized estimates of the direct effects of one factor on another. The R^2 values refer to the squared multiple correlation coefficients for the structural equations. For example, 51% of the variability in the "psychological" dimension was accounted for simultaneously by the direct effects of the "environment" and the "health" dimension scores, as well as the indirect effect of the "environment" score, mediated by the "health" score (Meuleners et al., 2003).

The SEM modeling found that "environment" had significant direct and indirect effects on the other four factors. Significant variables for the "environment" dimension included "the feeling of safety," "the home lived in," "the school the adolescent attends" and "the neighborhood." The "social" dimension had little effect on the other dimensions except "opportunities for growth and development." Meanwhile, "opportunities for growth and development" were significantly influenced by the "social," "health" and "psychological" dimensions. The "psychological" dimension also had a strong positive effect on "opportunities for growth and development" and a lesser effect on the "social" dimension (Meuleners et al., 2003).

In the next stage, the effects of covariates or personal characteristics on adolescent QOL and its five dimensions "physical health," "environment," "social," "psychological" and "opportunities for growth and development" were assessed using SEM (Meuleners and Lee, 2005). The variables age, control, chronic condition and perception of health were chosen based on literature review. Individual items constituting each of the five identified dimensions were not included due to the small sample size. Instead, composite regression scores from the five factor second-order CFA were used (Meuleners and Lee, 2005).

❷ *Figure 148-4* presents the fitted model. The standardized γ weights, indicating the strength of the relationship, showed several moderate associations between the personal characteristic variables and the QOL construct. In particular, "control" had a significant positive effect on the QOL construct ($\gamma = 0.43$, $p < 0.05$) and poorer "health" exerted a significant negative impact ($\gamma = -0.34$, $p < 0.05$). "Age" showed an inverse relationship but was not statistically significant. Support for the five dimensions to be included in adolescent QOL was also evident. All the factor loadings on the QOL construct were high (0.60–0.76) and significant at the 1% level. This analysis confirmed that adolescent QOL is a complex interplay between different factors (Meuleners and Lee, 2005).

7.4.3 Variations in QOL over a Six Month Period

It was of interest to examine how adolescent QOL varied over a 6 month period using overall QOL scores and the five dimension scores on "physical health," "environment," "social,"

■ Figure 148-2

Completely standardized solution to second-order CFA showing loadings and error variances for the 18 items, five underlying latent factors and a single factor. This figure presents the fitted model structure underlying adolescent QOL based on second-order confirmatory factor analysis, where η_1 to η_5 represent the 5 first-order factors, and ξ_1 represents the one second-order factor, QOL

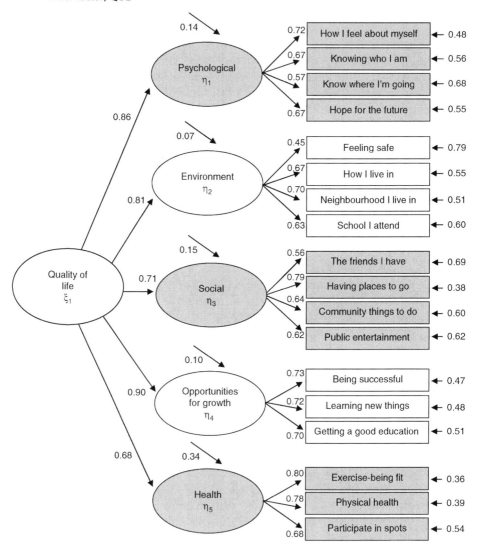

"psychological" and "opportunities for growth and development." A second identical questionnaire was sent to participants 6 months after they returned the initial questionnaire. Three hundred participants completed both questionnaires (Meuleners and Lee, 2003).

Overall QOL scores remained positive after 6 months though there was a significant decrease in the mean QOL score. ❷ *Table 148-2* shows the distribution of QOL scores at

■ Figure 148-3

Solution to recursive SEM, showing standardized direct effects and covariances. This figure shows the fitted recursive structural equation model of the five dimensions of adolescent QOL, where η_1 to η_5 represent the 5 first-order factors, and R^2 refers to the squared multiple correlation coefficients for the structural equations

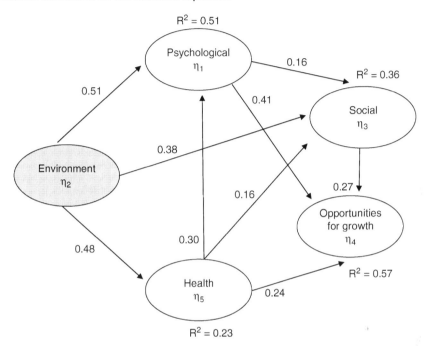

baseline and 6 months. It is possible the questionnaire timing could account for the decrease due to the change between winter and summer months in relation to school activities, sport and social activities. Univariate and multivariate tests on the five dimensions of QOL revealed significant changes in the "social," "physical health" and "opportunities for growth and development" scores for the combined data, however, the effect size scores were all minimal (Meuleners and Lee, 2003).

A longitudinal multilevel model was fitted to the data to determine the stability of the significant variables "age," "control," "opportunities" and "perceptions of health." It indicated that 62% of the variation in QOL was due to differences between individuals while 38% was due to within adolescent difference (time difference). Improved "control" and "opportunities" appeared to have a significant positive impact on QOL while increasing "age" and deteriorating "physical health" had the opposite effect (Meuleners and Lee, 2003).

7.5 Contribution to Adolescent QOL Research

This study provided valuable evidence about adolescent QOL in Australia. It focused on a wellness rather than an illness perspective (Raphael et al., 1996) and included

◘ Figure 148-4

Structural equation model of adolescent QOL. This figure shows the fitted structural equation model of the covariates and dimensions of adolescent QOL, where ξ_1 to ξ_4 represent the independent covariates with γ the corresponding effect on the QOL construct

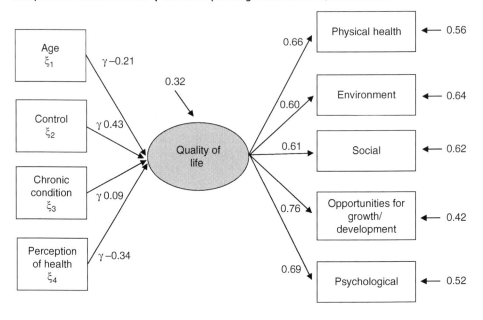

◘ Table 148-2

Distribution of QOL scores

QOL score[a]	Baseline $n = 363$	6 months $n = 300$
Very problematic (QOL < -1.5)	0(0%)	0(0%)
Problematic ($-1.5 \leq$ QOL < -0.5)	4(1%)	2(0.7%)
Adequate ($-0.5 \leq$ QOL < 0.5)	50(14%)	45(15%)
Acceptable (0.5 $\leq$ QOL $\leq$ 1.5	182(50%)	153(51%)
Very good (QOL > 0.5)	127(35%)	100(33.3%)
Mean (SD)	1.28(0.68)	1.18(0.69)

This table shows the distribution of QOL scores of Australian adolescents at baseline and 6 months. QOL score = (Importance score/3) × (Satisfaction score − 3)
[a]QOL score is an overall score based on the adolescent's rating of the importance of and satisfaction with each item

healthy adolescents in the sample. The study provided encouraging findings that WA adolescents, both with and without a chronic disease, reported their QOL positively (Meuleners et al., 2001).

Past research has highlighted the lack of definitive conceptualization of adolescent QOL (Wallander et al., 2001). This study provided validation for adolescent QOL in Australia to comprise five dimensions, namely, "physical health," "environment," "social," "psychological" and "opportunities for growth and development" (Meuleners et al., 2003).

Main results of the SEM indicated that the "environment" dimension has a significant direct and indirect effect on the other four dimensions (Meuleners et al., 2003). Other Australian research also reported associations between adolescent QOL and the environment including neighborhood, school and home factors (Chipuer et al., 2003; Meyers and Miller, 2004). Neighborhood and home factors are not always included in adolescent QOL or HRQOL instruments (Rajmil et al., 2004) despite their potential influence on QOL. The observed effect of the "psychological" dimension on the "social" and "opportunities for growth and development" dimensions highlights the importance of the role of psychological well-being in QOL and implies that public health practitioners should direct health promotion intervention towards this dimension.

The authors noted that alternative models could also fit the observed data equally well, resulting in a different interpretation of the measurement of QOL. To confirm the validity of the measurement model and interrelationships among the five dimensions, as well as the effects of the four covariates, replication with large samples was recommended (Meuleners and Lee, 2005; Meuleners et al., 2003).

This study was also unique due to its longitudinal design, providing insights into the determinants of adolescent QOL over a 6 month period. Very little is known about changes in QOL over time. The study highlighted the dynamic nature of QOL with 38% of observed variations being attributed to time, emphasizing the necessity of longitudinal study design to capture changes (Meuleners and Lee, 2003). The main finding from the multilevel modeling was the identification of covariates "physical health," "control," "opportunities," and "age" that affected the overall QOL scores over the 6 month period (Meuleners and Lee, 2003). "Physical health" and "age" are commonly acknowledged in the literature as being associated with QOL (Eiser and Morse, 2001; Vingilis et al., 2002), however, the finding provides support for the inclusion of potentially modifiable social determinants of heath, "control" and "opportunities."

Finally, the study showed that CFA and SEM methods are useful for developing hypothetical models and assessing the magnitude and direction of effects among identified factors. It has validated a generic questionnaire, the QOLPAV (Raphael et al., 1996) for measuring adolescent QOL in Australia.

7.6   Limitations

All participants were volunteers, possibly contributing to a self-selection or "healthy volunteer" bias. The sample was also relatively homogenous in their socioeconomic status, which was not a significant predictor of adolescent QOL in the study. The variable was measured based on residential postcodes which might not be sensitive enough to detect any significant relationship. There was also a higher prevalence of females in the study, which might contribute to the lack of observed difference in QOL between genders.

It is possible that relationships between the five identified dimensions of QOL are bi-directional but these could not be tested due to the small sample size (Meuleners et al., 2003). In addition, other emerging factors such as community activities, spiritual and coping styles (Eckersley et al., 2006; WHOQOL SRPB Group, 2006), were not included in the QOLPAV.

8   Conclusions and Future Research

Adolescent health information, including QOL, is important for health care researchers and policy makers. It captures the perspective of the individual and provides a holistic approach to the health and well-being of the general adolescent population. Recent developments in the area of adolescent QOL in Australia and worldwide are encouraging and have provided valuable information. Nevertheless, it remains a relatively new area and several gaps in research remain.

Although several instruments to measure adolescent QOL have been developed, few of these meet all the standards promoted by the WHO (WHO, 1994) and only one instrument was developed in Australia (Cummins, 1997). New instrument development or the modification and validation of internationally developed instruments would enhance adolescent QOL research in Australia. Consideration should also be given to emerging evidence on factors influencing adolescent QOL and how to best assess them. The WA study demonstrated the dynamic nature of adolescent QOL, yet the two survey time points of 6 months apart might not be sufficient to capture the apparent change in QOL. Future studies should use longitudinal designs that examine the stability of QOL and its potential determinants over a longer period, say, five time points over a 2 year period.

Aboriginal and Torres Strait Islanders and adolescents living in rural or remote areas were not included in the WA-based study (Meuleners et al., 2001). However, indicators of health and well-being have suggested that these adolescent groups are at risk of poorer QOL. For example, young indigenous Australians have higher rates of death, injury and some chronic diseases such as asthma and diabetes. They are also more likely to experience obesity, physical inactivity, smoking, imprisonment and lower educational attainment (AIHW, 2007). Similarly, young people living in remote areas have substantially higher rates of death and hospitalization for some health conditions, and are more likely to engage in certain risky health behaviors than their city counterparts (AIHW, 2007). The two groups are potential targets for future QOL research.

Finally, it is important to increase the awareness of health care researchers, health promotion professionals and policy makers about adolescent QOL. Information obtained from regular usage of the QOLPAV or another validated measure could form the basis of establishing an adolescent QOL database. This would be invaluable for further research and refinement of the instrument. Relevant factors that positively or negatively influence adolescent QOL are useful for the development of policy and intervention programs, monitoring the QOL status of the general adolescent population and identifying those at risk of low QOL. Putting QOL research findings into practice could enhance the overall health and QOL of adolescents in Australia.

Summary Points

- It is difficult to understand the health and well-being of the Australian adolescent population from traditional mortality and morbidity statistics. QOL measures the perspective of the adolescents themselves and can provide a holistic view of their health status.
- Researchers face various challenges because adolescent QOL is a relatively new field and the majority of existing literature is based on adults or the chronically ill.

- The unique dimensions of adolescent QOL are only just emerging in the literature. Several generic assessments of adolescent QOL have been developed in Europe and North America.
- One Western Australian-based study has contributed to the understanding of adolescent QOL in Australia. It reported that WA adolescents, both with and without a chronic disease, describe their QOL positively.
- The study provided initial validation for adolescent QOL in Australia to comprise the five dimensions, "physical health," "environment," "social," "psychological" and "opportunities for growth and development." It was further demonstrated through SEM that these dimensions were interdependent.
- The longitudinal design of the study revealed the dynamic nature of QOL and identified the potentially modifiable variables of adolescent "control" and "opportunities" as having a significant positive impact on QOL.
- Australian research should be directed towards the development of adolescent QOL measures based on the most current research or the modification and validation of internationally developed instruments.
- Aboriginal and Torres Strait Islanders and rural or remote adolescents are at particular risk of poor QOL in Australia so that future research should target these groups.
- It is recommended to use the findings for developing policy and health intervention programs, monitoring QOL status of the general adolescent population and identifying those at risk of low QOL.

References

Australian Institute of Health and Welfare. (2000). Australia's Health 2000 – The Seventh Biennial Health Report of the Australian Institute of Health and Welfare. AIHW, Canberra.

Australian Institute of Health and Welfare. (2003). Australia's Young People: Their Health and Well-being, cat. no. PHE 50. AIHW, Canberra.

Australian Institute of Health and Welfare. (2005a). 2004 National Drug Strategy Household Survey – Detailed Findings. Drug statistics series no. 16, cat. no. PHE 66. AIHW, Canberra.

Australian Institute of Health and Welfare. (2005b). A Picture of Australia's children, cat. no. PHE 58. AIHW, Canberra.

Australian Institute of Health and Welfare. (2007). Young Australians: Their Health and Wellbeing 2007, cat. no. PHE 87. AIHW, Canberra.

Bullinger M. (2002). Restor Neurol Neurosci. 20: 93–101.

Bullinger M, Schmidt S, Petersen C, Ravens-Sieberer U. (2006). J Public Health. 14: 343–355.

Chipuer HM, Bramston P, Pretty G. (2003). Soc Indic Res. 61: 79–95.

Coste J, Bouee S, Ecosse E, Leplege A, Pouchot J. (2005). Qual Life Res. 14: 641–654.

Cummins RA. (1997). Comprehensive Quality of Life Scale – Student (Grades 7–12): ComQol-S5, 5th ed. School of Psychology, Deakin University, Melbourne.

Drukker M, Kaplan C, Schneiders J, Feron FJ, van Os J. (2006). BMC Public Health. 6: 133.

Eckersley RM, Wierenga A, Wyn J. (2006). Flashpoints & Signpoints: Pathways to Success and Wellbeing for Australia's Young People. Australia 21, Australian Youth Research Centre, VicHealth, Melbourne.

Eiser C, Morse R. (2001). Arch Dis Child. 84: 205–211.

Fayers P, Machin D. (2000). Quality of Life: Assessment, Analysis and Interpretation. Wiley, West Sussex, England.

Hui EK. (2000). J Adolesc. 23: 189–203.

Hurrelmann K, Richter M. (2006). J Public Health. 14: 20–28.

Landgraf JM, Maunsell E, Speechley KN, Bullinger M, Campbell S, Abetz L, Ware JE. (1998). Qual Life Res. 7: 433–445.

Matza LS, Swensen AR, Flood EM, Secnik K, Leidy NK. (2004). Value Health. 7: 79–92.

Meuleners LB, Lee AH. (2003). Pediatr Int. 45: 706–711.

Meuleners LB, Lee AH. (2005). Qual Life Res. 14: 1057–1063.

Meuleners LB, Lee AH, Binns CW. (2001). Asia Pac J Public Health. 13: 40–44.

Meuleners LB, Lee AH, Binns CW, Lower A. (2003). Qual Life Res. 12: 283–290.

Meyers SA, Miller C. (2004). Adolescence. 39: 121–144.

Patrick DL, Edwards TC, Topolski TD. (2002). J Adolesc. 25: 287–300.

Rajmil L, Herdman M, Fernandez de Sanmamed MJ, Detmar S, Bruil J, Ravens-Sieberer U, Bullinger M, Simeoni MC, Auquier P. (2004). J Adolesc Health. 34: 37–45.

Raphael D, Rukholm E, Brown I, Hill-Bailey P, Donato E. (1996). J Adolesc Health. 19: 366–375.

Ravens-Sieberer U, Auquier P, Erhart M, Gosch A, Rajmil L, Bruil J, Power M, Duer W, Cloetta B, Czemy L, Mazur J, Czimbalmos A, Tountas Y, Hagquist C, Kilroe J. (2007). Qual Life Res. 16: 1347–1356.

Ravens-Sieberer U, Bullinger M. (1998). Qual Life Res. 7: 399–407.

Ravens-Sieberer U, Erhart M, Wille N, Wetzel R, Nickel J, Bullinger M. (2006). Pharmacoeconomics. 24: 1199–1220.

Ravens-Sieberer U, Gosch A, Abel T, Auquier P, Bellach BM, Bruil J, Dur W, Power M, Rajmil L. (2001). Soz Praventivmed. 46: 294–302.

Ravens-Sieberer U, Gosch A, Rajmil L, Erhart M, Bruil J, Duer W, Auquier P, Power M, Abel T, Czemy L, Mazur J, Czimbalmos A, Tountas Y, Hagquist C, Kilroe J. (2005). Expert Rev Pharmacoecon Outcomes Res. 5: 353–364.

Sapin C, Simeoni MC, El Khammar M, Antoniotti S, Auquier P. (2005). J Adolesc Health. 36: 327–336.

Schipper H. (1990). Oncology. 4: 51–57.

Schipper H, Clinch J, Olweny J. (1996). Quality of Life Studies: Definitions and Conceptual Issues. Lippincott-Raven, New York.

Smart D, Sanson A. (2005). Fam Matters. 70: 46–53.

Starfield B, Bergner M, Ensminger M, Riley A, Ryan S, Green B, McGauhey P, Skinner A, Kim S. (1993). Pediatrics. 91: 430–435.

Varni JW, Seid M, Rode CA. (1999). Med Care. 37: 126–139.

Vingilis ER, Wade TJ, Seeley JS. (2002). Can J Public Health. 93: 193–197.

Vogels T, Verrips GH, Verloove-Vanhorick SP, Fekkes M, Kamphuis RP, Koopman HM, Theunissen NC, Wit JM. (1998). Qual Life Res. 7: 457–465.

Wallander JL, Schmitt M, Koot HM. (2001). J Clin Psychol. 57: 571–585.

Ware JE, Jr. (2003). Arch Phys Med Rehabil. 84: S43–S51.

Waters E, Salmon L, Wake M. (2000). J Pediatr Psychol. 25: 381–391.

World Health Organization, Division of Mental Health. (1994). Measurement of Quality of Life in Children. MNH/PSF/94.5. World Health Organization, Geneva.

WHOQOL SRPB Group. (2006). Soc Sci Med. 62: 1486–1497.

Zullig KJ, Valois RF, Drane JW. (2005). Health Qual Life Outcomes. 3: 64.

149 Health-Related Quality of Life Among University Students

M. Vaez · M. Voss · L. Laflamme

1	*Introduction*	*2557*
2	*Student Quality of Life in Higher Education – a Transition*	*2558*
3	*Dealing with Stress as a University Student*	*2558*
4	*Student Quality of Life and Well-Being during the Years at University*	*2559*
5	*Students Concerns and Academic Performance*	*2559*
6	*Theoretical Perspective on Student Retention and Persistence*	*2561*
7	*University Student Health, Lifestyle and Quality of Life: a Cohort Study in Sweden*	*2561*
7.1	Student Questionnaire Surveys	2561
8	*Findings from Studies within the Project*	*2562*
8.1	First Year Student Health and Quality of Life- Cross Sectional Studies	2562
9	*Health and Quality of Life – from First to Third Year at University*	*2564*
9.1	Individual Changes in Health Status, Health Risk Behaviors and Perceived Stress	2564
9.2	Academic Performance	2564
10	*Health and Quality of Life at the First and the Final Academic Year*	*2565*
11	*Results*	*2566*
11.1	Self-Rated Psychological Health and General Health at Group Level	2566
11.2	Self-Rated Psychological Health and General Health at Individual Level	2566
11.3	Student Quality of Life in the First and the Final Year of Academic Life	2567
11.4	Associations to Current Quality of Life in the Final Academic Year	2568
12	*Conclusion*	*2570*
13	*Methodological Considerations*	*2572*
	Summary Points	*2572*

Appendix A: *2573*
Background 2573
Education 2574
Lifestyle 2574
Stress 2575
Physical Health 2575
Psychological Health 2575
General Health 2576
Quality of Life 2576

Abstract: Since the early nineties, universities in Sweden have witnessed a significant expansion in the number of students and now the university-student population constitutes a major part of the young adult population. To study at university has become a common choice for many young adults and as a consequence the student population has diversified in terms of age, gender, ethnical background and socio-economic profile. The transition to higher education has been recognized as a critical period in the formation of the life-pathways and in the establishment of adult behavior. In this context there is a growing interest in studying the impact of enrolment in higher education on the student quality of life and well being. In this prospective study of potential factors related to the student quality of life of 3000 first year full time students (in 1998/ 1999) at a large University in Sweden were followed during their education. The students have filled in three self-administrated questionnaire/covering aspects such as demographic, lifestyle, academics, health status and quality of life, at the end of 1999, 2001 and 2003. The findings emphasized that although, a high proportion of the students rated their health and quality of life as good and the persistence rate was relatively good during the years of university, there was a tendency for deterioration in self rated general and psychological health. This pattern was more pronounced among female students. The results also suggested that the students current quality of life in 2003 was strongly associated with self-rated psychological health, psychosomatic symptoms such as depression, concentration difficulties and perceived stress due to loneliness and doubts about the future. Greater attention should be paid to these factors, in particular by providing students with a work environment conducive to the reduction of stress.

1 Introduction

Conditions during higher education and on entry into working life are of great significance for differences in career opportunities, quality of life and health between men and women, and between social groups. In particular, the transition to college or university is a critical period in the formation of the life-pathways of young adults (Astin, 1984; Lu, 1994).

In countries like Sweden, choosing to study at university rather than immediately enter in the labor force is common – since there are relatively favorable economic conditions, low tuition fees, and access to study aid. To receive study support over a period of years, students must pursue their studies with a certain degree of success. Yet, it is intended that a person's social background and financial circumstances should not present a barrier. Further, access to university should not be influenced by where in the country a person lives. All people in Sweden up to the age of 50 can obtain study aid for university courses up to a maximum of 240 weeks (National Agency of Higher Education, 2000).

Since the early nineties, the Swedish Government has invested in higher education in a variety of ways. These include extending the number of places at university or college, establishing new universities, extending adult education, and developing post-high-school vocational training. These ventures, in combination with high unemployment rates in the second half of the nineties, resulted in a rapid expansion in the number of students enrolling in higher education. As a result, nowadays, studying at university is one of the major activities of the young-adult population.

Nonetheless, the composition of the student population is undergoing changes, with women constituting a majority and an increasing proportion of students with immigrant background or family responsibility. Even exchange students are on the increase. All the above implies that the student population cannot be regarded as a homogenous group with similar opportunities, living under the same conditions, and being offered challenges and career chances of equivalent value (National Agency of Higher Education, 2000).

2   Student Quality of Life in Higher Education – a Transition

There are reasons to expect that the years at college/university mark an important "rite of passage" for young adults (Pascarella and Terenzini, 1991). Whether people go to college/university immediately after high school, leave a full-time job to pursue an education, or work and study at the same time, they face at least some kind of life adjustment, usually substantial (Shield, 2002). The transition from adolescent-in-family to a university student involves considerable individual and contextual change in almost all areas of life, which may have implications for adult development and health status. Attending a university is an approved move towards personal independence, in particular from parental rules and restrictions. During their years at university, students will explore new interests, analyze innovative social norms, and also search for new social networks. They may seek to clarify their values and beliefs, learn a new set of behaviors, and create new identities and group affiliations (Latham and Green, 1997).

The time spent at university is likely to be a period not only of intellectual stimulation and growth, career development, but also of increased autonomy, self-exploration, discovery and social involvement. Students may go through changes in living arrangements, form a partnership, or have (maybe for the first time) responsibility for their own financial welfare (Beder, 1997). Students also have to cope with a new work environment, and the intellectual and relational demands it places on them.

In sum this life span is characterized by the high pressure of academic commitments, conflicting role demands, a rapidly changing environment, shifting between different circles of companions and social networks, financial pressures, and often a lack of time-management skills. Additionally, these years demand that individuals more closely define their own career interests, demonstrate performance, and present themselves as attractive on an increasingly competitive and individualistic labor market. At the same time, they have to show adaptive capacity when searching for balance and harmony between their various social roles. There is a sense in which they transfer between different worlds – the university on the one hand and of the family, the peer group, and (for some) a new relationship and the workplace on the other.

3   Dealing with Stress as a University Student

All these factors can generate a relatively high level of stress. This, in turn, has been an important subject in higher-education research for many years, largely because of the specificity of university life in terms of matters related to transitional and developmental issues. Earlier studies have shown that perceived high stress affects both health and academic performance and that those relationships are very strong (Bovier et al., 2004; Campbell et al., 1992; Hudd et al., 2000). Students with a high level of stress tend to perceive themselves as less healthy, to possess a lower level of self-esteem, and to be more prone to adopt a number of unhealthy lifestyles such as binge drinking, high tobacco consumption, drug use, and unsafe sex. A high level of stress has also been linked to a variety of negative outcomes, such as depression, anxiety, eating disorders, and suicide ideation (Dahlin et al., 2005; Ryan and Twibell, 2000).

Further, there is a variation in the behaviors and strategies that students use in order to cope with the above mentioned transitional and developmental issues. Some individuals change their situation immediately, some accept it, others look for more information, while still others restrain themselves from acting spontaneously (Ryan and Twibell, 2000).

Although many stress-related outcomes have been studied e.g., student retention, concentration difficulties, formation of unhealthy behaviors, and poor academic performance (Hirsch and Ellis, 1996; Pascarella and Terenzini, 1991; Seiman, 2005), little is know about how stress impacts on students' quality of life and well-being (Hudd et al., 2000; Disch et al.; 1999; Chow, 2005).

4   Student Quality of Life and Well-Being during the Years at University

In general, outcomes such as quality of life and well-being of young adults particularly university students have been described by a limited number of researchers. Despite the fact that several previous studies hade stated that psychological distress is elevated among university students, and may be significantly higher than in the general population (Stewart-Brown et al.; 2000), student quality of life and well-being and its determinant and changes during the period of enrolment have received only limited attention in work-environment and public health research internationally and nationally. On the other hand there is a substantial research literature addressing students' health-related behavior such as alcohol consumption and tobacco/drug use.

The scant research that has been done on the student well-being has tended to concentrate on selected segments of students such as medical students (Aktekin et al., 2001; Brimstone et al., 2007; Dahlin et al., 2005; Hojat et al., 2003; Rosal et al., 1997; Vitaliano et al., 1989). Most studies have addressed only the role of academic-related factors in explanation of health disorders and not included other type of factors related to student life outside the university, and have restrictive cross-sectional design. In sum, there is a lack of research on student well being and quality of life in a longitudinal perspective.

An improved understanding is essential in design and formation of higher education with superior quality. This area is significant either to examine how optional functioning and performance can be best obtained, and enhanced or to develop opportunity to exert a positive influence on the health of future generations through the assessment and reduction of the risks that may result in poor quality of life and well-being in later working life.

In recent years, there has been a public debate, even alarm, about a perceived increase in mental-health problems among university students (Adlaf et al., 2001; Rosal et al., 1997; Raj et al., 2000; Sharkin, 1997). This particularly applies to American students, but may also be of concern in other countries (Aktekin et al., 2001). Such concern has been aggravated by observations made by the staff of student health-care organizations – which have been assembled into bodies of longitudinal material, both nationally and locally. Among increasing problems are emotional and behavioral difficulties (Rosal et al., 1997), a range of psychological problems (O'Malley et al., 1990), and further problems related to developmental issues, relationships and academic skills (Benton et al., 2003). On the other hand, no significant changes have been observed in substance abuse, eating disorders, or chronic mental illness (Robbins et al., 1985).

5   Students Concerns and Academic Performance

An extensive body of literature has the common aim to identify student major concerns, needs and its relationship with academic functioning. As a result a wide range of different concern areas have been identified. The most commonly concerns are academic stress, financial issues, career planning and future employment, interpersonal and personal relationships, striking balance between studies, work and family, heavy workload and lack of feedback, pedagogical shortcoming, time management, housing conditions and emotional health. So far much effort has been devoted to understand the relationships between these concerns and student academic functioning sense by including a broad range of individual, social, cognitive and behavioral factors. The consequences of student concern and need in a quality of life and well-being sense are less researched.

Pritchard and Wilson (2003) found that both emotional (stress levels, depressive symptomatology, mood, fatigue, self-esteem, perfectionism, optimism) and social health factors were related (having a romantic relationship, type of residence, membership in various campus organization) to students performance and retention. According to this study which consisted of 218 undergraduate students, there was a significant correlation between emotional health and performance (grade point average GPA) regardless of gender. Moreover, students' emotional health was related to the intention to drop out of college. Conversely social health factors did not predict intention of student departure and social health components affected student's performance in less extant compared to emotional health (Pritchard and Wilson, 2003).

Disch et al. (1999) had employed a multivariate approach to examine the links between students concern and performance. The results highlighted that major sources of concern from most (1) to least (10) importance were issues related to (1) career and employment, (2) time management, (3) physical and mental health, (4) economy, (5) living, (6) sexual behavior, (7) crime and violence (8) learning style, (9) multicultural- gender related and (10) drug and alcohol consumption (Disch et al., 1999). These findings are in line with previous research conducted by Sax, Atin, Korn (1997) who found that while during the past 12 years student involvement in their academic studies has declined, students are more likely to be concerned with their career expectations and how the achievement of an academic degree will improve their prospective quality of life (Sax et al., 1997).

Several previous studies had examined the association between self-esteem, social support and student personal well-being. In the comparison of two separated college students samples (1984, 1992) Staats et al. (1995) found that despite the remaining impact of self esteem and social support on students well-being, several changes had ensued over the study period. Students in the sample 1992 had lower levels of subjective well-being, expectations and optimism about the future than students in the 1984 sample (Staats et al., 1995). Harlow and Newcomb (1990) identified several factors, namely purpose in life, intimate relationship, family and peer, perceived opportunity, health and work satisfaction which positively influenced young people's well-being and quality of life. On the other hand they showed that powerlessness and meaninglessness were two significant barrier factors of young peoples' quality of life (Harlow and Newcomb, 1990).

According to literature on student health the most frequent symptoms from which they suffer are depression, anxiety, sleeping problems, chronic fatigue, and back ache. Results from several studies indicated that the frequency of these symptoms has an influence on self-perception of health and students who have fewer symptoms tend to evaluate their own health significantly higher (Mechanic and Cleary, 1980, Piko, 2000). Further several studies demonstrated that mental and social well-being play an important roll in self-perception of global health and quality of life among young adults (Piko et al., 1997). In a study based on 691 students, Piko et al. (1997) found that the strongest predictor of self-perceived health among the students regardless of gender was psychological well-being. This is supported by several other studies.

6   Theoretical Perspective on Student Retention and Persistence

The impact of college/university on students has been viewed from different theoretical perspectives i.e., economic, psychological, organizational, educational and sociological. Examples of common conceptual models employed in this research area are given below.

Over time, several theories have been developed in order to investigate which factors play a key role in why some students leave and others persist to complete a degree. A major contribution to the study of students' attrition is made by Vincent Tinto's integration model (Seiman, 2005; Tinto, 1975; Tinto, 1993;). The model attempts comprehensively to incorporate the characteristics and procedures that influence students' decisions to leave college/university, and how these processes interact to result in attrition. The model includes different types of leaving behaviors, which are identified by Tinto as academic failure, voluntary withdrawal, permanent dropout, temporary dropout, and transfer.

Tinto has argued that academic and social integration are the most important predictors of college-student persistence. A match between the academic ability and motivation of the student and the social and academic qualities of the institution fosters academic and social integration into the university. According to his model, students who are not integrated into the university are more likely to develop low commitment, and this – in turn – will result in unsuccessful adjustment, thereby increasing the risk of dropout. According to Astin's theory of involvement the behavior that students engage in while attending higher education influence their outcome including persistence (Astin, 1984). Bean and Metzner (1985) hypothesize that one or several variables including academic attainment, intent to drop out, previous performance and educational aims and environmental factors is/are the predictors of older or non-traditional students departure decision. According to this theoretical model, environmental factors such as financial issues, the extent of employment, external support, family responsibility and opportunity to transfer have a greater influence on retention than academic related factors (Bean and Metzner, 1985).

Although Tinto's paradigmatic model is an important contribution to the literature on student departure, it does not reveal a complete understanding of the problem and student departure still remains as a major concern for institutions and faculty members.

7   University Student Health, Lifestyle and Quality of Life: a Cohort Study in Sweden

The data used in this study were drawn from the ongoing cohort study "University student health and quality of life." This cohort is one of the largest longitudinal studies within the university students in Sweden (Vaez et al., 2006a,b; Vaez et al., 2004; Vaez and Laflamme, 2003, 2008; Vaez, 2004). The project was initiated so as to follow up the development of university students' health status and quality of life during their enrollment years at the university, and the years of establishment on the labor market (See ❷ *Figure 149-1*).

7.1   Student Questionnaire Surveys

In early 1998, the proposed study was presented to the University's student health organization and to the committee with responsibility for quality assurance in education

☐ Figure 149-1

Study population and design. Three data collections by questionnaire, at Linköping University in Sweden, in 1999 (baseline), 2001(follow up I) and 2003 (follow up II)

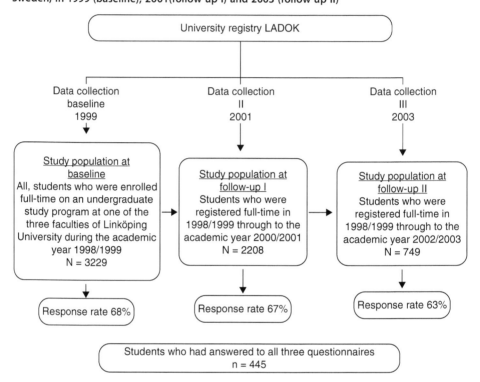

and other student-related matters. Students' health status was surveyed by means of a self-administered questionnaire. The questionnaire was developed during 1998 on the basis of a number of instruments previously employed in national investigations of issues related to student health. A preliminary version of the questionnaire was developed with the assistance of a group of higher-education/health professionals, student representatives, and members of the quality-assurance committee. After a pre-test on 70 students, the final questionnaire comprised 44 items. Most consisted of forced-response, multiple-choice questions. An overview of the variables considered in the full version of the questionnaire is presented in appendix A.

8   Findings from Studies within the Project

8.1   First Year Student Health and Quality of Life- Cross Sectional Studies

Health status. Our findings from the cross sectional studies of freshmen emphasized that the vast majority of students rated their health as good. The health concerns and problems that were identified included both physical and psychological factors and restriction on life activities, health-care seeking, use of prescription drugs and hospitalization was considerably more common for physical than for psychological problems. Gender differences were also observed in health care consumption due to either physical or psychological issues with a significant over-representation of female students. In addition a total of 46% of students reported that they had sought care, and also of those who sought care 6% had been hospitalized and 35% had consumed prescription drugs due to physical complaints during the past years. Women were significantly over-represented in all cases. Among first year students 5% reported that they sought health care due to psychological issues, and among those 4%, all of whom females, reported having been admitted to hospital during the previous year.

Further, in this study population, the most common symptoms/complaints were tiredness (35%), anxiety (24%), and concentration difficulties (22%) and symptoms related to psychological problems were more frequent among female than male students. Among the study population both physical and psychological self-rated health correlated strongly with general self-rated health, but the associations between them were not very strong – which suggests that they may capture different aspects of student life. Female students more frequently reported symptoms and had lower ratings of their self-rated health compare to their male peers.

Health-risk behaviors. The study populations' health-risk behaviors were comparable with those of other populations of university students internationally. Despite differences in the measures employed, the proportions of binge drinkers (40%) and tobacco users (24%) were similar to those observed in the USA (O'Malley et al., 1998; Wechsler and Kuo, 2000, 2003; Wechsler et al., 2001, 2002a,b) and in Eastern Europe (Steptoe and Wardle, 2001). We found that frequent drinking (2–4 times/week) and high consumption (7–9 glasses and > 10 glasses) were more common among male students, whereas occasional drinking (once a month) and low alcohol consumption (1–2 glasses and 3–4 glasses/occasion) were more common among female students. Of all respondents 24% reported use of tobacco, with more smokers than expected found among male students.

Perceived quality of life. When we studied first year student quality of life we found that regardless of gender the perceived current quality of life was more strongly associated with psychological self-rated health than with physical self-rated health. However, the males' average score on perceived current quality of life rating in 1999 were lower than those of females.

In a comparative study on health status and quality of life assessment of young adults aged 20–34 years, including freshmen (n = 1997 first year students, mean age 23) and those of their working counterparts (n = 947 subjects in full-time employment) we found that first-year university students had a lower score rating on their quality of life and self-rated health than their working peers. A possible confounder in relation to our result was the differences in age distribution between the groups compared. However the differences in rating of quality of life and self-rated health remained unchanged after required age adjustment. In the same study we also found that in both groups and both genders, mean ratings of current quality of life were higher than those of former quality of life and lower than those of expected. Other comparison made between the same groups revealed that first-year university students' health behaviors differed considerably from those of their working peers. Students smoked and used snuff in smaller proportions, they were not frequent drinkers but they drank higher quantities of alcohol than their working counterparts.

Stress. Our findings indicated that the most common stressors were, in descending order of importance, to "not coping academically," "poor finances," and the demands imposed by acceptance of "study aid" (which takes the form of student loans in Sweden), "extra-curricular activities," and "doubts about the future."

9   Health and Quality of Life – from First to Third Year at University

In the follow up studies, the study population consisted of 1,160 full-time students who had filled in each of two self-administered questionnaire (same questions) dealing with health status and quality of life at the end of 1999 and 2001. The aim of these studies were to describe changing pattern in health status and health behaviors over time and also to examined the role of perceived stress due to a range of academic and non academic factors on student academic performance. Assessments of stress, symptoms, and health were measured at the end of the first (1999) and third year of university (2001). The students' academic achievement was measured on the basis of whether they had been awarded their degree (about 55% of students on average) by the end of 2003. The total numbers of degrees awarded were taken from the University Registry (as of the end of November 2003).

9.1   Individual Changes in Health Status, Health Risk Behaviors and Perceived Stress

Our findings of individual changes from first to third year of university revealed that regardless of gender, the vast majority of students assessed their psychological and general health as good in both 1999 and 2001. The pattern was somewhat more pronounced for general than psychological health. Further, the occurrence of less-than-good psychological and general health was higher in 2001 compared to 1999. Deterioration in health assessment over time proved to be more important for psychological than general health. We also observed that binge drinking was much more common among males. 46% of male students were classified as binge drinkers at the end of 2001 (including binge drinkers in both 1999 and 2001 and new binge drinkers). Binge drinking became less frequent over time among both male and female students. The occurrence of binge drinking was almost 2.4% higher in 1999.

Further we found that the occurrence of smoking was 1.9% higher among females and 1.4% higher among males in 1999 compared to 2001. The proportion of smokers increased between 1999 and 2001 among female students (19%). Oral moist-snuff consumption is much higher among males in general. Use of snuff was higher in 2001 compared to 1999. These changes were more obvious among male students.

In the analyses of changing pattern in the sources of stress we found that the most common stressors were related, in descending order of importance, to "not coping academically," "poor finances" and the demands imposed by acceptance of "study aid," "extra-curricular" activities and "doubts about the future." Although the sources of stress in question did not change significantly between 1999 and 2003 in rank, the only, and easily understandable, exception was "doubts about the future," which were more a matter of concern towards the end rather than at the beginning of the university period.

9.2   Academic Performance

Few of the factors investigated had impact on the probability of being awarded a degree, but those from the first year at university that were significantly associated to degree success remain so in the third year. Furthermore we found that perceived high level of stress due to academic related factors such as "not coping academically" and "study support demands" were substantial barriers, in particular when combined with concentration difficulties. By contrast, perceived stress caused by non academic factors such as perceived inadequacy for the family and having family issues merge as incentives. Our findings emphasize that students aged 25 or older, females, and those enrolled in comparatively shorter programs (3 years) tend to have higher odds of obtaining a degree.

10 Health and Quality of Life at the First and the Final Academic Year

The data used in this study were extracted from the data set including 5 years follow up of university students. The study population consisted of those who were registered full-time in 1999 through the academic year 2003. In total 445 students filled in questionnaires in 1999, 2001 and 2003. The 26 students among the respondents who in 2003 stated that hey had left their study program or had taken a break from the original study program were excluded.

Accordingly, the current study is based on the responses of a total of 419 students. ❯ Table 149-1 presents distribution of students according to a number of socio-demographic characteristics.

■ Table 149-1
Socio-demographic characteristics of students in the cohort

Socio-demographic characteristics	Faculty of Arts and Sciences n (%)	Faculty of Health Sciences n (%)	Institutet of Technology n (%)	Total
Age at baseline (1999)				
18–20	19 (12.8)	4 (12.1)	56 (23.6)	79 (18.9)
21–24	72 (48.3)	20 (60.6)	158 (66.7)	250 (59.7)
25+	58 (38.9)	9 (27.3)	23 (9.7)	90 (21.5)
Gender				
Female	115 (77.2)	21 (63.6)	79 (33.3)	215 (51.3)
Male	34 (22.8)	12 (36.4)	158 (66.7)	204 (48.7)
Having parents with academic background				
Yes	69 (46.9)	21 (65.6)	142 (60.4)	232 (56.0)
No	78 (53.1)	11 (34.4)	93 (39.6)	182 (44.0)
Marital status in 2003				
Married/cohabitant	81 (55.1)	19 (57.6)	96 (40.7)	196 (47.1)
Unmarried	66 (44.9)	14 (42.4)	140 (59.3)	220 (52.9)
Living conditions in 2003				
Living alone	56 (37.6)	11 (33.3)	97 (40.9)	164 (39.1)
Living with others	93 (62.4)	22 (66.6)	140 (59.1)	255 (60.1)

The majority of the study group is 21–24 years old and living with others

11   Results

11.1   Self-Rated Psychological Health and General Health at Group Level

❯ *Table 149-2* demonstrates female and male students' health assessment at the first and final year of their study program. The results indicate that the majority of both groups of students

❑ Table 149-2

Health assessment at the first and the final academic year by female and male university students (at the group level with 95% confidence interval (95%))

Self-rated health	First academic year (1999)		Final academic year (2003)	
	Female	Male	Female	Male
Psychological health				
Good	81.2 (75.4–85.0)	89.1 (84.0–92.7)	76.4 (70.2–81.7)	87.1 (81.7–91.0)
Moderate	13.0 (9.1–18.2)	10.0 (6.5–14.9)	15.9 (11.5–21.4)	9.0 (5.7–13.7)
Poor	5.8 (3.3–9.8)	1.0 (0.3–3.6)	7.7 (4.8–12.1)	4.0 (2.0–7.6)
General Health				
Good	83.7 (78.0–88.1)	90.0 (85.1–93.5)	83.7 (78.0–88.1)	90.0 (85.1–93.5)
Moderate	13.0 (9.1–18.2)	9.5 (6.1–14.3)	10.1 (6.7–14.9)	6.5 (3.8–10.7)
Poor	3.4 (1.6–6.8)	0.5 (0.03–3.2)	6.3 (3.7–10.4)	3.5 (1.7–7.0)

The proportion of students who rated their psychological and general health as poor was significantly higher in 2003 than in 1999

rated their psychological and general health as good in the baseline and at follow-up while the proportion of women who rated their health (regardless of type) as good was lower compared to men in both the first and final year of academic life. The data at hand illustrate that the proportion of students who rated their health as poor was significantly higher in 2003 than in 1999. This pattern was somewhat more pronounced for general health than psychological health as well as for men compared to women.

11.2   Self-Rated Psychological Health and General Health at Individual Level

❯ *Table 149-3*, shows the distribution of student health assessment, both psychological and general health in their first year through to final academic year at the individual level for female and male, respectively. Regardless of gender and type of health assessment considered, the vast majority of the students rated their health as good in their first year of enrolment and the good health maintained 5 years later with a higher proportion of male students.

There was a tendency for deterioration in health (combining those who rated their health as good or moderate solely in 1999, but had lower ratings in 2003) over time was more pronounced for psychological health than for general health, and more pronounced among female students.

■ Table 149-3
Pattern in health assessment of female and male students over time of observations (1999 and 2003)

Female (n = 208)	Psychological health in 2003		
Psychological health in 1999	Good	Moderate	Poor
Good	142	19	8
Moderate	12	9	6
Poor	5	5	2
Female (n = 208)	General health in 2003		
General health in 1999	Good	Moderate	Poor
Good	153	14	7
Moderate	16	6	5
Poor	5	1	1
Male (n = 201)	Psychological health in 2003		
Psychological health in 1999	Good	Moderate	Poor
Good	159	13	7
Moderate	16	4	0
Poor	0	1	2
Male (n = 201)	General health in 2003		
General health in 1999	Good	Moderate	Poor
Good	166	11	4
Moderate	14	2	3
Poor	1	0	0

❯ *Table 149-3* shows the distribution of student health assessment, both psychological and general health in their first year through to final academic year at the individual level for female and male, respectively. Regardless of gender and type of health assessment considered, the vast majority of the students rated their health as good in their first year of enrolment and the good health maintained 5 years later with a higher proportion of male students

11.3 Student Quality of Life in the First and the Final Year of Academic Life

The mean score for all three time dimensions of quality of life was higher among men in comparison to women in the first year of education while this pattern changed somewhat in the final academic year. Female students rated their current and expected quality of life in the final year better than their male peers.

The mean scores of perceived quality of life in the first and the final academic year for females and males separately are illustrated in ❯ *Figure 149-2*. There was a tendency of an increased mean score of quality of life with time, i.e., both women and men had higher mean scores on current than former quality of life and higher scores on expected than current quality of life. This pattern appeared in both the first and the final year of academic studies.

■ Figure 149-2

Perceived quality of life. The mean scores of perceived quality of life (former, current and expected) measured by ladder scale in 1999 and 2003 by gender. The higher mean scores are indicative of better quality of life

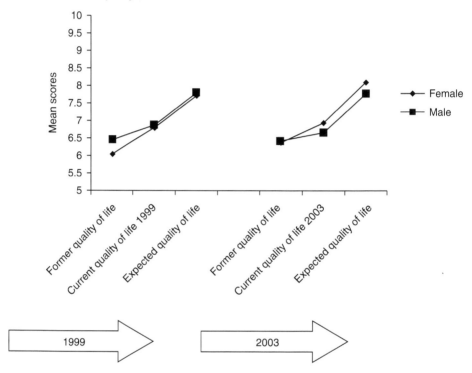

11.4   Associations to Current Quality of Life in the Final Academic Year

Bivariate Correlations was computed in order to study the pairwise associations between the current quality of life rated by student in the final academic year and all variables in the questionnaire. Kendall's tau-b statistics was used which measure the rank-order association between two scales or ordinal variables.

The ❷ *Figure 149-3* illustrated the significant correlations between current quality of life in 2003 and individual factors, life style, academic related factors, stressors, health assessment and symptoms. For an overview of included variables see Appendix A.

Significant correlations were notable between current quality of life in the final academic year and most of the sources of stress, health assessment and psychological symptoms. Among all significant correlations the strongest associations were found between current quality of life and self-rated psychological health followed by perceived depression, self-rated general health and perceived stress due to loneliness. No correlation coefficient was higher than −0.384.

■ Figure 149-3

(a). The significant correlations between current quality of life in 2003 and individual and lifestyle factors. (b). The significant correlations between current quality of life in 2003 and education-related factors. (c). The significant correlations between current quality of life in 2003 and perceived stress. (d). The significant correlations between current quality of life in 2003 and health assessment and symptoms. Correlation coefficient is a measure of linear association between two variables. The sign of the correlation coefficient indicates the direction of the relationship (positive or negative)

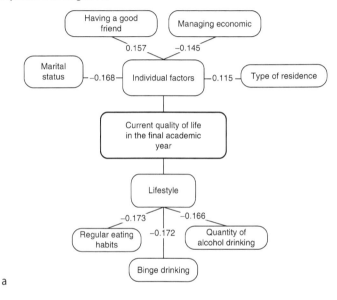

▣ Figure 149-3 (contined)

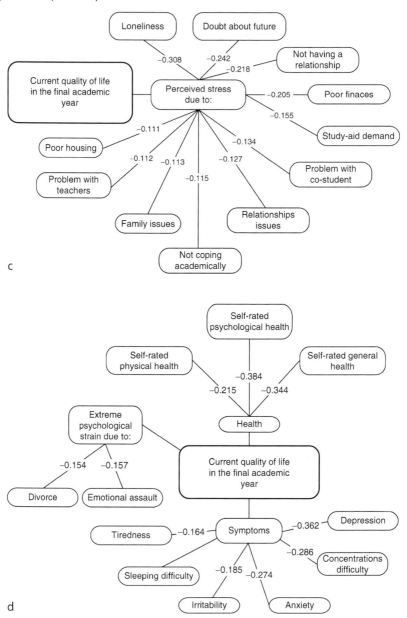

c

d

12 Conclusion

The longitudinal study discussed in this chapter considers student concerns health and quality of life during years at university. Follow-up of 3000 first year undergraduate students attending at 52 different study programs during their education is the first step that will hopefully lead not only to an increase in knowledge of students' health and quality of life at Linköping University but also to enhance visibility of students quality of life and well-being issues in higher education nation- and worldwide. Although, in this study a high proportion of students managed to complete their degree, rated their health and quality of life as good and were still enrolled full-time on a study program during the follow up; their health in general and psychological health in particular may be under threat. A lack of previous research focusing on student quality of life and well-being in a longitudinal perspective and also the fact that comparisons between university student and their working peers are uncommon makes it difficult to compare the results found here with those of other studies.

Our findings based on time comparative studies indicate that psychological health may be under threat in university-student populations, and the threat seems to be more pronounced among female students. The results also suggested that student current quality of life in 2003 were associated to lifestyle and academic factors only to a limited extent while strong correlations were found with psychological health and perceived psychosomatic symptoms such as depression and concentrations difficulty, perceived stress due to loneliness and doubt about the future. Furthermore we found that perceived stress due to not coping academically and due to study support demands are substantial barriers to students' academic achievement.

The findings from this cohort study contribute to the identification of sub-groups of students who are at particular risk of certain types of problems, and thereby can serve as a basis for initiation of interventions tailored for such groups. High alcohol consumption and binge drinking are examples of such problems, but other relevant issues include a variety of psychological disorders and sources of stress. More detailed psychological profiling of students might help to identify the individuals that might have difficulties psychologically to cope with stress. Changing students' coping styles is necessary, and should be a first priority.

Since there are indications that psychological health may be under threat in university-student populations, and since the students quality of life seems to be associated to health habits to only a limited extent, it might be time to switch focus in health studies from specific health-related habits – drinking, in particular – to those more generally related to life as a student. Understanding the manners in which the negative effects on health of stressors like "not coping academically," "doubts about the future," and "loneliness" can be counteracted may well help university students achieve their individual potentials, and develop into (even more) autonomous and responsible human beings.

The finding that academic achievement is associated, to some extent, by perceived stress and psychological symptoms during the years at university suggests that academic advisors should pay greater attention to these factors, in particular by providing students with a work environment conducive to the reduction of stress. From this point of view the productivity of students is extremely important to higher education systems and now it is more important than ever for universities and institutions to improve the rate of students' persistence and graduation. But productivity in higher education is not only concerned with increasing the number of places and ever facilitating access to university. The students' graduation rate is a key component in institutional economy and it is considered as a measure of quality of education. However attention needs to be paid to enhancing achievement and persistence (as performance indictors) in order to decrease the high rate of attrition, which is a major problem for many higher-education institutions.

13   Methodological Considerations

One set of limitations has to do with the content of the data-collection instrument itself. The questionnaire covers a wide variety of health disorders and health behaviors, but it does not investigate any single one of them in depth. The data at hand are also based on what respondents have knowledge of and remember about various health disorders, not on their medical records. Recall bias can be particularly important when the reference period used is as long as 1 year. As a consequence, it is possible that the current studies give a somewhat brighter picture of the health situation of students than is actually the case.

Self-reporting as a means of data collection can also be problematic. For example, with regard to alcohol consumption and tobacco use, problems of under-reporting or over-reporting of consumption may arise.

Further, the data in our studies on quality of life are based on a single measure taken from one global item rather than any global or specific scale. The inherent advantage of parsimony possessed by single measures is counterbalanced by a possible positive bias, implying that respondents may wish to present themselves as socially desirable. Another disadvantage of this approach, though of greater importance for the predictive value of longitudinal studies, is that brief questionnaires tend to lack sensitivity.

The findings here are based on information gathered from students in a variety of university programs, and are not restricted to any particular group. In this sense, they can be regarded as informative with respect to the health behaviors and the quality of life among university students more generally.

It is also possible that some of the students who did not respond to the questionnaires but were still enrolled full-time on a university program were in less good physical or mental shape than those who did. This also applies to individuals who had left their program since the beginning of the university year (reflecting a kind of "healthy student effect"). Further, it is not known whether the health status of students on single-subject courses (not included in the study) is better or worse than that of the study population as a whole.

The measure of "change" used in these longitudinal studies was based simply on two points. It cannot be regarded as a perfectly accurate representation of what happened "over time," or even allow us to assume that any change observed actually occurred during that period. Changes may be more sudden than they appear, and also closer to one point in time than another.

Summary Points

- The transition from adolescent-in-family to a university student involves considerable individual and contextual change in almost all areas of life simultaneously, which may have implications for adult development and health status.
- There is a lack of knowledge on student quality of life and well-being in a longitudinal perspective.
- There are indications that psychological distress is elevated and may be significantly higher among university students than in the general population.
- The scant research on student well-being has tended to concentrate on selected segments of students such as medical students. Most studies in the area have addressed only the role of academic-related factors in explanation of health disorders and (have) not included other type of factors related to student life outside the university.

- The most common symptoms/complaints, among first year Swedish students, were tiredness, anxiety and concentration difficulties.
- Female students more frequently reported symptoms and had a lower rating of their self-rated health compare to their male peers.
- The students perceived current quality of life was more strongly associated with psychological self-rated health than with physical self-rated health.
- The most common stressors reported by students were "not coping academically," "poor finances," and the demands imposed by acceptance of "study aid" (which takes the form of student loans in Sweden), "extra-curricular activities," and "doubts about the future."
- Perceived high level of stress due to academic related factors such as "not coping academically" and "study support demands" were substantial barriers for obtaining a degree, in particular when combined with concentration difficulties.
- The student current quality of life was significantly associated with, self-rated psychological health, perceived depression, self-rated general health and perceived stress due to loneliness.
- To identify sub-groups of students who are at particular risk of certain problems is essential for initiation of interventions tailored for such groups. High alcohol consumption and binge drinking are examples of such problems, but other relevant issues include a variety of psychological disorders and source of stress.
- Improvement of students' coping strategy is necessary, and should be a first priority.

Appendix A:

Background

- Type of study program (including 50 different study program)
- Students' age
- Student's gender: Female/male
- Country of birth
  - Sweden
  - Other Nordic country
  - Other European country
  - Other country
- Marital status
  Married/co-habiting, or not
- Living conditions
  - Living alone
  - Having a family of one's own,
  - Living with children without any other adult,
  - Living with parents or others
- Having children under age of 18: yes/no
- Type of residence
  - Student corridor
  - Student flat
  - Lodger
  - Tenement
  - Detached house
- Source of income during academic year and during summer break

- Study loan only
- Support from spouse/parents
- Income from paid employment
- Income from capital,
- Others
- Managing economy during student life (4- point scale from very good to very bad)

Education

- Satisfaction with study program with regard to: (5- point scale ranked from very satisfied to very unsatisfied)
  - Education content
  - Instructors
  - Examination form
  - Tuition form
- Education contribute to (4-point scale from not very much to very much):
  - Achieve/ a broad general knowledge/ an all-round education
  - Achieve work related knowledge and skills
  - Achieve a good study technique
  - Describe clear and comprehensible
  - Think critically and analytically
  - Independently seek knowledge
  - Analyze problems
  - Use computers and information technology
  - Cooperate/work together with others
  - Accept responsibility for ones own knowledge development
  - Achieve an increased self awareness
  - Understand people from a different cultural or ethnic background
  - Reflect over ones own valuation
  - Engage oneself in the social development
  - Understand theories of social and cultural differences between women and men
- Study program evaluation (4-point scale from very good to very bad)
- Choose same institution if redoing the degree (4-point scale: from definitive to definitive not)
- Having been exposed to violence, threats, sexual harassments at university

Lifestyle

- Frequency of physical activity (5-point scale from never to 4 times a week or more)
- Regular eating habits: yes/no
- Tobacco use: yes/no
- Frequency of alcohol consumption (5-point scale from never to 4 times a week or more)
- Quantity of alcohol consumption (5- point scale from 1–2 glasses to 10 ore more)
- Binge drinking (six or more glasses per same occasion)
- Participation in various spare time activities (yes/no)

- Frequency of spending time with friends, family (5-point scale from never to 4 times a week or more)
- Having a good friend (yes/no)

Stress

- Perceived stress due to: (4-point scale, from not at all stressed to highly stressed)
  - Loneliness
  - Doubt about future
  - Not having a relationship
  - Poor finances
  - Study-aid demand
  - Problem with co-student
  - Relationship issues
  - Not coping academically
  - Family issues
  - Problem with teachers
  - Poor housing
  - Inadequate for the family
  - Problem with friends
  - Extra-curricular activities
- Extreme psychological strain due to: yes/no
  - Divorce
  - Death in the family
  - Emotional assault
  - Sexual abuse
  - Illness/accident (self/family/close friends)

Physical Health

- Restriction of life activities due to:(4-point scale, from not at all to very much)
  - Illness
  - Accident
  - Disability
- Utilization of health services (yes/no)
- Hospitalization (yes/no)
- Use of prescription medicine (yes/no)
- Self-rated physical health (5-point scale from very good to very poor)

Psychological Health

- Psychological/psychosomatic symptoms (4-point scale, from not at all to very much)
  - Depression
  - Concentration difficulty
  - Anxiety
  - Irritability
  - Sleeping difficulty

- – Tiredness
- – Bad appetite
- – Headache
- – Upset stomach
- Restriction of life activities due to psychological illness (yes/no)
- Utilization of health services (yes/no)
- Hospitalization (yes/no)
- Use of prescription medicine (yes/no)
- Self-rated psychological health (5-point scale, from very good to very poor)

General Health

- Self-rated general health (5-point scale, from very good to very poor)
- Age-comparative self-rated health (5-point scale, from much better to much worse)

Quality of Life

- Quality of life current/1 year ago (former)/1 year from now (expected) (ladder scale) (Andrews and Withey, 1976)

The ladder question is introduced in the following way. "Here is a picture of a ladder. At the bottom of the ladder ('1') is the worst life you might reasonably expect to have. At the top ('10') is the best life you might expect to have. Where on the ladder is your life right now?

Question	Scale
	10
Where on the ladder is your life right now?	9
	8
	7
Where on the ladder was your life 1 year ago?	6
	5
	4
Where do you expect your life to be in 1 year from now?	3
	2
	1

References

Adlaf EM, Gliksman L, Demers A, Newton-Taylor B. (2001). J Am Coll Health 50: 67–72.

Aktekin M, Karaman T, Senol Y, Erdem S, Erengin H, Akaydin M. (2001). Med Educ. 35: 12–17.

Andrews F, Withey S. (1976). Social indicators of well-being: Americans' perceptions of life quality. New York, Plenum press.

Astin AW. (1984). J Coll Student Personnel. 25: 297–308.

Bean JP, Metzner BS. (1985). Rev Educ Res. 55: 485–540.

Beder SH. (1997). Addressing the issue of social integration for first year students. A discussion paper. UltiBASE.

Benton SA, Robertson JM, Tseng WC, Newton FB, Benton SL. (2003). Prof Psychol Res Pr. 34: 66–72.

Bovier PA, Chamot E, Perneger TV. (2004). Qual Life Res. 13: 161–170.

Brimstone R, Thistlethwaite JE, Quirk F. (2007). Med Educ. 41: 74–83.

Campbell RL, Svenson LW, Jarvis GK. (1992). Percept Mot Skills. 75: 552–554.

Chow HP. (2005). Soc indic Res. 70: 139–150.

Dahlin M, Joneborg N, Runeson B. (2005). Med Educ. 39: 594–604.

Disch WB, Harlow LL, Campbell JF, Dougan TR. (1999). Social indicators research 51: 41–74.

National Agency for Higher Education. (2000). Swedish Universities & University Colleges 1998/1999. Short Version of Annual Report. Stockholm.

Harlow LL, Newcomb M. (1990). Multivariate Behav Res. 25: 387–405.

Hirsch JK. Ellis JB. (1996). Coll Stud J. 30: 377–384.

Hojat M, Gonnella JS, Erdmann JB, Vogel WH. (2003). Pers Individ Dif. 35: 219–235.

Hudd S, Duamlo J, Erdmann-Sager D, Murray D, Phan E, Soukas N, Yokozuka N. (2000). Coll Stud J. 34: 217–226.

Latham G, Green P. (1997). The journey to University: a study of the first year experience. UltiBASE.

Lu L. (1994). Psychol Med. 24: 81–87.

Mechanic D, Cleary P. (1980). Prev Med. 9: 805–814.

O'malley K, Wheeler I, Murphey J, O'connell J, Waldo M. (1990). J Coll Student Dev. 31: 464–465.

O'Malley PM, Johnston LD, Bachman JG. (1998). Alcohol Health Res World. 22: 85–94.

Pascarella E, Terenzini P. (1991). How college affects students?. Jossey Bass, Sanfransisco.

Piko B, Baramas K, Boda K. (1997). Eur J Public Health. 7: 243–247.

Piko B. (2000). J Community Health. 25: 125–137.

Pritchard ME, Wilson GS. (2003). J Coll Student Dev. 44: 18–28.

Raj SR, Simpson CS, Hopman WM, Singer MA. (2000). Can Med Assoc J. 162: 509–510.

Robbins SB, May TM, Corrazini JG. (1985). J Couns Psychol. 32: 641–644.

Rosal MC, Ockene IS, Barrett SV, Hebert JR. (1997). Acad Med. 75: 542–546.

Ryan ME, Twibell RS. (2000). Int J Intercult Relat. 24: 409–435.

Sax LJ, Astin AW, Korn WS. Mahoney KM. (1997). The American Freshman: National norms for Fall 1996. Los Angeles, University of California, Higher Education Research Institute.

Seiman A. (2005). College student retention. Formula for student successed.: American council on education praeger.

Sharkin BS. (1997). J Couns Dev. 75: 275–281.

Shield N. (2002). Anticipatory socialization, adjustment to university life, and perceived stress: generational and sibling status. Social Psychology of Education 5.

Staats S, Annstrong-Stassen M, Partilo C. (1995). Soc Indic Res. 34: 93–112.

Steptoe A, Wardle J. (2001). Soc Sci Med. 53: 1612–1630.

Stewart-Brown SJ, Evans J, Petterson J, Petersen S, Doll H. (2000). J Public Health Med. 22: 492–499.

Tinto V. (1975). Rev Educ Res. 45: 89–125.

Tinto V. (1993). Leaving College: rethinking the cause and cures of student attrition. Chicago, The University of Chicago Press.

Vaez M. (2004). Health and Quality of Life during Years at University. Studies on their Development and Determinants. Public Health Sciences. Stockholm, Karolinska Institutet.

Vaez M, De Leon A, Laflamme L. (2006). J Prev Assess Rehabil. 26: 167–177.

Vaez M, Kristenson M, Laflamme L. (2004). Soc Indic Res. 221–234.

Vaez M, Laflamme L. (2003). J Am Coll Health. 4: 156–162.

Vaez M, Laflamme L. (2008). Soc Behav Personality. Int J. 36: 183–196.

Vaez M, Ponce De Leon A, Laflamme L. (2006b). WORK. 26: 167–177.

Wechsler H, Kuo M. (2000). J Am Coll Health. 49: 57–64.

Wechsler H, Kuo M. (2003). Am J Public Health. 93: 1929–1933.

Wechsler H, Lee JE, Kuo M, Seibring M, Nelson TF, Lee H. (2002a). J Am Coll Health. 50: 203–217.

Wechsler H, Lee JE, Nelson TF, Kuo M. (2002b). J Am Coll Health. 50: 223–236.

Wechsler H, Lee JE, Rigotti NA. (2001). Am J Prev Med. 20: 202–207.

Vitaliano P, Maiuro R, Russo J, Mitchell E. (1989). J Nervous Mental Disorders. 177: 70–76.

150 The Quality of Life and the Impact of Interventions on the Health Outcomes of Looked After and Accommodated Young People

D. Carroll · C. R. Martin

1   Introduction 2581

2   Looked after and Accommodated Children 2581

3   Children's Hearing System 2582

4   Community Care of Young People 2582

5   Health Inequalities 2582

6   Health Challenges 2583

7   Recognition and Intervention 2584

8   Quality of Life of LAAC 2584

9   Reliability 2584

10 Validity 2585

11 Most Commonly Used Quality of Life Assessment Scales 2586

12 Youth – Quality of Life Y-QOL 2587

13 QoL for Adolescents – Quality of Life Profile -Adolescent Version 2588

14 EQ-5D 2588

15 SF-36 2589

16 *Duke Health Profile – Adolescent Version (DHP-A)* *2589*

17 *Pediatric Quality of Life Inventory (PedsQL)* *2590*

18 *Child Health Questionnaire – Child Form (CHQ-CF)* *2590*

Summary Points *2591*

Abstract: The young people who are "looked after and accommodated" are high profile in all areas of public care including health, social care, criminal justice and education. They are an easily identifiable group with poor outcomes. Their complexity of need is such that there is a multiple agency and discipline approach, working to assess and address their poor outcomes. The use of ❷ quality of life tools to establish the profile of these young individuals would serve to inform the care the young people receive. This would address working from the child/adolescent perspective and serve to validate the interventions in this group and to assess the outcomes for evidence based practice to develop.

List of Abbreviations: *CHQ-CF*, child health questionnaire-child form; *DHP-A*, duke health profile-adolescent version; *EQ-5D*, euroqol-five dimensions; *HEBS*, health education board Scotland; *HRQoL*, health related quality of life; *LAAC*, ❷ looked after and accommodated children; *NHS*, national health service; *PedsQL*, pediatric quality of life inventory; *QoL*, quality of life; *SF-36*, short form-36; *STI*, ❷ sexually transmitted infections; *WHO*, World Health Organization; *Y-QOL*, youth-quality of life

1 Introduction

During the last century dramatic improvements in the health of Scotland's population have taken place, with life expectancy increasing and premature death from major killer diseases decreasing (NHS Health Scotland, 2006). We remain, however, at or near the top of the "league tables" of the major diseases of the developed world (Scottish Executive, 1999). Social inequalities and lifestyle factors such as poor diet, drug and alcohol misuse, poor dental health in children and lack of exercise are now increasingly working to negate the beneficial effects of advances in medical care (Scottish Executive, 1998).

It is becoming clear that many of the serious health problems of adult life are related to childhood health factors (Lamont et al., 1998) and that the effects of early abuse of children is related to health risk behavior and disease in adult life (Feletti, 1998). One of the major targets set for child health providers has therefore, been to look at the causes of poor health in children and to reduce inequalities in health care. The health of children and young people looked after by Local Authorities has been of particular concern.

2 Looked after and Accommodated Children

The term "Looked After and Accommodated Children (LAAC)," was introduced in the Children Act 1989, and refers only to those children in the public care system; living with foster carer's, in residential homes or residential schools, or with parents under care orders (Polnay, 2000). It is the responsibility of the Children's Hearing System in Scotland to make decisions with regards to the young persons brought before a hearing. It is they who take the decision to impose compulsory measures of care upon individuals. Anyone can refer a young person to the Reporter of the Children's Hearing but it is generally the police or social work that do so. There are a number of specific grounds for referral that must be met. These grounds include the child is:

1. Beyond the control of parents or other relevant persons
2. Exposed to ❷ moral danger

3. The victim of an offence including physical harm or sexual abuse
4. Likely to suffer serious harm or impairment through lack of parental care
5. Indulging in solvent abuse
6. Misusing alcohol or drugs
7. Guilty of committing an offence
8. Failing to attend school without reasonable excuse

3 Children's Hearing System

The Children's Hearing System has it own set of guidelines but all action needs to follow the legislative impositions of the Children's (Scotland) Act 1995.

The act has many sections relevant to the Hearing System. The three overarching principles of the act are worth noting as they allow us to form an understanding of the actions and thoughts behind any action taken by panel members at a hearing, without going into overly extensive detail of specific areas of the Children's (Scotland) Act 1995. The principles are:

1. The welfare of the child is paramount.
2. The views of the child must be taken into account.
3. No order principle. The children's hearing must be convinced that making any order is better than not making an order.

4 Community Care of Young People

The care of young people in the community can take various forms, for example, parents, foster care, children's home, residential care, secure care or other relatives who may be receiving local authority support to care for the child. Many young people have been in and out of the care system; with the average having had eight "homes" by the time they are 14 years old. These children and adolescents are placed in these care settings due to circumstances that those around them deem not suitable and their quality of life is such that an alternative place to stay and people to live with is sought.

In the 1995 Act, it is stated that children who are "looked after" should receive a standard of health good as all children of the same age in the same area. Despite this statement, the Department of Health report (1991) titled, "Patterns and Outcomes in Child Placements" stated that those young people in the care system come from highly disadvantaged social backgrounds and are likely to experience more serious health problems than the wider population. Brodie et al. (1997) adds further weight to this, arguing that even when compared to their peers from similar socially deprived backgrounds; the health outcomes for the group are poorer.

5 Health Inequalities

The overall ❷ health inequalities of LAAC when compared to children cared for at home with parents, has been known for some time, however until recently the main focus has been on the poor levels of educational attainment in LAAC (Philpott, 2004; Saunders and Broad, 1997), with health being lower on the agenda for both those responsible for care and LAAC themselves (Mather and Batty, 2000; Philpott, 2004).

Research has identified problems with service provision and the ❯ unmet health needs of LAAC (Bundle, 2001; Hill and Watkins, 2002; Holland et al., 2003; Philpott, 2004; Williams et al., 2001). The increasing body of evidence and the following debate amongst health and social care professionals has raised the profile of health needs in LAAC, and there is emergent recognition within government, local authorities and primary care providers (Holland et al., 2003) of the need to address these issues.

A number of studies (Ashton-key and Jorge, 2008; Brodie et al., 1997; House of Commons, Select Committee, 1998; Meltzer et al., 2003; Residential Care Project, 2004; Rivron, 2001; Smith, 2000; The Caroline Walker Trust, 2001), have highlighted the poor health outcomes of LAAC. They are less likely to have regular dental care, have undiagnosed chronic health problems including poor and uncorrected eyesight, significant weight problems, glue ear, incomplete immunization programs and courses of treatment. They are less likely to adopt healthy lifestyle choices resulting in smoking (Michell, 1997; The Residential Care Health Project, 2004) substance misuse (Smith, 2000), and sexually transmitted infections (The Residential Care Health Project, 2004). At least one in seven young women leaving care was either pregnant or had a baby (House of Commons, Select Committee, 1998; Teenage Pregnancy Unit, 2002). Mental health was highlighted as a particular concern with LAAC, having significantly higher incidences of mental health issues than children cared for at home (Bundle, 2001; Cocker and Scott, 2006; Hill and Watkins, 2002; House of Commons, Select Committee, 1998; McCann et al., 1996; Philpott, 2004; Scottish Executive, 2002a). The poor physical and mental health of these young people may in the long term compound the social and economic inequality they experience by reducing their ability to achieve in education, enter the work force, and function as a fully integrated member of society (Chambers et al., 2002).

6 Health Challenges

Health inequities are widespread despite the regular physical and mental health assessments undergone by LAAC. One of the issues raised was despite improvements in health assessment for LAAC leading to identification of health needs, there had been no standard or universal pathway for following up these issues (Hill and Watkins, 2002; Holland et al., 2003; Meltzer et al., 2000). The research evidence indicates the need for a highly specialized service to meet the needs of LAAC (Holland et al., 2005; Hill and Watkins, 2002; Meltzer et al., 2000).

Williams et al.'s (2001) study confirms the that LAAC have unmet health needs, that higher priority needs to be given to changes at a policy level and that community health practitioners need to take a more active role in reaching these vulnerable children. Acknowledging on entering the care system LAAC may present with poor physical health, as indicated by Mather et al. (1997), Bundle (2001), House of Commons Select Committee (1998), Saunders and Broad (1997), Philpott (2004), Hill and Watkins (2002), and Scottish Executive (2002b), thus a more structured approach to meeting the health needs of LAAC is required.

The importance of mental well-being is essential to physical health and cannot be reasonably separated, as stress or mental distress can also damage physical health. The World Health Organization defines health as "a state of complete physical, mental and social well-being and not merely the absence of disease or infirmity" page 1 (WHO, 1988). There is an acceptance that health is multi-dimensional when young people come into care system however, there are no standardized multi-dimensional measures used consistently in this group.

7   Recognition and Intervention

There have been considerable developments in the recognition of the poor heath outcomes for this group of young people. However, progress beyond being aware of health issues requires monitoring, as the interventions and resources are developed (Cocker and Scott, 2006). There is a need for standardized/universal tools that identify children and adolescents that are at risk of developing health problems. This would guide those providing health care to develop intervention and prevention strategies. There is much focus regarding the health of LAAC and young people there is a great need to monitor the health status of this population in general and make comparative longitudinal studies to establish what if any improvement in their outcomes have been achieved.

There is general consensus to recognize health in holistic terms rather than traditional health model, with respect to people's own perceptions, attitudes and expectations (Edwards et al., 2002). The WHO defines quality of life as people's "perceptions of their positioning in life in the context of the culture and value system in which they live and in relation to their goals, expectations, standards and concerns" (WHO QoL Group, 1994).

8   Quality of Life of LAAC

The quality of life of young people in the residential care system as Davidson-Arad et al. (2004), states has received little attention. This type of out of home placement is considered by many to be the least desirable (Davidson-Arad et al., 2004). For those interested in the young peoples perception of their quality of life as they enter, progress and leave the care system, the quality of life measures considered are generally viewed as a multi-dimensional construct, which include domains in physical, mental, social and psychological aspects of well-being and functioning from the young person's perspective (Hong et al., 2007). These dimensions built a profile of the young person to include moods, emotions, social support, autonomy, social acceptance and financial resources. However, it is the inter-relationships of these dimensions that affect the perceived quality of life (Hong et al., 2007). Nevertheless most authors in this field acknowledge a lack of information on health related quality of life for children and adolescents. This is both in terms of normative data and generic instruments for assessment.

9   Reliability

Some aspects of the adult quality of life tools are not relevant to children and adolescents. The emotional and cognitive stages of children and adolescents must be considered along with their reading ability (Hong et al., 2007). Tools that are mainly developed for adults would not be validated as this population have poor literacy skills. The health of young people is considerably different from that of adults. They are also less able to choose and control their own environment, less likely to articulate their concerns and troubles clearly.

Concerns about self reporting have been the subject of investigation by Varni et al. (2007) who have found that children and young people can provide reliable and valid responses across the age categories. Interestingly they report the ❯ reliability of children as young as 5 years old. However, Meuleners et al. (2002) in their study of the dimensions state that if the questions have a three point likert scales they are more likely to get ceiling and floor effects and consequently findings should be interpreted with caution. That said however children are reliable if you take their development stage into account (Hong et al., 2007). The reliability of young people was the subject of investigation when the HRQoL Kidscreen was used to see if there was a correlation between the QoL and the use of the health care services. It found it was related to their perceived HRQoL which reinforces the relevance of the young persons perceptions (Rajmil et al., 2006).

Bailey et al. (2002) report the health of LAAC within their sample as good, however these findings are based on a review of the child by a social worker and the researchers (also social care professionals) not by a health care professional. The reviewer would argue that the basis of what "good health" is may vary greatly between the two professional groups. It is not the perspective of the young people themselves. When staff rate the young persons quality of life as being better than the young persons rating this will have an impact on planning and care provision to meet the young persons needs. This leads to differences in the expectations of staff, which are not based on the reality of the young peoples needs.

The perspective that young people may rate their quality of life higher than staff may be attributed to the backgrounds that the young people come from. Their perception of their quality of life might be quite different from that of their peers; this would result in the voice of the young person driving the care. Edwards et al. (2002) states it is important that the adolescents can define what is important to their health and what will impact on their perceptions of their quality of life. Identifying the positive aspects of their quality of life and not just focusing on the deficits will direct those working with the young people to develop their resilience skills.

Age and gender are important factors to be considered when considering a quality of life tool (Ravens-Sieberer et al., 2007). It is recognized that young people as they get older rate their quality of life as poorer (Ravens-Sieberer et al., 2007). This is important when making longitudinal comparisons and evaluations on interventions. However, other studies have disputed the gender differences (Sweeting, 1995).

The method of administrate must be consistent whether it is postal, telephone or interview. This has been found to be more significant as the information becomes more personal, with postal and online seen as more confidential and anonymous (Raat et al., 2007) Raat et al. (2007) reported that on line there were fewer missing answers using this method over the paper method.

10   Validity

There are also cultural differences where this perspective of QoL being measured requires further investigation to ensure that the instruments can be validated and applicability to different adolescent populations (Wang et al., 2000). This is significant, as the stage of adolescence will have an impact in the policy and transition to adulthood within their culture. The autonomy of the young people within their culture and the age of adulthood may have an influence of the young person perceptions. Fuh et al. (2005) reported on the relevance of age.

Although these findings have been prevalent in a number of studies it is not a conclusive finding as Wang et al. (2000) found evidence of this in the Japanese population but not in the Chinese population of his study. The QoL instruments must be sensitive to cultural differences for example in his study of Chinese adolescents the family is rated highly, where this was not the case Taiwan (Fuh et al., 2005).

Questionnaires that are sensitive to cultural biases are essential in so far as the population of UK is becoming more diverse with Eastern Europeans settling in this country (The Scottish Government, 2008). The relevance of having an instrument that can be used in other European countries will allow for comparisons, which is important when considering the European laws on health and vulnerable groups.

There is an interest in specific groups of children and adolescents with health concerns however there is little in the research on the general population of adolescents. When making comparisons using the quality of life data it is vital that there is a comparative normative data. There is a lack of normative data and well-validated instruments this is particularly evident in assessing adolescents.

11   Most Commonly Used Quality of Life Assessment Scales

Kidscreen describes a series of quality of life tools for children and adolescents 8–18 years, suitable for cross-cultural use and to support comparisons. There are three versions, kidscreen 52, kidscreen 27 and kidscreen 10 which denotes the number of questions in the versions. The kidscreen was developed simultaneously in different countries. It can be used in national and international epidemiological studies to comparative data on children and adolescent population.

The self reported questionnaire is of the format of a five choice likert scale, which focuses on the past 2 weeks. There are parent/proxy versions available in all three measures. It is also sensitive to gender issues were girls have a self reported poor health in their adolescents years (Ravens-Sieberer et al., 2007).

Kidscreen 52 measures the frequency of a behavior or intensity of attitude across 10 dimensions. It is estimated that it will take 15–20 min to complete. The dimensions are:

Physical well-being (five items)
Psychological well-being (six items)
Moods and emotions (seven items)
Social support and peers (six items)
Parent relations and home life (six items)
Self –perception (six items)
Autonomy (six items)
School environment (six items)
Social acceptance bullying (three items)
Financial resources (three items)

Hong et al. (2007) argues for more extensive testing in clinical trials as comparisons between adolescents and children, noting that adolescents tend to report lower quality of life.

The kidscreen 27 was tested on a large population sample 22,877 for criteria ❯ validity. It is estimated to tale 10–15 min to complete. It has five domains:

◻ Figure 150-1

Diagrammatic representation of a uni-dimensional model of the SF-36. The uni-dimensional model of the SF-36 assumes the measured sub-scales contribute to an instrument along which represents a single overall dimension of quality of life

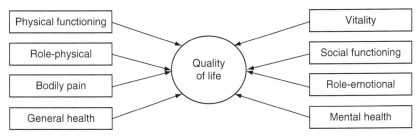

Physical well-being (five items) physical activity energy and fitness.

Psychological well-being (seven items) positive emotions, feeling well balanced, satisfaction with life. Parent relationship and autonomy (seven items) looks at the relationship with parents the atmosphere at home feeling of having enough and appropriate freedom, as well as their feelings in relation to financial resources.

Social support and peers (four items) examines their relationship with their peers.

School environment (four items) explores their perception of their own cognitive ability (Ravens-Sieberer et al., 2007).

This version has many of the advantages of the original kidscreen 52. It discriminates well between children and adolescents in good health to those in poor physical and mental health. Particularly so in the mental health as the kidscreen 27 focus on mental and social health. It also shows that socio-economic factors has a baring on health (Ravens-Sieberer et al., 2007).

Kidscreen 10. The 10 items provide a uni-dimensional index developed form the kidscreen 27. Provides a general HRQoL index score for monitoring and screening uses. It takes 5 min to answer the questionnaire (The Kidscreen group, 2004).

12   Youth – Quality of Life Y-QOL

This is an adolescent specific tool for generic health assessment of the quality of life. This self reported questionnaire is estimated to take 15 min to complete. The 57 questions take the format of the first 15 questions focus on the past 4 weeks in a five-scale answer option. The remaining questions are in an 11 point likert scale format "not at all" to "a great deal."

The four domains of this questionnaire focus on (1) self with domains of belief in self, being oneself, mental health, physical health, and spirituality. (2) Relationships, focusing on adult support, caring for others, family relations, freedom, friendships, participation, and peer relations. (3) Environment, focusing engagement and activities, education, neighborhood, monetary resources, personal safety, and view of the future. (4) General Quality of Life focusing on the young persons is enjoying life, feeling life is worthwhile, and being satisfied with ones life. Providing scores across the four domains and one overall score (Seattle quality of life group, 1997).

There was no significant differences were found between administering the questionnaire by mail or interview (Patrick et al., 2002).

□ Figure 150-2
Diagrammatic representation of a bi-dimensional model of the SF-36 specifying separable but correlated physical and mental quality of life domains. The bi-dimensional model of the SF-36 assumes the loading of four sub-scales on two separable but correlated dimensions of quality of life. These two higher order domains represent mental health and physical aspects of quality of life

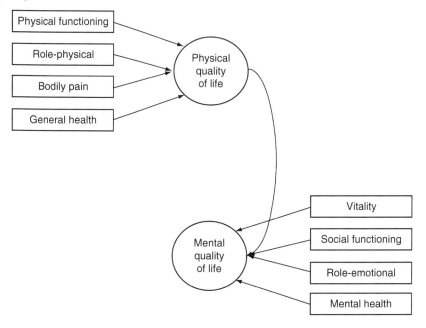

Davidson-Arad et al. (2004) in their Israel study of staff and residents QoL in residential care concluded that the staff did not have consistent responses demonstrating different perceptions from the young persons experiences. It raises many valid point for research here in the UK.

13   QoL for Adolescents – Quality of Life Profile -Adolescent Version

This 54 question, questionnaire focus on three domains "being, belonging and becoming" It has been tested on Canadian and Australian children (Meuleners et al., 2002).

It has not been assessed for adaptation of cross cultural and adaptations of language (Partick et al., 2002).

14   EQ-5D

Developed by the EuroQoL group. It is designed for self-completion and is it has the following dimensions mobility, self-care, usual activities, pain/discomfort and anxiety and depression. It has a three point style with no problems, some problems and sever problems. It is considered suitable for children age 12 year and over. A child version is currently being developed. This quality of life questionnaire focuses on "how is your health today?" (Oppe et al., 2007).

15 SF-36

The SF-36 is a multi-purpose, short-form health survey 36 questions. It has eight dimensions building a profile of functional health and well-being scores including physical and mental health. Has been used in some studies but is not specifically designed or validated with use in children or adolescents (Ware, 2008). The SF-36 is a particularly useful tool because of the abundance of research work conducted on it's measurement properties and the relationship of such measurements to dimensional structure and relationships. The evidenced-based associations between SF-36 sub-scale dimensions and higher order QOL factors are shown in ❯ *Figures 150-1–150-4.*

16 Duke Health Profile – Adolescent Version (DHP-A)

The 17 question self reported questionnaire is derived from the adult version of 64 questions for use with over 18 year old French population. It is easy to administer and distinguishes between boys and girls in the 12–19 age group (Hannh, 2005).

■ Figure 150-3
Diagrammatic representation of a bi-dimensional model of the SF-36 specifying uncorrelated physical and mental components within a higher order health quality of life domain. A more complex factor structure to the SF-36. This model assumes the SF-36 has the loading of four sub-scales on two separable but uncorrelated dimensions of quality of life. However, these uncorrelated domains are encapsulated within an overall dimension of health-related quality of life

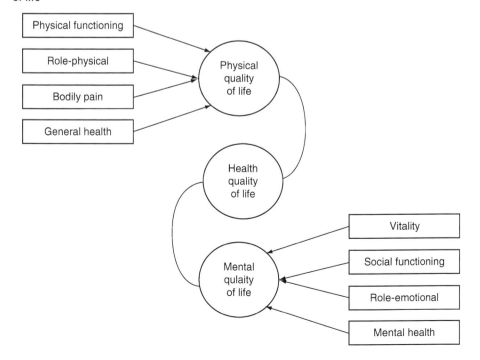

17   Pediatric Quality of Life Inventory (PedsQL)

This self reported questionnaire consist of a core scale of 23 items measuring the physical (8 items), emotional 95 items), social (5 items) and school (5 items) aspects of ❯ health-related quality of life in healthy and ill children and adolescents. It is estimated to take 4 min to complete with parent/proxy versions available (Varni, 2008).

18   Child Health Questionnaire – Child Form (CHQ-CF)

Developed in the USA then used in Australia, the Netherlands and Slavic countries. It has been translated into 21 languages and used in 32 countries. It consists of 87 questions in the domains of physical health, psychosocial health, impact of health problems.

The CHQ-CF has been used in clinical trials interested in chronic conditions such as asthma, epilepsy, undiagnosed pain, weight perceptions (Raat et al., 2002).

Disease specific instruments focus on the quality of life of chronically ill children and adolescents. In this client group the young people are classed as vulnerable with generally poorer health and health outcomes than their peers. However there is no tool that is designed specifically to measure the quality of life of young people that that vulnerable through neglect and abuse.

◼ Figure 150-4
Diagrammatic representation of a tri-dimensional model of the SF-36 specifying separable physical, mental and general well-being components within a higher order health quality of life domain. A still further complex factor structure to the SF-36. This model assumes a tri-dimensional structure to the SF-36 with uncorrelated sub-scale factors encapsulated within an overall dimension of health-related quality of life

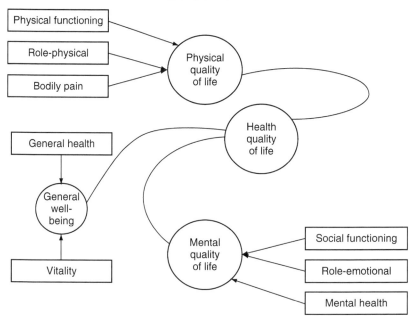

Summary Points

- QOL is an important issue in the assessment of LAAC.
- QOL tools may be useful in aiding to identify vulnerable children.
- To monitor the interventions experienced by children and adolescents in pubic care QOL measures offer an important outcome index.
- There are a number of measures of QOL that may be used in LAAC.
- There is a need for National record-keeping of LAAC in terms of QOL outcomes and the relationship of this important biopsychosocial domain to the development of significant pathology and psychopathology.

References

Ashton-key M, Jorge E. (2008). ADC online. http://adc.bmj.com/cgi/content/full/898/4/299

Bailey S, Thoburn T, Wakeham H. (2002). Child Family Soc Work. 7: 189–201.

Brodie I, Berridge D, Beckett W. (1997). Br J Nurs. 6: 386–390.

Bundle A. (2001). Arch Dis Childhood. 84: 10–14.

Chambers H, Howell S, Madge N, Ollie H. (2002). Healthy Care: Building an Evidence Base for Promoting the Health and Well-Being of Looked after Children and Young People. National Children's Bureau, London.

Cocker C, Scott S. (2006). J R Soc Promo Health. 126: 18–23.

Davidson-Arad B, Dekel R, Wozner Y. (2004). Soc Indic Res. 68: 77–89.

Department of Health. (1991). Patterns and Outcomes on Child Placement. HMSO. London.

Edwards T, Huebner C, Connell F, Patrick D. (2002) J Adolescence. 25: 275–286.

Feletti VJ. (1998). Am J Prevent Med. 14: 245.

Fuh J, Wang S, Lu S. (2005). Psychiat Clin Neuros. 59: 11–18.

Hannh T, Guillemiun F, Deschamps JP. (2005). Qual Life Res. 14: 229–234.

Health Education Board Scotland [HEBS]. (2001). Young People and Smoking. Cessation. A Report from Two Seminars. HEBS. Edinburgh.

Hill CM, Watkins J. (2002). Statutory health assessment for looked after children: What do they achieve? Child Care, Health and Development. 29(1): 3–13.

Holland S, Faulkner A, Periz-del-Aguila R, Connell D, Hayes S. (2003). Overview and Survey of Effectiveness of Interventions to National Assembly for Wales Sponsored Project. University School of Social Sciences, University of Wales College of Medicine, Morgannwg Health Authority, Cardiff.

Hong D, Yang J, Byun H, Kim M, Oh M, Kim J. (2007). J Korean Med Sci. 22: 446–452.

House of Commons Select Committee. (1998). Children Looked After by Local Authorities. http://www.esbhhealth.nhs.uk/publications/public_health/care.asp

Lamont DW. (1998). Public Health. 1998: 1.

Mather M, Batty D. (2000). Doctors for Children in Public Care. A Resource Guide Advocating, Protecting and Promoting Health. British Agencies for Adoption and Fostering, London, 12, pp. 85–93.

Mather M, Humphrey J, Robson J. (1997). Adopt Foster. 21: 36–40.

McCann J, James A, Wilson S, Dunn G. (1996). Br Med J. 313: 1529–1530.

Meltzer H, Gaward R, Goodman R, Ford T. (2000). Mental Health of Children and Adolescents in Great Britain. The Stationery Office, London.

Meltzer H, Gaward R, Goodman R, Ford T. (2003). The Mental Health of Young People Looked after by Local Authorities in England. The Stationary Office. London.

Meuleners L, Lee A, Binns C, Lower A. (2003). Qual Life Res. 12: 283–290, 2003.

Michelle M. (1997). Loud, sad or bad: young people's perceptions peer groups and smoking. Health Education Research. Vol. 12, No 1, p1–14.

NHS Health Scotland. (2006). Health Scotland Annual Report 2005–2006. Health Scotland. http://www.healthscotland.com/uploads/documents/2682-Annual%20Report_2362_11_2006.pdf

Oppe M, Rabin R, Charro F. (2007). EQ-5D User Guide version 1.0. EuroQoL Group.www.euroqol.org

Patrick D, Edwards T, Topolski T. (2002). J Adolescence. 25: 287–300.

Philpott M. (2004). Counsell Australia. 4: 4–7.

Polnay L. (2000). Child Family Soc Work. 7: 133.

Raat H, Landgaf JM, Bonsel GL, Gemke RJBJ and Essubi-Bot ML. (2002). Reliability and validity of the child health questionnaire-child form (CHQ-CF87) in Dutch adolescents population. Quality of Life Research. 11: 575–581.

Raat H, Mangunkusmo R, Landgraf J, Kloek G, Brug J. (2007). Qual Life Res. 16: 675–685.

Rajmil L, Alonso J, Berra S, Ravens-Sieberer U, Gosch A, Simeoni M, Auquier P. (2006). J Adolescent Health. 38: 511–518.

Ravens-Sieberer U, Auquier P, Erhart M, Gossch A, Rajmil L, Bruil J, Power M, Duer W, Cloetta B, Czemy L, Mauzur J, Czimbalmous Tountas Y, Hagquist C, Kilrow J. (2007). Qual Life Res. 16: 1347–1356.

Residential Care Health Project. (2004). Forgotten Children. Astron. Edinburgh.

Rivron M. (2001). A health promotion project for young people who are looked after. Adopt Fostering. 25: 70–71.

Saunders L, Broad B. (1997). The Health Needs of Young People Leaving Care. De Montfort University, Leicester.

Seattle Quality of Life Group. (1997). Youth Quality of Life-Research Version Instrument (YQOL-R). http://depts.washington.edu/yqol/instruments/YQOL-R.htm

Smith C. (2000). Improving the Health of Children Looked after by Local Authorities in Argyll and Clyde. Department of Public Health. Argyll and Clyde.

Sweeting. (1995). Soc Sci Med. 40: 77–90.

Teenage Pregnancy Unit. (2002). Cited in Big step 2001/02. Researching the Health of Young People in and Leaving Care in Glasgow. Executive Summary. www.thebigstep.org.uk

The Caroline Walker Trust – Expert Working Group. (2001). Eating Well for Looked after Children and Young People. Nutritional and Practical Guidelines. The Caroline Walker Trust.

The Kidscreen Group. (2004). Description of the KIDSCREEN-10 index. www.kidscreen.org

The Scottish Executive. (1998). Working together for a Healthier Scotland.

The Scottish Executive. (1999). Towards a Healthier Scotland: A White Paper on Health.

The Scottish Executive. (2002a). Joint Working Approach to the Delivery of Health Services. St Andrews House, Edinburgh.

The Scottish Executive. (2002b). Services for Young People with Problematic Drug Misuse. A Guide to Principles and Practice. Effective Interventions Unit. St Andrews House, Edinburgh.

The Scottish Government. (2008). Population and migration. The Scottish government statistics http://www.scotland.gov.uk/Topics/Statistics/Browse/Population-Migration.

Varni J. (2008). The Measurement Model for the Paediatric Quality of Life Inventory. http://www.pedsql.org/

Varni J, Limbers C, Burwinkle T. (2007). Health Qual Life Outcomes. 5: 1.

Wang X, Matsuda N, Ma H, Shinfuku N. (2000). Psych Clin Neuros. 54: 147–152.

Ware JE. (2008). SF-36® Health Survey Update. http://www.sf-36.org/tools/SF36.shtml

Williams J, Maddocks A, Jackson S, Cheung W-Y, Love A, Hutchings H. (2001). Arch Dis Childhood. 85: 280–285.

WHO. (1988). Ottawa Charter for Health Promotion. An International Conference on Health Promotion. WHO. Copenhagen.

WHO QoL (1994). cited by Edwards T, Huebener B, Connell F, Patrick D. (2002). J Adolescence. 25: 275–286.

151 Quality of Life Measures During the Menopause

G. D. Mishra · D. Kuh

1	*Introduction*	*2594*
1.1	Quality of Life	2594
1.2	Menopause	2595
1.2.1	Menopause, HRQOL, and Mid-Life Events	2595
1.2.2	Issues with Menopause-Related HRQOL Instruments	2595
1.3	Chapter Outline	2597
2	*Generic Quality of Life Instruments*	*2597*
2.1	Medical Outcomes Study Short Form 36 Items (SF-36)	2597
2.1.1	Psychometric Properties	2599
2.2	The World Health Organization Quality of Life-Brief (WHOQOL-BREF) Instrument	2599
2.2.1	Psychometric Properties	2600
2.3	Utian QOL (UQOL) Instrument	2600
2.3.1	Psychometric Properties	2601
3	*Menopausal Symptoms/HRQOL Instruments*	*2601*
3.1	Greene Climacteric Scale	2602
3.1.2	Psychometric Properties	2603
3.2	Women's Health Questionnaire (WHQ)	2603
3.2.1	Psychometric Properties	2604
3.3	Qualifemme	2605
3.3.1	Psychometric Properties	2605
3.4	Menopause-Specific QOL Questionnaire	2606
3.4.1	Psychometric Properties	2606
3.5	Revised MENQOL (MENQOL-Intervention) Questionnaire	2606
3.5.1	Psychometric Properties	2607
3.6	Menopause Rating Scale (MRS)	2607
3.6.1	Psychometric Properties	2607
3.7	Menopausal Quality of Life Scale (MQOL)	2608
3.7.1	Psychometric Properties	2609
3.8	MENCAV	2609
3.8.1	Psychometric Properties	2609
4	*Conclusion*	*2610*
	Summary Points	*2611*

Abstract: Menopause usually occurs sometime between 40–60 years and marks the end of the reproductive phase of a woman's life. The menopausal transition is associated with a wide range of symptoms, such as hot flushes and cold night sweats. However, the full impact on women's lives is difficult to disentangle from other concomitant changes, such as declining health, children leaving home, and the birth of grand children. Thus it is essential that researchers are able to use reliable and accurate instruments for assessing ❷ health related quality of life (HRQOL) and preferably ones that permit comparisons prior to, during, and after menopausal transition, as well as across populations.

Over the last three decades, numerous instruments have been developed to measure HRQOL during menopause, from simple checklists of symptoms to wide-ranging questions across several domains of psychosocial well-being. This review finds that although they all report good psychometric properties and are well documented, no single instrument has become pre-eminent in the field. The process of development is likely to continue since none of the instruments have met all the outstanding measurement issues, such as including questions for women on HRT or those using complementary and alternative medicine. It is hoped that as new scales evolve, these will exhibit a greater degree of convergence and compatibility.

Researchers should consider the benefits of using generic well-established measures of HRQOL and checklists of menopausal symptoms, with additional items used in a way that preserves compatibility. A robust and reliable instrument remains a highly worthwhile aspiration, since any findings, such as identifying successful management or coping strategies, would provide potentially invaluable information to communicate to women everywhere and help them prepare for this stage of life.

List of Abbreviations: *CAM,* complementary and alternative medicine; *HRQOL,* health related quality of life; *HRT,* hormone replacement therapy; *MENQOL,* menopause-specific HRQOL questionnaire; *MQOL,* menopausal quality of life scale; *MRS,* menopause-specific HRQOL questionnaire; *QOL,* ❷ quality of life; *SF-12,* short form 12; *SF-36,* short form 36; *UQOL,* Utian quality of life instrument; *VAS,* visual analogue scale; *WHQ,* women's health questionnaire; *WHOQOL_BREF,* World Health Organization quality of life-brief

1 Introduction

1.1 Quality of Life

The term health related quality of life (HRQOL) has been used in many different ways but there are unifying themes. There is general agreement that it is a multidimensional concept that focuses on the impact of a disease and its treatment on an individual in terms of their functioning in everyday life and their well-being. Another unifying theme is that the concepts forming these dimensions can be assessed only by subjective measures, and that they are evaluated by *asking the individual* (Fayers and Machin, 2000). HRQOL is distinct from general quality of life in that it relates to aspects of life that are likely to be correlated with health status and it is more sensitive to changes in health than general quality of life (Albert, 1998). Cella and Bonomi state that "health-related quality of life refers to the extent to which one's usual or expected physical, emotional and social well-being are affected by a medical condition or its treatment" (Cella and Bonomi, 1995). It is important to reiterate that an individual's well-being or health status cannot be directly measured, we are only able to make inferences from measurable indicators of symptoms and reported perceptions (Fairclough, 2002).

1.2   Menopause

The menopausal transition refers to the extended period of hormonal change in women that marks the end of their reproductive phase of life (McKinlay et al., 1992; van Noord et al., 1997). The worldwide average for menopausal age (that is the age at permanent cessation of menstrual periods) is around 51 years and usually occurs within the age range of 40–60 years. Menopause is reached when the follicular reserve is depleted to around 1,000, from a peak during fetal life of some 5 million follicles at 20 gestational weeks to 2 million at birth (Ginsberg, 1991). The experience of menopausal transition has been associated with a wide range of symptoms, including vasomotor symptoms such as hot flushes and cold night sweats, somatic symptoms such as headaches, muscle and joint pain, and psychological symptoms such as anxiety and depression (Hardy and Kuh, 2002; Kaufert and Syrotuik, 1981; Kuh et al., 1997; Mishra et al., 2003) (cf chapter by Amanda Daley, Helen Stokes-Lampard, Christine MacArthur).

1.2.1   Menopause, HRQOL, and Mid-Life Events

Cultural attitudes to the menopausal transition may influence the impact it has on a woman's life. Rather than being treated as a medical condition caused by hormonal changes, the menopause can be viewed as a natural transition encompassing changes that are part of the natural ageing process, including how a woman views herself and how she is viewed by society (Hunt, 2000). It may occur at a time that is concomitant with other biological, psychological, and social changes, such as declining health, children leaving home, the birth of grandchildren, marital tensions, or the death of parents. Hence, this time of complex psychological and physiological change renders it difficult to determine precisely the influence of menopausal transition on HRQOL over and above the impact of these other factors and life events (Zapantis and Santoro, 2003). These relationships are illustrated in ❷ *Figure 151-1*, adapted from the conceptual framework developed for HRQOL by Wilson and Cleary (1995).

HRQOL assessments are essential in the study of menopause and beyond just determining the impact of symptoms experienced during menopause. Also of interest is the way that duration of menopausal transition affects HRQOL or if women "adapt" to the transition, or recover once the transition is over. By assessing HRQOL prior to, during, and after menopausal transition with reliable and accurate instruments for HRQOL, then we may also measure how well women cope and whether any management strategies work.

1.2.2   Issues with Menopause-Related HRQOL Instruments

Unfortunately interpreting findings regarding the relationship between menopausal status and HRQOL has been hindered by issues related to the definition and measurement of HRQOL. There is a fundamental confusion of terminology by using "menopausal QOL," as denoted by the response to a checklist of specific symptoms experienced during ❷ peri- and ❷ post-menopause, to measure quality of life in general (Utian, 2007). Often these instruments were only intended to measure the extent of symptoms experienced by women during the menopause, such as problems with sleeping, from which the impact on HRQOL then seems to be inferred. Instead we need a series of measures for both menopausal symptoms and HRQOL for the general sense of well-being. These should be applicable to both before

◻ Figure 151-1

Relationships among factors during menopause in a health related quality of life conceptual model. The conceptual model was adapted from Wilson and Cleary [1995]. The direction of the arrow indicates the direction on the relationship

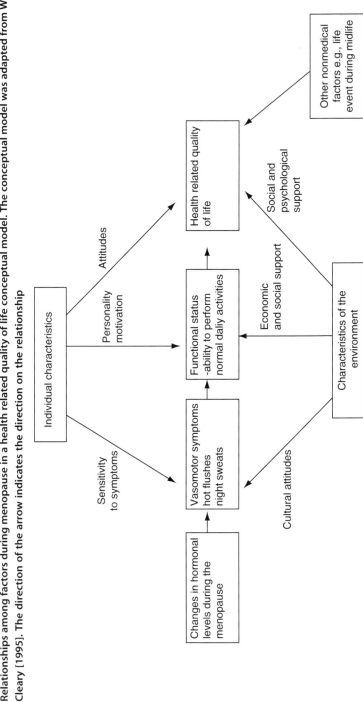

and after menopause. (Utian, 2007). Even with respect to the menopausal symptom inventories or scores, and more than two decades since the call for their harmonization (Greene, 1998), a wide variety of checklists are still in use; many on a national rather than international basis and using disparate assessment periods and scoring methods.

Last, there are issues concerning the coverage of the scores to the full population of women. Most of these symptom inventories were initially developed and validated on clinic and patient based samples of Western mid-aged women, and hence may have both a clinical and culturally specific focus. Women with hysterectomy or oopherectomy were usually excluded from the initial studies, so the list of menopausal symptoms may not be exhaustive. For women on hormone replacement therapy (HRT), very few scores have included possible negative side effects such as irregular bleeding, facial or body hair growth, voice deepening, and loss of hair from scalp as part of the assessment (Zollner et al., 2005). With the increase in popularity in the use of complementary and alternative medicine (CAM), researchers may also want to consider other possible side effects that could influence HRQOL. Bearing in mind the issue of harmonization, considerable further development of existing instruments may still be required to address all these issues.

1.3   Chapter Outline

The main aim of this chapter is to provide a comprehensive overview, though not an exhaustive list, of the HRQOL instruments available for the menopausal transition so that researchers can have a clear basis upon which to select either an existing instrument, or use it as a basis upon which additional study specific questions can be added. The first part provides an appraisal of three established generic HRQOL instruments; the second examines seven menopause symptoms inventories or checklists that may tap into certain HRQOL dimensions. Each is assessed on the basis of their extent of use, the domains they cover, their method of scoring, and their psychometric properties of coverage, ❷ validity, and ❷ reliability. We conclude with advice for practitioners in the selection and further development of menopause related HRQOL measures.

2   Generic Quality of Life Instruments

The three generic QOL instruments discussed here are the Medical Outcomes Study Short Form 36 items (SF-36) (Ware and Sherbourne, 1992), the World Health Organization Quality of life-Brief (WHOQOL-BREF) (The WHOQOL Group, 1998), and the Utian QOL instrument (Utian et al., 2002).

2.1   Medical Outcomes Study Short Form 36 Items (SF-36)

In 1992 SF-36 was developed during the Medical Outcomes Study (MOS) to measure generic health concepts relevant across age, disease, and treatment groups (McHorney et al., 1994; Ware and Sherbourne, 1992). The SF-36 includes one multi-item scale measuring each of the eight health concepts: physical functioning (PF, ten items); role limitations due to physical (RP) or emotional (RE) problems (4 items each); bodily pain (BP, 2 items); general health perceptions (GH, 5 items); vitality (VT, 4 items); social functioning (SF, 2 items); and emotional well-being or mental health (MH, 5 items) (❷ *Table 151-1*). In addition, there is a general health transition question, which asks: "Compared to 1 year ago, how would you rate your general health now?" There is also a global question about the respondent's perception of their health: "In general, would you say that your health is (excellent, very good, good, fair, poor)?" Most questions refer to the past four weeks, although some relate to the present. A few questions, such as for RP, take yes/no responses, while some, such as for PF items, have three categories (limited a lot, limited a little, not limited at all), and other items have five or six categories for responses. The SF-36 items and scales are scored so that a higher score indicates a better health state. Items and scales are scored in three steps: (1) recoding for the 10 items that require it; (2) computing scales and scores by summing across items in the same scale (raw scale scores); and (3) transforming raw scale scores to a 0–100 scale (transformed scale score). Physical and mental component summary scores can also be calculated for the eight SF-36 scales (Ware et al., 1993). Higher scores reflected better HRQOL status.

The SF-36 was constructed to achieve minimum standards of precision necessary for group comparisons in eight conceptual areas. It is intended to yield a profile of scores that would be useful in understanding population differences in physical and mental health status, the health burden of chronic disease and other medical conditions, and the effect of treatments on general health status.

◻ Table 151-1

Characteristics of the medical outcomes short form 36 (SF-36)

Items	Domains/health concepts	Assessment period	Psychometric properties
Fully phrased statements on health concepts (36 items) which can be completed by individuals over 14 years of age (McHorney et al., 1994)	1. Physical functioning (PF) (10 items)	Most of them refers to the past four weeks, though some relate to the present	*Reliability*
	2. Role limitations (RP) (4 items)		The median of the (test-retest) reliability coefficient exceeds 0.8 for all domains except for SF (0.76)
	3. Emotional problems (RE) (4 items)		
	4. Bodily pain (BP) (2 items)		
	5. General health perceptions (GH) (5 items)		*Internal consistency*
	6. Vitality (VT) (4 items)		Cronbach's alpha ranged from 0.73 to 0.96.
	7. Social functioning (SF) (2 items)		
	8. Emotional well-being/ mental health (MH) (5 items)		

2.1.1 Psychometric Properties

All estimates of score reliability exceed accepted standards for measures used in group comparisons. For each scale, the median of the reliability coefficients across studies equals or exceeds 0.8, with the exception of the social functioning scales (the median for this two-item scale is 0.76). The ❷ internal consistency estimates for the eight scales ranged from 0.73 to 0.96 with a median of 0.95, compared with a range of 0.6–0.8 and a median of 0.76 for the test-retest estimates in the UK population (McHorney et al., 1994).

In the SF-36 manual, Ware and colleagues reported that in tests of validity the SF-36 was able to discriminate between groups with physical morbidities, but the physical functioning subscale performed the best, and the mental subscale discriminated between patients with mental morbidities the best (Ware et al., 1993). However, the physical functioning scale, in common with many similar scales, poses questions about interpretation. Questions ask whether your health limits you in "vigorous activities, such as running, lifting heavy objects, participating in strenuous sports" or "walking more than a mile." It is not clear how those who have never participated in such activities should respond – their health many be severely impaired, and yet they should respond "No, not limited at all" and will therefore receive a score indicating better health functioning that might be expected.

The SF-36 can suffer from ceiling effects, whereby the data cannot take on a value higher than certain values, and therefore may not be responsive to the changes in the experience of symptoms or HRT use. In most cases, the distribution of each domain is highly skewed and does not follow the shape "standard" distribution. To overcome these problems, Rose et al. (1999) recommends the use of a dichotomous variable for each domain where having an having impaired health is defined if the score is lower that the 25th percentile for the appropriate age and gender.

Although the SF-36 does not contain any menopause specific symptoms nor has it been validated on women going though the menopause, it has been shown to be associated with HRQOL during the menopause (Avis et al., 2004; Kumari et al., 2005; Mishra et al., 2003). It can be administered at various stages from ❷ pre-, peri- to post-menopause to investigate how HRQOL changes as the women ages. Various "menopause QOL measures" have compared their scores with SF-36 in other to establish the psychometric properties of their instrument. An algorithm to deal with missing values for at most half the items is also provided. A shorter version, SF-12, (Ware et al., 1998) is also available for use which may be more practical if used in conjunction with other menopausal questions.

2.2 The World Health Organization Quality of Life-Brief (WHOQOL-BREF) Instrument

The 26-item WHOQOL-BREF was derived from data collected using the 100-item version (WHOQOL-100) instrument. It is developed to provide a short form QOL assessment that would be applicable cross-culturally (The WHOQOL Group, 1998). The 26 items of WHOQOL-BREF form the four domains of quality of life: Physical health (7 items), Psychological (6 items), Social relations (3 items), and Environment (8 items) (❷ Table 151-2). Each item is answered on a 5-point Likert scale and refers to the state experienced over the previous 4 weeks. Each domain is formed by summing up the scores for items corresponding to that domain. The three negative item scores are reversed so that higher scores reflected better QOL.

◘ Table 151-2

Characteristics of the World Health Organization quality of life-brief (WHOQOL-BREF) instrument

Items	Domains/health concepts	Assessment period	Psychometric properties
Fully phrased statements on health concepts (26 items)	1. General QOL (1 item)	All of them refers to the past four weeks	*Reliability*
(The WHOQOL Group 1998)	2. General Health (1 item)		The test-retest correlations ranged from 0.66 (Physical health) to 0.87 (Environment).
	3. Physical health (7 items)		*Internal consistency*
	4. Psychological (6 items)		Cronbach's alpha ranged from 0.66 (social relationships) to 0.96 (Physical health and Environment)
	5. Social relations (3 items)		
	6. Environment (8 items)		

The domain score is then transformed to take a value between 4 and 20. WHOQOL-BREF domain scores have been shown to have satisfactory psychometric properties (The WHOQOL Group, 1998).

2.2.1 Psychometric Properties

The reliability of the domains as measured by the test-retest correlations, administered 2–8 weeks apart, ranged from 0.66 (for physical health) to 0.87 (for environmental conditions). The estimates for internal consistency, or Cronbach alpha, ranged from 0.66 (for social relationships) to 0.80 (for physical health and environmental conditions). The instrument has also been shown to have good construct validity (Skevington et al., 2004).

This is a widely available and validated instrument which is able to assess global, rather than just health-related, QOL across different cultures. However the responsiveness of the instrument to detect a change in QOL is yet to be addressed. More recently a strategy to impute values for missing items has been proposed (Lin, 2006). As this instrument does not include menopausal symptoms or the side effects associated with the use of HRT or CAM, it may be administered in conjunction with menopausal symptoms checklist, in order to assess the QOL during the menopause.

2.3 Utian QOL (UQOL) Instrument

Utian and colleagues recognized that the presence or the absence of symptoms are just one of the sets of factors that may affect QOL during menopause (Utian et al., 2002). The UQOL

◼ Table 151-3

Characteristics of the Utian quality of life (UQOL) instrument

Items	Domains/health concepts	Assessment period	Psychometric properties
Fully phrased statements on symptoms and feelings (23 items)	1. Occupational (7 items)	All of them refers to the past month	*Reliability*
(Utian et al., 2002)	2. Health (7 items)		The test-retest correlations ranged from 0.77 (Emotional) to 0.87 (Sexual and Occupational).
	3. Emotional (6 items)		*Internal consistency*
	4. Sexual (3 items)		Cronbach's alpha ranged from 0.64 (Emotional) to 0.84 (Occupational)

measure consists of twenty three items on the four dimensions of quality of life: Occupational (7 items); Health (7 items); Emotional (6 items); and Sexual (3 items) (❯ *Table 151-3*). Each item in the UQOL questionnaire is answered on a 5-point Likert Scale, and each dimension of quality of life is scored by adding up items in that domain. Negative item scores are reversed so that higher scores indicate better HRQOL status.

2.3.1 Psychometric Properties

The reliability of the measure as demonstrated by the test-retest correlation, administered between three to seven days apart, was between 0.77 (for dimension Emotional) and 0.88 (for dimensions Sexual and Occupational). The estimates of internal consistency, Cronbach alpha, ranged from 0.64 (Emotional) to 0.84 (Occupational). The construct validity was demonstrated in relation to SF-36.

The UQOL instrument does not contain any symptoms specific to menopause, or the side effects of HRT use. It is not as widely used as some of the other generic QOL instruments and hence it performance cannot be evaluated in terms of its responsiveness to change in HRQOL. Furthermore, as some of the domain scales are composed of only a few items, missing values on more than one item could bias the results. We suggest that if this measure is used, then it should be done so in conjunction with a menopausal symptoms checklist (Utian, 2007).

3 Menopausal Symptoms/HRQOL Instruments

Although a few studies of menopause have used generic HRQOL instruments, such as the SF-36, (Avis et al., 2004; Kumari et al., 2005; Mishra et al., 2003) or a list of questions of the perceived changes in several dimensions (Mishra and Kuh, 2006), a number of instruments have also been developed specifically to examine menopause symptoms inventories or checklists that may tap into certain HRQOL dimensions. The seven instruments discussed here are the Green Climacteric Scale (Greene, 1998), Women's Health Questionnaire (WHQ) (Hunter, 1992), Qualifemme (Le Floch et al., 1996), Menopause-specific HRQOL Questionnaire (MENQOL) (Hilditch et al., 1996), Menopause Rating Scale (MRS) (Schneider et al., 2000b), Menopausal Quality of Life Scale (MQOL) (Jacobs et al., 2000), and the MENCAV questionnaire (Buendia et al., 2001).

3.1 Greene Climacteric Scale

The original Greene Climacteric scale, a 30-item self administered scale, was developed in 1976 (Greene, 1976). The items were mostly derived from Neugarten and Kraines (1965) meno-pausal check list which consisted of symptoms experienced by a group of peri-menopausal or climacteric women. Greene was one of the first to use factor analysis to establish independent domains of menopausal symptoms (Greene, 1976).

In 1998, Greene revised his original scale in order to reconcile the findings of seven factor analytic studies and meet the demand for a "communal and comprehensive measure" of menopausal symptoms (Greene, 1998). The revised scale, known as the standard climacteric scale, comprises 21 items forming three main domains and an item on sexual dysfunction: psychological symptoms (11 items); somatic symptoms (7 items); vasomotor symptoms (2 items); and loss of interest in sex. The first six items of psychological symptoms scale can be classified as the anxiety subscale, and the rest as the depressed mood subscale. Unlike many of the other scales, all items relate to the women's current experiences and have a 4-point Likert Scale: not at all (coded as 0); a little (1), quite a bit (2); and extremely (3). Scores for each scale or subscale are formed by summing across items in the same scale and an overall score for the Greene Climacteric Scale is calculated as the sum of all 21 items (❷ *Table 151-4*). Also it should be noted that higher scores indicate poorer HRQOL status.

◻ Table 151-4
Characteristics of the Green Climacteric scale (the Standard Climacteric scale)

Items	Domains/health concepts	Assessment period	Psychometric properties
Fully phrased statements on symptoms (21 items) (Greene 1998)	1. Psychological symptoms (11 items)	At the moment	*Reliability*
	• Anxiety subscale (6 items)		
	• Depressed mood subscale (5 items)		The test-retest correlations ranged from 0.83 (Vasomotor) to 0.87 (Psychological symptoms).
	2. Somatic symptoms (7 items)		
	3. Vasomotor symptoms (2 items)		*Internal consistency*
	4. Loss of interest in sex (1 item)		Not available

The standard Greene Climacteric Scale was constructed to be a "brief and standard measure" of the common climacteric symptoms. It has been used for comparison and replication purposes in studies of selected populations and as a quality of life measurement in an estrogen replacement trial (Ulrich et al., 1997). Greene also anticipated that, depending on the study hypotheses, researchers may supplement this scale by other measures assessing the characteristics of women.

3.1.2 Psychometric Properties

The reliability of the instrument exceeds the accepted standards for measures used in group comparisons. For each scale, the test-retest correlation was greater than 0.82. The validity is secured through the restricted inclusion of symptoms. Only those meeting the requirement of statistically significant factor loadings are included. Construct validity has been demonstrated in relation to life stress, bereavement, psychological, and HRT use. However in the 1998 paper, responsiveness of the scale was not assessed (Greene, 1998).

The Greene Climacteric Scale is a valid and widely used instrument. It has been replicated and applied in countries such as the Netherlands, Australia, and Ecuador. Studies confirm that the prevalence and intensity of climacteric symptoms as measured by the scale increase during the menopausal transition and stay high during the post-menopause (Barentsen et al., 2001). However, it could be used if augmented with a generic HRQOL measure and with questions on the effects of HRT and CAM use so that a comprehensive change in HRQOL for women in pre-, peri-, and post-menopause stage can be obtained. There remains an issue with accurately detecting effects since the climacteric items refer to current status, while the HRQOL items correspond to the experience over the previous month or 4 weeks.

3.2 Women's Health Questionnaire (WHQ)

In 1992, Myra Hunter published the WHQ instrument which was developed to assess mood and physical symptoms in women who may be experiencing concurrent hormonal and psychosocial changes (Hunter, 1992, 2000). It is intended to be completed by women aged 45–65 years both in the general population and clinical samples. It consists of a 36-item questionnaire rated on a 4-point Likert Scale (yes, definitely; yes, sometimes; no, not much; no, not at all) with all questions relating to the past few weeks. Factor analysis of the 36 items provided nine subscales: depressed mood (6 items); somatic symptoms (7 items); anxiety/fear (4 items); vasomotor symptoms (2 items); sleep problems (3 items); sexual behavior (3 items); menstrual symptoms (4 items); memory/concentration (3 items); attractiveness (3 items) (❷ *Table 151-5*). Item "I worry about growing old" was scored separately. These subscales reflect different aspects of emotional and physical self-reported health of mid-aged women. Items and scales are scored in two steps: (1) recoding of items where they are phrased positively rather than negatively; and (2) computing scales scores by summing across items in the same scale. Higher scores indicated poorer HRQOL status. The "attractiveness" scale accounted for a small proportion of the variance and is now generally omitted (Hunter, 2003).

■ Table 151-5

Characteristics of the women's health questionnaire (WHQ)

Items	Domains/health concepts	Assessment period	Psychometric properties
Fully phrased statements on symptoms and feelings (36 items) (Hunter 1992)	1. Depressed mood (6 items)	Past few days	*Reliability*
	2. Somatic symptoms (7 items)		The test-retest correlations ranged from 0.78 to 0.96
	3. Anxiety/fear (4 items)		
	4. Vasomotor symptoms (2 items)		*Internal consistency*
	5. Sleep problems (3 items)		
	6. Sexual behavior (3 items)		Cronbach's alpha ranged from 0.59 (sexual problems) to 0.84 (vasomotor symptoms).
	7. Menstrual symptoms (4 items)		
	8. Memory/concentration (3 items)		
	9. Attractiveness (3 items)		
	10. Worry about growing old (1 item) Note that this item is usually omitted		

3.2.1 Psychometric Properties

The test-retest reliability was conducted on women who repeated WHQ after 2 weeks. The test-retest correlations were above 0.75, ranging from 0.78 to 0.96, which suggests that the WHQ is reliable across a 2 week time interval (Hunter, 2003). The measure of internal consistency was reasonable and ranged from 0.59 (for sexual problems) to 0.84 (for vasomotor symptoms) (Hunter, 2003). The concurrent validity of psychological scales has been assessed by comparison with the 30-item General Health Questionnaire, which was found to have a 0.86 correlation with the depressed mood subscale (WHQ). Furthermore, this subscale inversely correlated with the SF-36 mental health subscale (−0.70) and with the SF-36 vitality scale (−0.65).

Recently Girod and colleagues have proposed a revised WHQ to be used in multi-centre, international studies that comprises 23 items across six domains: anxiety/depressed mood (7 items); well-being (4 items); somatic symptoms (5 items), memory/concentration (3 items); vasomotor symptoms (2 items); and sleep problems (2 items). It has two optional modules: sexual behavior (3 items); and menstrual symptoms (4 items) (Girod et al., 2006). They found that the psychometric properties of the 23-item WHQ were better than those of the original 36 items. The 23-item WHQ has been assessed with multinational data to establish the cross-cultural equivalence of linguistically adapted versions. It is subject to on-going assessment in terms of its reproducibility and responsiveness to change over time. We currently suggest that the original WHQ should still be used, with the shorter 23-item WHQ considered as an option for multi-national trials.

The application of the scale has been varied since the questionnaire measures a range of domains from vasomotor symptoms to psychosocial factors, general health, and ageing. It is a valid instrument that can be used in a cross-cultural setting. The scale has been applied not only to women going through the menopause as an outcome measure in clinical trials, but also in epidemiological studies with a population of healthy women. However it should be supplemented with a generic HRQOL measure and questions on the effects of HRT and CAM use so that a comprehensive change in HRQOL for women in pre-, peri-, and post-menopause stage can be obtained.

3.3   Qualifemme

In 1994 the original 32-item Qualifemme instrument was developed in French to measure the effect of menopausal hormone deficiency on the HRQOL of women (Le Floch et al., 1996). The initial items were selected from validated existing instruments such as the WHQ, McCoy Female Sexuality Index, and Nottingham Health Profile. The items were scored using a visual analogue scale (VAS). Item weighting was determined by a group of menopausal experts, thereby adding clinical experience to the instrument. A shorter version of Qualifemme was derived in 1996 that consisted of a 15-item scale (Le Floch et al., 1996). From principal component analyses, four subscales were identified: Climacteric (2 items); Psycho-social (5 items); Somatic (4 items); and Uro-genital (4 items) (❷ Table 151-6). Scales scores are computed by taking the product of the VAS score and weighting and then summing across items in the same scale.

3.3.1   Psychometric Properties

The test-retest reliability was conducted on women who repeated the Qualifemme instrument after four weeks. The correlation coefficients ranged from 0.84 to 0.98. The internal consistency was high as demonstrated by a Cronbach's alpha coefficient of 0.73. The five distinct factors explained 71.8% of the variance.

■ Table 151-6
Characteristics of the Qualifemme instrument

Items	Domains/health concepts	Assessment period	Psychometric properties
Fully phrased statements on symptoms (15 items) (Le Floch et al., 1996)	1. Climacteric (2 items)	At the moment	Reliability
	2. Psycho-social (5 items)		The test-retest correlations ranged from 0.84 to 0.98
	3. Somatic (4 items)		Internal consistency
	4. Uro-genital (4 items)		Cronbach's alpha was 0.73.

The Qualifemme has been used in a multi-centre study in France to compare HRQOL before and after the application of estrodial (Zollner et al., 2005). While it includes some items on the side effects of HRT use, no questions were asked about the use of CAM. This instrument should be supplemented with a generic HRQOL measure, and where appropriate, with additional questions on the effects of HRT and CAM use so that a comprehensive change in HRQOL for women in pre-, peri, and post-menopause stage can be obtained. Again there is an issue with accurately detecting effects since the Qualifemme items refer to current status, while the HRQOL items correspond to the experience over the previous month or 4 weeks.

3.4 Menopause-Specific QOL Questionnaire

In 1996 Canadian researchers published the Menopause-Specific Quality of Life questionnaire (MENQOL) (Hilditch et al., 1996). It was developed using data from women who have been between 2 and 7 years postmenopausal, who had an intact uterus, and who had not been on hormone therapy. Originally women were asked if they had experienced each of 106 menopausal symptoms or problems in the past month and if so to what extent they have been bothered by the symptom or problem (on a 7-point Likert Scale). Using the importance score method, which incorporates both the frequency and the extent that symptoms/problems were bothersome, 76 items were dropped. The resulting 30 items formed four domains: vasomotor (3 items); physical (16 items); psychosocial (7 items) and sexual (3 items), and global quality of life question. Each domain is scored separately in two steps: (1) item scores are recoded so that "not experiencing a symptom/problem" is scored as 1; "experiencing a symptom but not bothered by it" is coded as 2 while "being extremely bothered by the symptom" is coded as 8; and (2) computing scales scores by summing across items in the same scale. Higher scores indicate poorer HRQOL status. As with the WHQ instrument, since no overall score is available the relative contribution of each domain is unknown.

3.4.1 Psychometric Properties

The test-retest reliability was conducted on women who completed the MENQOL on two occasions 1 month apart. The intra-class correlation coefficients between factor scores were: 0.37 (vasomotor domain); 0.55 (quality of life question); 0.7 (sexual domain); 0.79 (psychosocial domain), and 0.81 (physical domain) (Hilditch, 1996). The author attributed systematic change in the vasomotor symptoms for the poor correlation across that domain (Hilditch et al., 1996). The scale has been used widely to measure health related quality of life in postmenopausal mid-aged women.

3.5 Revised MENQOL (MENQOL-Intervention) Questionnaire

In 2005 the MENQOL-intervention, a modified version of MENQOL, was developed to deal with some of the shortcomings of the original instrument such as the poor test-retest reliability of the vasomotor domain and the lack of an overall summary score (Lewis et al., 2005). It also aimed to incorporate both the positive effects of an intervention such as hormone replacement therapy use and any potential side effects. Lewis and colleagues made modifications to the MENQOL instrument by changing the questionnaire format, for example

◻ Table 151-7
Characteristics of the revised MENQOL questionnaire

Items	Domains/health concepts	Assessment period	Psychometric properties
Fully phrased statements on symptoms and feelings (32 items) (Lewis, 2005)	1. Vasomotor (3 items)	In the past month	*Reliability*
	2. Psychosocial (7 items)		The test-retest correlations ranged from 0.73 (Vasomotor) to 0.83 (Sexual).
	3. Physical (19 items)		*Internal consistency*
	4. Sexual (3 items)		Cronbach's alpha ranged from 0.72 (Sexual) to 0.88 (Physical).

wording was shortened in three items (Lewis et al., 2005). The MENQOL-intervention questionnaire also differs from the original questionnaire by asking the women about their experience over the last week as opposed to month (❯ *Table 151-7*).

3.5.1 Psychometric Properties

The MENQOL-Intervention questionnaire demonstrated good domain internal consistency and test-retest reliability. In particular, the intra-class correlation coefficient for the vasomotor domain had improved to 0.73, from 0.37 in the original instrument.

As the MENQOL instrument was developed for use by postmenopausal women, researchers would still need to supplement the questionnaire with a generic HRQOL measure and with additional questions on the effects of CAM use so that a comprehensive change in HRQOL for women in pre-, peri-, and post-menopause stage can be obtained.

3.6 Menopause Rating Scale (MRS)

The MRS was originally published in Germany in 1994 as a 10-item physician-completed questionnaire of menopausal symptoms or complaints (Hauser et al., 1994). A few years later it was converted into a standardized 11-item self-administered instrument (Schneider et al., 2000b). Women were asked to rate the severity of current symptoms experienced and each of the 11 items was assigned "0" (for no complaints) or up to "4" (for severe symptoms). From factor analysis of the items, the MRS creators defined three domains: psychological (4 items), somato-vegetative (4 items), and uro-genital symptoms (3 items) (❯ *Table 151-8*). Scores for each domain were formed by summing across items in the same scale and a global score was calculated as a total of all 11 items. Higher scores indicated poorer HRQOL status.

3.6.1 Psychometric Properties

Test-retest reliability was conducted on women who repeated the MRS questionnaire after eighteen months. The resultant Kappa statistics were low but nevertheless indicated a highly

◘ Table 151-8

Characteristics of the menopause rating scale (MRS)

Items	Domains/health concepts	Assessment period	Psychometric properties
Fully phrased statements on symptoms (11 items) (Heinemann et al., 2004)	1. Psychosocial (4 items)	At the moment	*Reliability*
	2. Somato-vegetative (4 items)		The test-retest correlations ranged from 0.84 (psychological score) to 0.89 (somatic score).
	3. Uro-genital symptoms (3 items)		*Internal consistency*
			Cronbach's alpha ranged from 0.65 (uro-genital score) to 0.87 (psychological score).

significant degree of agreement (p-value <0.001) between the factor scores over the 1.5 years: 0.26 (overall score); 0.25 (somatic symptoms); 0.30 (psychological symptoms); and 0.19 (uro-genital symptoms) (Schneider et al., 2000b). The concurrent validity of scales was assessed by comparison with the Kupperman Index which showed a good correlation, especially when the symptoms experienced tend to be either mild or very severe. The idiosyncratically named somato-vegetative subscale (which comprised of complaints of sweating, hot flushes, sleep problems, heart discomfort, and joint and muscular complaints) correlated with the physical component summary score of SF-36 (−0.48). The psychological factor correlated well with the mental component summary score of SF-36 (−0.73) (Schneider et al., 2000a).

The scale has been widely used to assess the severity of symptoms or complaints in mid-aged women (Heinemann et al., 2003). A recent review of the MRS instrument to evaluate its suitability for use across countries found that scale reliably measures the same phenomenon in women experiencing symptoms (Heinemann et al., 2003). The author found that it was possible to compare scale scores across Europe and North America but cautions against comparison of data from Latin America and Indonesia. While this instrument has the capacity to measure treatment effects, it does not cover all the dimensions of HRQOL or the negative effects of HRT or CAM use.

3.7   Menopausal Quality of Life Scale (MQOL)

A relatively new menopause-specific instrument was developed in 2000 by Jacobs and colleagues on the basis of interviews and focus groups with 61 women. It consists of 48 items which encompassed seven domains: energy (10 items), sleep (3 items), appetite (1 item), cognition (5 items), mood (12 items), social interactions (7 items), and symptom impact (10 items) (Jacobs et al., 2000). Participants rate the extent to which each statement was true using a six-point Likert Scale with responses ranging from "I am never like this" to "I am always like this." Standard scoring methods are applied to obtain an overall score. In addition women were also asked to rate their overall quality of life (GQOL) (❷ *Table 151-9*).

❏ Table 151-9
Characteristics of the menopausal quality of life scale (MQOL)

Items	Domains/health concepts	Assessment period	Psychometric properties
Fully phrased statements on symptoms (48 items) (Jacobs et al., 2000)	1. Energy (10 items)	At the moment	*Reliability*
	2. Sleep (3 items)		Not available
	3. Appetite (1 item)		*Internal consistency*
	4. Cognition (5 items)		Cronbach's alpha ranged from 0.69 (Energy) to 0.91 (Feelings).
	5. Mood (12 items)		
	6. Social interactions (7 items)		
	7. Symptom impact (10 items)		

3.7.1   Psychometric Properties

All items of this scale are highly inter-correlated with Cronbach's alpha ranging from 0.69 to 0.91 for the seven MQOL domains suggesting that the scale has reasonable internal consistency. The GQOL was correlated with each of the MQOL subscales (correlations ranging from 0.29 to 0.63) and with the overall MQOL (0.69). However, the seven domains are not stable as factor analysis on three sub-samples has resulted in different solutions (Jacobs et al., 2000). The domains were also highly correlated which results in multi-collinearity problems when they are used in regression models. This instrument does not cover the side effects of HRT or CAM use.

3.8   MENCAV

MENCAV was the first validated instrument in Spanish to measure HRQOL (Buendia et al., 2008). The scale is designed to measure women's physical, psychological, sexual, and social well-being in peri- and post-menopause. It was originally developed in 2001 and consists of 37-items designed to tap into five domains in peri- and post-menopausal women: physical health (10 items); mental health (9 items), partner relationship (4 items), social support (10 items) and sexual relations (4 items) (❷ *Table 151-10*). Participants rate each item on a 5-point Likert Scale from which scores were transformed into a 1–5 (worst-to-best) scale. Higher scores reflected better HRQOL status in women (Buendia et al., 2001).

3.8.1   Psychometric Properties

The test-retest reliability was conducted on women who completed the MENCAV on two occasions two weeks apart (Buendia et al., 2001). The intra-class correlation coefficients

◘ Table 151-10

Characteristics of the MENCAV scale

Items	Domains/health concepts	Assessment period	Psychometric properties
Fully phrased statements on symptoms and feelings (37 items) (Buendia et al., 2008)	1. Physical health (10 items)	In the past 4 months	*Reliability*
	2. Mental health (9 items)		
	3. Partner relationship (4 items)		The intra-class correlation coefficients ranged from 0.64 (physical health) to 0.75 (for partner relationship).
	4. Social support (10 items)		*Internal consistency*
	5. Sexual relations (4 items)		Cronbach's alpha ranged from 0.71 (sexual relations) to 0.91 (mental health).

between factor scores were: 0.64 (for physical health); 0.70 (for mental health); 0.71 (for sexual health); 0.75 (for partner relationship), and 0.74 (for social relationship).

All items of this scale are highly inter-correlated with Cronbach's alpha ranging from 0.71 to 0.91 for the five domains suggesting that the scale has reasonable internal consistency. The correlation between the total scores for each of the MENCAV dimensions and the assessments made by the experts were: 0.58 (for physical health), 0.76 (for mental health) and 0.87 (for total score). The correlation ranged from 0.28 to 0.47 for the remaining dimensions.

The MENCAV is one of the few instruments to take into account women's social and psychological well-being, as opposed to just symptoms. It is yet to be translated into and adapted to other languages. It may be used in conjunction with a comprehensive menopausal symptoms checklist, and items on the side effects of HRT and CAM use.

4 Conclusion

The last three decades have seen numerous instruments developed to measure HRQOL during menopause. These instruments have evolved, often building on earlier work and then adding or modifying questions to meet specific needs, from simple checklists of symptoms to wide-ranging questions across several domains of psychosocial well-being. Although they all report good psychometric properties that are well documented, there appears to be an ongoing process of development with no single instrument becoming internationally pre-eminent. A further reason for this process to continue is that none have met all the issues raised at the outset of this chapter, such as being appropriate to a representative sample of women from the population and specifically including questions for women with hysterectomy or on HRT. It is hoped that as new scales evolve, these will exhibit a greater degree of convergence and compatibility.

To provide some perspective for the future direction of these instruments, it is worthwhile to recall that while their objective is to measure how the menopausal transition affects

HRQOL, they need to look beyond these very specific research interests so as to be more widely accepted. Hence, researchers should be mindful of needing to cover research questions ranging from investigating changes in HRQOL from before, during and after the menopausal transition, to identifying successful management strategies or comparing the benefits and drawbacks of potential treatment options, such as HRT. Often it is crucial for effective research that it should be possible to place findings in their scientific context, for instance by being compared across populations and age groups. Therefore, at base the menopausal HRQOL instrument *should always comprise* a generic and well established QOL measure, that is complete and unaltered – even if for the sake of brevity it must used be in its short form, such as SF-12 or WHOQOL-BREF (Skevington et al., 2004; Ware et al., 1998). Immediately this provides a standard measure that will permit direct and accurate comparison of HRQOL with pre and postmenopausal women from cross-sectional studies or on a longitudinal basis.

The HRQOL measure can then be made menopause specific through the additional use of a checklist of menopause symptoms selected from one of the well established instruments. There is an added proviso: that ideally the symptoms ought to be assessed with respect to the same time period as the questions used in the HRQOL measure, otherwise any link sought between symptomology and HRQOL is rendered unnecessarily imprecise and uncertain. Hence for SF-12, this would mean that the presence of symptoms would be identified for over the last four weeks, rather than "at the moment" which is more commonly used in most symptom checklists. The questions from the symptoms checklist may then *be augmented with*, but not substituted by, specific questions that researchers wish to address or they feel have been incorrectly omitted. It is here that the instruments can be expanded so that they are appropriate for a representative sample of all women from the population, specifically they should ask about possible side effects of HRT. In another aspect of greater inclusiveness, it is clear that researchers are beginning to focus on the international usage of instruments and the need to design instruments that assess HRQOL in culturally meaningful ways and apply scientifically based methods for linguistic and cultural validation (Albert, 1998). It is also essential to provide guidelines regarding the clinical interpretation of scores and their responsiveness to changes in menopausal status and age to assist others in interpreting any results.

In summary, the perfect instrument for measuring HRQOL for all women during the menopausal transition probably does not exist, but much progress can be made if attention were paid to the essential principles of using generic well established measures of HRQOL and menopausal symptoms, with additional items used in a way that preserves compatibility. This remains a highly worthwhile aspiration, since any findings that derive from a robust, reliable and harmonized instrument, such as identifying a successful management strategy, would provide potentially invaluable information to communicate to women everywhere and help them prepare for this stage of life.

Summary Points

- The experience of menopausal transition has been associated with a wide range of symptoms, including hot flushes and cold night sweats, headaches, muscle and joint pain, anxiety, and depression.
- Menopause transition may occur at a time that is concomitant with other biological, psychological, and social changes which renders it difficult to determine precisely the

influence of menopausal transition on HRQOL over and above the impact of these other factors and life events.
- The instruments to measure HRQOL during menopausal transition range from simple checklists of symptoms to wide-ranging questions across several domains of psychosocial well-being.
- Although the instruments generally report good psychometric properties and some are well documented, there still appears to be an ongoing process of development, with no single instrument being pre-eminent in the field.
- It is recommended that menopausal HRQOL instrument should always include a generic and well established HRQOL measure, which can than be made menopause specific through the additional use of a checklist of menopause symptoms selected from one of the well established instruments.
- The provision of a guideline with regards to the clinical interpretation of the scores and their responsiveness to changes in menopausal status and age would be helpful in interpreting any results.

References

Albert SM. (1998). JAMA. 279(6): 429.

Avis NE, Assmann SF, Kravitz HM, Ganz PA, Ory M. (2004). Qual Life Res. 13(5): 933–946.

Barentsen R, van de Weijer PH, van Gend S, Foekema H. (2001). Maturitas. 38(2): 123–128.

Buendia BJ, Rodriguez SR, Yubero BN, Martinez VV. (2001). Aten Primaria. 27(2): 94–100.

Buendia BJ, Valverde Martinez JA, Romero SA, Ulla Diez SM, Cobo RA, Martinez VV. (2008). Maturitas. 59(1): 28–37.

Cella DF, Bonomi AE. (1995). Oncology (Williston Park). 9(11 Suppl): 47–60.

Fairclough DL. (2002). Design and Analysis of Quality of Life Studies in Clinical Trials. Chapman and Hall/CRC, Boca Raton, FL.

Fayers PM, Machin D. (2000). Quality of Life: Assessment, Analysis and Interpretation. Wiley, Chichester, UK.

Ginsberg J. (1991). BMJ. 302(6788): 1288–1289.

Girod I, de la LC, Keininger D, Hunter MS. (2006). Climacteric. 9(1): 4–12.

Greene JG. (1976). J Psychosom Res. 20(5): 425–430.

Greene JG. (1998). Maturitas. 29(1): 25–31.

Hardy R, Kuh D. (2002). Soc Sci Med. 55(11): 1975–1988.

Hauser GA, Huber IC, Keller PJ, Lauritzen C, Schneider HP. (1994). Zentralbl Gynakol. 116(1): 16–23.

Heinemann LA, DoMinh T, Strelow F, Gerbsch S, Schnitker J, Schneider HP. (2004). Health Qual Life Outcomes. 2: 67.

Heinemann LA, Potthoff P, Schneider HP. (2003). Health Qual Life Outcomes. 1: 28.

Hilditch JR, Lewis J, Peter A, van Maris B, Ross A, Franssen E, Guyatt GH, Norton PG, Dunn E. (1996). Maturitas. 24(3): 161–175.

Hunt S. (2000). Qual Life Res. 9: 709–719.

Hunter MS. (1992). Psychol Health. 7: 45–54.

Hunter MS. (2000). Qual Life Res. 9: 733–738.

Hunter MS. (2003). Health Qual Life Outcomes. 1: 41.

Jacobs PA, Hyland ME, Ley A. (2000). Br J Health Psychol. 5: 395–411.

Kaufert P, Syrotuik J. (1981). Soc Sci Med [E]. 15(3): 173–184.

Kuh DL, Wadsworth M, Hardy R. (1997). Br J Obstet Gynaecol. 104(8): 923–933.

Kumari M, Stafford M, Marmot M. (2005). J Clin Epidemiol. 58(7): 719–727.

Le Floch JP, Colau JC, Zartarian M, Gelas B. (1996). Contracept Fertil Sex. 24(3): 238–245.

Lewis JE, Hilditch JR, Wong CJ. (2005). Maturitas. 50(3): 209–221.

Lin TH. (2006). Pharmacoeconomics. 24(9): 917–925.

McHorney CA, Ware JE Jr., Lu JF, Sherbourne CD. (1994). Med Care. 32(1): 40–66.

McKinlay SM, Brambilla DJ, Posner JG. (1992). Maturitas. 14(2): 103–115.

Mishra G, Kuh D. (2006). Soc Sci Med. 62(1): 93–102.

Mishra GD, Brown WJ, Dobson AJ. (2003). Qual Life Res. 12(4): 405–412.

Neugarten BL, Kraines RJ. (1965). Psychosom Med. 27: 266–273.

Rose MS, Koshman ML, Spreng S, Sheldon R. (1999). J Clin Epidemiol. 52(5): 405–412.

Schneider HP, Heinemann LA, Rosemeier HP, Potthoff P, Behre HM. (2000a). Climacteric. 3(1): 50–58.

Schneider HP, Heinemann LA, Rosemeier HP, Potthoff P, Behre HM. (2000b). Climacteric. 3(1): 59–64.

Skevington SM, Lotfy M, O'Connell KA. (2004). Qual Life Res. 13(2): 299–310.

The WHOQOL Group. (1998). Psychol Med. 28(3): 551–558.

Ulrich LG, Barlow DH, Sturdee DW, Wells M, Campbell MJ, Nielsen B, Bragg AJ, Vessey MP. (1997). Int J Gynaecol Obstet. 59(Suppl 1): S11–S17.

Utian WH. (2007). Maturitas. 57(1): 100–102.

Utian WH, Janata JW, Kingsberg SA, Schluchter M, Hamilton JC. (2002). Menopause. 9(6): 402–410.

van Noord PA, Dubas JS, Dorland M, Boersma H, te Velde ER. (1997). Fertil Steril. 68(1): 95–102.

Ware JE, Kosinski M, Keller SD. (1998). SF-12: How to Score the SF-12 Physical and Mental Health Summary Scales. Quality Metric Inc, Lincoln, RI.

Ware JE Jr., Sherbourne CD. (1992). Med Care. 30(6): 473–483.

Ware JJ, Snow KK, Kosinski M, Gandek B. (1993). SF-36 Manual and Interpretation Guide. The Health Institute, New England Medical Center, Boston, MA.

Wilson IB, Cleary PD. (1995). JAMA. 273(1): 59–65.

Zapantis G, Santoro N. (2003). Best Pract Res Clin Endocrinol Metab. 17(1): 33–52.

Zollner YF, Acquadro C, Schaefer M. (2005). Qual Life Res. 14(2): 309–327.

152 Low Testosterone Level in Men and Quality of Life

S. Horie

1   Introduction 2616

2   Male Hypogonadism: Low T Levels 2616

3   Biochemistry of T 2618

4   Diagnosis of Male Hypogonadism 2619

5   Late Onset Hypogonadism 2620

6   Morbidities and Mortality Associated with Low T Levels 2622

7   Low Levels of Testosterone and Health-Related Quality of Life 2624

8   The Aging Males' Symptoms Scale (AMS) 2626

    Summary Points 2629

Abstract: The concept of age-related ❷ androgen deficiency in men, also termed ❷ late-onset hypogonadism (LOH), has opened up public awareness about men's health issues. Low testosterone levels can lead to depressed mood, sexual dysfunction, cognitive impairment, osteoporosis, cardiovascular disease, and metabolic syndrome. Low testosterone levels also affect health-related quality of life (QOL), impacting physical, social, emotional, cognitive, and sexual functioning. Use of generic questionnaires such as the Short-Form 36-Item Health Survey likely underestimates the impact of low testosterone levels on QOL. Other QOL scales that assess cognitive impact, sexual functioning, or body appearance need to be considered when assessing men with low testosterone levels. The ❷ Aging Males' Symptoms scale is the most frequently used scale to measure health-related QOL in aging males. Evidence points toward a high reliability and high validity of this scale to measure and to compare HRQOL of aging males.

List of Abbreviations: *ACTH,* adrenocorticotropine hormone; *AMS,* aging males' symptoms; *DHEA,* dehydroepiandrosterone; *DHT,* dihydrotestosterone; *FSH,* follicle-stimulating hormone; *GnRH,* gonadotropin-releasing hormone; *HRQOL,* health-related quality of life; *HSQ,* Health Status Questionnaire; *LF,* luteinizing hormone; *LOH,* late-onset hypogonadism; *QOL,* quality of life; *SF-12,* Short-Form 12-Item Health Survey; *SF-36,* Short-Form 36-Item Health Survey; *SHBG,* ❷ sex hormone binding globulin; *T,* testosterone

1   Introduction

Testosterone (T) and its metabolites play a crucial role in the health and development of males. During puberty, T is required for the development of male secondary sexual characteristics, stimulation of sexual behavior and function, and initiation of sperm production. In adult males, T is involved in maintaining muscle mass and strength, fat distribution, bone mass, red blood cell production, male hair pattern, libido and potency, and spermatogenesis (Bagatell et al., 1996) (❷ *Table 152-1*). Thus, decreasing levels of T cause symptoms that include sexual dysfunction, cognitive impairment, decreased energy, depressed mood, increased fat mass, muscle wasting (sarcopenia), anemia, and reduced bone mineral density (Bhasin et al., 2006) Low levels of T can also have an impact on physical, social, emotional, cognitive, and sexual functioning (Novak et al., 2002), all of which are key components of health-related quality of life (HRQOL) (Ware et al., 1992).

2   Male Hypogonadism: Low T Levels

The term *hypogonadism* is defined as the state of inadequate gonadal function, as manifested by deficiencies of T. ❷ Male hypogonadism has been categorized as *primary* or *secondary* (also termed *central*) based on the source of the disorder. Primary (hypergonadotropic) hypogonadism refers to testicular disorders and is characterized by low serum T despite high levels of follicle-stimulating hormone (FSH) and luteinizing hormone (LH). Causes of primary hypogonadism include genetic conditions, anatomic defects, infection, tumor, injury, and iatrogenic causes (surgery or certain medications). The most common genetic disorder resulting in primary hypogonadism in men is Klinefelter's syndrome, in which there is an extra sex chromosome, XXY. Secondary (hypogonadotropic) hypogonadism denotes a deficient release

◼ Table 152-1

Androgen target tissues

Testosterone
Brain
Bone
Pituitary
Kidney
Muscle
Submaxillary glands
Dihydrotestosterone
Germinal epithelium
Epididymus
Vas deferens
Prostate
Penis
Hair follicles
Sebaceous glands

This table lists the target tissues of androgen. Androgenic activity is mediated by testosterone (T) itself in certain tissues and primarily by dihydrotestosterone in others. In adult males, T is involved in maintaining muscle mass and strength, fat distribution, bone mass, red blood cell production, male hair pattern, libido and potency, and spermatogenesis

of gonadotropin-releasing hormone (GnRH) and is characterized by low–normal or low levels of FSH, LH, and T. Causes or manifestations of secondary hypogonadism include hyperprolactinemia (often secondary to pituitary adenoma), GnRH deficiency with anosmia (Kallmann syndrome), hypothalamic lesions or disorders, and pituitary lesions or disorders. Normogonadotropic hypogonadism denotes symptoms or signs of hypogonadism together with low serum T and normal LH levels. Conditions that may be associated with this type of hypogonadism include aging, type II diabetes mellitus, cancer, acquired immunodeficiency syndrome, liver cirrhosis, renal failure, hyperthyroidism or hypothyroidism, Cushing syndrome, protein-calorie malnutrition (and anorexia nervosa), morbid obesity and Parkinson's disease, as well as certain psychiatric disorders, including depressive disorders (Morley et al., 1979) (❷ *Table 152-2*).

In the aging population, T levels decrease but rarely to the levels seen in primary hypogonadism in young men. This decrease with age is associated with only a small increase in LH, except late in life (Morley et al., 1997). The prevalence of this type of hypogonadism has been estimated to be between 2 and 5% at 40 years of age and 30 and 70% by 70 years of age (Morley et al., 2003). With aging, there is a decrease in Leydig cells and the testicular response to stimulation with human chorionic gonadotropin. The negative feedback of T at the pituitary level increases with aging. There is a decreased pulse generation of GnRH. It is the combination of these factors that leads to the age-related decline in T levels. In men, LH and T are secreted in a pulsatile manner every 60–90 min in a diurnal rhythm, with peak levels occurring in the morning.

◘ Table 152-2

Major primary and secondary causes of hypogonadism

Primary
Klinefelter's syndrome
Mumps orchitis
Testicular trauma
Surgical disruption of testicular blood supply (e.g. Repair of inguinal hernia)
Irradiation of the testes
Cancer chemotherapy
Excessive heat
Malnutrition
Sickle cell disease
Secondary
Pituitary or hypothalamic tumor
Pituitary ablation secondary to surgery or radiation treatment
Hyperprolactinemia
Tumor of the adrenals or testes
Obesity
Hypothyroidism
Hemochromatosis
Primary or secondary
Hypercortisolemia
Occupational cause
Uremia
AIDS
Hepatic cirrhosis
Systemic illness
Medications

Hypogonadism is most frequently due to failure of testicular function (primary hypogonadism), usually involving the Leidig cells, but may also be due to failure of pituitary or hypothalamic function (secondary hypogonadism), or a combination of both

3   Biochemistry of T

The synthesis of T in men occurs primarily in the Leydig cells of the testes, with a small percentage produced in the adrenal cortex. T is synthesized through a series of five enzymatic reactions that convert cholesterol to T. The hypothalamus secretes GnRH, which stimulates the pituitary to secrete LH and FSH. In men, LH stimulates Leydig cells to produce T, and FSH acts on Sertoli cells, stimulating spermatogenesis. T can act directly on target cells, or it can be converted into its primary metabolites, dihydrotestosterone (DHT) and estradiol. Both T and DHT bind to the androgen receptor, but DHT has a higher affinity for the receptor and is therefore a more potent androgen. The 5α-reductase enzymes, which convert T to DHT, are

❏ Figure 152-1

Testosterone in the serum. Approximately 98% of T circulates in the blood bound to protein, of which approximately 60% is bound weakly to albumin and other proteins and 40% is bound with higher binding affinity to sex hormone binding globulin (SHBG)

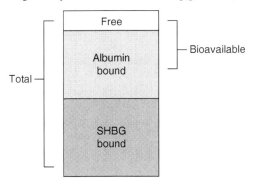

most abundant in prostate, skin, and reproductive tissues. The aromatase enzyme complex, which converts T to estradiol, an estrogen, is most abundant in adipose tissue, liver, and certain central nervous system nuclei (Mooradian et al., 1987). Approximately 98% of T circulates in the blood bound to protein, of which approximately 60% is bound weakly to albumin and other proteins and 40% is bound with higher binding affinity to sex hormone binding globulin (SHBG) (❷ *Figure 152-1*) (Bhasin et al., 1998). The remaining 2% is free or unbound. Because T bound to albumin is biologically available due to rapid dissociation, the fraction available to the tissues (also termed bioavailable T) is believed to be the free plus the albumin-bound T, consisting of approximately half of the total plasma T. Total T is generally measured by radioimmunoassay, which is a validated, standardized, and reproducible assay. However, because the level of the high-affinity binding protein SHBG increases with age (and therefore a greater percentage of the total T is bound to SHBG and is not available to the tissues), measuring total T may not be as useful in studies of aging populations. Bioavailable T can be calculated using measures of total T and immunoassayed SHBG concentrations. Free T can also be calculated using measurements of total T, albumin, and SHBG concentrations (Vermeulen et al., 1999). Salivary T measured by liquid chromatography mass spectrometry or enzyme-linked immunosorbent assay is a non-invasive, reliable substitute for serum calculating free or bioavailable T (Yasuda et al., 2008a). The reliability, precision, accuracy and analytical recovery of immunoassays designed to measure salivary T are now well documented, although salivary T levels are sensitive to the effects of blood leakage into the oral mucosa caused by microinjury.

4   Diagnosis of Male Hypogonadism

Male hypogonadism is diagnosed easily when the usual signs and symptoms of androgen deficiency are present or when the patient has a history of a predisposing condition (e.g., mumps orchitis, orchiectomy, radiation to the pelvis or head). Many studies have used the 300–350 ng/dL range of total T as a cutoff for identifying hypogonadal patients, although there is no clearly defined standard, and other factors such as SHBG, LH and FSH levels and the clinical presentation and physical findings are key in making a diagnosis of hypogonadism. The guidelines from a collaboration of the International Society of Andrology, the International Society for the Study of the Aging Male, and the European Association of Urology (Nieschlag et al., 2005) suggest that a diagnosis should be made only in men with signs and symptoms characteristic of hypogonadism and biochemical evidence of low serum T. The report of the Endocrine Society's Second Annual Andropause Consensus Meeting delineated three categories for consideration in screening and diagnosing hypogonadism in men older than 50 years: (1) total T less than or equal to 200 ng/dL: "diagnosis of androgen deficiency is confirmed. Rule out serious hypothalamic or pituitary disease in men with ❷ hypogonadotropic hypogonadism" prior to initiating T therapy; (2) total T levels greater than 200 but less than 400 ng/dL: recommend additional measures of T and further evaluation before considering T therapy; and (3) total T levels greater than 400 ng/dL: considered not to have T deficiency. Reference values for serum androgens are derived from serum levels in young men, because it is difficult to define normal values in elderly men owing to interactions between the effects of physiological aging and pathological processes that could have negative effects on androgen levels. In healthy, young eugonadal men, serum T levels range from 300 to 1050 ng/dL. Several lines of evidence show that T levels decline with age, particularly after 50 years (❷ *Figure 152-2*) (Morley et al., 1997; Harman et al., 2001; Snyder, 2001; Rhoden et al., 2004). Using a serum T level <325 ng/dL, the Baltimore Longitudinal Study of Aging reported that approximately 12, 20, 30 and 50% of men in their 50s, 60s, 70s and 80s, respectively, are hypogonadal (Harman et al., 2001) (❷ *Figure 152-3*). Longitudinal and cross-sectional studies have demonstrated annual T decrements of 0.5–2% with advancing age (Morley et al., 1997; Snyder, 2001; Vermeulen, 2001; Araujo et al., 2004). In the Baltimore Longitudinal Study of Aging, the average decline was 3.2 ng/dL per year among men age 53 years at entry (Harman et al., 2001). As for the prevalence of hypogonadism in the aging population, the Massachusetts Male Aging Study reported a prevalence of 12% at follow-up and an incidence of 12.3 per person-years (Araujo et al., 2004). The Hypogonadism in Males study, using a threshold level of <300 ng/dL, estimated a prevalence of 38.7% in men aged 45 years or older (Mulligan et al., 2006). Unlike the sharp, universal decreases in hormone levels observed in women with menopause, declines in circulating androgens in men with advancing age are gradual and variable. There is a progressive reduction in hypothalamic-pituitary-gonadal function in aging men; hence, serum T levels decline through both central (pituitary) and peripheral (testicular) mechanism (Seidman, 2003).

5   Late Onset Hypogonadism

The concept of age-related androgen deficiency in men, also termed late onset hypogonadism (LOH), has opened up public awareness to men's health issues. A joint statement from the International Society of Andrology, the International Society for the Study of the Aging Male, and the European Association of Urology defines LOH as "a clinical and biochemical syndrome associated with advancing age that is characterized by typical symptoms and a deficiency in serum testosterone levels that may result in significant detriment in the quality of life and adversely affect the function of multiple organ systems." Low T levels affect physical, mental, and sexual activities, manifesting as a loss of muscle mass and bone strength, increased body fat, decreased energy, less interest in sex, erectile dysfunction, irritability, and depression

◻ Figure 152-2

Longitudinal effects of aging on date-adjusted T and free T index. Linear segment plots for total T and free T index vs. age are shown for men with T and SHBG values on at least two visits. Each linear segment has a slope equal to the mean of the individual longitudinal slopes in each decade, and is centered on the median age, for each cohort of men from the second to the ninth decade. *Numbers in parentheses* represent the number of men in each cohort. With the exception of free T index in the ninth decade, segments show significant downward progression at every age, with no significant change in slopes for T or free T index over the entire age range. Reproduced from Harman et al. (2001) with permission

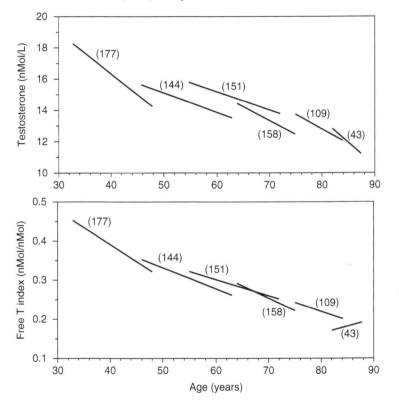

(Nieschlag et al., 2005). LOH is frequently reported as the result of an age-related decline in free and bio-available T. However, cross-cultural studies have shown that the pattern of age-related decline in male free T, as represented by salivary levels, is not a uniform characteristic of all populations. Indeed age patterns of T decline vary between populations representing different geographical, ecological, and cultural settings (Ellison et al., 2002). Middle-aged Japanese men had the lowest levels of salivary T compared with younger and older generations, presumably reflecting that middle-aged group had been exposed to the higher stress than younger and older groups in their working environment (Yasuda et al., 2007). The etiology of LOH is a complex matter involving cultural and socio-environmental issues as well as individual biological changes.

◘ Figure 152-3

Hypogonadism in aging men. *Bar height* indicates the percent of men in each 10-yr interval, from the third to the ninth decades, with at least one T value in the hypogonadal range, by the criteria of total T,11.3 nmol/L (325 ng/dL) (*shaded bars*), or T/SHBG (free T index), 0.153 nmol/nmol (*striped bars*). *Numbers above each pair of bars* indicate the number of men studied in the corresponding decade. The fraction of men who are hypogonadal increases progressively after age 50 by either criterion. More men are hypogonadal by free T index than by total T after age 50, and there seems to be a progressively greater difference, with increasing age, between the two criteria. Reproduced from Harman et al., (2001) with permission

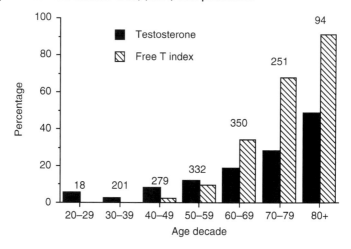

6   Morbidities and Mortality Associated with Low T Levels

Hypogonadism is associated with increased risk for mortality. A US study of men older than 40 years found that men with normal T levels (i.e., total T level of >250 ng/dL or 8.7 nmol/L) had a mortality rate of 20% compared with a rate of 35% in men with low T levels (mean follow-up was 4.30 years) (Shores et al., 2006). The association between low T levels and increased mortality was significant even after adjusting for age, comorbidity, and other clinical factors (Shores et al., 2006). In a prospective, population-based study, men whose total T levels were in the lowest quartile (<241 ng/dL) were 40% more likely to die than those with higher levels, independent of age, adiposity, and lifestyle. The low T-mortality association was also independent of the presence of metabolic syndrome, diabetes, and cardiovascular disease. In cause-specific analyses, low T predicted an increased risk of cardiovascular and respiratory disease mortality (Laughlin et al., 2008). Decreases in T levels or LOH can lead to depressed mood, sexual dysfunction, cognitive impairment, osteoporosis, cardiovascular disease, and metabolic syndrome (Nieschlag et al., 2005; Bhasin et al., 2006) (❷ *Table 152-3*). Depressed mood is a symptom often associated with hypogonadism, and T treatment has been shown to improve mood (Wang et al., 2004). A recent US study estimated a 2-year incidence of diagnosed depression of 21.7% for hypogonadal men and 7.1% for the control group (P = 0.01) (Shores et al., 2004). The study also found that as the severity of hypogonadism increased, so did the incidence of depression. In the Rancho Bernardo Study, depression rating scales were inversely related to bioavailable T levels irrespective of age, physical activity, or alterations in body weight (Barrett-Connor et al., 1999).

◻ Table 152-3

Key Features of late onset hypogonadism (LOH)

Decreased sex drive/libido
Erectile dysfunction
Loss of ejaculation
Infertility
Increased irritability
Decreased attention span
Depression
Reduced muscle mass and strength
Fatigue
Decreased bone mineral density
Less axillary and pubic hair
Reduced frequency of shaving
Small, soft testes
Gynecomastia
Vasomotor instability/hot flushes
Memory loss
Decline in well-being

Common symptoms of LOH are sexual dysfunction, cognitive impairment, decreased energy, depressed mood, increased fat mass, muscle wasting, anemia, and reduced bone mineral density

T appears to play a role in maintaining sexual function, especially libido, although androgen deficiency per se is infrequently the sole cause of erectile dysfunction in hypogonadal males, particularly elderly men (Vermeulen, 2001). Testosterone treatment has been shown to improve libido, sexual activity, nocturnal erections, sexual thoughts, and sexual satisfaction. It has been suggested that response to treatment may be correlated with severity of hypogonadism. In a recent study of androgen-deficient patients undergoing T replacement, reduced libido and lack of motivation and/or energy recurred when T reached approximately 280 ng/dL in patients with secondary (hypogonadotropic) hypogonadism and 337 ng/dL in patients with primary (hypergonadotropic) hypogonadism (Kelleher et al., 2004).

Cognitive performance, including mental-rotation tasks, is related to androgen levels across the normal range in healthy volunteers (Hooven et al., 2004). Low bioavailable T levels are correlated with poor cognition, especially visuospatial cognition (Moffat et al., 2002).

Male hypogonadism may also have cardiovascular and metabolic implications (Khaw et al., 2007). In the recent study on the prospective relationship between endogenous T concentrations and mortality due to all causes, cardiovascular disease and cancer, endogenous T concentrations are inversely related to mortality due to cardiovascular disease and all causes. Low T is associated with a number of cardiovascular risk factors, including increased body fat, insulin resistance, low levels of high-density lipoprotein, high cholesterol levels, and high levels of low-density lipoprotein (Shabsigh et al., 2005). Recent evidence suggests that hypogonadism is associated with metabolic syndrome (Kupelian et al., 2006), which is characterized by central obesity, insulin dysregulation, abnormal lipid profile, and borderline or overt hypertension. However, it is unknown whether metabolic syndrome is a cause of T deficiency or a consequence of it. The oxidative stress that occurs with hypogonadism may be a possible link between the decrease in T levels and the occurrence of metabolic syndrome and cardiovascular disease. Horie and his group showed that there was a weak inverse association between oxidative stress and salivary T levels in volunteers (Yasuda et al., 2008b). Moreover, T may serve as an antioxidant in vascular injury by stimulating endothelial replication and inducing endothelium-dependent vascular relaxation. Although it is not clear that the increased risk of cardiovascular disease and diabetes in patients with hypogonadism can be modified by T treatment, T treatment has demonstrated positive effects in the treatment of men with existing cardiovascular disease and has shown some beneficial effects on a number of the components of metabolic syndrome (Nieschlag et al., 2004).

7   Low Levels of Testosterone and Health-Related Quality of Life

Health-related quality of life (HRQOL) is a complex and abstract concept that includes physical, psychologic, social and other domains of functioning specific to a given health condition. It focuses on the ways in which a disease modifies the happiness and satisfaction of an individual. It generally has several domains, including symptoms, function, emotional stability, social functioning, and general satisfaction with life. In the case of male hypogonadism, decreased energy levels and impaired sexual performance appear to be the most important QOL areas. The negative impact of hypogonadism has on sexual function, energy levels, body composition, mood, and cognitive function is likely to affect QOL adversely. Recent investigations into the differences in QOL between men with hypogonadism and those without collected data from 24 men aged older than 50 years with low T levels (<200 pmol/L) and 24 age-matched controls. Differences in physical symptoms and vitality between the two groups were demonstrated, but no notable differences in mental health were seen (Finas et al., 2006). The study used the Short-Form 12-Item Health Survey (SF-12) and the psychological well-being and vitality components of the Short-Form 36-Item Health Survey (SF-36) as the measure of QOL. Horie and associates showed that middle-aged Japanese men had the lowest levels of salivary T and the worst QOL scores in relation to body pain, which may affect their overall QOL (Yasuda et al., 2007) (❷ *Figure 152-4*). Stress and other conditions that elevate circulating adrenocorticotropine hormone (ACTH) and cortisol levels lead to depressed T levels in men (Roy et al., 2003). A study also shows significant associations between salivary T levels and vitality on the SF-36 in healthy volunteers (Yasuda et al., 2008b). One study showed that decreased energy levels and impaired sexual function caused by the decrease in T have the greatest negative impact on QOL (Novak et al., 2002). The study identified seven key domains such as energy, emotional, social, social emotional, mental functioning, physical functioning and sexual functioning that should be included when assessing the impact of low T levels on QOL in elderly men. Further evidence of the effects of androgen deficiency on QOL comes from a study in men undergoing androgen deprivation therapy for prostate cancer (Potosky et al., 2001). Using the SF-36, the HRQOL was low after androgen deprivation therapy. The vitality domain scores of this questionnaire were particularly low along with the physical domain scores, which confirm that lack of energy is a particular issue in the QOL of men with low T levels (Yasuda et al., 2008b) (❷ *Figure 152-5* and ❷ *Table 152-4*).

◘ Figure 152-4

Decreased level of salivary testosterone in 40s–50s population in Japan. Salivary testosterone was measured in three age cohorts of adult Japanese men: 20s–30s, 40s–50s, and 60s+. Saliva samples were collected at 2-h intervals between 9:00 A.M. and 9:00 P.M. The mean salivary testosterone levels in the 40s–50s cohort were the lowest at almost every time-point among the healthy cohorts. Modified from Yasuda et al. (2008) with permission

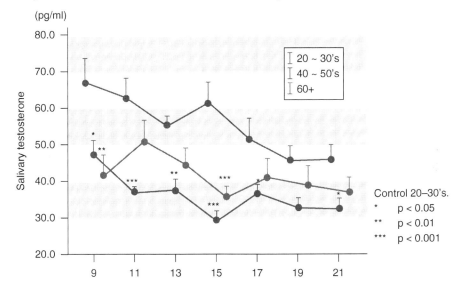

The effects of T replacement on HRQOL were examined in clinical studies (Nair et al., 2006; Emmelot-Vonk et al., 2008). A 2-year, placebo-controlled, randomized, double-blind study involving 87 elderly men with low levels of the sulfated form of dehydroepiandrosterone (DHEA) and bioavailable T used the Health Status Questionnaire (HSQ) to evaluate subjects' quality of life (Nair et al., 2006). The HSQ adds 3 questions to the SF-36 to provide a further assessment of emotional function. Subjects in the DHEA and T groups had no significant change in scores on the Physical Component Scale and the Mental Component Scale of the HSQ. Another double-blind, randomized, placebo-controlled trial of 237 healthy men between the ages of 60 and 80 years with a T level lower than 13.7 nmol/L was conducted in the Netherlands (Emmelot-Vonk et al., 2008). Participants were randomly assigned to receive 80 mg of T undecenoate or a matching placebo twice daily for 6 months. Evaluation of quality of life included SF-36 and the Questions on Life Satisfaction Modules. The Questions on Life Satisfaction Modules is a questionnaire translated from the *Fragen zur Lebenszufriedenheit* questionnaire according to the method described by Huber et al (Huber et al., 1988). The questionnaire is extended with a module on hypopituitarism (Herschbach et al., 2001) and divided in a general section, a health section, and a hormone section – the first two sections include eight items and the last section includes 16 items (resilience or ability to tolerate stress, body shape, self-confidence, ability to become sexually aroused, concentration, physical stamina, initiative or drive, ability to cope with your own anger, ability to tolerate noise and disturbance, weight, body size, sleep, self-control, memory or clear thinking, ability

■ Figure 152-5

The comparison of healthy middle-aged men and LOH patients. LOH patients had significantly lower testosterone levels than the healthy 40s–50s cohort at 11 A.M. (P = 0.016), 7 P.M. (P = 0.024) and 9 P.M. (P = 0.029) (*p < 0.05). In LOH patients, there was no circadian rhythm (Hotteling's Trace = 6.131, F = 3.061, P = 0.19). Modified from Yasuda et al. (2008) with permission

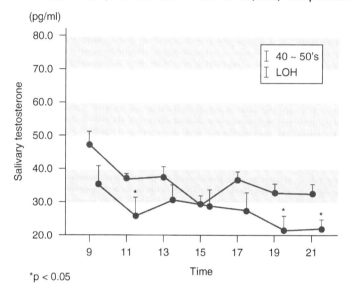

to relax, and social contacts). In that study, scores on the SF-36 did not improve with the use of androgen supplements. However, the Questions on Life Satisfaction Modules, a questionnaire developed to measure hormone deficiency-dependent QOL, showed modest beneficial results, especially on the item "resilience or ability to tolerate stress". These results raise the issue that use of generic questionnaires such as the SF-36 likely underestimate the impact of low T has on quality of life as they only cover specific domains (physical, emotional, and social) and do not include items such as cognitive impact, sexual functioning or body appearance, which are likely to be important determinants of HRQOL in this patient group. The limitation of using general questionnaires prompted the creation of more specific HRQOL scales to assess men with low T levels.

8   The Aging Males' Symptoms Scale (AMS)

Currently, the Aging Males' Symptoms (AMS) scale is the most frequently used scale to measure HRQOL in aging males ❷ Table 152-5 (Kratzik et al., 2005). The scale was designed and standardized as self-administered scale to (1) to assess symptoms of aging (independent from those which are disease-related) between groups of males under different conditions, (2) to evaluate the severity of symptoms over time, and (3) to measure changes pre- and post androgen replacement therapy. The development of the scale started with a listing of symptoms/complaints and a comparison of more than 200 variables in more than 100 medically

■ Table 152-4

Scores from the Short-Form 36-Item Health Survey (SF-36) for the 40s–50s cohort and the late-onset hypogonadism (LOH) patients

	Physical function	Role-physical	Body-pain	General health	Vitality	Social function	Role-emotional	Mental health
40'–50'	54.84 ± 2.79	55.11 ± 3.03	51.13 ± 7.39	52.54 ± 10.07	55.88 ± 6.40	51.62 ± 8.33	54.97 ± 2.19	53.32 ± 7.56
LOH	45.25 ± 7.56	37.77** ± 10.63	40.55** ± 7.24	35.42** ± 4.38	35.12** ± 7.92	32.43** ± 11.94	32.83** ± 16.26	39.37** ± 6.83

The scores for each domain of SF-36 v2 were significantly lower in LOH patients than in the 40s–50s cohort. Values given are Means ± SD

*P < 0.01, **P < 0.001 (Yasuda et al., 2008 with permission)

◻ **Table 152-5**

AMS Questionnaire

	none	mild	moderate	severe	extremely severe
Which of the following symptoms apply to you at this time? Please, mark the appropriate box for each symptom. For symptoms that do not apply, please mark "none".					
Symptoms: Score =	1	2	3	4	5
1. **Decline in your feeling of general well-being** (general state of health, subjective feeling)	☐	☐	☐	☐	☐
2. **Joint pain and muscular ache** (lower back pain, joint pain, pain in a limb, general back ache)	☐	☐	☐	☐	☐
3. **Excessive sweating** (unexpected/sudden episodes of sweating, hot flushes independent of strain)	☐	☐	☐	☐	☐
4. **Sleep problems** (difficulty in falling asleep, difficulty in sleeping through, waking up early and feeling tired, poor sleep, sleeplessness)	☐	☐	☐	☐	☐
5. **Increased need for sleep, often feeling tired**	☐	☐	☐	☐	☐
6. **Irritability** (feeling aggressive, easily upset about little things, moody)	☐	☐	☐	☐	☐
7. **Nervousness** (inner tension, restlessness, feeling fidgety)	☐	☐	☐	☐	☐
8. **Anxiety** (feeling panicky)	☐	☐	☐	☐	☐
9. **Physical exhaustion / lacking vitality** (general decrease in performance, reduced activity, lacking interest in leisure activities, feeling of getting less done, of achieving less, of having to force oneself to undertake activities)	☐	☐	☐	☐	☐
10. **Decrease in muscular strength** (feeling of weakness)	☐	☐	☐	☐	☐
11. **Depressive mood** (feeling down, sad, on the verge of tears, lack of drive, mood swings, feeling nothing is of any use)	☐	☐	☐	☐	☐
12. **Feeling that you have passed your peak**	☐	☐	☐	☐	☐
13. **Feeling burnt out, having hit rock-bottom**	☐	☐	☐	☐	☐
14. **Decrease in beard growth**	☐	☐	☐	☐	☐
15. **Decrease in ability/frequency to perform sexually**	☐	☐	☐	☐	☐
16. **Decrease in the number of morning erections**	☐	☐	☐	☐	☐
17. **Decrease in sexual desire/libido** (lacking pleasure in sex, lacking desire for sexual intercourse)	☐	☐	☐	☐	☐
Have you got any other major symptoms? Yes ☐ No ☐ If Yes, please describe: _____					

Severity of complaints: Scores: 17–26: No complaints; 27–36: few complaints; 37–49: moderate complaints; ≥50: severe complaints

well characterized males (older than 40 years). A factorial analysis was applied to establish the raw scale of complaints or symptoms that are not particularly related to diseases, treatment, social and other variables, but related to aging. Statistical methods were used to identify the dimensions of the scale and to reduce the number of items of the raw scale. Finally, 3 dimensions of symptoms/complaints were identified in the patient groups: a psychological, a somato-vegetative and a sexual factor that explained 51.6% of the total variance. The number of items of the scale was then reduced to 17. This final scale was applied to a large representative population sample of 992 German males to establish reference values for the severity of symptoms in males older than 40 years. International research during the recent years has contributed to the development of the AMS scale as a patient-reported outcome scale used in clinical studies in all age groups of men. Severity of complaints can be assessed by the total scores: Scores: 17–26: No complaints; 27–36: few complaints; 37–49: moderate complaints; 50: severe complaints.

Meanwhile, the AMS scale was internationally well accepted; it is now available in 21 languages (Heinemann et al., 2003), and can be downloaded from the internet at http:// www.aging-males-symptom-scale.info.

❯ *Figure 152-6* shows the effect of androgen supplementation on the scores of AMS for patients with LOH. The markedly altered HRQOL in androgen-deficient males shifted toward the "norm" of the male population after androgen treatment.

The currently available methodological evidence points toward a high reliability and high validity of the AMS scale to measure and to compare HRQOL of aging males over time or before/after treatment with androgen replacement therapy (Heinemann et al., 2006).

◻ Figure 152-6

The effect of androgen supplementation on the scores of the Aging Males'f Symptoms (AMS) for patients with late-onset hypogonadism (LOH). The markedly increased AMS scores in androgen-deficient males shifted toward the "norm" of the male population after androgen treatment (Horie, unpublished observation). Severity of complaints: Scores: 17–26: No complaints; 27–36: few complaints; 37–49: moderate complaints; 50: severe complaints

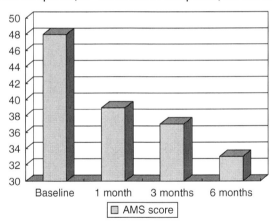

Summary Points

- Hypogonadism, the condition of low testosterone level in men, is associated with significant morbidities and has a negative impact on HRQOL.
- Decreased energy levels and impaired sexual performance appear to be the most important QOL areas in patients with low T levels.
- The negative impact of hypogonadism on sexual function, energy levels, body composition, mood and cognitive function is likely to adversely affect QOL.

- Currently, the AMS scale is the most frequently used scale to measure HRQOL in aging males.
- The AMS scale was designed and standardized as self-administered scale (1) to assess symptoms of aging, (2) to evaluate the severity of symptoms over time, and (3) to measure changes pre- and post androgen replacement therapy.
- Future studies that specifically address the burden that decreased level of T have on HRQOL using specific health-related questionnaires in adult men are needed.

References

Araujo AB, O'Donnell AB, Brambilla DJ, Simpson WB, Longcope C, Matsumoto AM, McKinlay JB. (2004). J Clin Endocrinol Metab. 89: 5920–5926.

Bagatell CJ, Bremner WJ. (1996). N Engl J Med. 334: 707–714.

Barrett-Connor E, Von-Muhlen DG, Kritz-Silverstein D. (1999). J Clin Endocrinol Metab. 84: 573–577.

Bhasin S, Bagatell CJ, Bremner WJ, Plymate SR, Tenover JL, Korenman SG, Nieschlag E. (1998). J Clin Endo Metab. 83: 3435–3448.

Bhasin S, Cunningham GR, Hayes FJ, Matsumoto AM, Snyder PJ, Swerdloff RS, Montori VM. (1006). Clin Endocrinol Metab. 91: 1995–2010.

Ellison PT, Bribiescas RG, Bentley GR, Campbell BC, Lipson SF, Panter-Brick C, Hill K. (2002). Hum Reprod. 17: 3251–3253.

Emmelot-Vonk MH, Verhaar HJ, Nakhai Pour HR, Aleman A, Lock TM, Bosch JL, Grobbee DE, van der Schouw YT. (2008). JAMA. 299: 39–52.

Finas D, Bals-Pratsch M, Sandmann J, Eichenauer R, Jocham D, Diedrich K, Schmucker P, Huppe M. (2006). Andrologia. 38: 48–53.

Harman SM, Metter EJ, Tobin JD, Pearson J, Blackman MR. (2001). J Clin Endocrinol Metab. 86: 724–731.

Heinemann LA, Moore C, Dinger JC, Stoehr D. (2006). Health Qual Life Outcomes. 4: 23.

Heinemann LA, Saad F, Zimmermann T, Novak A, Myon E, Badia X, Potthoff P, T'Sjoen G, Pöllänen P, Goncharow NP, Kim S, Giroudet C. (2003). Health Qual Life Outcomes. 1: 15.

Herschbach P, Henrich G, Strasburger CJ, Feldmeier H, MarĀn F, Attanasio AM, Blum WF. (2001). Eur J Endocrinol. 145: 255–265.

Hooven CK, Chabris CF, Ellison PT, Kosslyn SM. (2004). Neuropsychologia. 42: 782–790.

Huber D, Henrich G, Herschbach P. (1988). Pharmacopsychiatry. 21: 453–455.

Kelleher S, Conway AJ, Handelsman DJ. (2004). J Clin Endocrinol Metab. 89: 3813–3817.

Kratzik C, Heinemann LA, Saad F, Thai DM, Rücklinger E. (2005). Aging Male. 8: 157–161.

Kupelian V, Page ST, Araujo AB, Travison TG, Bremner WJ, McKinlay JB. (2006). J Clin Endocrinol Metab. 91: 843–850.

Laughlin GA, Barrett-Connor E, Bergstrom J. (2008). J Clin Endocrinol Metab. 93: 68–75.

Moffat SD, Zonderman AB, Metter EJ, Blackman MR, Harman SM, Resnick SM. (2002). J Clin Endocrinol Metab. 87: 5001–5007.

Mooradian AD, Morley JE, Korenman SG. (1987). Endocrine Rev. 8: 1–28.

Morley JE, Kaiser FE, Perry HM 3rd, Patrick P, Morley PM, Stauber PM, Vellas B, Baumgartner RN, Garry PJ. (1997). Metab Clin Exper. 46: 410–413.

Morley JE, Melmed S. (1979). Metabolism. 28: 1051–1073.

Morley JE, Perry HM 3rd. (2003). Clin Geriatr Med. 19: 507–28.

Mulligan T, Frick MF, Zuraw QC, Stemhagen A, McWhirter C. (2006). Int J Clin Pract. 60: 762–769.

Nair KS, Rizza RA, O'Brien P, Dhatariya K, Short KR, Nehra A, Vittone JL, Klee GG, Basu A, Basu R, Cobelli C, Toffolo G, Dalla Man C, Tindall DJ, Melton LJ 3rd, Smith GE, Khosla S, Jensen MD. (2006). N Engl J Med. 355: 1647–1659.

Nieschlag E, Behre HM, Bouchard P, Corrales JJ, Jones TH, Stalla GK,Webb SM,Wu FC. (2004). Hum Reprod Update. 10: 409–419.

Nieschlag E, Swerdloff R, Behre HM, Gooren LJ, Kaufman JM, Legros JJ, Lunenfeld B, Morley JE, Schulman C, Wang C, Weidner W, Wu FC. (2005). Eur Urol. 48: 1–4.

Novak A, Brod M, Elbers J. (2002). Maturitas. 43: 231–237.

Potosky AL, Knopf K, Clegg LX, Albertsen PC, Stanford JL, Hamilton AS, Gilliland FD, Eley JW, Stephenson RA, Hoffman RM. (2001). J Clin Oncol. 19: 3750–3757.

Rhoden EL, Morgentaler A. (2004). N Engl J Med. 350: 482–492.

Roy M, Kirschbaum C, Steptoe A. (2003). Ann Behav Med. 26: 194–200.

Seidman SN. (2003). World J Biol Psychiatry. 4: 14–20. View Record in Scopus | Cited By in Scopus (28).

Shabsigh R, Katz M, Yan G, Makhsida N. (2005). Am J Cardiol. 96: 67M–72M.

Shores MM, Matsumoto AM, Sloan KL, Kivlahan DR. (2006). Arch Intern Med. 166: 1660–1665.

Shores MM, Sloan KL, Matsumoto AM, Moceri VM, Felker B, Kivlahan DR. (2004). Arch Gen Psychiatry. 61: 162–167.

Snyder P. (2001). J Clin Endocrinol Metab. 86: 2369–2372.

Vermeulen A. (2001). Clin Endocrinol Metab. 86: 2380–2390.

Vermeulen A, Verdonck L, Kaufman JM. (1999). J Clin Endocrinol Metab. 84: 3666–3672.

Ware JE Jr., Sherbourne CD. (1992). Med Care. 30: 473–483.

Wang C, Cunningham G, Dobs A, Iranmanesh A, Matsumoto AM, Snyder PJ, Weber T, Berman N, Hull L, Swerdloff RS. (2004). J Clin Endocrinol Metab. 89: 2085–2098.

Yasuda M, Honma S, Furuya K, Yoshii T, Kamiyama Y, Ide H, Muto S, Horie S. (2008a). J Men Health Gender. 5: 56–63.

Yasuda M, Furuya K, Yoshii T, Ide H, Muto S, Horie S. (2007). J Men Health Gender. 4: 149–155.

Yasuda M, Ide H, Furuya K, Takashi Y, Nishio K, Saito K, Isotani S, Kamiyama Y, Muto S, Horie S. (2008b). J Sex Med. 5: 1482–1491.

153 Measuring Quality of Life in Macular Degeneration

J. Mitchell · C. Bradley

1   *Age-Related Macular Degeneration* 2634

2   *Measuring Quality of Life and Other Patient Reported Outcomes* 2636
2.1   Psychological Well-Being Instruments 2637
2.2   Health Status (HS) Measures 2637
2.3   Functional Status (FS) Measures 2638
2.4   Vision-Specific Functional Status (VF) 2638
2.5   Vision-Specific Individualized Quality of Life Measures 2639

3   *The Value of PROs* 2639

4   *MD-Specific Patient Satisfaction Measures Related to Quality of Life* 2640

5   *Validation of Questionnaires* 2641

6   *QALYs and Other Manipulations of PROs* 2642

7   *The Use of PROs* 2645

     Summary Points 2645

Abstract: ❯ Patient-reported outcomes are increasingly used in research and clinical practice in ophthalmology as in other medical specialties. ❯ Measures of health status, psychological well-being, ❯ functional status, and visual function are frequently referred to as quality of life (QOL) measures and have been used as such in research into macular degeneration (MD). However, such patient-reported outcomes do not measure QOL, although the constructs may be related to or influence QOL. When inappropriate or insensitive measures are used as QOL measures, the findings can be misleading and may lead to incorrect management of patients. Care is needed in the selection of patient reported outcomes (PROs) for use in research and clinical practice to ensure that they are appropriate for the intended purpose. In addition, PROs should be psychometrically validated, demonstrating qualities including face, content and construct validity, internal consistency and test-retest reliability and responsiveness.

❯ Utility values obtained using methods such as ❯ time trade-off and ❯ standard gamble are used to calculate ❯ quality adjusted life years and are frequently referred to as QOL measures. However, they do not measure QOL and give no impression of the ways in which MD or any other medical condition impacts on QOL. For older people, such as those with MD, the questions are particularly difficult to answer.

PROs have shown that MD has a considerable negative impact on the lives of people with the condition and on their families. The use of PROs is valuable in assessing the impact of clinical and rehabilitative interventions and other services for people with MD. Ideally a complementary combination of PROs would used for evaluation purposes to ensure considerate, individually tailored and effective management of this group of patients.

List of Abbreviations: *ADVS*, activities of daily vision scale; *CNV*, choroidal neovascularization; *DTSQ*, diabetes treatment satisfaction questionnaire; *EQ-5D*, EuroQOL 5-dimension questionnaire; *FS*, functional status; *HS*, health status; *HUI3*, health utility index 3; *MacSSQ*, macular service satisfaction questionnaire; *MacTSQ*, macular treatment satisfaction questionnaire; *MD*, macular degeneration; *NEI-VFQ*, National Eye Institute visual function questionnaire; *NICE*, National Institute for Health and Clinical Excellence; *PRO*, patient-reported outcome; *QALY*, quality adjusted life year; *QOL*, quality of life; *SF-36*, short form 36; *SG*, standard gamble; *TTO*, time trade-off; *VA*, ❯ visual acuity; *W-BQ12*, 12-item well-being questionnaire; *WHO*, World Health Organisation

1   Age-Related Macular Degeneration

Age-related macular degeneration (MD) is a chronic, progressive eye disorder that mainly affects people over the age of 50. It is the leading cause of blindness in the Western world in people over 60 years and the third most common cause of blindness globally after cataract and glaucoma (WHO, 2004). Recently it was estimated that, in the UK, with a population of 59 million, approximately 417,000 people have some degree of MD, of whom 214,000 have sufficient impairment for registration as partially sighted or blind (Owen et al., 2003). With increasing longevity in the population the prevalence of MD is likely to grow (Owen et al., 2003).

MD affects the most sensitive part of the retina, the macula. The condition leads to loss of central vision needed for activities requiring fine vision such as reading, driving and recognizing faces. Peripheral vision is usually retained but MD can impair proficiency in performing most activities in daily living and can make it more difficult for people to live independent lives. The effects of MD on vision are illustrated in ❯ *Figures 153-1– 153-3* (reproduced

◻ Figure 153-1
Scene as perceived with normal vision. The scene is clear and there is no distortion

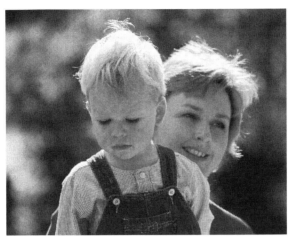

◻ Figure 153-2
Scene as observed with mild MD. Vision is blurred and there is some distortion

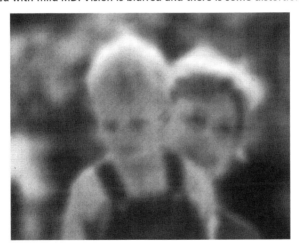

courtesy of The ❷ Macular Disease Society), which show a scene as perceived with normal vision, with mild MD and with moderately severe MD. In very severe cases central vision can be completely obliterated.

There are two types of MD. Dry MD (also called atrophic MD) accounts for about 85% of cases and generally develops slowly, often affecting both eyes simultaneously. Dry MD is characterized by fatty deposits behind the retina which cause the macula to thin and dry out. In general it causes less severe impairment than the more aggressive wet MD. Wet MD (also known as neovascular or exudative MD) is associated with rapidly deteriorating vision and severe impairment. It accounts for 90% of cases of severe visual impairment due to MD. Wet MD is caused by the growth of new blood vessels (a process known as choroidal

◘ Figure 153-3

Scene as observed with severe MD. The scene is very blurred and no detail is detectable in the centre of the picture

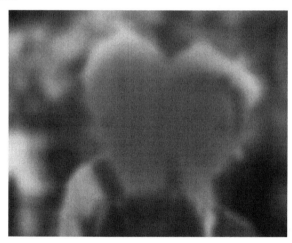

neovascularization [CNV]) behind the retina. These new blood vessels are weak and tend to leak, damaging the retinal cells and leading to scar tissue.

MD is a largely untreatable condition (❷ *Table 153-1*). Treatment is appropriate for a small percentage of people if they are diagnosed at an early stage with particular types of the wet form of the disease. Even then the treatment does not cure the condition but can limit its progress, at least for a time, although the newest treatments do offer some hope of improvement in vision for a proportion of patients. However, potential new treatments and rehabilitation interventions are continually being developed and tested.

2   Measuring Quality of Life and Other Patient Reported Outcomes

It is important that appropriate patient reported outcomes (PROs) are used in the evaluation of new interventions. Many PROs are routinely referred to as "quality of life (QOL) measures"

◘ Table 153-1

Key facts about macular degeneration (MD)

• MD is a progressive eye condition
• MD mainly affects people over 50 years of age and incidence increases with age
• MD is the leading cause of blindness in people over 60 in the western world
• MD damages the central part of the retina, the macula, which is needed for fine vision
• There are two types of MD. About 85% of cases are "dry MD," which develops slowly. Wet MD, progresses rapidly and, although it accounts for only about 15% of cases of MD, it is the cause of 90% of cases of severe vision impairment due to MD
• There is currently no treatment for dry MD. Wet MD can often be treated to halt progress of the condition. In some cases vision improves with treatment but there is no cure for MD

but this ubiquitous term is often misused and, when it is, data referred to as QOL data can be misinterpreted. This can lead to incorrect assumptions about the effects of intervention (Bradley, 2001) and may even result in the inappropriate management of patients.

Although a great deal of QOL research is carried out there is little agreement about the definition of QOL. The one we prefer, which guides our own measurement of quality of life, is:

▶ "Your quality of life is how good or bad you feel your life to be." (Bradley et al., 1999)

Implicit in this definition is that QOL is a subjective perception and that QOL means different things to different people. Although many so-called QOL measures allow people to indicate their own perceived levels of whatever aspect of life is being measured, many do not allow individuals to report the relevance or importance of that aspect of life for them (Bradley, 2001).

2.1   Psychological Well-Being Instruments

Psychological well-being instruments measure mood but they are often referred to as measures of QOL. People who feel depressed and anxious are unlikely to describe their QOL as good. However, people whose psychological well-being is good may nevertheless feel that their QOL is severely damaged by MD. Some well-being scales, such as the Beck Depression Inventory (Beck et al., 1961) measure only negative well-being (depression). Where people are not depressed to begin with, such a measure could show no improvement. Measures which also investigate positive well-being e.g., the positive well-being subscale of the 12-item Well-being Questionnaire [W-BQ12] (Mitchell and Bradley, 2001) which also measures energy and negative well-being (anxiety and depression), are more likely to detect improvement in psychological well-being.

2.2   Health Status (HS) Measures

Health status measures investigate subjective perceptions of health but unfortunately HS measures are often wrongly called QOL measures and this has caused great confusion and misleading conclusions (Bradley, 2001). HS is not QOL; although poor HS may be associated with impaired QOL, good HS does not indicate that QOL is good. HS measures such as the SF-36 (Ware et al., 1993) are unsuitable as indicators of the impact of eye conditions on QOL because most of the domains investigated (e.g., pain, energy, appetite) are not affected by visual impairment (Mitchell and Bradley, 2006). The SF-36, and the shorter subset, SF-12, have been found to be sensitive to age-related eye disease including MD in some work (Knudtson et al., 2005) but not in others (Childs et al., 2004; Stevenson et al., 2005) and found to be only minimally responsive to change in visual acuity (VA) in patients with CNV over a period of 2 years (Childs, 2004). The SF-12 was also found not to be responsive to change (Cahill et al., 2005). The health utility index (HUI-3) (Feeny et al., 2002) includes an item concerned with vision and, unsurprisingly, proved more sensitive to vision impairment (Espallargues et al., 2005) than the SF-12 and the EQ5D (Brooks, 1996) which investigates only five dimensions of health, none of which is vision. This disappointing performance of widely used HS measures in detailing impairment in people with MD and other eye conditions can be understood when it is appreciated that, for the most part, the general population do not think of problems with their eyesight when asked about their health. Patients may be registered blind with MD and still report that their health is excellent. If asked about their QOL they may nevertheless say it is badly affected by their MD. Quality of health is quite a different matter from QOL (Bradley, 2001) and this is particularly true for people with eye conditions, including people with MD. When the SF-36 and other HS measures show no impact of MD and are also wrongly referred to as QOL measures it may be mistakenly concluded that MD has no impact on QOL when all that has been shown is that MD has no impact on self-reports of health. The literature on MD abounds with studies that have used HS measures and wrongly referred to these as QOL measures (Mitchell and Bradley, 2006). It is essential that we recognize this problem and are not misled by the data.

2.3   Functional Status (FS) Measures

Functional status questionnaires investigate respondents' ability to carry out activities of daily living such as self-care and eating. They may contain some items that are relevant to vision but they do not particularly investigate vision-related activities (e.g., reading, watching TV). Generally they do not include psychological domains such as confidence or worry. They do not necessarily correlate well with objective measures of vision or with QOL because FS measures only ask what a person can do, not whether they want or need to do those things or how important they are to their QOL. Nevertheless, using the Instrumental Activities of Daily Living scale, Williams et al. (1998) demonstrated that, compared with visually unimpaired elderly people, patients with MD were 8 times more likely to report difficulty shopping, 13 times more likely to have difficulty managing finances, 4 times more likely to experience difficulties preparing meals, 12 times more likely to have problems using a telephone, and 9 times more likely to experience problems with light housework.

2.4   Vision-Specific Functional Status (VF)

Measures of visual function investigate vision-related tasks such as reading, writing, watching TV, recognizing faces or driving. They are usually correlated with standard measures of vision such as VA. However, they do not differentiate between what is relevant and what is irrelevant to individual respondents, or what is important to QOL and what is not, and therefore they are not true QOL measures, although they are frequently referred to as such (Slakter and Stur, 2005). The impact on QOL of loss of or deteriorating near vision would be greater for someone who spent a lot of time reading and doing embroidery than for someone who preferred listening to music and swimming. VF measurement has also been shown to be influenced by general health (Miskala et al., 2004). For example, the ability to prepare a meal may be affected by arthritis as well as by vision and, if the questionnaire does not specifically ask the respondent to consider only the effects of their vision on a task, co-morbidity may confound the scores and make results difficult to interpret. The Activities of Daily Vision Scale (ADVS) (Mangione et al., 1992) was found to discriminate between mild and severe MD (overall score, near vision, daytime driving and glare) but not between mild and moderate MD (Mangione et al., 1999).

The ADVS and some other VF measures investigate only visual function and do not include items relating to social or psychological functioning. Other VF measures, including the NEI-VFQ (Mangione et al., 1998), which has been well validated in the MD population, also investigates psychological aspects of visual impairment. As well as items pertaining strictly to function, the NEI-VFQ investigates social functioning, mental health and dependency.

It differentiates between different eye conditions, and overall score and relevant subscale scores are correlated with VA. It has been shown to be responsive to change in VA over time (Lindblad and Clemons, 2005), but this was in a large study over a long period of time. It remains to be seen if the NEI-VFQ is sufficiently responsive to detect change in smaller samples. For a more comprehensive review of measures of FS and VF used in studies of vision impairment see Mitchell and Bradley (2006).

2.5 Vision-Specific Individualized Quality of Life Measures

The MacDQOL is an individualized measure of the impact of MD on QOL (Mitchell and Bradley, 2004; Mitchell et al., 2005; Mitchell et al., 2008). The MacDQOL, modeled on the ADDQOL for diabetes (Bradley et al., 1999) (which in turn was influenced by the generic SEIQOL, McGee et al. (1991)) and developed alongside the RetDQOL for people with diabetic retinopathy (Woodcock et al., 2004), examines both impact and importance of each domain on QOL and allows for variability in the relevance of specific domains to individual respondents (see other chapter by Mitchell and Bradley, this volume for more detail on design and development). Impact and importance scores are multiplied to give weighted impact scores. The MacDQOL has two overview items (present QOL and MD-specific QOL) and 23 domain-specific items. It has been shown to differentiate between mild and moderate and mild and severe MD (measured by UK registration status: blind, partially-sighted or not registered) but, in common with visual function measures, not between moderate and severe. The overview items are also sensitive to severity of MD, the present QOL (generic) item less so than the MD-specific item, as would be expected. There are promising indications of the MacDQOL's responsiveness to change in a small sample (Mitchell et al., 2008), and some evidence that the MacDQOL is slightly more sensitive to VA impairment than the NEI-VFQ in a large multinational trial (Berdeaux et al., 2006). Measuring both the impact and the importance of a domain of life to QOL leads to considerable variability in scores and so it would not be surprising if correlations between the MacDQOL and measures of vision such as VA or contrast sensitivity were not as large as those between VA and vision function e.g., MacDQOL average weighted impact score correlates 0.45 with better eye distance VA (Mitchell et al., 2005), NEI-VFQ distance vision score correlates 0.65 with better eye distance VA (Mangione et al., 1998). This correlation between NEI-VFQ score and distance VA score would be expected to be high as with both measures the patients are being asked how well they can see. The MacDQOL measure captures the nature of the impact of MD on a person's life in a way that cannot be achieved with a vision function measure. If there is any loss of sensitivity to differences in VA, it is outweighed by the increased relevance of the QOL measure to the whole experience of MD including experience of any treatment and rehabilitation.

3 The Value of PROs

In the literature on MD, well-being, health status, functional status and visual function have all been referred to more or less inappropriately as QOL. We have argued that the use of such measures can be misleading, resulting in misinterpretation of findings. Nevertheless, PRO instruments other than QOL measures provide valuable data and, together, a variety of types of measure can give a fuller picture of the effect of MD on people's lives. Many PROs contain items which could appropriately be included in measures of more than one construct.

■ Figure 153-4

Venn diagram to show the relationship between PROs. The more the circles overlap, the stronger the relationship between constructs

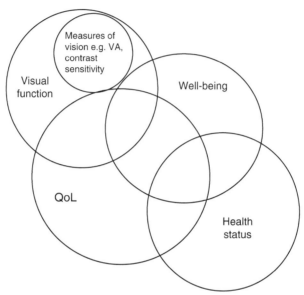

❯ *Figure 153-4* illustrates the complex relationship between different types of PRO. Some measures, such as most health status questionnaires (e.g., SF-36 (Ware et al., 1993); EQ5D (Brooks, 1996)) are clearly not helpful in evaluating the effects of MD. The SF-36 is a comprehensively validated and widely used measure and it may be that it is selected purely on the grounds of its ubiquity. If it is not expected to yield relevant results, however, it is an unnecessary burden on participants and is likely to give an underestimation of the benefits of an intervention designed to improve vision. In any study or clinical trial, careful thought must be given to the choice of measures to ensure that the data collected are the data that are required to answer the research question or investigate the effect of an intervention. A treatment for MD may result in enhanced visual function but, if the treatment is very unpleasant, has to be repeated regularly and is anticipated with trepidation by some patients and refused by others, then it might do substantial damage to QOL in spite of having the potential to improve visual function. The work reported here indicates that, in many cases, there is widespread confusion about the term "quality of life" and, generally, the choice of questionnaire indicates that it is defined inadequately. Choice of PRO instrument notwithstanding, measuring the impact of vision impairment is complicated by the involvement of a second eye and the interactions between the two eyes' visual status (Slakter and Stur, 2005).

4   MD-Specific Patient Satisfaction Measures Related to Quality of Life

The factors that contribute to QOL are many and varied. For people with MD, the way in which their condition is managed and treated is likely to impact on their QOL. Two measures have recently been developed to investigate MD patient satisfaction.

The MacSSQ (Bradley and Mitchell, 2006) is a measure of macular clinic service satisfaction. It is intended for use with MD patients, both newly diagnosed and returning. People with MD informed the content and design of the measure, which contains 35 items pertaining to a wide variety of aspects of clinic service. It is intended for use in eye clinics so that shortcomings in the service that may not be recognized or considered important by clinic staff may be highlighted. It is hoped that findings from such service evaluation may prompt changes in the clinics leading to increased patient satisfaction. ❯ Psychometric development and validation is being carried out on the MacSSQ in 2008.

The MacTSQ (Mitchell et al., 2007) is a measure of satisfaction with treatment for MD. It is modeled on the Diabetes Treatment Satisfaction Questionnaire (DTSQ) (Bradley, 1994; Bradley et al., 2007) which is widely used internationally. There are currently several possible treatments for wet MD and it is likely that the future will bring new developments in treatment for both wet and dry MD. The MacTSQ is a 16-item measure that investigates patient satisfaction with aspects of treatment including provision of information about the treatment, diagnostic tests, apprehension about the treatment, pain and side effects associated with the treatment, cost and convenience of treatment. It is anticipated that the measure will be valuable in clinical trials to assess the acceptability of treatments to patients. Psychometric development and validation of the MacTSQ will be conducted on data to be collected from clinical trials starting shortly.

5   Validation of Questionnaires

Measures of health status, functional status, visual function and well-being are not, in themselves, QOL measures. However, they are all concerned with aspects of life that may be important to QOL.

The value of questionnaire data collected depends on the psychometric properties of the measure. Psychometric properties that are regarded as important in a measure include those presented in ❯ Table 153-2 (Margolis et al., 2002). In addition to these psychometric properties, the burden placed upon respondents (length of questionnaire, complexity of language, relevance of the questions) and that on administrators should be considered. Where questionnaires are designed in one language and translated into other languages, linguistic validation is required, including cultural adaptation where needed. Forward and backward translations are necessary (preferably reviewed by the questionnaire author) to ensure that the translations have not introduced semantic discrepancies. Clinician review can be helpful and cognitive debriefing interviews with people who have MD are needed to ensure that the translated items and instructions are understood as intended. Psychometric evaluation of each language version is necessary, at least on first use, before analyzing data from multiple languages as one dataset.

The method of administration is a further consideration that is particularly important in visually impaired populations. Self-completion (pen and paper) has been found to elicit poorer scores than interview administration in some questionnaires but not in others (Mitchell et al., 2004). Where scores differ, using two implementation methods in one study may result in people with worse vision, and therefore having interview administration, under-reporting impairment compared with people self-completing the measure. This would confound the results. Generally it is better to use only one administration method in any one study.

◼ Table 153-2

Psychometric properties desirable in scales to measure patient-reported outcomes

Property	Definition	Considerations
Internal consistency reliability	The extent to which the items contribute to measuring the same construct (a reliability coefficient is calculated)	Only cases with complete data are valid for use in calculating internal consistency reliability
Test-retest reliability	The extent to which scores remain stable over time when no change has occurred (i.e., when there has been no change in vision, no treatment for MD or rehabilitation)	An appropriate time lapse between baseline and follow-up data collection is important. Two weeks is probably too short for patients to have forgotten their previous responses. Three months or more would be more appropriate
Content validity	The extent to which the topic of interest is comprehensively and appropriately investigated by the measure	It is important to involve patients in the design of a patient reported outcome measure in order to ensure content validity
Face validity	The extent to which the questionnaire appears to measure what it is intended to measure	Researchers designing questionnaires should consider the questions carefully and avoid ambiguity. Researchers considering the use of the measure should consider whether the items are suitable for their purposes
Construct validity	Hypotheses concerning the relationship of questionnaire scores to other measures (such as VA or contrast sensitivity) are tested	Ability to discriminate between levels of disease severity (e.g., between people who are registered blind, partially sighted or not registered) is important, particularly for a visual function measure, which would be expected to correlate strongly with disease severity
Responsiveness	Sensitivity to real change over time (e.g., deterioration in VA or contrast sensitivity)	Care is needed in deciding what constitutes significant change
Interpretability	The extent to which change scores can be interpreted and explained	Selecting the most appropriate PRO measure is critical. Health status and utility measures are not suitable for investigating quality of life, particularly for people with MD

Some psychometric properties are investigated using statistical procedures and others must be determined by examination of content and consideration of the design process

6   QALYs and Other Manipulations of PROs

A limitation of condition-specific or vision-specific measures of health status, functional status and QOL, even when they are interpreted appropriately, is that the scores are not comparable across diverse medical specialties. One use for outcome measures is to assess the relative cost-effectiveness of different treatments and to inform decisions concerning allocation of limited funds. Such a measure, that could be used across all medical conditions and allow direct comparison, would be an asset for health economists. One technique that is adopted increasingly to make such comparisons is utility assessment. Utility values (also called preference measures) are quantitative expressions of preference for given health states. A scale is used with utility values ranging from 0 to 1 where 0 represents death and 1 represents perfect health. Techniques used for eliciting this value include time trade-off (TTO) and standard gamble (SG). They are usually obtained during an interview using particular questions, which are shown in ❷ *Table 153-3*. The utility value obtained is used in conjunction with an estimate

□ Table 153-3

Standard gamble and time-trade off questions and utility calculations

Technique	Question(s) asked	Sample response
Standard gamble (SG)	A new treatment is available. When it works it always restores normal vision for the rest of your life but failure results in immediate death. The alternative to treatment is the certain continuation of your present visual status for the rest of your life. What percentage risk of death, if any, would you be willing to accept before refusing the treatment?	20% risk of death
SG utility calculation		1.0–0.2 = 0.8
Time trade-off (TTO)	How many more years do you expect to live	15 years
	Imagine that there is a new treatment for MD. It always works but it reduces the length of your life. How many of your remaining years would you be willing to give up if you could have this treatment and enjoy normal vision for the rest of your life?	3 years
TTO utility calculation		1.0–3/15 or 1–0.2 = 0.8

Participants are asked SG or TTO questions about a health state or medical condition and their responses are used to calculate utility values for that health state

of life expectancy to calculate Quality Adjusted Life Years (QALYs). QALYs are estimates of life expectancy in full health. One year of life in a health state rated as perfect health (utility value of 1) = 1 QALY. Two years of life in a health state with a utility value of 0.5 = 1 QALY. Cost per QALY can be calculated if the cost of treatment is known. Such costs can be calculated for any clinical intervention, and have been used by medical decision makers such as the UK National Institute for Health and Clinical Excellence (NICE) to make choices between treatments. Health economists argue that non-preference PROs correlate poorly with preference measures and so are not suitable for use in economic evaluation. It could be argued that preference measures, although convenient for calculating QALYs, do not correlate well with non-preference based QOL measures as they do not measure QOL.

A number of studies have reported utility values for MD using TTO or SG techniques e.g., Brown, Sharma, Brown et al. (2000a, b) and there has been reasonable concordance in the findings. Nevertheless the method has attracted criticism. For example, there is some debate about whose values are the most appropriate: patients', doctors' or those of the taxpaying general public (De Wit et al., 2000). The general public may be unaware of the impact of some medical conditions unless they themselves are affected by the condition. There can be marked differences in the values of patients, doctors and the public and the decision to use one group rather than another will therefore be likely to affect the results obtained. It has also been reported that demographic data may be more predictive in determining health state utilities than the health states themselves (Dolan and Roberts, 2002). Some studies have reported less than impressive response rates e.g., Brown et al. (2001). Others have not reported response rates (e.g., Brown et al., 2000c). TTO questions are often posed to MD patients during an eye clinic appointment while they wait to see the ophthalmologist following dilation of the pupils. Patients may feel vulnerable at this time and reluctant to express unwillingness to take part. When participants in a UK study were asked TTO questions during a telephone interview while they were in their own home, at a time convenient to them, response rates were a cause for concern (Mitchell and Bradley, 2005). A large proportion of people who did respond (38%) said they would trade no time for perfect vision. Unsolicited comments from participants indicated that they thought the questions ridiculous, too hypothetical or objectionable for religious or other reasons. People said they would not trade time because they were carers or because they wanted to see their grandchildren grow up. Nevertheless, it is likely that improvement in their MD would improve their QOL. There was no relationship between utility values and vision status (registration as blind, partially sighted or not registered) whereas, in the same study, vision status was significantly associated with MacDQOL scores. Another UK study (Hill et al., 2005) demonstrated that 50% of participants with varying severity of MD were not prepared to trade any time for perfect vision and, after removing scores where no time was traded, there was no relationship between TTO utility values and VA. It is likely that the questions posed in the TTO method would be particularly difficult for elderly people to answer given their shorter life expectancies. The comparability of TTO responses to questions about "perfect health" and those referring to "perfect vision" (see ❥ *Table 153-3* for wording of TTO questions) is doubtful. A person with poor vision and poor general health might view things differently from a person who has poor vision but otherwise good health.

Opinions differ as to whether utility values should be obtained from patients, health professionals or the tax-paying general public. Generally, the public overestimate the impact of medical conditions on QOL compared with patients but it has been shown that MD is an exception to this rule: both the public and health professionals report higher utility values for MD than do patients (Stein et al., 2003). This perhaps reflects an underestimation of the impact of the loss of central vision and an overestimation of the value of peripheral vision. Whatever the reason, a comparison of utility values across diseases when the utilities have been obtained from the public would mitigate against resources being allocated for treatment and rehabilitation of people who have MD.

Utility measures and QALYs are increasingly used to estimate so called "QOL" gains or losses. However, the QALY values obtained using TTO and SG methods are not measuring QOL (Slakter and Stur, 2005) and the measures give no impression of the ways in which MD impacts on people's lives. There are many reasons why a person may not want to relinquish any years of life in spite of serious visual impairment but this does not imply that they are content with the present situation or that their QOL would not be much better without their vision problems. When such measures are obtained from members of the public who have no awareness of living with MD the results are so far removed from the patients' experiences as to be completely irrelevant to QOL measurement. These inadequate and inappropriate measures and others like them have been the preferred instruments for "QOL" measurement and continue to be used uncritically in organizations such as the UK's NICE, dominated by health economists who are committed to such inferential methods of measurement, unaware of the importance of psychological factors and unaccustomed to listening to patients' accounts of their own experiences and descriptions of the impact of MD on their lives.

7 The Use of PROs

The use of QOL, well-being and vision function measures in assessing the value of changes to the services offered to people with MD will help to ensure that management of this group of patients is considerate, sensitive to individual needs and effective. Slakter and Stur (2005) asserted that, ideally, different trials should use the same measures to enable comparison of the effects. It would be premature to recommend a specific set of measures for use in all trials, as some of the instruments are relatively new, though it is clear that health status measures such as the SF-36 are of little relevance and utility values derived using TTO and SG methods are misleading and best avoided. A variety of visual function measures is available, with the NEI-VFQ being well established as a useful measure of visual function in MD. The W-BQ12 measure of well-being is psychometrically evaluated for people with MD (Mitchell and Bradley, 2001). There is growing evidence for the usefulness of the relatively recent MacDQOL measure of the impact of MD on quality of life which was developed specifically for people with MD (Berdeaux et al., 2006; Mitchell and Bradley, 2004; Mitchell et al., 2005; Mitchell et al., 2008) Such measures of well-being and quality of life are urgently needed in clinical trials in addition to measures of visual function in a context of continuing evaluation of their sensitivity to change in response to treatments and rehabilitation for MD.

It is well documented that MD has a damaging effect on many aspects of people's lives. The loss of central vision associated with MD impairs critical aspects of visual function including reading, driving, recognizing faces, watching TV and other near vision activities. Impaired visual function affects different people in different ways. Not all aspects of impairment will be important to all people with MD but evidence from studies using the MacDQOL shows that loss of visual function will affect all people with MD in some way. The extent to which MD impacts QOL will be influenced by individual lifestyles and personal characteristics as well as by factors such as social support, co-morbidity and access to rehabilitation services. The use of effective and appropriate patient-reported outcome measures in evaluating treatment, rehabilitation and management will be invaluable in the maintenance of good quality of life for people with MD.

Summary Points

- Macular degeneration is a chronic, progressive eye condition that mainly affects people over the age of 50. It is the leading cause of blindness in people over 60 years in the Western world. A minority of cases is treatable but this improves impaired vision for only a proportion of treated patients.
- Several different types of patient reported outcome measures, including measures of health status, psychological well-being, functional status and visual function are inappropriately used as measures of quality of life in the study of MD.

- When inappropriate PROs are used the findings may be misinterpreted and conclusions may be misleading.
- Utility measures, used in economic analysis, do not measure quality of life and give no flavor of the experience of living with MD.
- Care should be taken in the selection of PROs for use research and clinical practice so that relevant, psychometrically validated measures are used, enabling effective interpretation of the data.

References

Beck AT, Ward CH, Mendelson M, Mock J, Erbaugh J. (1961). Arch Gen Psychiatry. 4: 561–571.

Berdeaux G, Mesbah M, Bradley C. (2006). Value Health 9: A372–A373.

Bradley C. (1994). Bradley (ed.) C. Handbook of Psychology and Diabetes: A Guide to Psychological Measurement in Diabetes Research and Practice. Harwood Academic Publishers, Chur, Switzerland, pp. 111–132.

Bradley C. (2001). Lancet. 357: 7–8.

Bradley C, Mitchell J. (2006). Digest: J Macular Dis Soc. 2006: 31–34.

Bradley C, Plowright R, Stewart J, Valentine J, Witthaus E. (2007). Health Qual Life Outcomes. 5: 57.

Bradley C, Todd C, Gorton T, Symonds E, Martin A, Plowright R. (1999). Qual Life Res. 8: 79–91.

Brooks R. (1996). Health Policy. 37: 53–72.

Brown G, Sharma S, Brown M, Kistler J. (2000a). Arch Ophthalmol. 118: 47–51.

Brown GC, Brown MM, Sharma S. (2000b). Can J Ophthalmol. 35: 127–133.

Brown GC, Sharma S, Brown MM, Kistler J. (2000c). Arch Ophthalmol. 118: 47–51.

Brown MM, Brown GC, Sharma S, Kistler J, Brown H. (2001). Br J Ophthalmol. 85: 327–331.

Cahill MT, Stinnett SS, Banks AD, Freedman SF, Toth CA. (2005). Ophthalmology. 112: 144–151.

Childs AL. (2004). Am J Ophthalmol. 137: 373–375.

Childs AL, Bressler NM, Bass EB, Hawkins BS, Mangione CM, Marsh MJ, et al. (2004). Ophthalmology. 111: 2007–2014.

De Wit GA, Busschbach JJ, De Charro FT. (2000). Health Econ. 9: 109–126.

Dolan P, Roberts J. (2002). Soc Sci Med. 54: 919–929.

Espallargues M, Czoski-Murray CJ, Bansback NJ, Carlton J, Lewis GM, Hughes LA, et al. (2005). Invest Ophthalmol Vis Sci. 46: 4016–4023.

Feeny D, Furlong W, Torrance GW, Goldsmith CH, Zhu Z, DePauw S, et al. (2002). Med Care. 40: 113–128.

Hill AR, Aspinall P, Armbrecht AM, Dhillon B, Buchholz P. (2005). Int Congr Ser. 1282: 573–577.

Knudtson MD, Klein BE, Klein R, Cruickshanks KJ, Lee KE. (2005). Arch Ophthalmol. 123: 807–814.

Lindblad AS, Clemons TE. (2005). Arch Ophthalmol. 123: 1207–1214.

Mangione CM, Gutierrez PR, Lowe G, Orav EJ, Seddon JM. (1999). Am J Ophthalmol. 128: 45–53.

Mangione CM, Lee PP, Pitts J, Gutierrez P, Berry S, Hays RD. (1998). Arch Ophthalmol. 116: 1496–1504.

Mangione CM, Phillips RS, Seddon JM, Lawrence MG, Cook EF, Dailey R, et al. (1992). Med Care. 30: 1111–1126.

Margolis MK, Coyne K, Kennedy-Martin T, Baker T, Schein O, Revicki DA. (2002). Pharmacoeconomics. 20: 791–812.

McGee HM, O'Boyle CA, Hickey A, O'Malley K, Joyce CR. (1991). Psychol Med. 21: 749–759.

Miskala PH, Bressler NM, Meinert CL. (2004). Arch Ophthalmol. 122: 758–766.

Mitchell J, Bradley C. (2001). Qual Life Res. 10: 465–473.

Mitchell J, Bradley C. (2004). Qual Life Res. 13: 1163–1175.

Mitchell J, Bradley C. (2005). Int Congr Ser. 1282: 654–658.

Mitchell J, Bradley C. (2006). Health Qual Life Outcomes. 4: 97.

Mitchell J, Brose L, Bradley C. (2007). International Society for Quality of Life Research meeting abstracts. [www.isoqol.org/2007mtgabstracts]. The QLR Journal, A-120, Abstract 1150.

Mitchell J, Wolffsohn JS, Woodcock A, Anderson SJ, McMillan CV, ffytche T, et al. (2005). Health Qual Life Outcomes. 3: 25.

Mitchell J, Wolffsohn JS, Woodcock A, Anderson SJ, ffytche T, et al. (2008). Am J Ophthalmol. 146: 447–454.

Mitchell J, Woodcock A, Bradley C. (2004). Qual Life Res. 13: 1548 abstract.

Owen CG, Fletcher AE, Donoghue M, Rudnicka AR. (2003). Br J Ophthalmol. 87: 312–317.

Slakter JS, Stur M. (2005). Surv Ophthalmol. 50: 263–273.

Stein JD, Brown MM, Brown GC, Hollands H, Sharma S. (2003). Br J Ophthalmol. 87: 8–12.

Stevenson MR, Hart PM, Chakravarthy U, Mackenzie G, Bird AC, Owens SL, et al. (2005). Br J Ophthalmol. 89: 1045–1051.

Ware JE, Snow K, Kosinski M, Gaandek B. (1993). SF-36 Health Survey: Manual and Interpretation Guide. The Health Institute, New England Medical Center, Boston, MA.

WHO. (2004, 19.01.2006). Retrieved 12/03/2006, from http://www.who.int/mediacentre/factsheets.fs282/en

Williams RA, Brody BL, Thomas RG, Kaplan RM, Brown SI. (1998). Arch Ophthalmol. 116: 514–520.

Woodcock A, Bradley C, Plowright R, ffytche T, Kennedy-Martin T, Hirsch A. (2004). Patient Educ Couns. 53: 365–383.

154 Quality of Life Measures in the Elderly and Later Life

S. Evans

1   Introduction 2650

2   Conceptual and Definitional Issues 2651

3   Measuring the Quality of Life of Older People 2652

4   Reviewed Measures of QOL for Older People 2653

5   QOL Measures for Older People 2655
5.1 The Leipad 2656
5.2 Casp-19 2658
5.3 Multidimensional Quality of Life 2659

6   Culture Specific 2660

7   Studies Testing Specific Measures in Samples of Older People 2662

8   Domain Specific Measures of Components of QOL in Older People 2663

9   Conclusions 2663

    Summary Points 2664

Abstract: ❷ Quality of life (QOL) is a long established concept that has proliferated across professional and academic disciplines, and is applied extensively in clinical research and practice around the world, in many fields of healthcare. The term is associated with a wide range of theoretical models, approaches to measurement and measures, which in healthcare alone encompass generic, health-related and disease-specific models. This diversity contributes to a huge literature on the subject, which can be difficult to find one's way around, especially for the uninitiated. The purpose of this chapter is to review recent measures of quality of life for ❷ older people and to highlight their applicability for clinical research and evaluation. Distinguishing between measures of ❷ health status, functioning, HRQOL and QOL as it is generally understood, the content and psychometric properties of existing measures are considered in order that readers can make informed choices about the concepts and measures that are of relevance to them.

List of Abbreviations: *BSQ*, brief screening questionnaire; *EQ5D*, Euroqol 5D; *FAI*, functional assessment inventory; *GHQ20*, general health questionnaire-20; *GQLQ*, geriatric quality of life questionnaire; *HRQOL*, health related quality of life; *HUI3*, health utilities index 3; *IADL*, instrumental activities of daily living; *LSES*, life satisfaction in elderly scales; *MFAQ*, multidimensional functional assessment questionnaire; *MQOL*, multidimensional quality of life; *NHP*, nottingham health profile; *PGCMAI*, philadelphia geriatric center multilevel assessment; *PGI*, patient generated index; *QOL*, quality of life; *QOLP-SV*, quality of life profile – seniors version; *QuiLL*, Quality in later life; *RGT*, repertory grid technique; *SEIQOL*, self evaluation of individual quality of life; *SELF*, self evaluation of life; *SF-36*, short form 36; *SIP*, sickness impact profile; *WB*, wellbeing; *WHOQOLOLD*, World Health Organization QOL Old; *WI*, wellness index

1 Introduction

Quality of life (QOL) is a long established concept that has proliferated across professional and academic disciplines. The term is associated with a wide range of theoretical models and measures, perhaps because the intuitive and global appeal of the concept (along with its in exactitude) encourages a variety of conceptual interpretations (Oliver et al., 1996) that in turn attract interest from different fields; alternatively it might be that the interest from within different disciplines has encouraged the development of alternative or complementary conceptual models. The multiple-interpretations of the meaning of life quality have led to claims that QOL is difficult to conceptualize and operationalize, but despite these persistent albeit largely unfounded assertions the concept is applied extensively in clinical research and practice around the world, in many fields of healthcare. The relevance of QOL to clinical research, ❷ service evaluation and monitoring, and individual care and treatment planning for older people has been outlined in the previous chapter of this handbook, which also highlights how the concept is valued, especially by those in receipt of health and social care services. Nevertheless, the concept can be a difficult one to study and understand for several reasons. The lack of clarity in definition has, as we have seen in the previous chapter led to a variety of approaches to measurement, which in healthcare alone encompasses generic (as in domain based measures that cover many aspects of life), health-related and disease-specific models. The variety of definitions, conceptualizations, models and measures contribute to a huge literature on the subject, which can be difficult to find one's way around, especially for the uninitiated. For example, searches for the term in the ❷ Medline database generate 4.5 million citations currently, while the same search of all of the major literature databases generates over 7 million (7,139,415) citations; most of these publications relate to clinical research, but less than 20,000 focus on older people (19,318). One of the problems associated with the study of QOL is that the intrinsic appeal and popularity of the concept often leads authors to assert associations with life quality in their Abstract, even though the study does not measure the concept, a practice that is reflected in the fact that to date fewer than one-thousand of the publications relating to older people refer to "measures" or "instruments." While this reduces the burden of reviewing measures of quality of life for older people, it still leaves a considerable field to review, especially for those who are not versed in measurement and psychometric properties. The purpose of this chapter therefore, is to review the measures of quality of life specifically designed for use with older people as identified in the recent literature (from 1998 to 2008), in order to clarify for hard pressed clinicians and other health and social care professionals the utility and applicability of existing measures for clinical research and evaluation; little consideration is given to the QuiLL (Quality of Life in Later Life) measure (Evans et al., 2005) however, as this is the subject of the previous chapter.

2   Conceptual and Definitional Issues

Issues relating to the definition of life quality generally concern the purpose, focus and content of measures. In its widest sense, the expression quality of life encompasses all aspects of human life, including each person's material, physical, social, emotional, psychological and spiritual well-being, and multidimensional generic quality of life measures such as those introduced in studies of general populations in America (Andrews and Withey, 1976; Campbell et al., 1976) aim to capture all of these aspects of life quality. In contrast, in the health sector there has been a tendency to focus more narrowly on those aspects of life that can be attributed directly to illness or treatments (Namjoshi and Buesching, 2001; Spiro and Bosse, 2000) using ❷ health-related quality of life (HRQOL) or disease-specific QOL measures that were developed to relate to specific disease entities. In this arena the terms health status, functioning, HRQOL and QOL are often used interchangeably, but each term has subtle and important differences in respect of their dimensionality, perspective and scope (Bergner, 1989), as outlined in ❷ Table 154-1, which need to be considered when choosing an evaluation tool.

❏ Table 154-1
Defining Life Quality

Health status refers specifically to the state of physical and mental health and often incorporates the patient's perspective of these attributes.
Functioning relates to one's capacity to perform everyday activities associated with daily living (e.g., cleaning and cooking) and independence (e.g., personal care) and to engage in social activities.
Health-related Quality of Life concentrates on the effects of illness on physical, psychological and social aspects of life.
Quality of Life extends its focus beyond the health domain and the effects of illness to incorporate a wide range of human experiences. A distinguishing characteristic of QOL measures is that they incorporate user values, judgments and individual preferences (Gill and Feinstein, 1994).

❷ *Table 154-1* defines QOL and related but distinct concepts that are often confused with one another

It is important to recognize at the outset that there is now a degree of controversy about the use of the term health-related QOL, and concerns about the appropriateness of the use of HRQOL measures in evaluations of healthcare systems and interventions. Cummins et al. (2004) has argued that HRQOL instruments should not be regarded as valid measures of life quality as they do not reflect the common understanding of the term quality of life. He has even gone so far as to recommend that HRQOL measurement be abandoned in favor of three separate forms of assessment, namely medical symptoms, ❷ subjective well-being and specific dimensions of psychological ill-being.

Michalos (2004) has taken a similar stance, arguing that there are good reasons for carefully distinguishing between the concepts of health and quality of life, and for not interpreting Short Form-36 (SF-36) scores for instance (Ware, 1997) as a measure of life quality, as is done commonly; we would agree on this point, as the SF36 was designed as a measure of health-status and not QOL and as such reflects an altogether different concept. Nevertheless, while Michalos (2004) agrees that we might all be better off if the term "❷ health-related quality of life" was simply abandoned, he realizes that this is unlikely to happen. Therefore, he has recommended that researchers (and anyone involved in clinical and service evaluations) be much more careful in their usage of the phrase "quality of life," as well as in their interpretation of measures that purport to assess whatever the phrase is supposed to designate.

Cameron et al. (2006) have made a similar argument for caution in the conceptualization and understanding of the alternative term "well-being," the subjective form of which was one of the three proposed forms of assessment advocated by Cummins et al. (2004). Their argument is supported by the earlier works of Spiro and Bosse (2000), in which the distinction between HRQOL and well-being (WB) was examined in the ❷ Veteran's Administration Normative Aging Study; the study indicated that HRQOL and WB were only moderately correlated and factor analyses that produced a four-factor solution loaded HRQOL and WB scales on separate factors. These results led the authors to suggest that HRQOL and WB while conceptually related have only a modest degree of overlap.

3   Measuring the Quality of Life of Older People

Despite the concerns about the use of health-related concepts as indicators of QOL and WB, the literature includes a diverse range of approaches to measurement that one needs to be able to distinguish between when studying QOL in older populations.

The first distinction is between general measures that were designed for use with all population groups, such as the 15 instruments reviewed by Haywood et al. (2005a; which they refer to as generic measures) and older-people specific measures such as the 18 instruments reviewed by Haywood et al. (2005b). This classification is not entirely straightforward however, as some generic measures have since been adapted (e.g., the WHOQOLOLD and the Veteran SF36) to ensure that they are valid and reliable when used with older people (e.g., Bergland and Wyller, 2006; Duffy et al., 2005; Hoe et al., 2005; Ip et al., 1999); others like the Lancashire Quality of Life Profile – Residential (Mozley et al., 2004) have been modified for use with older people in different care settings. Such adaptations are reviewed in more detail later in this chapter; those that are labeled as QOL but relate to other concepts such as affect or morale are not included (e.g., Ranzijn and Luszcz, 2000).

Secondly, one can distinguish between measures of health status, functioning and HRQOL, and QOL itself (see ❷ Table 154-1).

A third distinction can be made between multi-dimensional measures that include items such as psychological well being, activities of daily living or spiritual well-being, and domain structured measures. Many domain based indicators have been adapted from instruments that were originally designed for use in general population surveys and tend to cover many different aspects of life in objective and subjective terms. In contrast to these measures that aim to assess objective and subjective circumstances across several domains, others focus specifically on one aspect of life such as leisure activity (Nilsson and Fisher, 2006) or friendship (Hawthorne, 2006).

Finally, one can also distinguish between standardized measures that ask the same questions of all respondents, and individualized measures that focus specifically on those aspects of life identified as important by the individual e.g., the Schedule for the Evaluation of Individual Life Quality (SEIQOL) or Patient Generated Index (PGI). Similarly, one might want to consider culturally specific measures, such as the QOL measures for older people in Hong Kong and Taiwan developed by Chan et al. (2004) and Ku et al. (2008) respectively.

While the emphasis in this chapter is on standard, older-people specific measures, the properties of individualized and generic measures are also summarized.

4   Reviewed Measures of QOL for Older People

Reviews of available quality of life measures (e.g., Kliempt et al., 2000) tend to include disease-specific measures and generic instruments that are actually health status measures, alongside quality of life scales. Recent reviews of QOL in older people by Haywood et al. have added to the confusion as their foci are on health (2005a), health status (2005b) and self-reported health incorporating quality of life, health related quality of life and health status (2006) respectively. The diversity of instruments purporting to measure life quality is illustrated in the latest review by Haywood et al., (2006), which included 20 generic (two of which had been adapted for older populations) and 25 older-people specific self-assessed, multi-dimensional measures of health status and quality of life.

Haywood et al. (2006) reported that older-people specific measures had been subject to fewer evaluations than the generic measures. Of the 20 generic measures reviewed, 13 were able to demonstrate reliability, validity and responsiveness, which are all essential properties for robust measurement. The Short-Form 36 (SF36) was the one that was thought to have the most supporting evidence about use with older populations, both in terms of the number of evaluations (n = 76) and the quality of evidence about its measurement properties. The Nottingham Health Profile (NHP), Sickness Impact Profile (SIP) and EuroQol 5D (EQ5D) were also considered to have a reasonable evidence base (Haywood et al., 2005a, 2006), although the SIP may be considered impractical for routine use in clinical or operational practice given that it includes 136 items. While each of the four measures were considered to be valid, reliable and responsive to change they also all have a strong emphasis on health status assessed in terms of energy, pain, mobility, functioning, anxiety and depression etc rather than life quality itself; little consideration is given to social aspects of life, with only the NHP including domains relating to recreation and pastimes, social interaction and work (although the EQ5D does have an item on usual activities). As such none of these generic measures would be deemed suitable QOL indicators by Cummins et al. (2004), Michalos (2004) and Cameron et al. (2006), and on the basis of the definitions outlined in ❷ Table 154-1 we would tend to agree. Their focus on health status rather than life quality is illustrated clearly by the comments of Haywood et al. (2005a, p 1651) in their recommendation of the SF36 for use where "a detailed and broad assessment of health is required", and the EQ-5D where "a more succinct assessment is required, particularly where a substantial change in health is expected." The suitability of such measures for evaluations of life quality is drawn into further doubt by recent evidence that generic health status measures such the SF-36, the health utilities index 3 (HUI3), and the EQ-5D do not capture the effects of sight loss on quality of life (Chakravarthy, 2006). Potential users of the SF36 who are only interested in health status rather than life quality might still want to consider new evidence (Hann and Reeves, 2008) suggesting that the factor structure of the physical and mental component scales of the measure vary significantly by disease condition.

Of the older-people specific measures only 5 of the 21 ❷ standard measures were thought to have demonstrated reliability, validity and responsiveness to change; these included the OARS (Older Americans Resources and Services) Multi-dimensional Functional Assessment Questionnaire (MFAQ), the Philadelphia Geriatric Centre Multi-level Assessment (PGCMAI), the Quality of Life Profile – Seniors Version (QOLPSV), the Quality in Later Life assessment (QuiLL) and the Self-evaluation of Life (SELF) (Haywood et al., 2006). Nevertheless, the authors considered that the evidence base was strongest for the MFAQ, the Functional Assessment Inventory (FAI), the QOLPSV and the CARE, largely on the basis that they had been the subject of more evaluative papers (even though most evaluations for the CARE and the QOLPSV were based on the same studies). Readers should consider the practicality of using the CARE either in research or evaluation at the outset however, given that in its original form it includes 1,500 items and even the CORE-CARE and SHORT-CARE include 329 and 143 items respectively. Potential users should also be aware that neither the CARE nor the FAI has demonstrated responsiveness to change, an attribute that is fundamental to the ability to evaluate the impact of treatment and care in ❷ longitudinal studies. Although the MFAQ, FAI and CARE do include items relating to economic and social resources, social resources and social needs respectively the emphasis is very much on functioning, which we would argue make these measures inadequate for the measurement of life quality as defined in ❷ Table 154-1.

Haywood et al. (2006) found less supporting evidence for using subjective indicators of life quality in elderly populations, on the basis that most instruments had only been included in one evaluation or the reporting of evidence was considered rather basic, and three of the six measures that included some subjective component had not demonstrated responsiveness to change. Nevertheless, three measures had demonstrable reliability, validity and responsiveness to change: the Self-evaluation of Life Scale (SELF), which is a HRQOL measure that includes an assessment of social satisfaction; the Quality in Later Life (QuiLL), which assesses domain-specific and global life quality in objective and subjective terms; the QOLPSV, which examines importance and enjoyment of physical, psychiatric and spiritual being and community, physical and social belonging, and hopes, goals and aspirations for leisure and practical activities, and personal growth.

Worryingly none of the four individualized measures were considered to have demonstrated reliability, validity and responsiveness. Only the Patient Generated Index (PGI) modified for older people had proven reliability, but the validity and responsiveness of this measure had not been demonstrated. The Geriatric QOL Questionnaire (GQLQ) was the only individualized measure to have proven responsiveness, but this measure while valid had no proven reliability. Similarly, the Repertory Grid Technique (RGT) and the Schedule for the Evaluation of Individual Quality of Life (SEIQOL) Direct Weighting for Frail Elderly, while valid instruments of life quality could not demonstrate reliability or responsiveness to change (Haywood et al., 2006). Therefore, on the basis of these findings one would have to question the appropriateness of using individualized measures in studies of older people, particularly given that aggregation to a group level is also somewhat difficult.

All of this illustrates the importance of examining the relevance of the content of QOL measures in the context of the purpose of the investigation, and of selecting measures that are fit for purpose, whether that be for research or clinical practice (Cameron et al., 2006; Haywood et al., 2006; Michalos, 2004). For instance the MFAQ is particularly strong, and therefore appropriately used in relation to the measurement of activities of daily living, but might be considered less useful when seeking to assess the impact of illness and disease on life generally. Similarly, although the LEIPAD (De Leo et al., 1998), which is reviewed in more detail in the next section, is presented as a quality of life measure, life satisfaction forms only one part of this multidimensional instrument that covers a wide range of types of data that may or may not be pertinent to one's particular requirements. Whatever the purpose, one needs to consider the reliability and validity of any measure in order to ensure robust measurement in a consistent way, of the concept that one thinks one is measuring. While all of the older-people specific measures have proven validity, two lack evidence of reliability – the Brief Screening Questionnaire and the Geriatric Quality of Life Questionnaire (Haywood et al., 2005b, 2006) – and so should be treated with some caution. Clinicians and researchers need also to consider the stability and responsiveness of measures, particular when examining changes in status over time, in order that changes that occur can be detected, but also that stability is demonstrated where no changes have taken place. In order to help readers identify easily the measures that might best suit their requirements, the characteristics of the five older-people specific measures that appear to be reliable, valid and responsive to change are presented in ❷ *Table 154-2*.

Readers might also want to consider using instruments for which the content has been informed or determined by older-people themselves, as these might have greater face validity than other measures, given that their content reflects older peoples' own definitions and interpretations of life quality. Instruments of this type include the GQLQ, the CASP-19, the QOLPSV, the QuILL and the WI, although we are disinclined to recommend the GQLQ given its lack of reliability, and would suggest only using the CASP-19 and WI in cross-sectional studies given that their responsiveness has not been established. A final consideration might be the flexibility of administration: seven older people-specific measures can be administered either as self-complete questionnaires or in interviews, namely the BSQ, CASP-19 (reviewed in detail in the next section), QOLPSV, QuILL, SENOTS and WI, although only the QuILL and QOLPSV have demonstrated reliability, validity and responsiveness in any way.

5   QOL Measures for Older People

In this section we consider the development and properties of two older people-specific measures that are either used frequently in studies of life quality for this population group, and others that have been reported on since 2006. We have included instruments that have been developed specifically for use in certain cultures and settings, but have excluded those relating to the measurement of QOL in people with dementia (whether patient focused or proxy measures) as QOL in dementia is the subject of another chapter in this handbook.

◻ Table 154-2

Classification of robust older people-specific measures

Measure	Content	Concepts
MFAQ	120 items: Multi-dimensional measure including activities of daily living, economic resources, mental health, physical health, social resources, service use and service need	Functioning
		Service use
		Service need
PGCMAI	147 items: Multi-dimensional measure including physical health, activities of daily living, self-management, morale, perceived environment, social interaction, time use. Mid-length version (67 questions) and short version (48 questions) also available	Health status
		Functioning
		QOL (some aspects)
QOLPSV	Full: 111 items; Short: 54 items; Brief 27 items: Multi-dimensional assessing importance and enjoyment in nine areas: physical, psychological and spiritual being; community, social and personal engagement; aspirations for practical and leisure activities and personal growth	QOL
QuiLL	27 items: Domain based measure assessing objective circumstances and subjective ratings for nine life domains: family, finances, how one spends one's day, living situation, safety, social life, health and mental health, self (independence, influence on life), and global and general life quality	QOL
SELF	54-item: physical disability, symptoms of aging, self-esteem, social satisfaction, depression, and personal control	Functioning (physical, emotional, and social function)

MFAQ multi-dimensional functional assessment questionnaire; *PGCMAI* Philadelphia geriatric center multi-level Assessment; *QOLPSV* quality of life profile – seniors version; *QuiLL* quality in later life assessment; *SELF* self-evaluation of life

5.1   The Leipad

The LEIPAD [Its name is an acronym deriving from the first two of the three most involved universities: LEIden (the Netherlands), PADua (Italy), and Helsinki (Finland)] is one such measure (De Leo et al., 1998) that was developed to provide a shorter and more clinically acceptable multidimensional measure of quality of life than had been available previously. The authors argued that existing scales were over-long, required extensive training, and did not cover cognitive function; moreover existing instruments had not been validated for use in a wide variety of institutional and community settings. Their rationale for a new measure was that older people experience various adverse life events that make their physical, mental, emotional and social well-being more closely interrelated than in other age groups, although the evidence for this assertion was not provided. Because cognition may be impaired they also argued that this needs to be a component part of any QOL measure for older people. In support of these arguments the authors cited studies that advocate a multidimensional approach to include psychological constructs such as self-esteem, personality and morale.

In contrast we would suggest that if necessary cognition be assessed separately using a validated measure of that construct in order that its impact on QOL can be determined, rather than confusing the two concepts by assimilating cognition into a QOL assessment.

The original version of the instrument comprised of 37 items – that were either created ad hoc or taken from existing questionnaires – covering ten areas relating to self-perceived physical health, mental health, emotional health status, self-esteem, expectations for the future, activities of daily living (including the Instrumental Activities of Daily Living [IADL]), interpersonal and social functions, recreational activities, financial position, and religiousness/spirituality. The third version of the instrument (which was also reviewed by Haywood et al., 2006) consists of 49 items, 31 of which are grouped into 7 core instrument scales relating to cognitive function, depression/anxiety, life satisfaction, physical function, self-care, sexual function and social function. Eighteen other items borrowed from already available instruments were also included to facilitate assessments of how factors such as personality characteristics and social desirability might influence an individual's score, or were developed ad hoc to measure self-esteem and anger; these can be grouped into five "moderator scales."

The Physical Function Scale is composed of five items that examine the elderly person's perception of his or her physical status at the time of the interview. The Self-Care Scale consists of six items that analyze ability to perform daily activities without the help of others. As might be expected these scales had acceptable internal consistency demonstrated by Cronbach alphas of 0.74 in both cases (conventional levels of acceptability are in the range of 0.7–0.9; Streiner and Norman, 1995). The Depression and Anxiety Scale is composed of four items that examine subjective feelings of anxiety and participants' perceptions of feeling depressed; the alpha coefficient was 0.78. The Cognitive Functioning Scale deals with problems concerning such functions as ability to concentrate, feelings of confusion, and memory problems; the alpha coefficient was also acceptable at 0.79. Clearly then, these health related subscales can be considered reliable at least in so much as they are internally consistent, but are they valid indicators of QOL. Again, this depends on the definition that one favors, but Cummins et al. (2004) would argue that according to conventional definitions in the literature none of these LEIPAD scales relate to components of quality of life; rather, on the basis of the definitions in ❯ *Table 154-1*, the scales are simply indicators of health status and functioning.

Nevertheless, the LEIPAD does encompass measures that relate more specifically to conventional understanding of the term QOL, but unfortunately the internal consistency of scales for these less clinical aspects of the LEIPAD measure fell below conventionally acceptable levels. This might be explained by the disparate nature of the individual items included within these scales: for instance, the social function scale, which has an alpha coefficient of 0.61, mixes objective indicators relating to the presence of friends and confidantes with indicators of satisfaction with these aspects of life; similarly the life satisfaction scale, which also has an alpha of 0.61, includes six items relating to leisure (one item) and finances (two items), along with satisfaction with life now compared to the past, how things will go in the future, and the extent to which expectations stand in the way of doing or initiating future things. The inclusion in this scale of items requiring completely different frames of judgment is likely to have resulted in a low internal consistency. Although the authors deemed the internal consistency of these scales to be "sufficient," considering that the items related to different ❯ life domains, we would suggest that they demonstrate that the scales are not necessarily measuring one construct.

The "moderator" scales (relating to self-esteem, anger, social desirability, faith in God and self-perceived personality disorders) that were included to explain any variation in functioning and satisfaction items, also did not reach acceptable levels of internal consistency (the highest alpha was 0.63). In fact, as a result of further testing the authors have decided to abandon these moderator scales "because they do not seem to have a determining effect on the quality of life of elderly people," possibly because these scales were not measuring the individual constructs that they purported to measure.

The fact that the Haywood review (Haywood et al., 2006) focused on self-reported health (including QOL, HRQOL and health status) might explain their perception that the LEIPAD has demonstrable reliability and validity, as the health scales were indeed reliable, whereas the social function and life-satisfaction scales were not. Similarly, the factor structure of the instrument reflected psycho ➋ social functioning on the one hand and physical functioning on the other and the LEIPAD has demonstrated satisfactory concurrent validity with other physical function and mental health scales. Nevertheless, these results suggest that this instrument might be better suited as a measure of health status, functioning or HRQOL than of QOL itself. The fact that the LEIPAD has no demonstrable responsiveness to change (Haywood et al., 2006) makes it best suited to cross-sectional studies of this type.

The development and use of this scale illustrates well the need for conceptual clarity and understanding of what constitutes quality of life and what components contribute to it. There is a sense in which the LEIPAD is not a QOL measure at all, nor even a measure of HRQOL even though its multidimensionality encompasses physical health, activities of daily living and some subjective appraisals, as the latter are confined to one domain only and require judgments of a very different order (e.g., satisfaction with leisure and finance compared to a rating of the difference between current and future life satisfaction). Potential users should also consider evidence from a review of measures (Courtney et al., 2003) which led the authors to argue that an overemphasis on physical functioning in scales supposed to measure QOL could result in an unnecessarily negative picture of the actual QOL of older people.

Several authors (including ourselves) have recognized the need to consider QOL more broadly including Hyde et al. (2003), who found that many of the early measures described as QOL instruments:

▶ *were actually measures of health designed to uncover the extent of illness and frailty amongst the older population... However, whilst health continues to be an important determinant of QOL in older age it can no longer be considered a sufficient proxy. Quality of life measures that are designed for use in this age group need to be broader than health alone (p 191)*

5.2   Casp-19

In response, Hyde et al. (2003) sought to develop a new measure that was theoretically sound, based on the concept of needs satisfaction. Their measure, which captures four domains: control, autonomy, pleasure, and self-actualization was piloted in focus groups, in a self-completion pilot study, and in cognitive interview testing. The initial 22-item scale was included in a postal questionnaire of 286 people aged 65–75 years, distributed in two mail-outs 14 days apart that eventually achieved a 92% response.

These data were used for data reduction and ➋ psychometric testing purposes, producing a final 19-item scale (CASP-19), which includes four sub-scales. The subscales for pleasure and self actualization have good internal consistency (alpha coefficients of 0.75 and 0.77 respectively), but control (alpha 0.59) and autonomy scales (alpha 0.65) failed to reach acceptable levels. Concurrent validity was assessed against the Life Satisfaction Index-wellbeing. Although a positive association was found between the two scales (r = 0.6, p = 0.01) they shared only 36% of the variance, suggesting that the CASP-19 does not capture all aspects of life satisfaction. In addition, the CASP-19 items are entirely subjective and are likely to be highly correlated with measures of affect and mood, but such associations were not tested or controlled for in the development of the scale. Therefore, although the CASP-19 extends its focus beyond that of health-related measures, it does not appear to assess QOL in the way that is generally understood by the research community (Cummins et al., 2004). In addition, as reported by Haywood et al. (2006) the responsiveness of the CASP-19 has not been established, which limits its utility to cross-sectional studies.

Kreitler and Kreitler (2006) also criticized the majority of the better-known and commonly used QOL measures because they focused largely on the domain of physical health. They say that

▶ *this bias is unwarranted in view of the fact that physical disorder is, for better or worse, neither the most common state of human beings nor the only domain justifying assessment of QOL (p 8)*

On this basis the authors presented a new measure for assessing quality of life – the Multidimensional Quality of Life (MQOL) – and described its derivation, characteristics, structure and applications.

5.3 Multidimensional Quality of Life

The authors sought to move away from the measurement of health status and function and aimed to develop an instrument that focused on the person as a whole, looking beyond the disease and physical or mental symptoms from which he or she may be suffering. The content was informed by 490 interviews involving older people and three subsequent development phases: the first draft was piloted and respondents were asked to comment on the comprehensiveness and adequacy of items; data reduction and item-total reliability was undertaken on data for a revised version (n = 500); finally, reliability and validity was tested for the final 60-item measures based on a survey of 755 individuals.

This 60-item self-report tool covers various themes that on the basis of factor and cluster analyses relate to 17 scales and constitute five factors. The instrument includes items relating to worries about health, mobility, functioning at work or at study, eating and appetite, living conditions, family functioning and communication, entertainment, being successful, independence, memory and concentration, loneliness, anger, despair, unhappiness, hopefulness, joy, fear, sense of estrangement, self-esteem, sense of coherence, helplessness, strength and coping etc. It has been applied with thousands of individuals, in English, Hebrew, Russian and Arabic, and is reported as being adequate for healthy and physically or mentally sick individuals, under regular or challenging circumstances.

Tests of internal consistency and test-retest reliability in these three groups indicate that the measure itself and its subscales are reliable (internal consistency alphas of 0.76 – 0.90; test-retest correlation coefficients 0.69–0.92, and 0.72–0.86 for subscales). Concurrent validity, as tested against non older-people specific measures such as the SF36 (correlation 0.68–0.77 in three population groups), SIP (r = 0.75) and NHP (r = 0.73–0.88) suggested that the MQOL measures the same construct, which are commonly used as indicators of HRQOL but were actually designed as measures of health status or functioning. It seems somewhat strange that the authors chose to assess validity against the same health focused measures that they had criticized rather than more generic measures. It would appear therefore that the MQOL does not measure QOL in the way defined in ❷ *Table 154-1*, or in the way commonly accepted within the broader QOL research community (Cummins et al., 2004), and at best can only be described as a HRQOL indicator. As the responsiveness of the MQOL was not tested, the MQOL is only suitable for cross-sectional studies.

6   Culture Specific

All of the measures reviewed so far in this chapter were developed in Western societies for use in Western populations and do not necessarily match ideas about QOL in other parts of the world. For this reason a number of culture specific QOL measures have been developed.

Chan et al. (2004) set out to develop an instrument to address the need for a culturally relevant measure of quality of life for Chinese older people living in Hong Kong. It is an example of a measure which starts from the perception of older people themselves rather than clinical or research experts. The first stage of the research involved four focus groups in which older people reflected on how they interpreted the term "quality of life" followed by a content analysis resulting in a 100-item questionnaire. The focus groups were categorized as: working-class young-old; working-class older-old; middle-class young old; and middle-class older-old. The young-old were aged between 65 and 74 years, the older-old, 75 or above. The resulting questionnaire was reviewed by a panel of experts and the items were refined and reduced to 86 indicators, to which a further 25 items were added relating to socio-demographic background. The participants took "life quality" (a rather literary term in Chinese) principally to mean "life satisfaction," "happiness" or "a good life."

The next stage involved a representative survey resulting in 1,616 successful interviews with people aged 60 + living in the community (74% response rate). The data came from the Hong Kong General Household Survey. Analyses indicated that 21 items should be retained, forming six domains (subjective well-being, health, interpersonal relations, achievement-recognition, finance and living conditions, although finance and living conditions were assessed as single items). The importance of subjective well-being to other domains was ascertained by multiple regression and the results showed that all the domains accounted for 54% of subjective well-being. The overall QOL scale has a respectable Cronbach alpha of 0.72 with its domains ranging from 0.65 (which is slightly below the acceptable standard) to 0.77. The item-total correlation for each scale ranged from 0.31 to 0.71, suggesting that no items dominated nor were unrelated to the scale measure. While, each of the six domains were correlated significantly with the overall score, the association with achievement-recognition (not reported) and living conditions ($r = 0.56$) was low. Unusually, rather than being compared with an existing measure of life quality, validity was assessed against six individual items that were expected to (and did) correlate highly (general QOL and laughing a lot), moderately (joining in group activities and concern for important social matters) and not at all (family responsibility and demanding a lot of others). This approach might have been necessitated by the uniqueness of this culturally sensitive measure, but we are not convinced of the appropriateness of this approach. The measure's stability was determined appropriately in test-retest reliability analyses and the scale and domain scales were stable ($r = 0.68$–0.74; gamma 0.67 and 0.69; all $p < 0.001$) but responsiveness to changes over time was not assessed. It is not clear to what extent the instrument has been used to assess QOL specifically in other

Chinese communities, and Shek and Lee (2007) suggest that QOL data in Hong Kong are seldom compared with QOL data from other places, which seems rather like a missed opportunity.

Ku et al. (2008) have argued that subjective well-being has emerged as a key indicator in aging studies (Stathi et al., 2002). Because it is likely that eastern cultures carry different life values they developed and tested robustly the Chinese Aging Well Profile for measuring subjective well-being in Chinese adults over 50 years of age. The approach taken was to confirm or disconfirm content from the psychometrically established Aging Well Profile developed for a UK and European population (Stathi and Fox, 2004) while allowing new content reflecting local culture and values to be included.

A total of 210 lower order themes, 21 sub-dimensions, and 7 dimensions were identified through the inductive coding and categorizing process. Interviewees also revealed that physical activity could contribute to their well-being through positive influences on several key dimensions of subjective well-being, including "physical," "psychological," "developmental" and "social" well-being. These dimensions were (1) "physical" well-being: the extent to which you feel you have maintained a strong, healthy body and an energetic lifestyle, free from pains and illnesses; (2) "psychological" well-being: the extent to which you feel you maintain cognitive function and you feel positive towards daily life rather than negative; (3) "developmental" well-being: the extent to which you feel you are able to develop yourself, pursue self-growth and take care of yourself; (4) "material" well-being: the extent to which you feel you do not need to worry about financial situations; (5) "spiritual" wellbeing: the extent to which you feel your life is meaningful and you are supported by your beliefs towards life or spirituality; (6) "environmental" well-being: the extent to which you feel you are satisfied with the political situation, government's social welfare services, living environment, and leisure life; and (7) "social" well-being: the extent to which you feel you are able to maintain a close relationship with your family and friends and provide support to others in the community. Meaning of life and religious beliefs were said to be of significance, but were omitted from the instrument.

It is evident from these descriptions that the bulk of this measure is concerned with physical and psychological well-being, rather than the accepted domains of general quality of life measures. The single environmental well-being scale encompasses disparate social life domains, as does the social well-being scale. Tests of convergent/divergent validity were based on comparisons with the Satisfaction with Life Scale, Rosenberg's Self-Esteem Scale, and Positive and Negative Affect. As one might expect the environmental scale was not highly correlated with other measures of physical and psychological well being and had the lowest Cronbach alpha in subsequent testing (although still acceptable at 0.80); its path coefficients were also the only ones to fall below 0.4 in the modeling stages. While test-retest reliability analyses demonstrated the stability of the measure, responsiveness to changes over time was not examined.

There are two general issues that we have already touched upon, which the development and testing of this measure reveal (impressive and rigorous though these are). The first is that the predominant orientation of the measure is towards psychological well being and the high correlation with affect scores might suggest that the Chinese Aging Well Profile is measuring affect or affect related items. The second is that the social content of the measure is relatively thin in relation to the commonly accepted domains in QOL measures, being confined to two of the seven scales.

Nevertheless, the measure is of interest because of some of the clues it gives to the cultural differences that might be important when measuring life quality. According to the qualitative results, Chinese older people appear to have different attitudes to western populations concerning independence and interdependence aspects of subjective well-being. For instance, some participants reported that they "do not wish to rely on others" and "do not wish to cause or increase burden on offspring," but others suggested that "when my children grow up, they can stay with us. That is my best hope." Others expressed the view that ". . . taking care of aged parents is an offspring's obligation. . . ."

The authors indicated that these findings are similar to those on the "interdependent self" (Markus and Kitayama, 1991) and to socially oriented cultural conceptions of subjective well-being (Lu and Gilmour, 2006). Autonomy and independence are emphasized in the West unlike Taiwan and other parts of East Asia where individuals are seen as closely connected, and interdependent; they argue that this represents a "collectivist" culture. Indications that Taiwan remains a collectivist society in spite of modernization (Lu and Kao, 2002) come from the higher proportion of co-residence (67.8%) among Chinese aged 50 and over in Taiwan and the fact that the majority of their financial support comes from their children (51.7%).

7   Studies Testing Specific Measures in Samples of Older People

Bergland and Wyller (2006) validated an instrument consisting of five items and first used in the Nord-Trondelag Health Survey (HUNT-5), as a measure of HRQOL in a population of elderly women living at home. Both the General Health Questionnaire-20 (GHQ-20) and the HUNT-5 questionnaire were completed by 307 women. The psychometric properties of the instrument were acceptable but the items related largely to subjective well being in aspects of health and mental health and as a consequence were very highly correlated with GHQ scores. As a HRQOL measure this seems to have little to offer above other measures in this age group.

Efklides et al. (2006) adapted the Questionnaire Quality of Life in Epilepsy QoLIE-89 RAND for use with older adults suffering from chronic diseases. The QOLIE-89 inventory comprises 89 items that measure 17 topics relating to physical health and functioning, cognition, and social behavior, for which Cronbach alphas range from 0.6 to 0.9. Discriminant validity was established between healthy and unwell groups, but the instrument did not differentiate between three chronic illness groups. Further work on the measure was recommended.

Lau et al. (2005) explored the cross-cultural equivalence of the Personal Wellbeing Index, which was developed to measure subjective well-being. Three age groups, one over 65 years, were recruited in Hong Kong and Australia. There were only 60 people over 65 in each of the samples. The authors reported that the PWI had good psychometric performance in terms of its reliability, validity and sensitivity, which were comparable in both countries. The item "satisfaction with own happiness" was found to contribute significantly to the scale's psychometric performance in Australia but not in Hong Kong. The authors suggested that cultural differences in the concepts "satisfaction" and "happiness" may be responsible for this finding. The mean score for the Australian sample fell within the established range of 70–80, on a scale from 0 to 100. The Hong Kong population, however, fell below this range, and again cultural response bias was identified as a possible explanation for the difference.

Duffy et al. (2005) examined the utility and reliability of the Salamon-Conte Life Satisfaction in the Elderly Scales (LSES) in measuring life satisfaction in elderly ❷ nursing home residents in comparable samples in the UK (n = 100) and the USA (n = 207). The LSES was convenient and easy to administer by trained interviewers. Reliabilities on the original eight factor scale were high with Cronbach alpha's of 0.92 for the US sample and 0.90 for the UK sample. When the results were compared, a shorter five-factor scale emerged which gave comparable results in both countries.

8 Domain Specific Measures of Components of QOL in Older People

Rather than focus on QOL generally, or its health-related approach some studies have focused on specific aspects of social quality, and a number of domain specific measures have been developed for use with older people. Recent examples include measures of leisure activities and social isolation. Nilsson and Fisher (2006) developed an instrument to assess leisure activity in older people in four areas: interest, performance, motivation, and well-being. The psychometric properties of the instrument were good, although it was only tested on a relatively small number of volunteers in rural Sweden. Hawthorne (2006) developed a measure of social isolation that is relatively shorter and user friendly. The psychometric properties are very good and it measures six important dimensions of isolation from other people. There was a strong association between isolation and mental ill health in Hawthorne's data.

9 Conclusions

Over the past 20 years or more the field of quality of life measurement has become a diverse and specialized field. The growth in the number of measures has been substantial, and many more measures can be expected to be created that relate specifically to older people and to individual life domains. This will provide a considerable range of possible outcomes tools with which to evaluate the efficacy and effectiveness of targeted interventions with older people.

There is a need, as different authors have argued (Albert et al., 2001; Rabins and Black, 2007) for the selected measures to be fit for purpose. That is, they need to conceptually and practically cover items that relate to the intervention in question and that are capable of revealing any change that takes place. Interventions need to be fit for purpose also, and it would not come as a surprise to find that those that are not aimed at improving QOL are not likely to improve it. Rabins and Black (2007) remind us of an important caveat, which is that, under certain circumstances QOL should be considered as a ❯ secondary outcome for treatments so that where other outcomes measures show no difference in impact in different groups of patients, if the QOL of one group is superior to the other, then that one should be selected as the treatment of choice. In other cases, where the intervention is aimed at the improvement of QOL, QOL measures should be used as the primary outcome.

In this chapter we have reviewed the properties of a range of measures, distinguishing between health status, functioning, HRQOL and QOL as it is generally understood, in order that readers can make informed choices about the concepts and measures that are of relevance to them.

Summary Points

- Most measures of QOL that are used in evaluations of clinical services and treatment interventions were not designed specifically for use with older people.
- The literature on Quality of Life for older people includes measures that relate to health status, functioning, health-related quality of life and QOL defined more broadly.
- Most measures were developed in the Western world and culture specific measures or items might be necessary in other areas of the world.
- It is essential to choose a measure that is fit for purpose, in terms of content and psychometric properties taking account of the requirements of the study and the nature of the intervention being evaluated.
- Only five older-people specific measures have demonstrable reliability, validity and responsiveness: three of these capture health status and/or functioning (MFAQ, PGCMAI and SELF) and two are based on the broader conceptualization of life quality (QOLPSV and QuiLL).

References

Albert SM, et al. (2001). Am J Geriat Psychiat. 9: 160–168.

Andrews FM, Withey SB. (1976). Social Indicators of Well-Being: Americans Perceptions of Quality of Life. Plenum, New York.

Bergland A, Wyller TB. (2006). Soc Ind Res. 77: 479–497.

Bergner M. (1989). Med Care. 27(suppl): S148–S156.

Cameron E, Mathers J, Parry J. (2006). Crit Pub Health. 16: 347–354.

Campbell A, Converse P, Rogers WL. (1976). The Quality of American Life: Perceptions, Evaluating and Satisfactions. Russell Sage, New York.

Chakravarthy U. (2006). BMJ. 333(7574): 869–870.

Chan ACM, Cheng S, Chi I, Ho SSY, Phillips DR. (2004). Soc Ind Res. 69: 279–301.

Courtney M, Edwards H, Stephan J, O'Reilly M, Duggan C. (2003). Aus J Ageing. 22: 58–64.

Cummins RA, Lau ALD, Stokes M. (2004). Expert Rev Pharmacoeco Out Res. 4: 413–420.

De Leo D, Diekstra RFW, Lonnqvist J, Trabucchi M, Cleiren MHPD, Frisoni GB, Della Buono M, Haltunen A. (1998). Behav Med. 24: 17–27.

Duffy M, Duffy JA, Kilbourne W, Giarchi G. (2005). Clin Gerontologist. 28: 17–28.

Efklides A, Varsami M, Mitadi I, Economidis D. (2006). Soc Ind Res 76: 35–53.

Evans S, Gately C, Huxley P, Smith A, Banerjee S. (2005). QoL. Res. 14: 1291–1300.

Gill TM, Feinstein AR. (1994). JAMA. 272: 619–626.

Hann M, Reeves D. (2008). QoL. Res. 7: 413–423.

Hawthorne G. (2006). Soc Ind Res. 77: 521–548.

Haywood K, Garratt A, Fitzpatrick R. (2005a). QoL. Res. 14: 1651–1668.

Haywood K, Garrett A, Fitzpatrick R. (2005b). J Eval Clin Prac. 11: 315–327.

Haywood KL, Garratt AM, Fitzpatrick R. (2006). Expert Rev Pharmacoeco Out Res. 6: 181–194

Hoe J, Katona C, Livingston G, Room B. (2005). Age Ageing. 34: 130–135.

Hyde M, Wiggins RD, Higgs P, Blane DB. (2003). Aging Ment Hlth. 7: 186–194.

Ip W-, Kwan Y-, Pong GTY, Troutt MD. (1999). J Soc Serv Res. 25: 43–56.

Kliempt P, Ruta D, McMurdo M. (2000). Revs Clin Gerontol. 10: 33–42.

Kreitler S, Kreitler MM. (2006). Soc Ind Res. 76: 5–33.

Ku P, Fox KR, McKenna J. (2008). Soc Ind Res. 10.1007/s11205-007-9150-2, published on-line.

Lau ALD, Cummins RA, McPherson W. (2005). Soc Ind Res. 72: 403–430.

Lu L, Gilmour R. (2006). Asian J Soc Psychol. 9: 36–49.

Lu L, Kao S. (2002). J Soc Psychol. 142: 45–59.

Markus HR, Kitayama S. (1991). Psychol Rev. 20: 568–579.

Michalos Alex C. (2004). Soc Ind Res. 65: 27–72.

Mozley C, Sutcliffe C, Bagley H, Cordingley L, Challis D, Huxley P, Burns A. (2004). Towards Quality Care: Outcomes for Older People in Care Homes. Ashgate, Aldershot.

Namjoshi MA. Buesching DP. (2001). QoL. Res. 10: 105–115.

Nilsson I, Fisher AG. (2006). Scand J Occ Ther. 13: 31–37.

Oliver JPJ, Huxley PJ, Bridges K, Mohammed H. (1996). Quality of Life and Mental Health Services. Routledge, London.

Rabins PV, Black BS. (2007). Int Psychogeriat. 19: 401–407.

Ranzijn R, Luszcz M. (2000). Int J Aging Hum Devel. 50: 263–278.

Shek DT, Lee BM. (2007). Sci World J. 7: 1222–1229.

Spiro A, Bosse R. (2000). Int J Aging Hum Devel. 50: 297–318.

Stathi A, Fox KR, McKenna J. (2002). J Aging Phys Act. 10: 79–92.

Stathi A, Fox KR. (2004). J Aging Phys Act. 12: 300.

Streiner DL, Norman GR. (1995). Health Measurement Scales: A Practical Guide to Development and Use. Oxford University Press, Oxford.

Ware JE. (1997). SF-36 Health Survey. Manual and Interpretation Guide (2nd. edn). The Health Institute, New England Medical Centre, Nimrod, MA.

155 Cochlear Implant Outcomes and Quality of Life in the Elderly

S. R. Saeed · D. J. Mawman

1	Introduction	2668
1.1	Prevalence of Hearing Loss in the Elderly	2668
2	Cochlear Implantation in the Elderly and Quality of Life	2669
	Summary Points	2672

Abstract: Cochlear Implantation is an established safe and effective treatment for patients with severe-profound sensori neural hearing loss. Demand for implants in the UK has increased over time partly as a result of the population living for a longer time and ❷ life expectancy is also increasing. The prevalence of severe-profound hearing loss in the 60–80 year old age group is estimated to be 1.3% rising to 16.8% in the over 80 year old group and so the demand for ❷ cochlear implants in this group of patients is higher.

The evaluation of the clinical effectiveness of cochlear implantation in the elderly population utilizes tests of speech discrimination ability and the outcome scores are compared to the scores of younger patients. The studies find that there is no significant difference in outcomes between the two groups (p > 0.05).

Health related quality of life questionnaires administered to elderly patients show a statistically significant benefit when the pre operative health status is compared to the post operative health status (p < 0.001).

In conclusion the evidence indicates that cochlear implantation in elderly patients will allow them to gain significant hearing and quality of life benefits that are comparable to the benefits that younger patients experience. These outcomes should encourage ❷ healthcare purchasers to ensure that funding is allocated for implantation in the elderly population.

List of Abbreviations: *AB*, Arthur Boothroyd; *BKB*, Bamford Kowal Bench; *CID*, Central Institute for the Deaf; *CNC*, consonant vowel consonant; *CUNY*, City University New York; *GBI*, ❷ Glasgow Benefit Inventory; *GHSI*, ❷ Glasgow Health Status Inventory; *HINT*, Hearing in Noise Test

1 Introduction

The population of Great Britain has been living longer over the past 20 years, but this additional longevity has not necessarily been lived in good health. Life expectancy and healthy life expectancy (expected years of life in good or fairly good health) both increased between 1981 and 2001, with life expectancy increasing at a faster rate than healthy life expectancy.

Life expectancy is higher for females than for males. In 2001 the life expectancy at birth for females was 80.4 years compared with 75.7 years for males. However, life expectancy for males has been increasing faster than for females. There was an increase of 4.8 years in male life expectancy between 1981 and 2001. For females the corresponding increase was 3.6 years.

The gap in healthy life expectancy between males and females is smaller than for total life expectancy. In 2001, healthy life expectancy at birth was 67.0 years for males and 68.8 years for females, a gap of 1.8 years.

The difference between life expectancy and healthy life expectancy can be regarded as an estimate of the number of years a person can expect to live in poor health. In 1981 the expected time lived in poor health for males was 6.5 years. By 2001 this had risen to 8.7 years. Females can expect to live longer in poor health than males. In 1981 the expected time lived in poor health for a female was 10.1 years, rising to 11.6 years in 2001.

1.1 Prevalence of Hearing Loss in the Elderly

The National Study of Hearing estimated that there were almost nine million deaf and hard of hearing adults in the UK. The study also showed that the majority of hearing loss occurs in older people with 6.6% of the UK population aged 16–60 experiencing a degree of ❯ deafness, compared with 46.9% of people 61–80 years old and 93.2% of people over 81 years old (Davis, 1995).

Age related hearing loss occurs because of gradual changes in the entire auditory system. Such changes may occur in the central auditory pathways or be due to ❯ presbyacusis caused by degenerative changes in the inner ear. Additionally specific diseases of the ear such as end stage otosclerosis and Meniere's disease may cause severe loss of inner ear function. Sensorineural hearing loss also can occur as a result of hereditary factors, various systemic disorders such as autoimmune diseases and as side effects of certain drugs such as cytotoxic medication and the aminoglycoside antibiotics.

Presbyacusis also may be in part caused by changes in the blood supply to the ear due to heart disease, hypertension, diabetes and other vascular disorders. The hearing loss may be mild, moderate, severe or profound.

It is estimated by the Royal National Institute for Deaf People that there are approximately 613,000 severely or profoundly deaf adults in England and Wales. The prevalence of hearing loss increases with age, with 3% of those over 50 years of age and 8% of those over 70 being severely to profoundly deaf. It is likely that these figures will increase in line with the current ageing population.

The prevalence of severe to profound deafness in the elderly population is the most important consideration in terms of both service provision and funding of cochlear implants in the UK. By far the most important effect on the prevalence of hearing impairment within the population is the age group with occupational group and occupational noise exposure having major effects (Davies, 1989). ❯ Table 155-1 illustrates the prevalence of hearing loss as a function of age. The data are derived from the National Study of Hearing 18–80 age group and studies of the age 80 and over group (Davies et al., 1992).

◻ Table 155-1
Estimated percentages of the UK population who are deaf or hard of hearing

UK	16–60 years old (%)	61–80 years old (%)	Over 81 years old (%)
Mild deafness	4.6	28.1	18.4
Moderate deafness	1.6	16.5	57.9
Severe deafness	0.2	1.9	13.2
Profound deafness	0.1	0.4	3.6
All degrees of deafness	6.6	46.9	93.2

Summary of estimated percentage of adults in the UK who have a hearing impairment from mild to profound, depending on age

2 Cochlear Implantation in the Elderly and Quality of Life

In light of the changing demographics of the population with respect to age, and the expansion of the availability and utility of cochlear implantation, most established implant programs are managing an increasing number of elderly candidates and recipients. Over the last two decades there has been an explosion of cochlear implant medical and basic science literature. Much of this has related to pediatric and adult outcomes with little reference to this intervention in the elderly.

However, in the last 10 years as implant programs have expanded, issues around cochlear implant safety, effectiveness and quality of life in the elderly has lead to an emergent literature.

Waltzman and colleagues posed the question as to whether the accepted observation that reduced global speech understanding and processing in the elderly would comprise benefit from a cochlear implant in the elderly (Waltzman et al., 1993). They reported the outcomes of 20 recipients aged 65–85 years and found that post-operative testing showed significant improvements in auditory performance and quality of life, concluding that the elderly can process the new auditory code delivered by an implant. Similarly, the Mayo clinic group observed that of 56 consecutive patients implanted between 1988 and 1994, fourteen individuals were over the age of 65 years and several remained in gainful employment with their cochlear implant (Facer et al., 1995). Kelsall and colleagues described one of the earliest reports comparing the elderly group to the remaining adult implant recipient population (Kelsall et al., 1995). This paper compared 28 patients aged 60–80 years to a matched group of younger adult recipients. In the elderly group, 65% were able to recognize voices over the telephone and 80% described improved quality of life and self-confidence. A smaller French multicenter study also compared their elderly group with the younger adult recipients (Shin et al., 1997). Whilst the numbers were small (18 patients over the age of 60 years), the study showed comparable outcomes between the two groups. This finding was corroborated by the House Ear Clinic who recognized that despite age related changes in the auditory system and prolonged duration of deafness, cochlear implantation in the over 65 years age group conferred audiological and quality of life benefit (Buchman et al., 1999). Labadie and colleagues in 2000 concluded that age alone should not be part of the decision making process when assessing cochlear implant candidacy (Labadie et al., 2000). They compared 20 younger adults (mean age 46.9 years) with an older group of 18 (mean age 71.5 years) and found no significant difference in operative time, length of hospitalization, monosyllabic word test and sentence recognition between the two groups following cochlear implantation.

In a larger group of older implant recipients, the Baltimore group undertook a retrospective analysis of 47 individuals aged between 50 and 80 years (Francis et al., 2002). The patients were assessed at 6 and 12 months post implantation. The gain in health utility in this group correlated with a favorable cost per ❷ quality adjusted life-year in addition to the expected improvements in speech perception scores. This represents an important observation as the issue of ❷ cost effectiveness of cochlear implantation in the older individual was discussed in detail. However, the Baltimore group had defined the older adult as 50 years of age or older for the purposes of their study. A higher age threshold was utilized by Chatelin and colleagues who defined their elderly group as aged 70 years or over (Chatelin et al., 2004). Sixty-five such implant recipients were studied and their outcomes compared to 101 randomly selected younger implant patients. The elderly group showed a significant improvement in auditory performance tests when compared to the pre-implant assessment but fared less favorably than the younger group. The authors postulate that this may be a reflection of the higher age threshold in the group studied and these individuals were more likely to have implant outcomes that were subject to age related degenerative changes such as loss of spiral ganglion cells (auditory nerve) and central vasculo-degenerative changes. In addition, no difference in surgical complications was found between the two groups, an observation corroborated by Haensel et al. in their study of 26 implanted individuals over the age of 65 years (Haensel et al., 2005). In the same year, the Antwerp group attempted to address the quality of life issue in elderly cochlear implantation (Vermeire et al., 2005). They compared 64 younger adult recipients with 25 patients implanted aged 70 years or over. Quality of life assessment included the Hearing Handicap Inventory for Adults and the Glasgow Benefit Inventory (GBI). The post-operative audiological performance improved in both groups but more so in the younger adults. However, the quality of life outcomes were similar for the two groups, confirming the observations of the Baltimore group. ❷ *Table 155-2* summarizes the studies cited with respect to the number of elderly implant recipients in each study and the age range studied.

◻ Table 155-2

Studies investigating cochlear implantation in elderly patients

Study	Number of recipients	Age range in years	Comparison with younger group
Waltzman et al., 1993	20	65–85	No
Facer et al., 1995	25	55+	No
Kelsall et al., 1995	28	60–80	Yes
Shin et al., 1997	18	60+	Yes
Labadie et al., 2000	16	65+	Yes
Francis et al., 2002	47	50–80	No
Chatelin et al., 2004	65	70–91	Yes
Haensel et al., 2005	26	65+	Yes
Vermiere et al., 2005	25	70+	Yes
Orabi et al., 2006	34	65–80	Yes

Cochlear implant studies in elderly patients illustrating the number and age range of patients and whether the outcomes for the study group was compared to a group of younger patients

Finally, the report from the Manchester Cochlear Implant Programe in 2006 studied the auditory performance, surgical complications and quality of life outcomes in a group of 34 consecutive cochlear implant recipients aged 65 years and over (Orabi et al., 2006). In keeping with the reports cited above, this group of patients showed a marked improvement in auditory tests when compared to the pre-implant condition (Bamford-Kowal Bench sentences, Arthur Boothroyd word test and City University of New York sentence tests). The outcomes were comparable to the outcomes from the younger adult implant recipients from the same programme, though the median BKB sentence scores were lower when the groups were tested in the presence of background noise. This may represent poorer central auditory processing in the older group.

Two-thirds of the elderly group in this study had associated co-morbidity such as cardiovascular or pulmonary diseases but the surgical complications were not significantly different from the younger adult group. There are several reasons for this. Firstly, cochlear implantation is invariably undertaken by experienced otologists who draw on their expertise to minimize the surgical and anesthetic time for the procedure. Secondly, as the scalp and mastoid are static anatomical areas, the operation is not particularly painful unlike chest, abdominal or limb surgery which may be associated with ambulatory and respiratory difficulties in the post-operative period. Thirdly, modern anesthetic techniques allow controlled hypotensive anesthesia with reduced bleeding without compromising cardiac and cerebral perfusion.

In keeping with previous studies, the Manchester group of elderly patients demonstrated improvements in the quality of life measures studied which included the Glasgow Health Status Inventory (GHSI) and Glasgow Benefit Inventory (GBI). In addition this report compared the pre-implantation patient expectation profile with the realization of expectations post implantation and found that the patient's expectations from the outcome of implantation was invariably realized. ❷ *Table 155-3* summarizes the audiological data in the two largest more recent studies cited and ❷ *Table 155-4* summarizes the quality of life data in the Manchester study.

❑ Table 155-3

Pre and post operative speech discrimination outcomes

Study	Pre-operative audiological outcome measures	Audiological outcome measures at 12 months or longer	Statistical comparison with younger adult group
Chatelin et al., 2004	CNC words 9%	CNC word 36%	p = 0.03
	CID sentences 17%	CID sentences 62%	p = 0.07
	HINT sentences 18%	HINT sentences 62%	p = 0.07
Orabi et al., 2006	BKB sentences 0%	BKB sentences 73%	p > 0.05
	CUNY sentences 4%	CUNY sentences 95%	p > 0.05
	AB words 11%	AB words 50%	p >0.05

Speech discrimination scores indicating the improvement in performance between the pre and post operative test sessions and the comparison of results with the younger adult group

❑ Table 155-4

Pre and post operative health related quality of life outcomes (GHSI) and cochlear implant benefit (GBI)

Quality of life measure	Pre-implantation	Post-implantation	Statistical analysis
Overall GHSI	44 (25–68)	60 (50–88)	P < 0.001
Overall GBI	-	45 (15–90)	P = 0.058

The GHSI questionnaire illustrates a significant improvement in health related quality of life benefit after implantation

Summary Points

- Cochlear implantation is an established cost-effective intervention for selected children and adults with severe to profound sensorineural deafness.
- As life expectancy in the developed world continues to increase, most implant programmes are assessing increasing numbers of elderly individuals as potential implant recipients.
- The current evidence shows that such patients gain significant benefit in terms of auditory performance after implantation with a low surgical morbidity that is comparable to the younger adult group.

- Several reports in the literature have also shown the quality of life benefit to these patients who often experience increasing social isolation as a consequence of their hearing loss.
- ❯ Healthcare providers and purchasers should not use age alone as a factor in determining the potential recipient's candidacy for cochlear implantation.

References

Backous DD, Dowell R, Manrique M, Waltzman S, Haynes DS, Garcia-Gomez JM. (2007). Ear Hear. 28(2): 128S–129S.

Buchman CA, Fucci MJ, Luxford WM. (1999). Ear Nose Throat J. 78(7): 489–494.

Chatelin V, Kim EJ, Driscoll C, Larky J, Polite C, Price L, Lalwani AK. (2004). Otol Neurotol. 25(3): 298–301.

Davis A, Stephens D, Rayment A, Thomas K. (1992). Br J Audiol. 26: 1–14.

Davis A. (1995). Hearing in adults. Whurr Publishers, London.

Davis AC. (1990). Acta Otolaryngol Suppl. 476: 23–31.

Davis AC. (1989). Int J Epidemiol. 18(4): 911–917.

Djalilian HR, King TA, Smith SL, Levine SC. (2002). Ann Otol Rhinol Laryngol. 111: 890–895.

Facer GW, Peterson AM, Brey RH. (1995). Ann Otol Rhinol. 166: 187–189.

Francis HW, Chee N, Yeagle J, Cheng A, Niparko JK. (2002). Laryngoscope. 112(8 Pt 1): 1482–1488.

Gates GA, Mills JH. (2005). Lancet. 366(9491): 1111–1120.

Herzog M, Mueller J, Milewski C, Schoen F, Helms J. (2000). Adv Otorhinolaryngol. 57: 393–396.

Kelsall DC, Shallop JK, Burnelli T. (1995). Am J Otol. 16(5): 609–615.

Labadie RF, Carrasco V, Gilmer CH, Pillsbury H. (2000). Otolaryngol Head Neck Surg. 123: 419–424.

Labadie RF, Carrasco VN, Gilmer CH, Pillsbury HC 3rd. (2000). Otolaryngol Head Neck Surg. 123(4): 419–424.

Marcincuk MC, Roland PS. (2002). Geriatrics. 57(4): 44, 48–50, 55–56 passim.

Mosnier I, Bouccara D, Ambert-Dahan E, Herelle-Dupuy E, Bozorg-Grayeli A, Ferrary E, Sterkers O. (2002). Ann Otolaryngol Chir Cervicofac. 121: 41–46.

Nakajima S, Iwaki S, Fujisawa N, Yamaguchi S, Kawano M, Fujiki N, Naito Y, Honjo I. (2000). Adv Otorhinolaryngol. 57: 368–369.

Orabi AA, Mawman D, Al-Zoubi F, Saeed SR, Ramsden RT. (2006). Clin Otolaryngol. 31(2): 116–122.

Pasanisi E, Bacciu A, Vincenti V, Guida M, Barbot A, Berghenti MT, Bacciu S. (2003). Clin Otolaryngol. 28: 154–157.

Shin YJ, Fraysse B, Deguine O, Valés O, Laborde ML, Bouccara D, Sterkers O, Uziel A. (2000). Otolaryngol Head Neck Surg. 122: 602–606.

Sterkers O, Mosnier I, Ambert-Dahan E, Herelle-Dupuy E, Bozorg-Grayeli A, Bouccara D. (2004). Acta Otolaryngol Suppl. 552: 64–67.

Vermeire K, Brokx JP, Wuyts FL, Cochet E, Hofkens A, Van de Heyning PH. (2005). Otol Neurotol. 26(2): 188–195.

Waltzman SB, Cohen NL, Shapiro WH. (1993). Otolaryngol Head Neck Surg. 108(4): 329–333.

http://www.rnid.org.uk/information_resources/about-deafness/statistics

http://www.rnid.org.uk/information_resources/fact-sheets/

http://www.fda.gov

http://www.statistics.gov.uk

156 Back Pain and Quality of Life in Elderly Women

K. Zhu · R. L. Prince

1	*Introduction*	2676
2	*Prevalence of Back Pain in Elderly People*	2676
3	*Prevalence of Back Pain in Elderly Australian Women*	2677
3.1	Prevalence of Back Pain at Baseline	2677
3.2	Prevalence of Back Pain at Follow-Up	2677
4	*Back Pain and Physical Function in Elderly Women*	2678
5	*Back Pain and Health Related Quality of Life in Elderly Women*	2679
6	*Back Pain and Risk of Mortality*	2682
7	*Conclusions*	2684
	Summary Points	2684

Abstract: ❯ Back pain is one of the most common musculoskeletal symptoms affecting the elderly population. The ❯ prevalence of back pain in elderly people is not known with certainty, but is likely to range between 13% and 49%. Back pain is associated with reduced quality of life and physical function in the elderly. Our 5-year study with 1,484 community dwelling Australian women aged 70–85 years showed that 22% women suffered from daily back at baseline and this rate increased to 27% 5 years later. Compared to those with infrequent (<1/month) back pain, women with daily back pain had significantly lower quality of life physical component score and reduced physical function as assessed by the ❯ Timed Up and Go test (TUAG) and the ❯ Barthel Index at both baseline and 5 years. New or more frequent back pain at 5 years was also associated with greater reduction in the quality of life physical component score and mobility compared to baseline. Daily back was associated with 103% higher risk of mortality after adjustment for baseline age in this population. In conclusion, frequent back pain is a serious health problem in elderly women. Management of back pain and health conditions related to back pain are likely to be important in the maintenance of functional independence and well-being of elderly women.

List of Abbreviations: ❯ *ADL*, activity of daily living; *HR,* ❯ hazard ratio; *HRQOL,* ❯ health related quality of life; *MCS*, mental component score; *OPAQ*, osteoporosis assessment questionnaire; *PCS*, physical component score; ❯ *SF-36*, medical outcome study short form-36 questionnaire; *TUAG*, timed up and go test

1 Introduction

Musculoskeletal conditions are a major cause physical limitation and therefore reduced quality of life in the elderly. With the aging of population the prevalence of these conditions is expected to rise dramatically. Back pain is one of the most common musculoskeletal symptoms affecting the elderly population. The prevalence of back pain in elderly people is likely to range between 13 and 49%. ❯ Health related quality of life (HRQOL) is a multidimensional concept characterizing the health of individuals according to specific dimensions, namely physical, social, emotional and functional well being. In this chapter, we described the prevalence of back pain in elderly women, the association between back pain and quality of life and physical function, and the association between back pain and mortality risk.

2 Prevalence of Back Pain in Elderly People

The prevalence of back pain in elderly people is not known with certainty. A review of literatures suggested that it is likely to range between 13 and 49% (Bressler et al., 1999). In the United States, a study with 1,037 elderly people aged 68–100 years old showed that 48.6% of them experienced back symptoms including pain, aching or stiffness in the past year and 22.3% had back symptoms on most days (Edmond and Felson, 2000). This study also showed that the prevalence was higher among women then men (52.7% vs. 41.6% for in the past year; 25.6% vs. 16.5% for on most days) and back symptoms on most days are more common in the lower back (23.6%) then in the mid or upper back (8.5%). In Australia, a survey conducted in Sydney with 1,527 people aged 65 years and above showed that 49.7% women and 42.7% men had back problems at the time of survey (March et al., 1998). In Canada, back problems have been ranked as the third and fourth leading cause of chronic health problems in women and men aged over 65 years, respectively (Goel et al., 1996).

3 Prevalence of Back Pain in Elderly Australian Women

To understand the magnitude of the problem in community dwelling elderly Australian women, the prevalence of back pain was evaluated in 1,484 elderly women aged 70–85 years living in Perth, Australia who participated in the Calcium Intake Fracture Outcome Study (CAIFOS), a 5-year double blinded, placebo controlled calcium supplementation study (Prince et al., 2006). These subjects were recruited using a population-based approach in which a random selection of women (n = 24,800) over the age of 70 on the electoral roll in Western Australia received a letter inviting them to join the study. Over 98% of women of this age are on the Western Australia electoral roll. Of the 4,312 women who responded to a letter, 34% joined the study. Although patients entering into the study had a higher social class than the general population of this age, disease burden and pharmaceutical consumption was similar to data obtained from the whole populations of this age (Bruce et al., 2002). Subjects were excluded if they had significant current illness (0.8%) or were receiving bone active agents including calcium supplements (25%). Information on back pain frequency and site was collected by a questionnaire at baseline and 5 years. In the questionnaire, subjects were asked to tick one of the following five categories that best describes the frequency of the pain they experience at the lower back or upper back over the previous year: (1) never, (2) less than once a month, (3) once a month to once a week, (4) once a week to once a day, and (5) once a day or more. Frequency of back pain was scored based on the frequency of pain occurring at the site (lower or upper back) with the higher frequency of pain.

3.1 Prevalence of Back Pain at Baseline

Among the 1,484 study subjects, 1,029 (69.3%) reported back pain at baseline, 515 (34.7%) had lower back pain only, 73 (4.9%) had upper back pain only and 441 (29.7%) had pain at both sites. For the 441 subjects had pain at both sites, 109 subjects had more frequent back pain at the lower back than the upper back, 63 subjects had more frequent back pain at the upper back than the lower back and 269 subjects had back pain at the same frequency at both sites. As there were no significant differences between the "no pain" group and the "pain <1/month" group in any outcome variables examined, these two groups were grouped together as "infrequent pain." For similar reasons, the "pain 1/month – 1/week" group and the "pain 1/week – 1/day" group were grouped together as "frequent pain." There were 751 (50.6%), 410 (27.6%) and 323 (21.8%) subjects had infrequent, frequent and daily back pain, respectively.
    The demographic differences between the three back pain categories are shown in ❯ *Table 156-1*. Women with daily back pain were heavier and had lower socio-economic scores compared with women with infrequent back pain. Women with daily back pain also had lower levels of physical activity. With increased back pain frequency, the percentage of subjects who had prevalent spine fracture and used analgesia increased significantly.

3.2 Prevalence of Back Pain at Follow-Up

At 5 years, of the 1,484 patients recruited into this study, 65 (4.4%) subjects had died, 242 (16.3%) subjects were lost to follow up and back pain and clinical data were obtained from the remaining 1,177 subjects. Those who were not available for review at 5 year (20.7%) were slightly older and had a slightly higher percentage of subjects who had daily back pain at baseline. Compared to baseline, a significantly higher proportion of subjects suffered more

◻ Table 156-1

Characteristics of subjects by baseline back pain frequency

	Infrequent (<1/month)	Frequent (1/month–1/day)	Daily (≥1/day)
Baseline demographics			
Number (%)	751 (50.6)	410 (27.6)	323 (21.8)
Age, years	75.3 ± 2.7	75.0 ± 2.7	75.1 ± 2.7
Socio economic status score[a]	5 (3–6)	5 (3–6)	4 (3–6)[b]
Weight, kg	67.4 ± 11.8	68.7 ± 12.1	71.4 ± 14.4[b,c]
Height, cm	158.9 ± 5.7	158.7 ± 6.1	158.8 ± 6.4
Body mass index, kg/m²	26.7 ± 4.4	27.3 ± 4.5	28.4 ± 5.6[b,c]
Physical activity, kcal/day[a]	121.3 (43.5–214.5)	103.8 (0–190.5)	92.6 (0–188.9)[b]
Analgesia use, n (%)[d]	147 (19.6)	135 (32.9)	170 (52.6)
Spine fracture, n (%)[d]	8 (1.1)	10 (2.4)	11 (3.4)

Data are mean ± SD unless stated otherwise (Source: Zhu et al. (2007). Spine. 32:2012–2018. Reproduced with permission)

[a]Median and IQR

[b]Significantly different from that of the infrequent pain group, $P < 0.05$

[c]Significantly different from that of the frequent pain group, $P < 0.05$

[d]Percentage of subjects with conditions increased significantly with increased pain frequency, $P < 0.05$

frequent back pain at 5 years, with 26.9% compared to 21.8% of subjects experiencing daily back pain. Individual level change in back pain frequency over the 5 years is presented in ❯ *Table 156-2*. About half of those with infrequent or daily back pain remained in the same category 5 years later, but only approximately one third of those with frequent back pain remained in the same category with about third improving and a third deteriorating.

In summary, back pain is a significant problem in community dwelling elderly Australian women aged 70–85 years, with 28% and 22% of them at baseline suffering from frequent (1/month – 1/day) and daily back pain (≥1/day), respectively, and 24% and 27% of them suffering from frequent and daily back pain at 5 years, respectively. About half of those with daily back pain at baseline still had it 5 years later. Similar to the findings of the study with elderly Americans (Edmond and Felson, 2000), it was found that lower back pain was a more common problem than upper back pain.

4 Back Pain and Physical Function in Elderly Women

Back pain is one of the major caused of physical limitation and a number of studies have demonstrated that back pain is related to decreases in physical function in elderly people (Edmond et al., 2005; Liu-Ambrose et al., 2002; Melzer et al., 2005). A study with 11,392 community-living people aged 50 years and over showed that high levels of back pain when walking was associated with mobility disability based on reported difficulty walking a quarter of a mile (402 m) (OR = 2.58; 95% CI 1.83–3.63) (Melzer et al., 2005). In a study with 444 elderly women aged 72–96 years old, having back symptoms on most days was associated with

◼ Table 156-2

Status at 5-year follow-up by baseline back pain frequency

Baseline back pain status	5-year back pain status				
	Infrequent (n = 573)	Frequent (n = 287)	Daily (n = 317)	Died (n = 65)	Lost to follow-up (n = 242)
Infrequent	423	116	75	26	111
(n = 751)	(56.3%)	(15.4%)	(10.0%)	(3.5%)	(14.8%)
Frequent	117	120	91	18	64
(n = 410)	(28.5%)	(29.3%)	(22.2%)	(4.4%)	(15.6%)
Daily	33	51	151	21	67
(n = 323)	(10.2%)	(15.8%)	(46.8%)	(6.5%)[a]	(20.7%)[a]

Data are the number of subjects and the % of each row (Source: Zhu et al. (2007). Spine. 32:2012–2018. Reproduced with permission)

[a]Significance tests for differences in mortality and follow-up rates showed that the rates for daily back pain were significantly higher than those for infrequent and frequent back pain, P < 0.05

most functional limitations, for example, the relative risk of having difficulty standing in one place for about 15 min was 4.26 (95% CI 2.17, 8.38), difficulty walking ½ mile 2.70 (95% CI 1.40, 5.22) and difficulty stooping, crouching or kneeling 1.92 (95% CI 1.23, 3.01) (Edmond et al., 2005). In a study with 93 community-dwelling women aged 65–75 yeas old with osteoporosis, back pain explained 9% of the variance in balance and 13% of the variance in functional mobility (Liu-Ambrose et al., 2002).

In our study with elderly Australian women, activity of daily (ADL) living was assessed by the Barthel index, a 10-item scale of self-care ADL ability; with a maximum score of 100 represents maximum ability (Mahoney and Barthel, 1965). Subjects' mobility functioning was measured by the Timed Up and Go Test (TUAG), which required the subjects to be timed whilst getting up from a standard height chair, walking 3 m, turning, returning to the chair and sitting down again (Podsiadlo and Richardson, 1991). Pain medication was not consumed on the day mobility testing was measured. At both baseline and 5 years, with increased back pain frequency, the percentage of subjects who had Barthel ADL score less than 100 increased significantly, indicating that back pain is related to difficulties in performing activity of daily living (❯ Table 156-3). Increased back pain frequency was also associated with reduced mobility as measured by the TUAG test both at baseline and 5 years (❯ Table 156-3). In women who had both baseline and 5 years data available, those who experienced more frequent back pain at 5 years had significantly greater increases in TUAG time (+23.0 ± 2.0%) compared to baseline than those who did not experience more frequent back pain (+18.1 ± 0.9%). In summary, these data indicated that back pain is associated with reduced mobility and ability to perform activity of daily living in elderly women.

5   Back Pain and Health Related Quality of Life in Elderly Women

The suffering and physical limitation caused by back pain lead to reduced health related quality of life (HRQOL) in elderly people. HRQOL is a multidimensional concept

■ Table 156-3

Activity of daily living and mobility by back pain frequency at baseline and 5 years

	Infrequent (n = 751, 573)[a]	Frequent (n = 410, 287)	Daily (n = 323, 317)
Barthel activity of daily living score, %			
Baseline[b]			
100	83.6	77.8	72.8
90–99	16.4	21.0	25.7
<90	0	1.2	1.5
5 years[b]			
100	81.0	72.0	69.7
90–99	17.9	27.3	26.8
<90	1.1	0.7	3.5
Timed up and go, seconds			
Baseline	9.6 ± 2.4	10.0 ± 3.1[c]	10.7 ± 3.1[c,d]
5 years	10.7 ± 2.6	11.7 ± 4.6[c]	12.6 ± 4.4[c,d]

Data are mean ± SD or percentage as stated
[a]Subject numbers for baseline and 5 years, respectively
[b]Percentage of subjects with Barthel score below 100 increased significantly with increased pain frequency, $P < 0.001$
[c]Significantly different from that of the infrequent pain group, $P < 0.05$
[d]Significantly different from that of the frequent pain group, $P < 0.05$

characterizing the health of individuals according to specific dimensions, namely physical, social, emotional and functional well being and is commonly assessed by subject questionnaires. There are two types of questionnaires: general and disease specific. In our study with the elderly Australian women, HRQOL was assessed by a general questionnaire, the Medical Outcome Study Short Form-36 (SF-36) questionnaire. This SF-36 questionnaire consists of 36 questions that inquire about the general heath status of subjects. This questionnaire is made of 8 domains of Physical Functioning, Role-Physical, Bodily Pain, General Health, Vitality, Social Functioning, Role-Emotional and Mental Health which are summarized in two main composite scores: the physical component score (PCS) and mental component score (MCS) (Ware, 1996). This questionnaire has been validated for use in Australia (Australian Bureau of Statistics, 1991) and we derived the SF-36 summary statistics PCS and MCS from the eight domains using Australian normative data (Australian Bureau of Statistics, 1991). Very low scores for PCS indicate severe physical dysfunction, severe social and role disability, distressful bodily pain, frequent tiredness and unfavorable evaluation of health status. Very low scores of MCS indicate frequent psychological distress, and severe social and role disability due to emotional problems.

At baseline and 5 years, quality of life decreased with increasing back pain frequency as shown by the decreased scores of the eight domains and decreased physical and mental component scores of the SF-36 (❯ *Table 156-4*). In women who had both baseline and 5 years data available, those who experienced more frequent back pain at 5 years had significantly greater reduction in the physical component score but not mental component score of Quality of life compared to baseline than those who did not experience more frequent

◼ Table 156-4

SF-36 Quality of life by back pain frequency at baseline and 5 years

	Infrequent	Frequent	Daily
Baseline (n)	751	410	323
PF	77.2 ± 19.2	68.3 ± 21.6[a]	58.1 ± 24.2[a,b]
PR	79.1 ± 33.2	67.0 ± 39.1[a]	53.0 ± 42.9[a,b]
BP	80.9 ± 20.2	64.7 ± 20.0[a]	47.1 ± 20.2[a,b]
GH	78.5 ± 15.1	73.9 ± 15.9[a]	65.7 ± 19.9[a,b]
VT	71.0 ± 16.0	63.4 ± 18.0[a]	56.9 ± 20.1[a,b]
SF	91.2 ± 17.0	85.5 ± 21.4[a]	80.6 ± 23.9[a,b]
RE	82.2 ± 32.3	75.4 ± 36.4[a]	68.8 ± 40.8[a]
MH	82.6 ± 13.5	78.9 ± 14.4[a]	76.6 ± 16.4[a,b]
PCS	48.7 ± 7.9	43.7 ± 9.0[a]	37.5 ± 10.3[a,b]
MCS	54.0 ± 7.8	52.6 ± 8.9[a]	52.0 ± 10.2[a]
5-years (n)	573	287	317
PF	71.1 ± 22.2	61.1 ± 23.6[a]	47.2 ± 24.3[a,b]
PR	66.8 ± 39.3	57.1 ± 41.6[a]	33.4 ± 39.9[a,b]
BP	77.8 ± 22.0	63.8 ± 20.6[a]	43.1 ± 20.7[a,b]
GH	75.7 ± 16.5	70.8 ± 16.5[a]	61.0 ± 20.0[a,b]
VT	66.6 ± 17.8	61.0 ± 19.0[a]	50.9 ± 20.1[a,b]
SF	86.9 ± 20.5	85.4 ± 22.4	75.0 ± 26.4[a,b]
RE	77.3 ± 35.5	75.8 ± 36.5	68.4 ± 41.6[a,b]
MH	81.8 ± 13.4	79.6 ± 15.6	75.5 ± 17.3[a,b]
PCS	44.0 ± 10.1	39.9 ± 10.9[a]	34.5 ± 11.3[a,b]
MCS	53.9 ± 8.7	52.5 ± 9.5	52.1 ± 10.9[a]

Data are mean ± SD. PF physical functioning; RP role physical; BP bodily pain; GH general health; VT vitality; SF social functioning; RE role emotional; MH mental health; PCS physical composite score; MCS mental composite score

[a]Significantly different from that of the infrequent pain group, P < 0.05
[b]Significantly different from that of the frequent pain group, P < 0.05

back pain after accounting for baseline values, age, 60 months incident spine fracture and calcium supplementation group (❯ Table 156-4).

A few previous studies also showed that back pain is associated with reduced quality of life in elder people (Rabini et al., 2007; Silverman et al., 2005). In a study with 42 men (mean age 45.5 ± 15.8 years) and 66 women (mean age 60.1 ± 23.8 years) with quality of life assessed by the SF-36 questionnaire, the scores of the eight domains of patients with back pain were 9–50 units lower compared with the healthy population (Rabini et al., 2007). In a study with 471 postmenopausal women with osteoporosis, the health related quality of life was assessed by an osteoporosis specific questionnaire, the Osteoporosis Assessment Question-naire (OPAQ) (Silverman et al., 2005). Compared with those who did not have back pain at baseline, the 172 subjects who had back pain has significant lower OPAQ dimension scores for physical function (No pain 87.8 ± 14.4; Pain 76.0 ± 19.2), emotional status

■ Table 156-5

Changes in quality of life according to change in back pain status over 5 years

	Baseline (mean ± SD)		Percentage change since baseline at 5 years (mean ± SE)	
	Frequency reduced or unchanged (n = 895)	Frequency increased (n = 282)	Frequency reduced or unchanged (n = 895)	Frequency increased (n = 282)
SF-36 physical component score	45.4 ± 9.6	45.2 ± 9.6	−6.0 ± 0.7	−16.7 ± 1.3[a]
SF-36 mental component score	53.7 ± 8.5	53.1 ± 8.7	0.7 ± 0.9	3.2 ± 1.5

[a]Significantly different from that of the frequency reduced or unchanged group after adjustment for baseline values, age, 60 months incident spine fracture and calcium supplementation group, P < 0.05 (Source: Zhu et al. (2007). Spine. 32:2012–2018. Reproduced with permission)

(No pain 72.0 ± 14.6; Pain 62.5 ± 18.4), symptoms (No pain 67.9 ± 17.5; Pain 53.3 ± 19.9), and social interaction (No pain 65.9 ± 15.2; Pain 62.0 ± 15.7) (P < 0.05). Prevalent back pain was also associated with lower overall HRQOL score (P < 0.01). Of 429 women completed the questionnaire at baseline, 12 months and at study termination (median follow-up duration 19 months), 88 experienced new or worsen back pain, which was associated with significant greater reduction in OPAQ dimension scores for physical function, emotional status, symptoms, and social interaction (P < 0.05) as well as overall HRQOL score (P < 0.01) (Silverman et al., 2005).

One of the major purposes of health and social policy in old age is to increase quality of life of elderly people. As back pain is a cause of reduced quality of life, it would be important to manage back pain and health conditions related to back pain in order to maintain quality of life of elderly women.

6 Back Pain and Risk of Mortality

Pain is not only related to suffering and reduced quality of life, but also could be a sign of underlying medical conditions, which is associated with the longevity. Therefore, an investigation of the influence of back pain and mortality risk is of clinical interest. A few studies on the association of back pain and mortality risk in elderly people have failed to show any association (Heliovaara et al., 1995; Jacobs et al., 2005; Kareholt and Brattberg, 1998). However, in a 13 years prospective study with Finnish farmers aged 30–66 years at baseline, back pain in the year before baseline has been shown to be related to increased risk of dying of ischemic heart disease (Penttinen, 1994). Furthermore, a recent study of elderly Americans showed that a summary score of physical symptoms including back pain as one of the symptoms was a significant independent predictor of death at 1 year (Sha et al., 2005).

We evaluated the association between back pain frequency and risk of mortality in elderly Australian women. All cause of death data were obtained from the Hospital Morbidity Data System accessed via the Data Linkage Unit of the Health Department of Western Australia.

■ Figure 156-1

Cox proportional hazard analysis of time to death. Analysis adjusted for baseline age and calcium supplementation. HR 1.27 (95% CI 0.70–2.32) for frequent pain compared to infrequent pain, HR 2.03 (95% CI 1.14–3.60) for daily pain compared to infrequent pain (Source: Zhu et al. (2007). Spine. 32:2012–2018. Reproduced with permission)

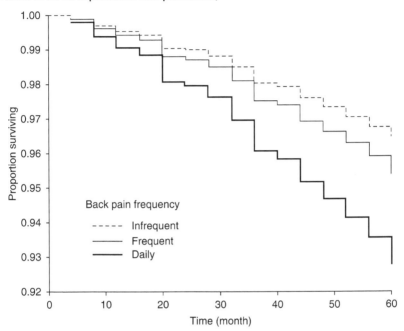

The all cause of death data were also ascertained from death certificates from the Registrar of Births Marriages and Deaths available for all deaths over 5 years. After 5 years, 65 subjects had died. Among those with daily back pain at baseline, the crude mortality rate was higher than those with infrequent back pain at baseline (6.5% vs. 3.5%) (❯ *Table 156-2*). Subjects with daily back pain had a risk of death that was double that of subjects with infrequent back pain after adjustment for baseline age (Hazard Ratio (HR) 2.03, 95% CI 1.14–3.60) (❯ *Figure 156-1*). Further adjustment for baseline cardiovascular risk factors including baseline BMI, smoking history, analgesia use, diabetes, cardiovascular disease, hypercholesterolemia and hypertension and physical activity level had little influence on the effect (Cardiovascular risk factors adjusted HR 1.85, 95% CI 1.00–3.43; Physical activity level adjusted HR 1.93, 95% CI 1.08–3.43).

These findings suggested that daily back pain is related to a higher mortality risk in this population. The fact that the mortality effect was reduced but not removed by adjustment for cardiovascular risk factors suggests that these risk factors may account for some of the association. One mechanism may relate to the fact that atherosclerosis has been postulated to be involved in the etiology of back pain through reducing blood flow to bone and soft tissue in the back (Kauppila, 1995). In patients with lower back pain, atherosclerotic calcifications of the abdominal aorta and occluded lumbar and/or middle sacral arteries were more frequently presented than age-matched controls (Kauppila et al., 2004; Kurunlahti et al., 1999). A 25-year population based cohort study has shown that advanced atherosclerosis was associated with increased risk for the development of disc degeneration and the occurrence of back pain (Kauppila et al., 1997). More recent studies have suggested that inflammation might be a common factor in back pain and heart disease (Banks and Watkins, 2006). Another mechanism of the association between mortality and back pain may relate to the association with decreased physical activity level and decreased mobility. When the Cox regression model was adjusted for physical activity level, the HR of daily back pain for mortality was attenuated but not removed. As mentioned earlier, increased Timed Up and Go, a reliable and valid test for quantifying functional mobility (Podsiadlo and Richardson, 1991), were associated with increase back pain frequency. This reduction in physical activity may be associated with increased weight with it deleterious consequences on cardiovascular disease.

7 Conclusions

In conclusion, our study demonstrates that frequent back pain is a serious health problem in elderly women, which not only lead to reduced quality of life and physical function, but also is associated with increased risk of mortality. Management of back pain and health conditions related to back pain are likely to be important in the maintenance of functional independence and well-being of elderly women.

Summary Points

- Back pain is one of the most common musculoskeletal symptoms affecting the elderly population. The prevalence of back pain in elderly people is not known with certainty, but is likely to range between 13 and 49%.
- More than twenty percent of community dwelling elderly Australian women suffered from daily back pain and about half of those with daily back pain at baseline still had it 5 years later.
- Back pain is associated with reduced quality of life and physical function.
- New or worsen back pain is associated with greater reduction in quality of life and physical function.
- Daily back pain was associated with 103% greater risk of mortality in community dwelling elderly Australian women.

References

Australian Bureau of Statistics. (1991). National Health Survey: Musculoskeletal Conditions. ABS, Canberra.

Banks WA, Watkins LR. (2006). Pain. 124: 1–2.

Bressler HB, Keyes WJ, Rochon PA, Badley E. (1999). Spine. 24: 1813–1819.

Bruce DG, Devine A, Prince RL. (2002). J Am Geriatr Soc. 50: 84–89.

Edmond SL, Felson DT. (2000). J Rheumatol. 27: 220–225.

Edmond SL, Kiel DP, Samelson EJ, Kelly-Hayes M, Felson DT. (2005). Osteoporos Int. 16: 1086–1095.

Goel V, Iron K, Williams JI. (1996). Goel V, Williams JI, Anderson GM, Blackstein-Hirsch P, Fooks C, Naylor CD (eds.) Patterns of Health Care in Ontario. The ICES Practice Atlas. 2nd ed. Canadian Medical Association, Ottawa, pp. 5–26.

Heliovaara M, Makela M, Aromaa A, Impivaara O, Knekt P, Reunanen A. (1995). Spine. 20: 2109–2111.

Jacobs JM, Hammerman-Rosenberg R, Stessman J. (2005). J Am Geriatr Soc. 53: 1636–1637.

Kareholt I, Brattberg G. (1998). Pain. 77: 271–278.

Kauppila LI. (1995). Lancet. 346: 888–889.

Kauppila LI, McAlindon T, Evans S, Wilson PW, Kiel D, Felson DT. (1997). Spine. 22: 1642–1647.

Kauppila LI, Mikkonen R, Mankinen P, Pelto-Vasenius K, Maenpaa I. (2004). Spine. 29: 2147–2152.

Kurunlahti M, Tervonen O, Vanharanta H, Ilkko E, Suramo I. (1999). Spine. 24: 2080–2084.

Liu-Ambrose T, Eng JJ, Khan KM, Mallinson A, Carter ND, McKay HA. (2002). Osteoporos Int. 13: 868–873.

Mahoney FI, Barthel DW. (1965). Maryland State Med J. 14: 661–665.

March LM, Brnabic AJ, Skinner JC, Schwarz JM, Finnegan T, Druce J, Brooks PM. (1998). Med J Aust. 168: 439–442.

Melzer D, Gardener E, Guralnik JM. (2005). Age Ageing. 34: 594–602.

Penttinen J. (1994). Br Med J. 309: 1267–1278.

Podsiadlo D, Richardson S. (1991). J Am Geriatr Soc. 39: 142–148.

Prince RL, Devine A, Dhaliwal SS, Dick IM. (2006). Arch Intern Med. 166: 869–875.

Rabini A, Aprile I, Padua L, Piazzini DB, Maggi L, Ferrara PE, Amabile E, Bertolini C. (2007). Eura Medicophys. 43: 49–54.

Sha MC, Callahan CM, Counsell SR, Westmoreland GR, Stump TE, Kroenke K. (2005). Am J Med. 118: 301–306.

Silverman SL, Piziak VK, Chen P, Misurski DA, Wagman RB. (2005). J Rheumatol. 32: 2405–2409.

Ware J. (1996). Spilker B (ed.) Quality of Life and Pharmacoeconomics in Clinical Trials. 2nd ed. Lippincott-Raven, Philadelphia, PA, pp. 337–345.

157 Measuring Quality of Life at the End of Life

L. A. Roscoe · D. D. Schocken

1	Introduction	2688
2	Quality-of-Life Domains Relevant to the End-of-Life Context	2689
2.1	Quality of Life and Quality of Care	2689
2.2	Patient Preferences and Individual Differences	2691
2.3	Self-Report Data	2691
2.4	Proxy Data	2692
3	Measuring Quality of Life at the End of Life	2692
3.1	Clinimetric Tools and Research Measures	2693
3.2	Quality of Life of Cancer Patients	2693
3.3	Disease-Specific Quality of Life Measures	2693
3.4	Quality of Life Measures Appropriate Across Disease Conditions	2694
3.5	Quality of Care at the End of Life	2697
4	Hospice Care and Quality of Life at the End of Life	2698
4.1	Barriers to Hospice Care	2699
5	Barriers to Research with Dying Patients	2699
6	Conclusions and Future Directions	2700
	Summary Points	2701

© Springer Science+Business Media LLC 2010 (USA)

Abstract: For patients near the ❷ end of life, quality of life becomes an even more central goal of care than for patients for whom recovery is expected. While patient quality of life is essentially an individual matter and a reflection of a particular patient's goals, experiences, values and preferences for treatment, there is considerable agreement about what domains are relevant. Domains that comprise patient quality of life at the end of life generally include: trusting one's physician, avoiding a prolonged dying experience, attaining a sense of closure, avoiding being a burden to family members, managing pain and other symptoms, and maintaining open communication.

The characteristics of quality of life measures useful in this context are described, and seven quality of life measures with demonstrated reliability and validity in the end of life context are discussed. The domains that comprise quality of care at the end of life overlap the domains of quality of life; thus three measures of quality of care at the end of life are also described. Since patients nearing the end of life are often debilitated and unable to respond to measurement instruments, the benefits and risks of using ❷ proxy data for patient quality of life measurements are summarized. The influence of ❷ hospice care on patient quality of life is summarized, as well as the difficulties of conducting research in this patient population. The chapter concludes with suggested directions for future research.

List of Abbreviations: ❷ *HIPAA*, Health Insurance Portability and Accountability Act; ❷ *HQLI*, Hospice Quality of Life Index; ❷ *MQLS*, McMaster Quality of Life Scale; ❷ *MQOL*, McGill Quality of Life Questionnaire; ❷ *MQOL-CSF*, McGill Quality of Life Questionnaire-Cardiff Short Form; ❷ *MVQOLI*, Missoula-VITAS Quality of Life Index; ❷ *QODD*, Quality of Dying and Death; ❷ *TIME*, Toolkit of Instruments to Measure End of Life Care

1   Introduction

Patient quality of life has become a central goal of care at the end of life. Patients used to die relatively quickly of infectious diseases, but now patients in industrialized nations are far more likely to die of chronic progressive illnesses whose courses are characterized by periods of decline and stability (Bradley et al., 2000; Teno and Dosa, 2006). Such illness trajectories are accompanied by prolonged periods of functional dependence, and are marked by a number of decisions about how, when, and if to continue treatment to prolong life. When interventions to cure a patient's disease become futile or overly burdensome, the goals of care change. Patient quality of life becomes more important than seeking to cure the disease. Thus, the measurement of quality of life at the end of life has received increased attention in both clinical practice and in the research literature.

This chapter will first review the domains that are generally agreed to comprise patient quality of life at the end of life. Measures of quality of life that are reliable and valid in the end-of-life context are described next, including some related measures of quality of care at the end of life. The influence of hospice care on patient quality of life at the end of life will be summarized, as well as a discussion of the difficulties of conducting research on patients near the end of life. Final observations about measuring patients' quality of life at the end of life conclude the chapter.

While each patient near the end of his or her life must be treated as a unique and particular individual, there are some overall characteristics of patients near the end of life that may be helpful to keep in mind, particularly for researchers and clinicians new to this patient population. ❷ *Table 157-1* summarizes these characteristics.

◻ Table 157-1

Key characteristics of patients at the end of life

Patients typically have a prognosis of 6 months or less of life
Patients may be coping with a range of symptoms that vary in severity, distress, and prevalence
Patients may reside in a variety of settings that may influence their quality of life and/or the measurement of their quality of life (home, nursing home, hospital, or hospice)
Patients retain the right to make their own decisions about research participation and clinical decision making
Suffering at the end of life is a multi-dimensional construct that may include physical symptoms, mental distress, unresolved family issues, or spiritual anguish
Patients at the end of life may find meaning and benefit in research participation, even if it is unlikely to be of direct benefit to them

2 Quality-of-Life Domains Relevant to the End-of-Life Context

Quality of life at the end of life is a subjective concept that should reflect each patient's goals, values, and preferences for medical treatment. However, studies that have identified domains associated with quality of life in the context of life-limiting illness reveal remarkable consistency among patients in the U.S. Seriously ill people with limited life expectancy tend to identify the following correlates of quality of life: trust in one's physician, avoidance of a prolonged dying experience, attainment of a sense of closure, not being a burden to family members, adequate support to remain at home, symptom relief, and open communication (Heyland et al., 2006). These domains are also consistent with results from focus groups, interviews, and expert opinion that preceded the development of measurement tools (Patrick et al., 2001; Steinhauser et al., 2000, 2001; Stewart et al., 1999). Other investigators have added domains such as the importance of maintaining social connectedness and strengthening relationships with family and friends (Emmanuel et al., 2000; Johansson et al., 2006; Kutner et al., 2007); managing life while ill or maintaining a sense of control (Johanson et al., 2006); or attention to spiritual issues (Cohen et al., 1996; Emmanuel et al., 2000; Kutner et al., 2007). Quality of life domains for patients near the end of life are summarized in ❯ *Table 157-2*.

2.1 Quality of Life and Quality of Care

In the context of patients with limited life expectancy, quality of life becomes a goal of treatment, as well as a component of the measurement of the quality of end-of-life care (Roila and Cortesi, 2001). There is significant overlap between the domains identified for patient quality of life at the end of life and of quality of care at the end of life. Singer and colleagues (1999) identified the following domains of quality of care derived from patient interviews: receiving adequate pain and symptom management, avoiding inappropriate prolongation of dying, achieving a sense of control, relieving burden, and strengthening relationships with loved ones. Quality end-of-life care supports patients' quality of life, therefore, quality of life represents a significant outcome indicator to evaluate the quality of care and the efficacy of interventions aimed at symptom management.

◼ Table 157-2

Quality of Life Domains for Patients At the End of Life

Reference	Dimensions	Methodology
Singer et al. (1999)	pain and symptom management avoiding prolonged dying sense of control relieving burden strengthen relationships with loved ones	Patient interviews
Stewart et al. (1999)	physical comfort and emotional support shared decision-making advance care planning focus on individual spiritual needs coordination of care	Literature and expert review
Emanuel et al. (2000)	patient-clinician relationship social connectedness care giving needs psychological support spirituality/religiousness personal acceptance sense of purpose clinician communication	Patient interviews
Steinhauser et al. (2000, 2001)	pain and symptom management preparation for death sense of completion decisions about treatment treated as whole person remaining mentally aware having funeral planned relieving burden helping others being at peace with God decisions about life-sustaining treatment dying at home meaning of death	Interviews with patients, bereaved family members, physicians and other care providers
Patrick, Engelberg and Curtis (2001)	symptom management and personal care preparation for death moment of death family relationships treatment preferences honored whole person concerns	Interviews with patients with and without chronic and terminal conditions
Heyland et al. (2006)	trust and confidence in physicians avoiding prolonged dying experience honest communication preparation for death closure support to remain at home symptom relief	Focus groups with experts and patient interviews

◻ Table 157-2 (continued)

Reference	Dimensions	Methodology
Johansson et al. (2006)	maintaining ordinariness of life maintaining a positive life alleviating suffering maintaining significant relationships managing life while ill	Focus group
Kutner et al. (2007)	physical symptom management functional status psychological symptom management interpersonal relationships/social interaction environment impact of care giving spiritual/existential outlook preparation for death	Prospective cohort study

2.2 Patient Preferences and Individual Differences

Although there is considerable agreement concerning domains of quality of life at the end of life, a patient's experiences, beliefs, expectations, perceptions, culture, and preferences may influence the relative importance of these domains. For example, some patients may not want to die at home, and may equate prolonging their time at home with becoming a burden to family members. As patients approach death, some domains may be emphasized more than others. Functional status has long been a hallmark of quality of life, although function is perhaps less relevant to patients nearing the end of life than are other domains such as attention to spiritual issues or attainment of closure (Massaro and McMillan, 2000; McMillan, 1996a).

The meaning of various domains may also change as patients get closer to dying. Social well-being may change meaning from how much the respondent is able to engage in social activities deemed "normal" for a well person, to meaning how much of a burden the respondent feels he or she is on the family, friends, and health care providers in their social network (Schwartz et al., 2005). It is important to note that quality of life at any stage of life's journey must include both the avoidance of negative outcomes, such as pain, as well as pursuit of more positive outcomes, such as maintaining social connectedness (Kane et al., 1997; Lawton, 1991). Most important overall is the relief of suffering (Rummans et al., 2000), recognizing that the source of suffering may be multi-focal.

2.3 Self-Report Data

Patient-derived taxonomies are important in the development of quality-of-life measures, and use of self-report data is the goal (Massaro and McMillan, 2000). For example, in contrast with domains derived from expert opinion, patient-derived descriptions of quality end-of-life care are simpler and more straightforward, more specific, and less bound by established concepts for which measurement scales are available (Singer et al., 1999). In the patient-derived taxonomy, rather than a general label such as "psychological," the patient perspective speaks of "achieving a sense of control;" rather than "social," of "relieving burden" and "strengthening relationships."

Patients near the end of life, however, often cannot provide information as their diseases progress, and it is often necessary to rely on family caregivers as informants. Systematic bias may be created if data are reported only by patients who are less impaired; likewise, missing data from debilitated patients weakens the scientific rigor of studies that attempt to validate or utilize measures of patient quality of life at the end of life. While patient self-report may be the ideal, in this population it is often necessary to rely on the reports of proxies such as family caregivers, or health care providers (Fowler et al., 1999).

2.4　Proxy Data

In their review of the use of proxy reports about the quality of life of terminally ill cancer patients, Tang and McCorkle (2002) found at least moderate agreement between family members and patients regarding patients' quality of life. The bias introduced by the use of family informants was generally of a modest magnitude. When discrepancies existed, without exception, family caregivers held a more negative view of patients' quality of life than did patients. In two studies comparing quality-of-life scores of hospice patients and caregivers, correlations were weak to moderate (r = 0.39–0.55) with caregivers tending to underestimate the quality of life reported by the patients (McMillan and Mahon, 1994; McMillan, 1996b). Kutner and colleagues (2006) concluded that proxy responses appeared to be a fair substitute for patient responses when patient self-report data were unavailable. Taken in sum, proxy responses appear both valid and reliable.

3　Measuring Quality of Life at the End of Life

The field of research into palliative and end of life care has grown in recent years with the emergence and increased utilization of standardized tools for assessing quality of life and the parameters of quality of care at the end-of-life (Schwartz et al., 2005). Massaro and McMillan (2000) specify characteristics of quality-of-life measures appropriate in the end of life context; ❯ Table 157-3 provides a summary of these characteristics.

Several types of questionnaires are available to measure health-related quality-of-life, but may not be appropriate in the end-of-life context (Donnelly, 2000; Massaro and McMillan, 2000; Steinhauser et al., 2002; Teno et al., 1999). Questionnaires that are used for patients receiving active treatment have several limitations when used to assess the quality-of-life of

◻ Table 157-3

Characteristics of quality of life instruments appropriate in the end-of-life context

Instruments should:
Be multi-dimensional; all aspects of quality of life that are affected by life-limiting illnesses should be included;
Provide subjective data obtained via self-report data from patients;
Be useful in the setting in which they will be used; and
Have demonstrated validity and reliability.

Adapted from: Massaro and McMillan, 2000

patients who have progressive diseases and are dying. For example, questionnaires used to assess the quality of life for cancer patients enrolled in clinical trials often give increased weight to physical domains of functioning, the salience of which may be lessened as life expectancy decreases. Also many questionnaires used in clinical trials don't capture the existential or spiritual domain that may increase in importance as death approaches (Cohen et al., 2001).

3.1 Clinimetric Tools and Research Measures

Quality-of-life measures appropriate for use in the end-of-life context can further be described as those that are appropriate for clinical decision making (❷ clinimetric tools) and those that demonstrate the required psychometric properties essential for research (Schwartz et al., 2005). Clinimetric tools evaluate a phenomenon such as patient quality of life by assessing the occurrence of multiple, heterogeneous attributes, such as symptoms that affect the phenomenon, and may create scores by summing a set of ratings (Wright and Feinstein, 1992). In contrast, ❷ psychometric tools measure an underlying construct by assessing attributes that are relatively homogeneous and are affected by changes in the latent construct. All measurement tools have to be relevant to the populations to which they are applied, and should be responsive to clinically important changes; thus the tools that are described in detail below generally have both clinical utility and validity in a research context.

3.2 Quality of Life of Cancer Patients

Just as most hospice patients of past years were cancer patients, most instruments developed to measure quality of life at the end of life were initially developed based on the experience of cancer patients, especially those enrolled in clinical trials (Massaro and McMillan, 2000; McMillan, 1996a). An early quality of life measure for use by physicians assessing patients with terminal cancer was developed by Spitzer and colleagues (1981). Although designed specifically for end-stage cancer patients, it is included here since it has served as a useful benchmark for determining construct validity for other quality of life measures developed for use with patients across end-stage conditions. Physician interviews of patients assessed the domains of activity, living, health, support and outlook on life. Patients used a 3-point scale (0–2) to rate each item, yielding quality-of-life scores from 0 to 10. The Quality of Life Index (QLI) is reported to have adequate internal consistency and acceptable inter-rater reliability when tested by 150 physicians' interviews with 879 patients with cancer of varying stages.

3.3 Disease-Specific Quality of Life Measures

Specific instruments have been developed in recent years to capture the unique experiences of other patient populations at the end of life, notably measures assessing the quality of life for end-stage dialysis patients and transplant patients. For example, Montazeri et al. (1998) report that over 50 instruments have been developed to measure the quality of life of end-stage lung cancer patients. Gentile et al. (2003) described three disease-targeted instruments developed for end-stage kidney patients undergoing dialysis and two specific disease-targeted instruments for renal transplant patients. Such disease-targeted instruments may be more sensitive to the needs of a specific population.

3.4   Quality of Life Measures Appropriate Across Disease Conditions

The instruments described below have demonstrated their reliability and validity across patient disease conditions, and have proven reliable and valid in an end-of-life setting. Measures of quality of life at the end of life that may be used across end-of-life settings and patient populations are described below; their characteristics are summarized in ❂ *Table 157-4*.

❏ Table 157-4

Characteristics of measures of quality of life at the end of life

Instrument	Reference	Dimensions	Self-Report?	Length	Validity	Reliability
Quality of Life Index (QLI)	Spitzer et al. (1981)	Activity Living Health Support Outlook on life	Yes	5 items	Inter-rater reliability r = 0.81	α = 0.78
Hospice Quality of Life Index (HQLI)	McMillan and Mahon (1994)	Psychosocial Functional Social/Spiritual well-being	Yes	28 items	Content validity assessed by hospice experts r = 0.83	α = 0.88
McGill Quality of Life Questionnaire (MQOL)	Cohen et al. (1995)	Physical symptoms Psychological symptoms Outlook on life Meaningful existence	Yes	16 items	Strong significant correlation with single item measures of quality of life	α = 0.70 Cohen et al. (1997)
McGill Quality of Life Questionnaire-Cardiff Short Form (MQOL-CSF)	Lua et al. (2005)	Physical Psychological Outlook Meaning	Yes	8 items	Correlation between MQOL-CSF and analogous MQOL items (r = 0.48–0.73)	α = 0.46–0.86
McMaster Quality of Life Scale (MQLS)	Sterkenberg et al. (1996)	Physical Non-physical	Yes	32 items	Concurrent validity assessed by correlation with Spitzer QLI (r = 0.70) and correlations with staff ratings (r = 0.50)	α = 0.80, total scores α = 0.60 physical α = 0.79 non-physical

□ Table 157-4 (continued)

Instrument	Reference	Dimensions	Self-Report?	Length	Validity	Reliability
Missoula-VITAS Quality of Life Index (MVQOLI)	Byock and Merriman (1998)	Symptoms Function Interpersonal Well-being Transcendence	Yes	25 items	Correlations with global quality of life item, r = 0.43 (Byock and Merriman 1998) r = 0.35 Schwartz et al. (2005)	α = 0.77 (Byock and Merriman, 1998) α = 0.71 (Schwartz et al., 2005)
QUAL-E	Steinhauser et al. (2002)	Life completion Symptoms impact Relationship w/health care provider Preparation	Yes	25 items	Convergent and discriminant validity demonstrated with multiple comparison measures (Steinhauser et al., 2004)	α = 0.83 overall (Steinhauser et al. 2002) α = .080, life completion α = 0.87, symptoms impact α = 0.71, relat w/health care provider α = 0.68, preparation (Steinhauser et al., 2004)

Hospice Quality of Life Index (HQLI). The HQLI is a 28-item patient self-report questionnaire (McMillan and Mahon, 1994). Items cover three major categories: psychosocial, functional, and social/spiritual well-being. Each item is rated on a 0–10 scale, resulting in total scores ranging from 0 to 280 (indicating lowest to highest quality of life). Reliability and validity analyses were initially conducted with 68 patients enrolled in hospice and their caregivers, and hospice experts evaluated the items to assess content validity. Further psychometric tests (McMillan and Weitzner, 1998) using data from 255 hospice patients revealed high reliability for the total scale.

McGill Quality of Life Questionnaire (MQOL). The MQOL is a 16-item self report measure that assesses four domains: physical symptoms, psychological symptoms, support/outlook on life, and existential/meaningful existence (Cohen et al., 1995). Patients are asked to assess their condition over the past two days using a scale from 0 to 10, where 0 indicates "very bad," and 10 indicates "excellent." This instrument differs from most others in three ways; the existential domain is measured, the physical domain is important but not predominant, and positive contributions to quality of life are measured. Cohen and colleagues (1997) conducted a validation study with eight palliative care services, the results of which showed that the MQOL demonstrated strong evidence of construct validity through correlations with a single-item measure of quality of life and with Spitzer's Quality of Life Index (Spitzer et al., 1981) and internal consistency.

McGill Quality of Life Questionnaire-Cardiff Short Form (MQOL-CSF). An 8-item short form of the MQOL was developed from the original version. The McGill Quality of Life Questionnaire-Cardiff Short Form (MQOL-CSF) was tested in palliative care patients including 56 out-patients, 48 hospice patients, and 86 in-patients (Lua et al., 2005). The MQOL-CSF demonstrated moderate to high internal consistency, and moderate to strong correlations between items in the short form and analogous items in the MQOL. The MQOL-CSF reduces respondent burden (average completion time was 3.3 min) and demonstrated favorable psychometric properties in the palliative care population.

McMaster Quality of Life Scale ❷ *(MQLS).* The MQLS consists of 32 items that measure physical and non-physical (emotional, social, and spiritual) domains (Sterkenberg, King and Woodward, 1996). Patients use a 7-point scale to rate each item, and family members and medical staff complete a parallel form. Concurrent validity was assessed by correlation with Spitzer and colleagues (1981) QLI and with staff ratings. The MQLS demonstrates high overall reliability among palliative care patients in both in-patient and out-patient settings. Some of the content areas have too few items to be used as scales, so the MQLS is best divided into physical and non-physical subscales; both subscales demonstrated acceptable internal consistency. Validation studies correlated ratings of different raters (patient, family, staff members) and found systematic differences; thus the authors concluded that substituting family or staff ratings for patient ratings should be avoided.

Missoula-VITAS Quality of Life Index ❷ *(MVQOLI).* The MVQOLI is a 25-item patient-centered index that weights each of five quality of life dimensions (symptoms, function, interpersonal, well-being, and transcendence) by its importance to the respondent (Byock and Merriman, 1998). Some items are single statements to which patients indicate agreement on a Likert-type scale, and others are presented as two contrasting statements from which patients select the best description of their situation. The MVQOLI was administered to 257 patients enrolled in ten community-based hospices, and demonstrated acceptable internal consistency, but only modest correlation of the total score with patient-reported global quality of life assessments.

Psychometric and implementation studies conducted on end-stage renal patients on dialysis, hospice patients, and long-term care patients revealed similar results, and Schwartz and colleagues (2005) concluded that the measure may be more appropriate for clinical decision making that for research. The MVQOLI was particularly useful in stimulating communication about the psychosocial and spiritual issues important to life closure, although it is somewhat long and complex for seriously ill patients to complete.

❷ *QUAL-E.* The QUAL-E asks respondents to rate the importance of 25 items in four domains using a 5-point Likert-type scale: life completion, symptoms impact, relationship with health care provider, and preparation for death. The QUAL-E has been validated with data from 200 seriously ill patients with either end-stage cancer, congestive heart failure, end-stage renal disease, or chronic obstructive pulmonary disease. This initial validation study yielded a final instrument with an additional domain of affective social support, and demonstrated high overall reliability (Steinhauser et al., 2002). Further psychometric studies (Steinhauser et al., 2004) confirmed a four-domain structure with high reliability: life completion, symptoms impact, relationship with health care provider, and preparation for death. The QUAL-E employs empirically derived domains of demonstrated importance, is acceptable to seriously ill patients, and has demonstrated acceptable psychometric properties, including acceptable correlations with other quality of life measures.

3.5   Quality of Care at the End of Life

As mentioned previously, there is considerable overlap between dimensions that measure the quality of life of dying patients and the quality of care that dying patients receive. Three assessment instruments that primarily assess quality of care at the end of life are discussed below, and their characteristics are summarized in ❷ *Table 157-5*.

Toolkit of Instruments to Measure End of Life Care (TIME). Teno and colleagues have developed and validated interview protocols for bereaved family members of patients who died in hospitals, nursing homes, or under hospice care (Teno et al., 2001a). Bereaved family members respond to interview questions assessing eight domains of care: decision-making, advance care planning, closure, coordination, achieving control and respect, family emotional support, self-efficacy and an overall rating of satisfaction (measured by a 5-point, "excellent" to "poor" scale). A validation study (Teno et al., 2001b) conducted with 156 family members whose loved ones died in either an outpatient hospice service, a consortium of nursing homes,

■ Table 157-5

Characteristics of measures of quality of care at the end of life

Instrument	Reference	Dimensions	Self-Report?	Length	Validity	Reliability
Toolkit of instruments to measure end of life care (TIME)	Teno et al. (2001a)	Decision-making Advance care planning Closure Coordination Control/Respect Emotional support Self-efficacy Overall satisfaction	No-interviews with bereaved family members	53 questions	Correlation w/overall satisfaction r = 0.44–0.52 Teno et al. (2001b)	α = 0.58–0.87 Teno et al. (2001b)
Quality of death and dying (QODD)	Curtis et al. (2002)	Symptom management Patient preferences Satisfaction with care	No-interviews with bereaved family members	31 questions	Satisfactory cross-sectional validity	α = 0.89
Quality of end-of-life care and satisfaction with treatment scale (QUEST)	Sulmasy et al. (2002)	Availability of medical staff Attentiveness to patient Satisfaction with care	Yes	15 items	Correlation with related satisfaction with care measure r = 0.38–0.47	α = 0.88–0.93

or a hospital revealed a range of internal consistency scores for the subscales, and moderate correlations with the overall rating of satisfaction.

*Quality of Dying and Death*❷ *(QODD).* The QODD is a 31-item structured interview with bereaved family members after a patient's death (Curtis et al., 2002). Bereaved family members are asked to report and rate the quality of the dying experience in the decedent's last seven days, or if the patient was unconscious or unresponsive throughout the last seven days, over the last month before death. Respondents rate each item on a scale from 0 to 10, where 0 = "a terrible experience," and 10 = "an almost perfect experience." A total score is calculated by adding the scores on all items and dividing by the number of items answered; this mean score is then multiplied by 10 to construct a scale from 0 to 100, with higher scores indicating a better quality of dying and death.

The QODD assesses the following domains: symptom management, patient preferences, and satisfaction with care. The QODD was initially validated using 205 after-death interviews with bereaved family members. The QODD demonstrated high internal reliability, and the total score demonstrated good cross-sectional validity (Curtis et al., 2002). The QODD was also applied in a community sample and a sample of hospice enrollees (Patrick et al., 2003). How well patients' symptoms were controlled in the community sample and how well patients' preferences were followed and treatments were explained in the hospice sample were associated with higher quality dying.

*Quality of End-of-Life Care and Satisfaction with Treatment Scale*❷ *(QUEST).* The QUEST is a clinimetric instrument that has demonstrated utility in assessing quality and satisfaction with care of hospitalized patients at the end of life (Sulmasy et al., 2002). The QUEST utilizes two subscales (9 items) that assess the availability of medical staff and attentiveness to the individual patient based on the work of Matthews and Feinstein (1989), as well as 6 items that relate to satisfaction with care. Respondents use a 5-point Likert-type scale ranging from "never" to "always" in response to each item. Analysis of responses from 30 hospitalized in-patients revealed modest correlations with a somewhat related measure of satisfaction with care. Data from 206 hospitalized patients with do-not-resuscitate orders or their surrogates revealed good internal consistency.

Each of the measurement instruments described above can provide relatively reliable and valid assessments of the quality of life for patients near the end of life. Researchers and clinicians should evaluate respondent burden, whether patients or proxies are available to respond, and the domains of relevance to the patient and context when choosing the appropriate measure.

4   Hospice Care and Quality of Life at the End of Life

Maintaining quality of life at the end of life requires a multi-dimensional approach that emphasizes physical, psychological, practical, social, and spiritual domains. The care required to enhance the quality of life of dying patients is probably best orchestrated by physicians working collaboratively with the full range of available physical, psychological, social and spiritual interventions (Rummans et al., 2000). Such multi-disciplinary care for dying patients may be best exemplified by hospice care, although multidisciplinary palliative care consultations are increasingly available and effective in improving quality of life for hospitalized patients near the end of life (Griffin et al., 2007). Hospice care has traditionally been provided by physicians, nurses, social workers, chaplains, volunteers and others in the patient's home, supported by a family caregiver. Hospice care can also be provided to nursing home patients when contractual relationships exist between hospice agencies and long-term care facilities (Miller et al., 2000), and is also available in residential hospice houses, and in-patient hospital units. Hospice care is available in the United States for patients who meet eligibility criteria – generally that death is expected within six months. Some hospice agencies require patients to forego curative therapies, although nearly half of U.S. hospices permit patients to combine therapeutic and palliative treatments while under hospice care (Schonwetter et al., 2006).

Hospice care addresses many patient and family concerns and has been demonstrated to enhance quality of life at the end of life; in fact many hospice patients report a relatively stable quality of life despite progressive deterioration in physical status as death approaches (Cohen et al., 2001; Miller et al., 2000; Rummans et al., 2000; Steele et al., 2005). Bereaved family members typically report very high satisfaction with the quality of care provided by hospices. Connor and colleagues (2005) reported results from a total of 29,292 respondents who were family members of recently deceased patients under hospice care; on average respondents rated their overall satisfaction with care as 47.1 on a 50-point composite scale of five satisfaction measures.

4.1   Barriers to Hospice Care

Barriers to hospice care include societal-level barriers such as taboos to discussing death and dying, as well as organizational, professional, family, and individual barriers (Roscoe and Schonwetter, 2006). Efforts should continue to extend the length of stay for eligible patients, to ensure that patients and families benefit from the full scope of available hospice services. In addition, outreach efforts to underserved populations are important. Physician and public education, improving prognostic guidelines, and extending insurance coverage for hospice services can improve patient quality of life at the end of life.

5   Barriers to Research with Dying Patients

Dying patients present unique challenges for physicians and other health care providers whose goals are to maintain patient quality of life despite approaching death and progressive deterioration. This patient population also presents challenges to researchers who study quality of life at the end of life (McMillan and Weitzner, 2003; Moody and McMillan, 2002). These potential difficulties are summarized in ❷ Table 157-6.

Patients with life-limiting illnesses may be too debilitated to participate in research, or may find some interview or questionnaire formats too burdensome to complete. Family caregivers and health care professionals may be overly protective of their family members or dying patients, many of whom may find meaning and purpose in participating in research. Attrition is also a problem, as dying patients may not live long enough to participate in longitudinal or intervention studies. McMillan and Weitzner (2003) suggest that researchers seek ways to collect data that provides only minimal disruption to the agency or care facility, familiarize clinical staff with the importance of the study, and minimize burden to patients, including using proxies for data collection when necessary. It is crucial that research on dying patients continues, and that clinicians and researchers work with patients and families to address these difficulties.

◘ Table 157-6

Difficulties in end-of-life research

HIPAA (Health Insurance Portability & Accountability Act) versus Informed Consent
HIPAA is designed to protect patients' privacy, and some health care organizations use it to prevent contacts with patients; if researcher cannot inform patients about a study, patients cannot make an informed decision to participate or not
Debilitated Patients
Need to understand patient's experience and minimize burden of participation and still insure that sufficient data are collected
Over-protective Caregivers
Some family caregivers protect patients from research participation; should patients be protected from making decisions?
Over-protective Staff
Some clinical staff don't support clinical research or think that research is appropriate with patients near the end of life, and thus block access to patients
Longitudinal Data
Patients at the end of life often don't live long enough to participate in longitudinal studies; result is missing data
Data Integrity
Balance patient/family goals with research and/or clinical data collection

Adapted from: McMillan and Weitzner, 2003; Moody, McMillan, 2002

6 Conclusions and Future Directions

There are several acceptable measures of quality of life for patients near the end of life; however, all of the instruments described here can benefit from further refinement and study. There is no one tool that is ideal for all dying patients.

Researchers and clinicians must balance the need for valid and reliable measurement tools with the interests of patients. Evaluations and measurement of quality of life at the end of life should assess the domains of critical importance and relevance to patients, not what is most convenient or easiest to measure. Quality of life is a unique and subjective assessment for a particular patient at a vulnerable point in time. Our search for measurement tools that can efficiently and predictably assess the quality of life of patient populations must be balanced by the recognition that what constitutes quality of life at the end of life is unique to each individual patient and family. Attempts to introduce weighted items to account for patient preferences also introduce additional response burden. However, to be useful indicators of patient quality of life, measurement tools must account for what is of most importance to a specific individual.

While the biases introduced by the use of family members or other proxies when patients are too debilitated to respond have been described, the difficulties of conducting research and clinical assessments on dying patients cannot be overlooked. At the end of life, the patient and family caregivers together become the relevant unit of analysis, and efforts should continue to develop ways to minimize the bias introduced by proxy respondents. Similarly, research conducted with dying patients may also be biased since patients enjoying a better quality of life may be most inclined or able to participate. Research attention should be devoted to developing ways to reduce respondent burden so that the needs of debilitated patients are also taken into account.

Context and environment are also factors that deserve further attention. Patients dying at home may have different requirements or quality of life concerns than patients dying in institutional settings such as hospitals or nursing homes (Teno et al., 2004). In these settings, institutional norms and practices may constrain patient quality of life, and our measurement tools should be responsive to these realities. Similarly, while it may be desirable to have measurement tools that are appropriate for patients dying from a variety of diseases, disease-specific measures may be more appropriate for developing care plans to maximize patient quality of life.

In summary, the measures described here can be useful and valid tools for assessing patient quality of life at the end of life. Quality of life is a critical outcome measure that aids in the design of care plans for dying patients, and it is important to continue to refine our abilities to measure it. The goal should be to maximize optimal quality of life for all patients at the end of life.

Summary Points

- For patients near the end of life for whom further intervention is deemed futile or overly burdensome, quality of life becomes an even more central goal of care than for patients for whom recovery is expected.
- While quality of life at the end of life is a subjective concept that should reflect each patient's goals, values, and preferences for treatment, there is considerable agreement about the relevant domains.
- Domains that comprise patient quality of life at the end of life include: trusting one's physician, avoiding a prolonged dying experience, attaining a sense of closure, avoiding being a burden to family members, managing pain and other symptoms, and maintaining open communication.
- Several quality of life measures that have demonstrated their reliability and validity in the end of life context are available and can be used across patient disease conditions and contexts (hospital, nursing home, hospice, home care).
- Since patients near the end of life are often debilitated and may be unable to respond to questionnaires or interviews, proxy reports from family members familiar with the patient's condition may be used; proxy reports generally underestimate patient quality of life.
- The domains that comprise quality of care at the end of life overlap with quality of life measures; several measures to assess quality of care at the end of life exist in the literature and generally consist of interviews with bereaved family members.
- Hospice care for eligible patients near the end of life has demonstrated its ability to improve patient quality of life, but remains under-utilized.
- There are barriers to conducting research with patients near the end of life, which include dying before the conclusion of the study, being too debilitated to participate in research, and the protectiveness of professional and family caregivers toward patients who are dying.

References

Bradley EH, Fried RR, Kasl SV, Idler E. (2000). Annu Rev Gerontol Geriatr. 20: 64–96.

Byock IR, Merriman MP. (1998). J Palliat Med. 12: 231–244.

Cohen SR, Boston P, Mount BM, Porterfield P. (2001). Palliat Med. 15: 363–371.

Cohen SR, Mount BM, Bruera E, Provost M, Rowe J, Tong K. (1997). Palliat Med. 11: 3–20.

Cohen SR, Mount BM, Strobel MG, Bul F. (1995). Palliat Med. 9: 207–219.

Cohen SR, Mount BM, Tomas JJN, Mount LF. (1996). Cancer. 77: 576–586.

Connor SR, Teno J, Spence C, Smith N. (2005). J Pain Symptom Manage. 30: 9–17.

Curtis JR, Patrick DI, Engelberg RA, Norris K, Asp C, Byock I. (2002). J Pain Symptom Manage. 24: 17–31.

Donnelly S. (2000). Curr Oncol Rep. 2: 338–342.

Emmanuel LL, Alpert HR, Baldwin DC, Emanuel EJ. (2000). J Palliat Med. 3: 419–431.

Fowler FJ, Coppola KM, Teno JM. (1999). J Pain Symptom Manage. 17: 114–119.

Gentile S, Delaroziere JC, Fernandez C, Tardieu S, Devictor B, Dussol B, Daures JP, Berland Y, Sambuc R. (2003). Nephrologie. 24: 293–301.

Griffin JP, Koch KA, Nelson JE, Cooley ME. (2007). Chest. 132: 404S–422S.

Heyland DK, Dodek P, Rocker G, Groll D, Gafni A, Pichora D, Shortt S, Tranmer J, Lazar N, Kutsogiannis J, Lam M for the Canadian Researchers, End-of-Life Network (CARENET). (2006). CMAJ. 174: 627–633.

Johansson CM, Axelsson B, Danielson E. (2006). Cancer Nurs. 29: 391–399.

Kane RA, Caplan AL, Urv-Wong EK, Freeman IC, Aroskar MA, Finch M. (1997). J Am Geriatr Soc. 45: 1086–1093.

Kutner JS, Bryant LL, Beaty B, Fairclough DL. (2007). J Pain Symptom Manage. 34: 227–236.

Kutner JS, Bryant LL, Beaty B, Fairclough DL. (2006). J Pain Symptom Manage. 32: 300–310.

Lawton MP. (1991). A multidimensional view of quality of life in frail elders. In Birren JE, Lubben JE, Rowe JC, Deutchman DE (eds.) The Concept and Measurement of Quality of Life in the Frail Elderly. Academic Press, San Diego.

Lua PL, Salek S, Finlay I, Lloyd-Richards C. (2005). Qual Life Res. 14: 1669–1681.

Massaro T, McMillan S. (2000). Int J Palliat Nurs. 6: 429–433.

Matthews DA, Feinstein AR. (1989). J Gen Intern Med. 4: 14–22.

McMillan SC. (1996a). Cancer Control. 3: 223–229.

McMillan SC. (1996b). Oncol Nurs Forum. 8: 1221–1228.

McMillan SC, Mahon M. (1994). Qual Life Res. 3: 437–447.

McMillan SC, Weitzner M. (1998). Cancer Pract. 6: 282–288.

McMillan SC, Weitzner M. (2003). Onol Nurs Forum. 30: 123–129.

Miller SC, Mor V, Gage B, Coppola K. (2000). Annu Rev Gerontol Geriatr. 20: 193–223.

Montazeri A, Gillis C, McEwen J. (1998). Chest. 113: 467–481.

Moody L, McMillan SC. (2002). Nurs Res. 51: 129–133.

Patrick DL, Engelberg RA, Curtis JR. (2001). J Pain Symptom Manage. 22: 717–726.

Patrick DL, Curtis JR, Engelberg RA, Nielsen E, McCown E. (2003). Ann Intern Med. 139: 410–415.

Roila F, Cortesi E. (2001). Ann Oncol. 12: S3–S6.

Roscoe LA, Schonwetter RS. (2006). J Palliat Care. 22: 46–50.

Rummans TA, Bostwick JM, Clark MM. for the Mayo Clinic Cancer Center Quality of Life Working Group. (2000). Mayo Clin Proc. 75: 1305–1310.

Schonwetter RS, Roscoe LA, Nwosu M, Zilka B, Kim S (2006). J Palliat Med. 9: 638–645.

Schwartz CE, Merriman MP, Reed G, Byock I. (2005). J Palliat Med. 8: 121–135.

Singer PA, Martin DK, Kelner M. (1999). JAMA. 281: 163–168.

Spitzer WO, Dobson AJ, Hall J, Chesterman E, Levi J, Shepherd R, Battista RN, Catchlove BR. (1981). Chronic Dis. 34: 585–597.

Steele LL, Mills B, Hardin SR, Hussey LC. (2005). Am J Hosp Palliat Care. 22: 95–110.

Steinhauser KE, Bosworth, Clipp EC, McNeilly M, Christakis NA, Parker J, Tulsky JA. (2002). J Palliat Med. 5: 829–841.

Steinhauser KE, Christakis NA, Clipp EC, McNeilly M, Grambow S, Parker J, Tulsky JA. (2001). J Pain Symptom Manage. 22: 727–737.

Steinhauser KE, Clipp EC, Bosworth HB, McNeilly M, Christakis NA, Voils CI, Tulsky JA. (2004). Palliat Support Care. 2: 3–14.

Steinhauser KE, Clipp EC, Tulsky JA. (2002). J Palliat Med. 5: 407–414.

Steinhauser KE, Christakis NA, Clipp EC, McNeilly M, McIntyre L, Tulsky JA. (2000). JAMA. 284: 476–482.

Sterkenberg CA, King B, Woodward CA. (1996). J Palliat Care. 12: 18–25.

Stewart AL, Teno JM, Patrick DL, Lynn J. (1999). J Pain Symptom Manage. 17: 93–108.

Sulmasy DP, McIlvane JM, Pasley PM, Rahn M. (2002). J Pain Symptom Manage. 23: 458–470.

Tang ST, McCorkle R. (2002). Cancer Investigat. 20: 1086–1104.

Teno JM, Byock I, Field MJ. (1999). J Pain Symptom Manage. 17: 75–82.

Teno JM, Clarridge BR, Casey V, Welch LC, Wetle T, Shield R, Mor V. (2004). JAMA. 291: 88–93.

Teno JM, Dosa D. (2006). CMAJ. 174: 643–644.

Teno JM, Casey VA, Welch LC, Edgman-Levitan S. (2001a). J Pain Symptom Manage. 22: 738–51.

Teno JM, Clarridge B, Casey V, Edgman-Levitan S, Fowler J. (2001b). J Pain Symptom Manage 22: 752–758.

Wright JC, Feinstein AR. (1992). J Clin Epidemiol. 45: 1201–1218.

158 Quality of Life Measures in the Elderly and the Role of Social Support in Elderly Chinese

L. Zhang · R. Hunter · C. Shao

1   *Introduction* *2706*

2   *Main Text* *2707*
2.1   The Development of Quality of Life Assessment in Elderly Chinese 2707
2.2   Application of the GQOL-EC Questionnaire – A Joint Product of the Chinese
      Medical Association, the Elderly Medical Association, and the Epidemiology
      Study Group in Elderly Chinese 2709
2.3   Application of Foreign Quality of Life Measures and Related
      Instruments in Elderly Chinese 2712
2.4   Evaluation of Indicators of Quality of Life in Elderly Chinese 2713
2.5   Social Support of the Elderly in China 2717
2.6   The Problems and Prospects in Research on Quality of Life and Social
      Support in Elderly Chinese 2718

      Summary Points *2718*

      Annex 1 .... *2719*
      The Proposed Standard and Content on GQOL-EC (Draft) 2719

Abstract: China has stepped into an ageing society. Factors such as it's massive population, rapidly evolving societal structure and still developing economy make China's situation unique. The elderly Chinese person faces a number of difficulties, with an ageing body and reduced physical strength on the one hand, and reduced adaptability to their social surroundings and diminishing ❷ social support. Therefore, it is now more important than ever to evaluate the quality of life and social support in elderly Chinese people.

At present, tools for evaluating quality of life and social support in the elderly can be divided into those used in China and those used internationally, without either China or the international community taking advantage of what the other has to offer. Better understanding of these assessment tools could fundamentally enhance and improve the quality of life and social support in elderly Chinese people, and may have a wider impact on the economy and strengthen the nation.

List of Abbreviations: *GDS*, geriatric depression scale; *GQOL-EC*, geriatric quality of life investigation and evaluation criterion in China; *GQOLI*, generic quality of life inventory; *HRLQS*, health relative life quality scale; *Katz ADL*, activities of daily life; *Lanton IADL*, instrumental activities of daily life; *LSIA*, life satisfaction index A; *LSIB*, life satisfaction index B; *LSIZ*, life satisfaction index Z; *LSR*, life satisfaction rating scale; *MOS SF-36*, medical outcome study 36-item short form; *MUNSH*, Memorial University of Newfoundland Scale of Happiness; *PGC*, Philadelphia Geriatric Center Morale Scale; *QOL*, quality of life; *SAS*, self-rating anxiety scale; *SES*, the self-esteem scale; *SEIQOF*, schedule for evaluation of individual quality of life; *SSRS*, social support rating scale; *UCLA*, UCLA loneliness scale; *WHO QOL-BREF*, World Health Organization Quality of Life Brief

1   Introduction

In the twentieth century improvements in public health and medicine, universal vaccination, use of antibiotics, and the development of treatment for chronic diseases all prolong human life expectancy greatly. The Increase in life expectancy over the last 100 years is equivalent to or greater than the total summation of that for the four previous millennia, from the Bronze Age to the end of nineteenth century. China is a developing country with a large population, and has stepped into an aging society. In 2000, the population of those over 60 years of age in China rose to nearly 130 million (10% of the total population in China), which accounts for 20% or more of the world's total elderly population. The population aged 65 and above is over 93 million (7% of the total population in China), and population aged 80 and older is more than 13 million (14% of the 65-and-older population in China), which is rising at an average speed of 3% per year. Therefore, China's ageing population has several distinctive features such as its rapid growth, large absolute numbers and a still developing economy. So far, it is hard to make a complete and scientific evaluation on the health status of China's elderly. Under the influence of the traditional medical model, the health of the people has been interpreted as "absence of disease and disability," with mortality and life expectancy taken as the most important measurements of health. Research shows that the prevalence of chronic disease in nine provinces and municipalities in elderly Chinese is 59%, and the incidence of new illness over a 2 weeks period is 19%. The annual hospitalization rate in the elderly is 7.62%. Because of illness and disability, around 20% of the elderly have impaired mobility and may spend prolonged periods of time bed-bound. Around 4% are completely dependent on others as carers. The elderly suffer mainly from chronic and degenerative diseases, with similar prevalence of the same common illnesses across the various regions. Therefore, the health and well-being of elderly Chinese people is seriously affected by physical illness and co-morbidity, with reduced mobility and ability to adapt to surroundings. Along with the more simplistic data regarding mortality and disease morbidity, medical professionals and scholars in various countries have agreed that quality of life measures can also be used as objective indicators of health status in a population. Since the 1970s and 1980s, the use of quality of life measures has gradually increased in gerontology, especially in research. Our group has been researching quality of life in the elderly since the mid-1980s. In the early 1990s, the International Research Institute of the Quality of Life was set up, and the first national seminar on the quality of life was held in Beijing, China in 2000, which effectively promoted the study on the quality of life in elderly Chinese people.

2 Main Text

2.1 The Development of Quality of Life Assessment in Elderly Chinese

The quality of life in the elderly is a product of their physical health, psychological well being, levels of independence, their social network and living environment. The evaluation of quality of life in elderly Chinese is in a developing stage. As yet there is no widely recognized definition for quality of life in elderly Chinese, and there is no unified framework for assessment. Feng Litian and Dai Xingyi were the first to conduct a comprehensive and systematic study on the quality of life in the elderly in the book, Quality of Life Study of the Chinese Population, which established a basic framework for understanding factors involved in the quality of life of older persons. However, more in-depth study is needed to assess and influence quality of life.

In 1995, building on work by S. R. Walker and D. R. Patrick, Professor Guo (1995) of Zhejiang Medical University proposed a model to understand quality of life in the elderly with four main components: the internal body and the internal spirit, external material and external spirit. The Internal body refers to the physical health of the individual, and whether they have the ability to continue to participate in social activities and engage in domestic life. The internal spirit refers to their psychological state, their emotional state and whether they are optimistic, and general happiness and self-satisfaction. Their remaining intellect is also important, in particular their memory and attention span, and whether they can adapt socially. The external spirit refers to the financial income, ❷ housing, savings, actual standard of living, couples living conditions and medical care available and so on. The external spirit refers to family relations, neighborhood relations, and relations with their leaders and colleagues, care from their sons and daughters, free-time hobbies, and general satisfaction with their current situation (Guo, 1995). The overwhelming majority of clinicians and academics believe that quality of life is a multidimensional concept that includes both subjective feelings and an objective evaluation of ones situation. The environment, community, neighborhood, family and income are objective indicators of quality of life, but these alone do not fully determine quality of life.

In 2002, Professor Yang Zhongxin of Shenzhen University put forward his model where quality of life in the elderly population in China has 10 determinants (Yang, 2002):

1. Quality of the economic life, in particular levels of income, the consumption structure and the consumption levels.
2. Quality of the family life. This is determined largely by the standing of the elderly person in the family and interpersonal relations, as well as their physical condition.
3. Quality of the relationship with their partner.
4. Quality of health.
5. Quality of the education available to the patient, as whether formal or more commonly informal, this is good for the mental health of the recipient and helps keep the elderly person in touch with society.
6. Quality of the life interests, meaning participation in hobbies and activities to entertain people and bring pleasure to their lives.
7. Quality of working life, as being able to continue work has a beneficial effect on the quality of life of the elderly person and also a knock on economic benefit for society.
8. Quality of the environmental life. The elderly are more dependent on their environment than other age groups, and are very much affected by their housing, social and living environment.
9. Quality of the political life. The elderly often consider politics an emotive topic, and can draw a great deal of satisfaction from political harmony and seeing their leaders respected and supported by society.
10. Quality of the humanistic life. Dating right back to the origin of China's cultural era, a strong sense of respect for the elderly and a need to provide for and care for the elderly is engrained into Chinese culture. There were several acts passed by previous dynasties to protect the elderly, many of which are still upheld today. The elderly are revered by younger generations to some extent, and they often derive great spiritual strength from this.

Based on this model, and combining it with the current level of Chinese economic and social development, and the research on ageing, Minister Duoji Cairang suggested in the 2002 National Countermeasures Conference on Improvement of the Quality of Life in the Elderly (Duoji, 2002), "The quality of life in the elderly is a product of the existing state of the elderly in the material, spiritual, physical condition and social environment, and their feelings of self-worth under these conditions."

Domestic research on the quality of life in elderly persons is done mostly via questionnaires and surveys, and the applied questionnaires or scoring systems used in different fields varies along with differing definitions and concepts of quality of life. At present, measurement tools used by researchers to study quality of life in the elderly are divided into two categories.

1. The quality of life of elderly questionnaire (GQOL-EC) formed by the Chinese Medical Association.
2. International current quality of life and related measurement scales.

The application of Western measurement scales must take into account cultural background, the state of physical health and psycho-social status. The final application of the measurement tables is then dependent on a strict scientific method. However, designing quality of life questionnaires for the elderly is fraught with problems, and this inevitably hinders the development of reliable scales for measurement and evaluation of the quality of life in elderly Chinese persons (Li et al., 2003).

2.2 Application of the GQOL-EC Questionnaire – A Joint Product of the Chinese Medical Association, the Elderly Medical Association, and the Epidemiology Study Group in Elderly Chinese

The study of quality of life as a cross-disciplinary field of research using economics, sociology and demographics started late in China. Epidemiology of elderly Chinese began in 1958, and in mid-1980s 20,841 elderly people in 9 major cities were surveyed. The work was carried out to investigate the quality of life in elderly. With the ongoing development of life science and the persistent efforts of some relevant researchers, the draft recommendation of Geriatric Quality of Life Investigation and Evaluation Criterion in China (GQOL-EC) (Yu et al., 1996) was established in 1994 by the Geriatric Epidemiology Group of the Chinese Medical Association with reference to quality of life assessment in China and abroad.

GQOL-EC includes five fields and 11 survey items. The basic conditions include age, sex, education, occupation and marital status. The physiological conditions include somatic health conditions which consist of a physical examination, assessment of the five sensory modalities, 16 biochemical/hematological indices and also assessment of levels of self care and nutrition. The psychological conditions include positive and negative emotional status and how these are affected by life events. The economic conditions include economic income and expenditure. The social conditions include housing, living conditions, social conditions and medical care etc. Evaluation criteria include 11 items surveyed which are rated from 1 to 3 (3 being good and 1 being poor). Quality of life scores are then assessed as good, medium and poor, respectively each for 30–33 points, 22–29 points, and 11–21 points. (See Annex 1 for contents of the GQOL-EC questionnaire.)

Since the GQOL-EC was evaluated and validated (Sun et al., 2003; Zhang et al., 2001a), most Chinese domestic research on quality of life in the elderly has been based on this. Subsequently assessment of quality of life in the elderly using the GQOL-EC has spread across Guangzhou, Guizhou and Hainan in the south (Jiang et al., 2007; Ning et al., 1999; Xiao et al., 1997; Zhong et al., 1998), Beijing and Jilin in the north (Tao et al., 1997), Shanghai and Suzhou in the east (Zhang et al., 2003a), Xinjiang in the west and Chengdu, Yinchuan, Henan, Shanxi, Shaanxi in the middling (Cheng et al., 2004; Shi et al., 1998; Wang et al., 2001a). The total number of surveyed persons was nearly 30,000 people. At the same time, partial completion of the survey was carried out on the elderly population in rural areas (Song et al., 2004; Tang et al., 2001; Xu and Ou, 1998; Xu et al., 2003; Yang, 2007; Yang et al., 2000). It suggested that the quality of life in rural elderly people should be considered and improved. The mysteries surrounding longevity in the elderly Chinese were also discussed and analyzed (Jiang et al., 1999; Lin et al., 2000; Lv et al., 1999; Zheng et al., 1998; Zhu et al., 1995). The quality of life was also assessed in special elderly populations such as the elderly in minority groups, the very elderly, persons in residential accommodation and those in overcrowded accommodation (He et al., 2002; Yuan et al., 2000; Zhou et al., 2003) (❯ Figure 158-1 and ❯ Table 158-1).

Currently GQOL-EC looks at characteristics thought to be important in China and is primarily constructed to assess elderly Chinese people. It is therefore limited in its usefulness in certain regions of China and abroad, and in certain special populations. Since it has not yet been evaluated abroad it cannot be widely used internationally. Meanwhile, partial limitation still exists in the questionnaires. For example, the standard of economic income survey is still ratified according to national income and price levels in 1994, which fell short of the current economic living standard and needs adjusting.

◘ Figure 158-1

The distribution of the QOL survey in elderly Chinese using GQOL-EC

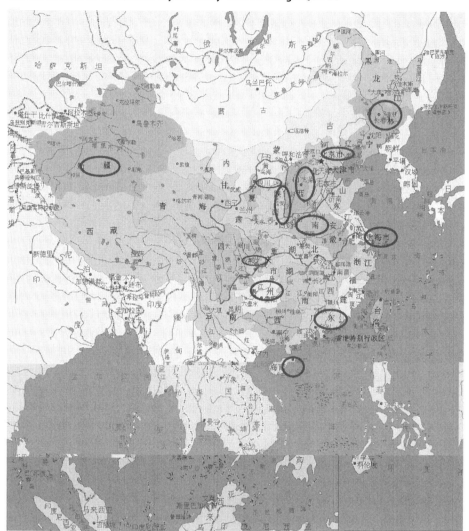

In the field of gerontology research, in addition to the GQOL-EC, another assessment tool known as the GQOLI was established by Li Lingjiang (Li et al., 1995). This has four parameters including physical health, mental health, social functioning and material living conditions. It has 16 main categories and 64 items overall. The HRLQS was designed by Wang Kai (Wang and Li, 1998). This has been well validated in rural areas and has four components including physical function, emotional balance, cognitive ability and social function. The attitude to ageing questionnaire (Li et al., 2003), the coping with the elderly questionnaire (Lu et al., 2000), and self-edited elderly mental health questionnaire (Wu et al., 2003) are all assessment questionnaires, but with no subsequent research done to validate them.

■ Table 158-1

The quality of life ranking of elderly people in different cities as assessed by different authors using the GQOL-EC

	Zhou et al. (2003)			Xu et al. (2003)			Wang et al. (2001a)			Zheng et al. (1998)			Jiang et al. (2007)		
	good	medium	poor	good	medium	poor	good	medium	poor	good	medium	poor	good	medium	poor
Total	23.3	56.0	20.7	24.9	69.8	5.3	19.8	65.0	15.2	10.0	45.0	45.0	27.6	51.1	21.3
Health status	31.5	51.7	16.8	35.1	46.4	18.5	30.8	44.5	24.7	20.0	50.0	30.0	28.9	50.6	20.5
Living habits	47.4	48.7	3.9	47.1	50.5	2.2	22.1	61.6	16.3	26.0	51.0	23.0	27.2	57.7	15.1
Activities of daily living	58.2	27.6	14.2	92.5	7.5	0	37.6	60.1	2.3	21.0	49.0	30.0	76.8	12.9	10.3
Family harmony	52.2	28.5	19.4	25.9	66.7	7.4	54.4	38.8	6.8	53.0	43.0	4.0	63.6	22.8	13.6
Living Condition	65.5	27.6	6.9	47.7	48.5	3.8	27.4	63.9	8.7	33.0	45.0	22.0	48.9	39.8	11.3
Economic status	27.2	32.8	40.0	66.9	32.2	0.9	29.3	35.0	35.7	26.0	60.0	14.0	44.0	38.0	18.0
Nutritional status	53.0	39.2	7.8	89.1	10.9	0	40.3	39.9	19.8	25.0	67.0	8.0	52.2	30.6	17.2
Mental health	49.1	37.9	12.9	41.5	55.8	2.7	24.3	66.2	9.5	20.0	56.0	24.0	39.2	21.8	39.0
Social interaction	54.3	33.6	12.1	46.9	47.1	6.0	19.8	59.3	20.9	14.0	48.0	38.0	31.6	47.1	21.3
Life satisfaction	30.2	33.6	36.2	38.3	51.3	10.4	23.2	65.4	11.4	38.0	51.0	11.0	33.8	58.9	7.3
Physical examination	39.2	38.4	22.4	41.8	54.5	3.7	26.3	60.8	12.9	19.0	40.0	41.0	34.9	49.4	15.7

The evaluation criteria include 11 lines of enquiry, of which each good item will score three points, medium scores two points, and poor scores one point. The 11 areas assessed comprised Health Status, Living Habits, Activities of Daily Living, Family Harmony, Living Condition, Economic Status, Nutritional Status, Mental Health, Social Interaction, Life Satisfaction and Physical Examination. Quality of life scores were assessed as good, medium or poor, respectively each for point scores ranging from 30 to 33, 22 to 29, and 11 to 21 points respectively. GQOL-EC: Geriatric Quality of Life Investigation and Evaluation Criterion in China

2.3   Application of Foreign Quality of Life Measures and Related Instruments in Elderly Chinese

In order to integrate with the international scientific community, Chinese scholars began to adopt the current relevant international instruments to study Chinese elderly persons (Li et al., 2002; Zhang et al., 2001a). The current international quality of life measures can be divided into two types, general instruments and special instruments. General instruments are used to measure aspects common to all persons. Quality of life measures in common use include the MOS SF-36, Euro QOL, WHO QOL, SEIQoF and so on. The special instruments are designed for special populations such as those with a particular disease. The majority of contemporary research tends to use an approach combining both general and specific measures of QOL.

Foreign measurement instruments have come forth in the evaluation of QOL as there is a lack of these in China. In nearly 10 years, lots of documents have been involved in linguistic and cross-cultural translation, as many of the measures of health and QOL use English. Translating the foreign measurement instruments into Chinese is a unique challenge. However, quality of life is socially, economically, and culturally dependent, and is deeply rooted in peoples cultural backgrounds and value systems. So Chinese versions of QOL measures must be culturally adapted then tested for reliability and validity.

MOS SF-36 has been evaluated through studies in China for feasibility, reliability and validity, and has been used successfully in elderly Chinese (Chen et al., 2005; Li et al., 2004; Liu et al., 2001; Zhang et al., 2001, 2004). It consists of 36 items, and measurements are simple and quick, but its content is broad. Therefore, SF-36 is more widely applied in China than other international instruments. It is mainly used to assess the overall health status with eight health dimensions, including physical functioning, physical limitations, bodily pain, general health, vitality, social functioning, emotional limitations and mental health.

Surveys using the SF-36 on elderly Chinese in Tianjin (Tian et al., 2003), Beijing and Inner Mongolia Baotou City pastoral area (Wang et al., 2001b; Zhang et al., 2001) in north of China, the rural elderly in Changchun City in the northeastern China (Feng et al, 2005), the elderly persons in Xi'an in Midwest China (Zhang et al., 2003), the aged in rural Hubei Province in the west (Zhu et al., 2006), the elderly in Suzhou in the east (Zhang et al., 2003), the elderly in Kaifeng City in the central part of China (Wang et al., 2001a), the elderly in Shenzhen (Jiang et al., 2003) and Li ethnic minority in Wuzhishan City in south of China, respectively. The cumulative number of people surveyed is nearly 10,000. Since there are so many regions and topography is complex and individual differences large, the large-scale investigation on the measurement instrument is still underway so as to obtain a reliable tool and to establish genuine data for the Chinese population (❷ *Figure 158-2* and ❷ *Table 158-2*).

Application of other foreign common instruments in China is less than that of MOS SF-36, and they are only adopted in reports of partial areas. For example, WHO QOL-BREF which includes several fields of physiology, psychology, environment and social relations has only been used to survey the urban elderly in Beijing, Ningxia, Jilin City and Chuxiong City in Yunnan Province (Ding et al., 2007; Dong et al., 2007), and has also been used to evaluate the quality of life and factors affecting it in the rural elderly in Jining City (Wang, 2007), the special elderly populations in Nantong City and in mining areas (Lu et al., 2007).

Health and Sanitation System Responsiveness questionnaire (Mann - Whitney U) provided by WHO includes four indicators, including body function, spiritual and psychological function, economic and cultural factors, and social abilities and adaptability. The instrument has been used in a report in Honan province (Shi et al., 2002). In addition,

■ Figure 158-2
The distribution of the QOL survey in elderly Chinese using SF-36

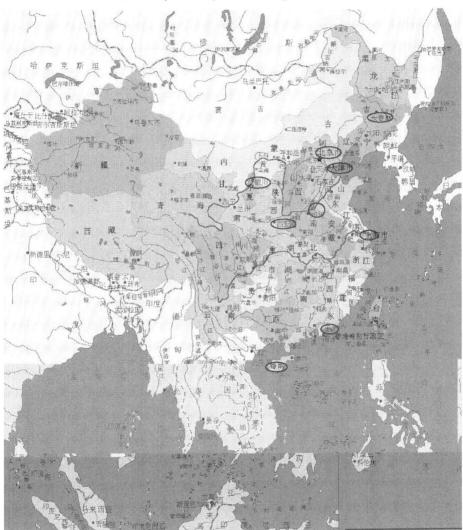

some specific instruments have been used to research certain areas by different groups, such as FLIC by Napi and Rosowbressan, Katz ADL, Lanton IADL, PGC, GDS, SAS, MUNSH, LSR, LSIA and LSIB, etc.

2.4 Evaluation of Indicators of Quality of Life in Elderly Chinese

The QOL indicators of elderly Chinese are important tools to quantitatively describe and measure quality of life. Design of the QOL indicators of older persons must follow scientific and practical principles. It has three practical principles. The characteristics in each of the

■ Table 158-2

The quality of life in Chinese elderly using MOS SF-36

	City					Village	
	Jiang et al. (2003)	Zhang et al. (2003b)		Tian et al. (2003)	Feng et al. (2005)	Zhu et al. (2006)	
		Suzhou	Xian			Special	General
Physical function	70.9 ± 24.1	74.6 ± 20.7	67.8 ± 26.0	66.4 ± 31.1	69.9 ± 9.4	57.5 ± 27.3	71.7 ± 24.7
Role – physical	78.0 ± 36.0	63.2 ± 40.7	44.8 ± 42.9	59.9 ± 45.0	61.9 ± 5.5	30.4 ± 41.1	45.2 ± 42.9
Bodily pain	81.2 ± 19.2	68.0 ± 21.1	67.0 ± 23.1	73.2 ± 27.9	40.4 ± 3.6	58.2 ± 27.7	65.6 ± 28.5
General health	57.8 ± 15.8	53.1 ± 23.4	48.9 ± 21.5	69.3 ± 28.3	52.4 ± 4.8	35.7 ± 23.1	52.3 ± 24.4
Vitality	63.2 ± 16.9	70.9 ± 19.2	67.0 ± 20.7	79.1 ± 18.3	59.9 ± 5.4	49.7 ± 24.8	64.1 ± 24.7
Social function	82.9 ± 34.5	76.6 ± 22.6	68.2 ± 28.4	67.9 ± 44.1	48.8 ± 8.7	69.9 ± 30.3	77.5 ± 24.5
Role – emotional	76.6 ± 12.3	71.9 ± 38.4	58.7 ± 43.4	68.1 ± 23.3	75.2 ± 10.4	36.7 ± 39.3	50.8 ± 41.7
Mental health	73.7 ± 14.3	68.9 ± 15.5	69.4 ± 15.6	57.1 ± 23.5	49.9 ± 5.3	54.3 ± 25.5	69.3 ± 23.6

Each of the scores was expressed as a value between 0 and 100, with higher scores representing better health. The eight domains are collapsed to create two global components, a physical component score and a mental component score. Scores on the Physical Component Summary are associated with high scores on the Physical Function, Role-Physical, Bodily Pain and General Health scales and low scores on the Role-Emotional and Mental Health scales. For the Mental Component Summary, positive weights are placed on the Mental Health, Role-Emotional, Social Function and Vitality scales, whereas substantial negative ones are placed on the Physical Function and Role-Physical scales. SF-36 Short-Form 36 categories of indicators should reflect the full range of characteristics of the elderly persons life, i.e. it must be complete in its assessment of the index systems; It must allow collection of data and statistical analysis. Within each index system it must provide a comprehensive analysis of the conditions. There are also three scientific principles. The choice of a variable can accurately reveal the characteristics of the quality of life in the elderly. The associated indicators should be clearly defined. The analysis should be conducted using established mathematical and statistical principles.

The basic nature of the living needs in elderly can be divided into the following three categories: quality index of material life, spiritual life and social life (Li, 2003).

1. Quality index of material life. This reflects the elderly population's material living conditions, taking into account the quality of living, food, transportation, medical care and other basic aspects and its impact on quality of life. It includes seven indicators:
   (i) Quality index of living, which reflects living conditions of older persons. This includes factors such as whether they own their own home and whether their home is detached or terraced.
   (ii) Quality index of meals, which refers to their dietary intake and its nutritional content.
   (iii) Quality index of travel, which reflects whether the elderly person has access to, or owns their own vehicle for transport, and of course whether they are able to use their vehicle independently and have the economic capacity to fund its upkeep.
   (iv) The index of owning household appliances, meaning whether the elderly person or their family living with them posses basic household appliances such as washing machines and refrigerators and the like.
   (v) The index of owning modern communications equipment, which is an indicator of whether the elderly person possesses basic communication tools, such as home telephone and/or mobile telephones and other modern communications tools. These are important for strengthening interpersonal communication within their social network, in particular strengthening links with friends, relatives and public service agencies. This benefits physical and mental health of the older person, and helps access health services in a timely manor when needed.
   (vi) The index of owning computer equipment, which refers to the indicators of both ownership of computer equipment and the ability to operate it. Computer network equipment in particular the internet effectively shortens the distance between the elderly person and their immediate social circle. It also potentially allows extensive contact with the rest of society and can act as a learning resource, facilitating understanding of politics and current affairs. This can improve both mental and physical health.
   (vii) The index of basic medical treatment protection, which refers to indicators of medical care available. This takes into account both convenience and how accessible these services are, as well as what can be afforded from a financial perspective. Combined study with the two together is the "basic guarantee index for medical treatment." Whether the elderly person has basic protection in terms of medical treatment available is often a major psychological concern to the elderly.
2. The quality index of spiritual life reflects the spiritual life of the older person, which is directly related to whether the elderly are living a peaceful and happy life, and their general sense of well-being. The quality of the spiritual life is important not only for health and

longevity, but also impacts on the wider social group's spiritual life. It contains four quantitative indicators.

   (i) Index of participation in cultural entertainment, which reflects the ability of the elderly to participate in recreational and cultural activities, and is one of the basic components of the spiritual life of the elderly person. The degree of participation of the older person in various cultural and entertainment activities involves the following basic elements and conditions. The first is the arena in which the cultural activities occur and how accessible they are to the elderly person. The second is the cultural disposition of the elderly. The third is the condition of their health.

   (ii) The index of seeking knowledge. This index reflects whether the elderly participate in scientific and cultural learning in order to acquire knowledge. This index reflects not only the desire and enthusiasm to pursue new knowledge, but encompasses their general outlook in terms of keeping in step with the developments around them. This can be a very rewarding pursuit for the elderly.

   (iii) The index of fostering taste. This is an index reflecting the quality of life in the elderly in developing hobbies and "self-taste," raising living standards around them, and living a peaceful and happy life after retiring. This is another basic constituent of the spiritual life. Self-taste refers to gardening, raising grass, agriculture, fish farming, and craftwork process etc, and broadly includes anything in which the elderly can participate to enjoy themselves.

   (iv) The index of spiritual independence incorporates independence from others and freedom from psychiatric illness, in particular depressive illness.

3. Quality index of social life. The social life is not only important for the elderly to continue social contact, but also an important way to reaffirm their own values and achieve new goals through social practice. Core factors affecting social life are marriage and family life. This is assessed using five indicators.

   (i) The index of personnel resource development. This index reflects the continued employment and re-employment conditions of some older persons. The elderly are a rich human resource, and possess a wide range of abilities. Societal recognition of the great importance of developing this resource is key to promoting and accelerating socio-economic development.

   (ii) The index of personal development. This index takes into account that some elderly people with technical expertise still make their contributions to society in their own professional fields. Often elderly people with professional expertise are accessed by others in their field although without being formally employed as such.

   (iii) The index of elderly people with spouses. This index studies the marital situation of the elderly person. The situation of an elderly person with a spouse is completely different from that of the elderly living alone. The loss of a spouse is often the worst shock in the life of the aged person. Hence this index has an important bearing on quality of life.

   (iv) The index of divorced or widowed elderly. This index analyzes the cause of missing spouses, which is usually death or divorce.

   (v) The index of family harmony. This refers to how well the elderly person can get along with family members happily and harmoniously. As families can be considered cells of society, the quality of family life has important social significance.

2.5   Social Support of the Elderly in China

Any society finds it difficult to meet the demands of the aging population. China has built a social endowment support network system which is expected by the elderly and is afforded by China's current socio-economic status. The reform of the Chinese social pensions system is an urgent affair. Social support refers to kinds of social assistance and services available to the elderly community in various forms (Chen and Pan, 2000). It is of great significance both to provide a buffer for the elderly and to help maintain their quality of life.

Currently, SSRS, MUNSH, UCLA, SES and PGC are generally adopted to evaluate the relevant factors to determine the social situation and quality of life in the elderly. It is found that with increasing age, the social support available to the elderly declines. The main effect of social support is to provide a buffer system for the elderly and to improve their mental health. More support and comfort from family members can significantly improve the mental health and subjective well-being of the elderly. At the same time, support to their children from the elderly can improve their own positions in the family, and establish mutual support within the family which also has a positive effect on the mental health of the elderly person (Wang et al., 2004; Yue et al., 2006).

Difference in social support, especially in the form of more social contacts and close interpersonal relationships, results in the elderly feeling more supported psychologically and spiritually. The elderly with sound marriages and couples living together have distinctively higher quality of life than that of divorced, widowed or elderly living alone, whether measured subjectively or objectively. This is related to increased emotional loneliness and reduced social contact in those who are now single for whatever reason (Xiang et al., 1998).

The support received by the elderly and the availability of social support are correlated to age, level of education, income, and housing area. The elderly worry about four aspects of their social support network. Firstly, the majority of elderly people worry about medical needs and whether they will be met, and whether they have adequate pension provisions. Secondly, they fear being a burden to their children due to their physical decline and increasing dependency. Third, they worry that the so-called "generation gap" between them and younger people could cause psychological isolation, and make the elderly lose their social contact and support from their children. Fourth, they worry that the rising pace of social change may result in trouble for the economy and societal upheaval in general. Therefore, elderly people have various concerns and needs which are material, social and spiritual (Chen, 1999; Wang et al., 2007).

Based on the above, there are several fundamental changes that ought to be made to improve quality of life for the elderly. Firstly, the availability of health care should be improved. Second, there is an urgent need for government funding for an adequate pensions system. Third, the provision of social services in the community should be established and improved so as to help less wealthy elderly people, and make less independent elderly people less dependent on their family for help. Fourth, the establishment of a state-based pension supplemented by a community care system to complement any private pension and care provided by the family. Finally, the government needs to concentrate on strengthening and consolidating the family pension system, and promote the concepts of respect for and caring for the elderly by the younger generation. Thus, the "trinity" of the old-age security system should be comprised of support from the family as ever, social services in the community, and the old-age pension.

2.6 The Problems and Prospects in Research on Quality of Life and Social Support in Elderly Chinese

The aging of the population is the dominant demographic trend in twenty-first century China, which will inevitably have a profound impact on social development. For the sustained development of our society, addressing the aging of the population is a challenge and an opportunity.

1. The elderly population in China has ❷ ten characteristics such as ethnicity, region, traditions, ethics, religion, management, psychology, diet, sociality and entertainment. Starting with these "characteristics" (Yang, 2002), first of all, and looking at the different factors which constitute quality of life in elderly, characteristics which correlate with a good quality of life can be identified both in China and throughout the world. Second, from analysis of quality of life in elderly Chinese, it can be established how quality of life in the elderly develops and changes in China so as to reduce unrealistic competition with that of older persons in Europe and the United States. Third, it is easy for foreign scholars and governments to directly understand the quality of living in the elderly in China for comparison to the elderly elsewhere. Finally, this allows the Chinese government the opportunity to make informed decisions when formulating policies on the elderly population, improving the social security system, strengthening community cultural development, and generally furthering the cause of the elderly. Therefore, the definition of and constituents of quality of life in the elderly and the development of systems for its evaluation will undoubtedly become a hotspot in future.

2. The issue of the "❷ Empty-nest" (Mu, 2007) is a factor impacting on the psychological state of the elderly more and more in this ageing society. In the last 10 years, the trend towards the empty family nest is increasing; in 1993, the proportion of empty nest families in China was only 16.7% of all families with elderly persons, and in 2003 it rose to 25.8%. In some big cities the issue of the empty family home is especially prominent. It is necessary to carry out longitudinal studies to monitor quality of life in the elderly over time to provide a scientific basis for the building of community services, endowment institutions and other social support networks.

3. The aging of the population in China occurs on a poorly developed socio-economic background. This gives rise to problems such as a "rapid outbreak" of an elderly population, ageing of the people before being allowed the opportunity to become financially secure, and a serious shortage of pension resources. The study of quality of life in older persons can be used for the development of resources to help the older person, but also to fully tap the potential physical and mental resources of the elderly, especially the elderly as a human resource.

Summary Points

- The quality of life in elderly Chinese is a product of their material, spiritual, and physical condition, as well as their social environment, and their feelings of self worth within that environment.
- The current domestic research on quality of life in elderly Chinese is mostly based on GQOL-EC.

- In order to become compatible with international research in this field, Chinese scholars used the MOS SF-36 to evaluate the quality of life in elderly Chinese.
- The QOL indicator of elderly Chinese can be divided into the following three categories: quality index of material life, spiritual life and social life.
- There are various aspects of social support of older persons, such as financial and material needs, spiritual and social needs.

Abundant material life, good health and longevity, a rich cultural life, a comfortable living environment and harmonious family relations are the needs of the elderly in pursuit of a good quality of life. The above results show that the creation of "a society for all, regardless of age" needs further consensus and painstaking efforts of the whole society. Developing the economy and strengthening the nation is the fundament to all. Only in this way, can we fundamentally enhance and improve the quality of life for the elderly.

Annex 1

The Proposed Standard and Content on GQOL-EC (Draft)

In October of 1994, Chinese Medical Association Society's Geriatric epidemiology study group meeting recommended investigating the quality of life of older persons in the country's conditional areas. The survey content and evaluation criteria are as follows.

1. Health Status

A good status refers to being asymptomatic, with no illness or abnormality impacting on normal physiological function, having no obvious chronic disease, being able to read newspapers with or without vision correction, listening to day-to-day dialogue, functional capacity with regard to activities of daily living such as housework being good, normal intelligence and having no emotional or psychiatric illness such as depression.
The middling refers to those with occasional symptoms, deformity, chronic disease, seeing and hearing not affecting daily life, being competent for some housework, and needing some care.
The poor refers to those with diseases, deformities, chronic illness, seeing and hearing difficulties affecting daily life, loss of the ability to work, dependent on others for care to live, poor intelligence, and depression.

2. Living Habits

A good status refers to not being addicted to tobacco and alcohol, daily participation in light labor and regular exercise, often participating in cultural and recreational activities, daily having a sleep for 7–8 h, going to bed and waking up regularly, and dreams being fewer.
The middling refers to smoking less than 10 cigarettes daily and drinking less than 100 ml of alcohol (spirit), sometimes participating in labor, sport, cultural and recreational activities, sleep being less than 7 h, going to bed and waking up irregularly, and dreams being more common.
Poor refers to being addicted to tobacco and alcohol, not participating in labor, sport, cultural and recreational activities, suffering from frequent insomnia and taking sleeping pills.

3. Activities of Daily Living

This includes self-care and daily living activities such as eating, dressing and undressing, washing and combing, going to bed and getting out of bed, going to the lavatory, having a bath, locking up a door and closing a window, shopping, managing money and things, going to hospital, going upstairs and downstairs, walking 250 m.
Good refers to those who can perform the above activities entirely.
    The middling refers to those who can complete some of the above activities.
    Poor refers to those who can not undertake these activities.

4. Family Harmony

    Good refers to harmonious family relationships.
    The middling refers to reasonable family relationships.
    The poor refers to non-harmonious family relationships.

5. Living Conditions

    The good refers to housing area (bedroom) $\geq 4\ m^2$, cohabiting or living alone with their spouses in a room, alone, with running water and flush toilets, washing equipment, gas, heating, home security, no noise, no pollution.
    The middling refers to housing area being less than $4\ m^2$, two or three generations cohabiting, toilets and water supply being communal, having gas, not having bath equipment and heating, safety being sub-optimal, noise and pollution being light.
    The poor refers to above three generations cohabiting or not having formal housing, having no bathing facilities, no gas, no heating, shelter being unsafe, noise and pollution being serious.

6. Economic Status

    The good refers to per capita income being more than 500 RMB.
    The middling refers to per capita income being 200–500 RMB.
    The poor refers to per capita income being less than 200 RMB.

7. Nutritional Status

The good refers to not being particular with food, the three major nutrients and calories being reasonable, eating fruits and vegetables everyday, quantity and time for three meals being fixed, and body weight being normal.
The middling refers to the total calories being still appropriate but the three major nutrients proportion being unsuitable, eating vegetables and fruits less, two meals daily or time and quantity for meals not being fixed, body being slim or overweight.
    The poor refers to being particular with food, the total calories being inadequate or excessive, the three major nutrients being unreasonable, eating less or even not eating vegetables and fruits, time and quantity for meals not being fixed, emaciation or obesity.

8. Mental Health

    Evaluation of Mental Health has 33 items which are divided into three groups.
    Group 1 refers to encountering 17 negative incidents over the past 3 years, including retirement, serious illness or injury to self or their spouses, discord with spouses, death of spouse, children's life being frustrated or serious illness/death, discord with their children, the

death of parents, the death of friends, moving house or changing of minder, discord with neighbors, economic difficulties, significant property losses, legal disputes, and serious natural disasters.

Group 2 refers to those encountering 10 positive and negative psychological feelings, such as low energy, feeling useless, diminished happiness, often feeling suppressed, feeling demotivated or very positive after completing something they had wanted to do, feeling redundant or being ignored, desire for contact with other people or not, and often feeling alone.

Group 3 refers to those encountering any of six things to worry about, including economic difficulties, overcrowded housing, difficulties in medical care, lack of care, family discord and price increases.

Good mental health refers to those with not more than two negative events which have not affected the emotion, having four positive psychological feelings, having nothing to worry about at present.

The middling mental health refers to those with not more than five negative events, with minimal impact on emotion, having two to three positive psychological feelings, and having only one to three negative psychological feelings and things to worry about.

The poor mental health refers to those with ore to five negative events with significant impact on the emotion, more than six negative feelings and more than three things to worry about.

9. Social Interaction

Good refers to those having regular conversation with family members, friends and neighbors together with regular participation in collective activities.
The middling refers to occasionally participating in the above activities.
The poor refers to not participating in the above activities.

10. Life Satisfaction

Eleven items are included in life satisfaction such as economic status, food and clothing, accommodation, marital life, sports, entertainment and cultural life, treatment by their children, family harmony, health status, medical care, family life, and interpersonal relationships. For each of the above items, satisfaction results in a score of three points, sub-satisfaction scores two points, and dissatisfaction scores one point. The total satisfaction score is from 30 to 33 points, total sub-satisfaction score is from 22 to 29 points, and total dissatisfaction score is from 11 to 21 points.

11. Physical Examination

Good physical ability: Weight, blood pressure, sight and hearing are normal. More than 50% of teeth are healthy. Sitting and standing can be completed five times within 30 s. Hands can extend and be put behind the neck.
Medium physical ability: Obesity with borderline hypertension. Sight and hearing are poor but do not impact on daily life; a small number of healthy teeth is left, but their function is poor; sitting and standing can be completed one to four times within 30 s. Hands can extend but cannot be put behind neck.
Poor physical ability: Body is emaciated or obese, suffering from high blood pressure. Vision, hearing, and dental condition have affected their daily lives. Sitting and standing cannot be completed within 30 s. Hands cannot extend or be put behind neck.

Evaluation of physical ability includes 11 factors, of which each good item will get three points, medium scores two points, and poor scores one point. Quality of life scores were assessed as good, medium and poor, respectively for scores of 30–33 points, 22–29 points, and 11–21 points.

References

Chen C. (1999). J Soc Sci Hunan Normal Univ. 28(4): 19–26.

Chen C, Pan Z. (2000). J Soc Sci Hunan Normal Univ. 29 (6): 25–31.

Chen R, Liao D, Li X, Xie C, Feng Q, Li Y. (2005). J Guangxi Med Univ. 22(2): 237–239.

Cheng X, Gao X, Gao H. (2004). China Health Educ. 20 (4): 376–377.

Ding G, Ma J, Shen C. (2007). J Commun Med. 5(13): 16–18.

Dong L, Du R, Xu L. (2007). J Beihua Univ (Nat Sci). 8(3): 258–261.

Duoji C. (2002). http://www.shrca.org.cn/text/readnews.

Feng X, Li J, Li Z, Mei S, Zhang S, Wang X, Mu D. (2005). Chinese J Gerontol. 25(11): 1333–1334.

Guo Y. (1995). Med soc. 8(4): 25.

He B, Li X, Yu G (2002). J Chinese Phys. 4(4): 393–395.

Jiang J, Sun G, Zhang C. (1999). Chinese J Gerontol. 19 (3): 129–130.

Jiang B, Xu T, Liao M, Yi G, Liu C, Sun Y. (2003). Chin Ment Health J. 17(5): 291–293.

Jiang W, Lin T, Li M. (2007). Guangdong Med J. 28(7): 1162–1163.

Li Y. (2003). J Sichuan Administr College. 3(1): 53–57.

Li X, Guo J. (2003). Soc Med Sec. 20(4): 154–158.

Li L, He W, Yang D, Zhang Y, Wu K, Luo Y, Huang J, Zhang B, Liu J, Liao J. (1995). Chin Ment Health J: 9(5)227–231.

Li L, Wang H, Shen Y. (2002). Chin J Prevent Med. 36 (2):109–113.

Li C, Wu Z, Li J. (2003). Chin Ment Health J. 17(1): 47–49.

Li D, Xu T, Wu D, Wang Z. (2004). Chinese J Rehabilit Med. 19(7): 515–517.

Lin Y, Jiang X, Wang R. (2000). Chinese J Gerontol. 20 (2): 65–66.

Liu Z, Li N, Ren X, Li J, Zhang J, Sun D. (2001). J West China Univ Med Sci. 32(1): 39–42.

Lu K, Jiang Q, Zhu Y. (2000). Chin Ment Health J. 14(2): 93–95.

Lu R, Zhao Y, Qv C. (2007). Chinese Remedies Clinics. 7(9): 700–701.

Lv T, Zhang Z, Lv D, Zhang Q. (1999). Chin J Prevent Control Chronic Non-Commun Dis. 7(5): 224–225.

Mu G. (2007). South China Populat. 17(1): 33–36.

Ning H, Luo C, Zhang Q, Zhu Y, Wu S, Liang H, Zhang X. (1999). Chin J Prevent Control Chronic Non-Communicable Dis. 7(4): 168–170.

Shi J, Zhang S, Yang Y, Guo D, Fan D, Zuo Y, Yu P. (1998). Chin J Epidemiol. 19(1): 15–17.

Shi X, Wang A, Li Y, Xie J. (2002). China Pub Health. 18 (9): 1095–1096.

Song X, Wang A, Chen X, Tan K, Zhen J. (2004). Chin J Nat Med. 6(2): 74–76.

Sun Y, Jiang B, Xu T, Huang L, Zeng Y, Zhong S. (2003). Pract Prevent Med. 10(4):476–478.

Tang X, Jiao J, Wu C. (2001). Chin J Rehabilit Theory Pract. 7(2): 76–83.

Tao G, Liu X, Chen F, Wu Q, Zhang J, Ji X, Lin N, Zhang B, Li X, Liu L, Che J, Wang X. (1997). Chinese J Gerontol. 17(4):197–198.

Tian L, Wang C, Zhou L, Xu B, Deng D. (2003). J Bethune Military Med College. 1(1): 29–31.

Wang L. (2007). J Jining Med College. 30(1): 66–67.

Wang K, Li B. (1998). Chin J Health Statist. 15(5): 9–13.

Wang Y, Wang Z, Xing Y, Tian A, Ma Y, Zhang W, Kong J, Wang S. (2001a). Academic J Kaifeng Med College. 20(1): 76–78.

Wang S, Li L, Wei L, Ma S, Chen Z, Zhang H. (2001b). Chin J Behav Med Sci. 10(3): 246–247.

Wu Z, Li J, Xu S. (2003). Chin J Gerontol. 23(11): 713–715.

Wang D, Dong Y, Zhou L, Shen J. (2004). Acta Psychologica Sinica. 36(1): 78–82.

Wang S, Xia Y, Xiao Q, Shao J, Dai Y, Sheng S. (2007). China J Health Psychol. 15(5): 454–456.

Xiang F, Mao H, Tang Y, Ai L, Shi X. (1998). Health Psychol J. 6(3): 354–355.

Xiao L, Zhong H, Li Z. (1997). Pract Geriat J. 11(6): 263–265.

Xu T, Ou Q. (1998). Chin J Epidemiol. 19(1):9–11.

Xu T, Jiang B, Sun Y, Huang L, Lu T, Liu J. (2003). Chin J Geriat. 22(7): 427–429.

Yang Z. (2002). Shenzhen University J (Humanities and Social Science). 19(1): 60–66.

Yang M. (2007). J Commun Med. 5(15): 61–63.

Yang J, Pan J, Tao Q. (2000). Guizhou Med J. 24(5): 315–316.

Yu P, Yang C, He H. (1996). Chin J Geriatr. 15(5): 320.

Yuan A, Chen Y, Lv C. (2000). J High Altitude Med. 10 (1): 55–57.

Yue C, Wang D, Li L. (2006). Chin J Clin Rehabilit. 10 (18): 53–55.

Zhang l, Huang J, Fan F, Li L. (2001a). Chin J of Behav Med Sci. 10(6): 601–603.

Zhang H, Lv Z, Wang S, Chen Z, Zhang C, Qi L, Tian Z, Wu J. (2001b). J Baotou Med College. 17(4): 262–264.

Zhang L, Shao C, Fan F, Huang J, Li L. (2003a). Chinese J Gerontol. 23(5):272–274.

Zhang L, Huang J, Li L, Wang B, Wang A. (2003b). J Fourth Mil Med Univ. 24(13): 1236–1239.

Zhang L, Shao C, Wang B, Long Y, Zhang Z, Li L. (2004). Chin J Geriat. 23(2): 112–114.

Zheng Z, Zhu H, Wang Z. (1998). Chinese J Gerontol. 18 (4): 193–194.

Zhong H, Xiao L, Li Z. (1998). Chin J Nurs. 33(6): 314–317.

Zhou Y, Liu L, Guo Z, Huo Q. (2003). J Ningxia Med College. 25(1): 19–21.

Zhu Z, Zhao G, Ou Q. (1995). Chinese J Gerontol. 15(1): 12–14.

Zhu J, Wang W, Mao Z, Li B, Mi Y. (2006). Chin J Rehabilit Med. 21(2): 149–151.

159 Quality of Life in Elderly Dyspnea Patients

A. Hooshiaran · F. van der Horst · G. Wesseling · J. J. M. H. Strik ·
J. A. Knottnerus · A. Gorgels · A. Fastenau · M. van den Akker ·
J. W. M. Muris

1	*Introduction*	**2726**
1.1	Definition and Prevalence	2726
1.2	Differential Diagnosis	2727
2	*Evaluation and Measurement of Dyspnea*	**2729**
2.1	Evaluation	2729
2.2	Measurement	2730
2.3	Short-Term Intensity Tools	2731
2.4	Situational Dyspnea Tools	2732
2.5	Impact Tools	2732
3	*Impact of Dyspnea on Quality of Life*	**2734**
3.1	Definition	2734
3.2	Interactions	2734
3.3	Measurement	2736
4	*Dyspnea Management and Rehabilitation*	**2737**
4.1	Pulmonary Rehabilitation	2738
4.2	Cardiac Rehabilitation	2739
4.3	Psychosocial Supports	2740
4.3.1	Self Management	2740
4.3.2	Nutritional Intervention	2742
4.3.3	Occupational Therapy	2742
	Summary Points	**2742**

Abstract: ❷ Dyspnea is a subjective term. Psychosocial or cultural parameters may influence the reaction of individuals to a certain sensation of breathing discomfort. The context in which dyspnea occurs can also impact its perception. Most of underlying diseases of dyspnea are progressive, frustrating and debilitating and their influence permeates every aspect of the patient's life. In most elderly patients with chronic dyspnea, the specific cause of the dyspnea is usually elusive and because of coexistence of multiple causes a specific treatment is not available; so treatment should be aimed at symptom relief.

Research literature concerning dyspnea as a symptom in the elderly is scarce, although much has been written about specific diseases that may cause dyspnea, especially ❷ chronic obstructive pulmonary disease (COPD) and chronic heart failure (CHF). As the prevalence of these conditions increases with advancing age, dyspnea becomes an important cause of decrease in ❷ quality of life and morbidity in the elderly. To get a better view of this impact we need standardized means to quantify dyspnea. There are several objective instruments available to measure dyspnea. Much of them focus on quantifying the functional consequences of dyspnea, such as decreased activity, which have the potential to dramatically impact quality of life and translate into impairment and disability.

In this chapter diagnostic procedures and measurement of dyspnea and its consequences are discussed. Furthermore, current evidence based effective methods to manage and rehabilitate elderly patient with dyspnea are summarized.

List of Abbreviations: *ABG*, arterial blood gas; *ADL*, ❷ activities of daily life; *BDI*, baseline dyspnea index; *BNP*, brain natriuretic peptide; *CAD*, coronary artery disease; *CCQ*, ❷ clinical COPD questionnaire; *CHF*, chronic heart failure; *CHQ*, chronic heart failure questionnaire; *COPD*, chronic obstructive pulmonary disease; *CRP*, cardiac ❷ rehabilitation program; *CRQ/ CRQ-D*, chronic respiratory questionnaire/-dyspnea subscale; *CXR*, chest X ray; *ECG*, electrocardiography; *FEV1*, forced expiratory volume in 1 s; *HRQOL*, health related quality of life; *KCCQ*, kansas cardiomyopathy clinical questionnaire; *MBS*, modified borg scale; *METs*, metabolic equivalent tasks; *MLHF*, minnesota living with heart failure; *MRC*, medical research council; *MVO2*, myocardial volume oxygen (consumption); *NFPD*, non-fearful panic disorder; *NYHA*, New York heart association; *OT*, occupation therapy; *PFSDQ/PFSDQ-M*, pulmonary functional status and dyspnea questionnaire/-modified; *QLQ- QOL*, quality of life; *SF-36*, short-form 36-item questionnaire; *SGRQ*, St. George's respiratory questionnaire; *SHF*, quality of life questionnaire in severe heart failure; *SIP*, sickness impact profile; *SOLQ*, seattle obstructive lung disease questionnaire; *TDI*, transition dyspnea index; *VAS*, visual analogue scale; *WHO*, World Health Organization

1   Introduction

1.1   Definition and Prevalence

Dyspnea is a common symptom which is defined as abnormal or uncomfortable breathing in the context of what is normal for a person according to his or her level of fitness and exertional threshold for breathlessness (Morgan and Hodge, 1998). It occurs in healthy individuals as well, e.g., during intense emotional states and heavy labor or exercise.

Many patients describe their feeling as, "breathlessness," "tightness" "suffocating" "inability to take a deep breath," or simply "I can't get enough air." In contrast to pain and cough, for which specific receptors and neural pathways have been identified, the mechanisms that underlie the sensation of dyspnea remain poorly understood. So far no specialized dyspnea receptors have been identified. It seems clear that its mechanisms are multifactorial. In ❯ *Table 159-1* some key features of dyspnea are summarized.

◼ Table 159-1
Key facts of dyspnea

Dyspnea, or the patient's subjective perception of shortness of breath, is a common, function-limiting symptom found in patients with a wide variety of diagnoses.
Psychosocial or cultural factors may influence the perception of dyspnea by the patients.
Smoking is an important risk factor for many heart and lung diseases which can cause dyspnea.
Although breathlessness can be evaluated with various instruments, the most effective dyspnea measurement tool for patients with chronic lung disease or for measuring treatment effectiveness remains uncertain.
As the underlying diseases progress, dyspnea begins to have an impact on every aspect of patient's life.
The treatment of dyspnea is best directed at the underlying cause (if known).
Cardiac and pulmonary rehabilitation programs are also evidence-based treatments for patients with chronic dyspnea.

This table lists the key facts of dyspnea about its definition, measurement and treatments

To gain a better understanding of the dyspnea experience, we need to make a difference between respiratory "sensation" (the neural activation resulting from stimulation of a peripheral receptor), and "perception" (the reaction of the individual to the sensation). Dyspnea is a subjective term. Psychosocial and cultural factors may influence the reaction of individuals to a certain sensation of discomfort. Cultural or language differences may also result in patients using different words to describe the same experience.

The context in which a sensation occurs can also impact the perception of the event. The sensation experienced by an individual during maximal exercise will evoke very different reactions than the same sensation occurring at rest. Understanding the physiological and emotional factors may help health care providers to make a better approach and management for those with a faulty warning system (American Thoracic Society, 1999).

There are no precise data on the prevalence of dyspnea. The actual scope of the problem varies among clinical settings, underlying disease(s) and patient subgroups. Decrease in quality of life is a decisive factor for dyspnea patients to visit a physician. In general practices, dyspnea was found as chief complaint in 3.0–3.8% of patients who were older than 65 years (Thoonen and van Weel, 2002). In an ambulatory setting the prevalence of dyspnea was 3.7% (Kroenke and Mangelsdorff, 1989). Morbidity associated with dyspnea can range from minor to disabling.

1.2 Differential Diagnosis

The differential diagnosis of dyspnea includes respiratory, cardiac and psychiatric conditions. As a result, diagnosing the cause of the dyspnea is a difficult task, complicated by the variety of (patho-) physiological and psychological processes that play a role in the origin of the sensation of dyspnea. To make it easier we can divide the differential diagnosis into four general categories: cardiac, respiratory, mixed cardiac and respiratory, and noncardiac/non-respiratory (❯ Table 159-2).

❑ Table 159-2
Differential diagnosis of dyspnea

Cardiac	Mixed
– Congestive heart failure (right, left, biventricular)	– COPD with pulmonary hypertension and cor pulmonale
– Coronary artery disease	– Acute and chronic pulmonary emboli
– Myocardial infarction	– Trauma
– Dilated and hypertrophic cardiomyopathy	
– Valvular dysfunction	
– Left ventricular hypertrophy	
– Pericarditis	
– Arrhythmias	
Respiratory	**Non cardiac/non respiratory**
– Malignancy	– Metabolic conditions (e.g., acidosis)
– COPD	– Pain
– Asthma	– Neuromuscular disorders
– Restrictive lung disorders	– Otorhinolaryngeal disorders
– Hereditary lung disorders	– Anxiety and depression
– Pneumonia	– Panic disorder
– Pneumothorax	– Hyperventilation
– Pulmonary edema	– Iatrogenic (medical, surgical)
– Interstitial lung diseases	– Anemia
– Pulmonary circulation defect	– Chest wall deformities
– Gas exchange abnormalities	– Deconditioning (reduced peripheral muscle force)
– Upper airway obstruction	– Obesity
– Pleural effusion	

This table lists the differential diagnoses that underlie dyspnea: cardiac, respiratory, mixed and non cardiac/non respiratory

In most elderly patients with dyspnea there is obvious clinical evidence of disease of the heart and/or lungs. The difficulty in the distinction between cardiac and pulmonary dyspnea may be due to the coexistence of diseases involving both organ systems. Since presence of impairment in one system in the presence of the other has important diagnostic and therapeutic implications, knowledge about the concomitant prevalence is clinically important.

Major causes for dyspnea in the elderly are heart failure and COPD, but studies on the prevalence of heart failure in COPD patients or vice versa are scarce. However, it seems that the combined presence is rather common (Rutten et al., 2006). Up to one third of elderly patients with ❯ congestive heart failure (CHF) have coexistent COPD and one fifth of elderly patients with known COPD, have unrecognized concomitant CHF (Havranek et al., 2002). The risk for developing CHF is 4.5-fold greater in elderly patients with COPD compared with age-matched controls (Curkendall et al., 2006).

Dyspnea can also occur as a somatic manifestation of hyperventilation or panic attacks or even psychiatric disorders, such as panic disorder and depression. In the 1980s, the concept of "non-fearful panic disorder" (NFPD) was introduced by Beitman and defined as intense episodes of discomfort without either fear of dying, going crazy or losing control, but including at least four other "somatic" panic attack symptoms (Beitman et al., 1987; Fleet et al., 2000). NFPD seems to be a variant of panic disorder (PD) and has a chronic course similar to PD. NFPD is therefore a common problem in for example cardiological practice.

Disease processes that involve the chest wall, respiratory muscles, lung parenchyma, upper or lower airways, and pulmonary arteries or veins are also capable of causing dyspnea. Dyspnea is also increasingly regarded as an important outcome of both medical (e.g., drug treatment in chronic obstructive pulmonary disease, heart failure, weaning from mechanical ventilation) and surgical (e.g., lung volume reduction surgery) intervention trials.

Dyspnea can influence aspects of life in the suffering persons. To optimally enhance quality of life and to identify persons most vulnerable to this symptom, it is important to investigate how to assess dyspnea, how other symptoms and coping are related to dyspnea, and what the consequences of dyspnea are, especially on quality of life.

2   Evaluation and Measurement of Dyspnea

2.1   Evaluation

Dyspnea should be evaluated systematically, and a thorough history and physical examination and baseline tests of heart and lung function are necessary to establish a complete database. Although the mechanisms for dyspnea are not fully known, health care practitioners need to be able to evaluate and monitor dyspnea in their patients in order to help them to achieve the highest possible functional outcome.

The patient who has chronic shortness of breath may be more difficult to diagnose because the dyspnea typically develops over weeks to months or even years. Patients adapt their activities in response to the dyspnea so the severity may not be apparent.

As impairment, dyspnea reduces a patient's activity tolerance, which can lead to functional limitation and disability. Physicians must be able to examine the patient thoroughly, evaluate the cause of dyspnea, and use the information acquired to guide therapeutic interventions.

Dyspnea, like hunger or thirst, is largely a sensation that often arises from multiple sources of information rather than from stimulation of a single neural receptor. In addition, the severity of dyspnea as well as the qualitative aspects of unpleasant breathing experiences varies widely among patients (American Thoracic Society, 1999).

Despite the importance of evidence-based medicine, much of medical decision-making relies on clinical judgment; a process when a relevant evidence base is unavailable. Diagnostic tests serve to reduce uncertainty about a diagnosis or prognosis in a particular individual. It helps the physician to decide how to manage best the individual's condition and improve their quality of life. Not only laboratory tests and procedures but also the history and the physical examination can be considered as a part of the battery of diagnostic tools. Practitioners and therapists need to take a comprehensive history and examine the patient to identify impairments that can cause dyspnea and limit physical activity tolerance. When evaluating a patient with shortness of breath, one should also determine the time course over which the symptom has become manifest; acute shortness of breath (over a period of hours to days, subacute presentation (over days to weeks), chronic presentation (over month to years).

Additional testing in chronic dyspnea should be targeted in attempt to answer specific questions which arise by history and physical examination (❷ *Table 159-3*). A string of special studies may be required for diagnosis of dyspnea.

◻ Table 159-3

Diagnostic tests for identifying cause of dyspnea

Imaging techniques	CXR, Ventilation/Perfusion lung scanning, Ultra sound, MRI, Chest CT scan, Fluoroscopy, Gallium scan
Cardiac evaluations	ECG, Echocardiography, BNP, Holter monitoring, Thallium scanning, Cardiac catheterization, Radionuclide ventriculography, maximal oxygen uptake
Pulmonary evaluations	Standard spirometry, body Plethysmography, gas dilution techniques, Exercise testing, Gas diffusion techniques, Provocation test, Pulse oximetry, ABG, Myocardial oxygen consumption (MVO2)
Psychological assessments	Mental status exam, anxiety assessment

CXR: Chest X Ray; MRI: Magnetic Resonance Imagination; ECG: Electrocardiography; BNP: Brain Natriuretic Peptide; ABG: Arterial Blood Gas

Dependent on the patient's history and physical examinations we can use many useful instruments to diagnose the underlying cause of dyspnea. This table summarizes four types of diagnostic tests for identifying underlying diseases

2.2   Measurement

In evaluating the patient's impairments, two of the major outcomes are symptoms (usually dyspnea), and activity levels (functional status). Since dyspnea is a subjective sensation, it also can be a normal response to exercise (at high altitudes and after vigorous intensity) and is difficult to quantify. Depending on the underlying diseases, dyspnea is often associated with other common symptoms such as cough, anxiety, fatigue and pain. These symptoms are usually studied together, and caregivers are often asked to assess all of them using various types of analog or graphic rating scales.

The assessment of dyspnea during cycle ❷ ergometry or treadmill walking gives caregivers an opportunity to link symptoms to explanatory variables. In planning interventions for dyspnea, it is important to assess the degree of distress the dyspnea causes for the patient.

When dyspnea is quantified through standardized means, it is critical to know what that particular questionnaire, survey or instrument has captured, as not all dyspnea tools measure the same thing or are interchangeable. On the other hand, we must be sure about what we need to measure. For example, in a certain patient while the frequency of dyspnea may increase over time, the intensity may not increase.

Much of dyspnea measurement focuses on quantifying the secondary responses, particularly behavioral ones such as decreased activity. Few instruments attempt to quantify an individual's perception of these distinct sensations. In addition, secondary physiological responses are those that have the potential to dramatically impact quality of life and translate into impairment and disability (Meek, 2004).

There are several objective instruments available to measure dyspnea (❯ *Table 159-4*). Practitioners, nurse practitioners and physical therapists would be advised to familiarize with several measurement tools and try to apply an appropriate tool to a given patient. Some of the instruments are not only to be used as an instrument to measure the current/present state of dyspnea, but they can be used to evaluate treatment strategies (medication, rehabilitation program). Some instruments require patient subjective awareness and proper cognitive function, others are observations. Practical questionnaires are self administered, easy to understand by patients and quick to complete.

◻ Table 159-4

Categories of dyspnea tools and their measurements

Groups of tools	Set up	Time recall	Scaling
Short-term intensity			
MBS	Self administrated	Currently	0–10
VAS	Self administrated	Currently	0–100
Situational			
MRC	Self administrated	Long term	1–5
BDI/TDI	Rater associated	Currently	0–12
Impact			
CCQ	Self administrated	Last week	0–6
CRQ	Rater associated	Last 2 weeks	1–7
PFSDQ	Self administrated	Today, currently	0–12
NYHA	Rater associated	Long term	1–4

MBS: Modified Borg scale; VAS: Visual Analogue Scale; MRC: Medical Research Council dyspnea scale; BDI: Baseline Dyspnea Index; TDI: Transition Dyspnea Index; CCQ: Clinical COPD Questionnaire; CRQ: Chronic Respiratory Questionnaire; PFSDQ: Pulmonary Functional Status and Dyspnea Questionnaire; NYHA: New York Heart Association
To quantify the sensation of dyspnea we can use different types of questionnaires. Some of them are self-administrated and others need the rater's impression. This table summarized three groups of tools (short-term intensity, situational and impact tools) differentiated into set up, time recall and scaling

2.3   Short-Term Intensity Tools

These are excellent measures of dyspnea with exercise in a laboratory setting. Less is known about their responsiveness to change following intervention.

The Borg scale is particularly suited for the laboratory evaluation of dyspnea under controlled exercise conditions. In 1970 Borg was the first who described a scale ranging from 6 to 20 to measure perceived exertion during physical exercise. The scale was modified from its original form to a 10-point scale with verbal expressions of severity anchored to specific numbers.

The Visual Analogue Scale (VAS) consists of a line, usually 100 mm in length, placed either horizontally or vertically on a page, with anchors to indicate two extremes of the sensation of dyspnea. Scoring is accomplished by measuring the distance from the bottom of the scale (or left side if oriented horizontally) to the level indicated by the subject.

Because such an assessment is clearly highly subjective, it has most value when looking at change within individuals, and less value for comparing across a group of individuals at one time point. Thus, some caution is required in handling such data (American Thoracic Society, 1999).

2.4 Situational Dyspnea Tools

These tools quantify dyspnea in relation to a standard set of activities such as walking on level ground or up a hill. Situational measures are less able to capture rapid change in current states or treatments that have rapid effects.

The Medical Research Council Scale (MRC) is a rating system indicating dyspnea associated with walking that produces a single score. Individuals are assigned to one of five grades, based on their difficulty with mobility. The MRC does not measure dyspnea intensity itself, except as it relates to activities. It is recommended that the use of the MRC dyspnea scale be considered when evaluating an individual whose history indicates that they experience breathlessness during physical activities. Other uses of the MRC include allocation of individuals for intervention (Ciccone et al., 2003).

In 1984 Mahler et al. developed a scale to assess dyspnea using a multidimensional format to measure the associated effort and resultant impairment. The baseline dyspnea index (BDI) was designed to rate the severity of dyspnea at a single point in time, and the transition dyspnea index (TDI), to note changes from the baseline assessment. Each index rates three different categories: magnitude of task, magnitude of effort, and functional impairment. Each category has five grades ranging from severe to unimpaired.

The Baseline Dyspnea Index (BDI), like the MRC, is a rater evaluation of dyspnea associated with activities. The rating includes the magnitude of the task, and effort to perform the task.

The MRC and BDI/TDI are situational measures; both are completed as part of an interview with the respondent and the rater's impression is recorded. They are generally easy to use and will capture intermediate to prolonged changes.

Again, a limitation in using them is the rating or assignment of dyspnea associated with activities. This linkage of dyspnea with activities is useful to standardize for comparison purposes, but makes it impossible to separate activity level from dyspnea intensity. Thus, their use in evaluating dyspnea following any intervention must take this into consideration (Meek, 2004).

2.5 Impact Tools

In the past decade a number of tools have been developed that evaluate the overall impact of diseases on quality of life. Some of these impact tools have items intended to evaluate severity of dyspnea, but they are generally less specific to the symptoms.

The Clinical COPD Questionnaire (CCQ) is a short and simple tool for patients with COPD to evaluate the impact of disease on their health status. It arose from general practice where it was recognized that clinicians need a simple instrument to identify not only the clinical status of the respiratory system, but also functional needs, activity limitations and emotional dysfunctions in the patient.

CCQ is a self administered disease specific questionnaire which includes ten items rated on six-point scale covering symptoms, functional state and mental state of the patients. It can also be useful in clinical trials and other research studies to evaluate the adequacy of clinical management and to assess the effect of interventions. However the CCQ is not intended to assess patient's ❯ well-being or the impact of the disease on their wellbeing, moderate to high correlations is found between the CCQ and prominent quality of life measuring instruments which indicates convergent validity. Furthermore, the CCQ scores are highly correlated with the MRC scale (van der Molen et al., 2003).

The CRQ (Chronic Respiratory Questionnaire) is a 20-item, disease-specific quality of life questionnaire, which has been extensively used. The CRQ is interviewer-administered and contains four subscales (dyspnea, fatigue, emotional function and mastery) rated on a seven-point scale. The CRQ has been widely tested as a measure of dyspnea with several different types of interventions, including pulmonary rehabilitation inspiratory muscle training, and inhaled steroids (Covey et al., 2001; Hanania et al., 2003). The dyspnea subscale (CRQ-D) measures the severity of dyspnea in the past 2 weeks during five activities of daily living (ADL) chosen by the patient as being important in his or her daily life.

The tool has been successfully used in many situations to capture intermediate and prolonged changes and provides a unique approach to quantifying the impact of dyspnea (Meek, 2004).

The PFSDQ (Pulmonary Functional Status and Dyspnea Questionnaire) is a disease specific, self-administered impact tool consisting of 164 items which evaluates dyspnea and activity levels in patients with pulmonary impairment. The PFSDQ has been shown to be responsive to prolonged change, and to intermittent change following pulmonary rehabilitation. The PFSDQ provide a unique measure of the impact of dyspnea as it is linked to specific activities.

But there were some concerns about completeness of the data obtained and length of the questionnaire which could create measurement difficulties, interference with results and limit the instrument's use. As a result, it was desirable to modify the PFSDQ to a new version that would have a limited amount of missing data and could be used more easily.

The PFSDQ is modified by reducing the number of activities evaluated to 40, standardizing scaling formats, and adding a fatigue component. Findings suggest that the PFSDQ-M demonstrates internal reliability and good validity estimates. Dyspnea and activity scores appear responsive to physiologic changes in lung function over time (Lareau et al., 1998).

Many other tools are available for the measurement of breathlessness but there is no single instrument that encompasses all the components of the sensation of breathlessness. Different measures cover one or more dimensions or aspects of breathlessness. Therefore the assessment tool should be chosen for the specific question being asked.

The New York Heart Association (NYHA) classification is a four-point, semiquantitative, rater administered index to assess functional status of patients with heart failure, regarding the level of their maximal physical activity. NYHA classification is widely accepted because of its correlation with quality of life. Especially when measured serially over time, it provides a means of tracking disease progression and quality of life in response to therapeutic interventions. The NYHA classification has been challenged, because of the absence of the factor time (i.e., the duration an individual is able to perform a given amount of exercise), and the inaccuracy to make the distinction between classes II and III (Apostolakis and Akinosoglou, 2007). Because of the interindividual differences in interpreting the NYHA classification, potential hazards may be present regarding the resulting clinical decision making process (Kubo et al., 2004).

A proposed objective classification could be based on the measurement of METs (Metabolic Equivalent Tasks) produced by a patient during exercise. In patients not being able to exercise this problem could be overcome by a new classification, based, for example, on a scale that measures the amount of oxygen the heart can provide to the musculature at rest (MVO2: Myocardial Volume Oxygen in ml/kg/min).

3   Impact of Dyspnea on Quality of Life

3.1   Definition

Quality of life (QOL) refers to the patient's ability to enjoy normal life activities. It is a broad concept defined in different ways and includes varying areas of life. Unlike standard of living, quality of life is not a tangible concept, and therefore cannot be measured directly.

In gerontological studies, quality of life contains two distinct domains; Health Related Quality of Life (HRQOL) and non-health related or environmental quality of life (Spilker and Revicki, 1999).

HRQOL originates from the WHO definition of health: "Health is a state of physical, mental, social well-being and not merely the absence of disease or infirmity" (Anderson and Burckhardt, 1999). It encompasses domains of life directly affected by changes in health which minimally include:

- Functional status (e.g., whether a patient is able to manage a household, uses the telephone or dress independently)
- Mental health or emotional wellbeing (e.g., depressive symptoms, positive affect)
- Social engagement (e.g., involvement with others, engagement in activities)
- Symptom states (e.g., pain, shortness of breath, fatigue)

Non-health-related QOL domains include:

- Natural and the created environment (i.e., economic resources, housing, air and water quality, community stability, access to the arts and entertainment)
- Personal resources (i.e., the capacity to form friendships, appreciate nature, or find satisfaction in spiritual or religious life). These factors affect health-related QOL but, unlike health-related QOL domains, are less likely to improve with appropriate medical care (Albert et al., 2002)

3.2   Interactions

Dyspnea and fatigue caused by cardiac and/or pulmonary diseases influence all aspects of life in elderly patients suffering from them. These symptoms and their effect on activity levels are important factors in HRQOL.

Research literature concerning dyspnea as a symptom in the elderly is scarce, although much has been written about specific diseases that may cause dyspnea, especially COPD and heart failure. As the prevalence of these conditions increases with advancing age, dyspnea becomes an important cause of morbidity in the elderly.

Although extensive data do not exist on the prevalence of dyspnea in the elderly population, a review of the medical literature indicates prevalence in the range of 17–38% based on surveys of adults at different ages (Mahler et al., 2003).

In another research a high prevalence of dyspnea is found among patients >70 years of age, with 55% of participants in the postal survey (MRC). Three months later in the same research, of those who completed the extended questionnaire (BDI) during the home interview, 71% reported dyspnea symptoms. Dyspnea showed a positive association with age. In addition, dyspnea was associated with poorer physical and mental health, more anxiety and depressive symptoms, impaired daily functioning, and lower happiness. Dyspnea measured with BDI and MRC was also a predictor of death within a period of 8 years when age and gender were controlled for in the analysis. Especially in the case of death due to cardiovascular or lung disease, the more dyspnea complaints, the greater the mortality risk (Huijnen et al., 2006). These findings are in accordance with those of another study (Tessier et al., 2001).

Dyspnea during exertion is a frequent complaint most commonly associated with a cardiac or respiratory disease, but it might also be due to other less frequent causes. In studies on clinical elderly outpatients, the relation between pulmonary function and quality of life has been shown to be weak (Peruzza et al., 2003). Findings concern the fact that pulmonary function in elderly patients is hardly related to the SIP (the Sickness Impact Profile) scores of quality of life. Otherwise, dyspnea has an especially strong relation with the quality of life measurements, which is an indication of the substantial impact dyspnea has on patients' daily life (Schrier et al., 1990).

In elderly patients with CHF, pathophysiologic variables including those commonly used to assess cardiac structure and function (e.g., left ventricular end-diastolic dimension, ejection fraction) and neurohormonal activation (e.g., brain natriuretic peptide) do not have a direct effect on a patient's quality of life. In elderly patients with CHF, although prognosis in patients with normal systolic function is better than patients with systolic dysfunction, there are no considerable differences in quality of life between patients with diastolic and systolic dysfunction. The same amount of symptoms, functional disability and psychosocial impairment exist in both populations (Jaarsma et al., 1999).

Several interrelated variables intervene between a patient's pathophysiology and quality of life. Therefore, the correlation between pathophysiologic variables and quality of life is not expected to be strong or predictive (Rector, 2005).

As the underlying disease progresses with age, patients with dyspnea experience a progressive deterioration and disability. These patients seek medical attention because of symptoms, particularly dyspnea, and impaired ability to function, which clearly impact on an individual's HRQOL.

Symptoms, functional status and HRQOL may follow different trajectories. This discordance between physiologic and health outcomes, results from a complex interaction of these variables (e.g., changes in health expectations, activity levels and physical ❷ deconditioning). Exertional dyspnea often causes patients to unconsciously reduce their daily activities to reduce the intensity of their distress; this can lead to deconditioning which, in turn, further increases dyspnea. These confusions preclude for example using the NYHA classification as a reliable tool to measure functional status of the CHF patients (Kubo et al., 2004). As a result, the clinical assessment should include not only the intensity of dyspnea but also activity limitation because of the disease.

Dyspnea in elderly patients may be influenced also by emotional and mood components. The relationship between dyspnea and depression still remains unclear but we can argue that older subjects with a depressed mood tend to emphasize dyspnea, and a dyspneic patient tends to be more depressed due to his functional restriction (Peruzza et al., 2003). Given the complexity of relationships and intricacy of quality of life per se, it is difficult to make accurate inferences about a patient's quality of life from typical symptom, functional, and psychologic assessments. These relationships are roughly showed in ❷ *Figure 159-1*.

◻ Figure 159-1

Conceptual model of relationships between dyspnea and other components which affect QOL. changes in QOL are not only dependent on dyspnea and its underlying diseases, but also on impaired ability, psychological components and their mutual interactions. According to this model underlying disease has no direct impact on QOL

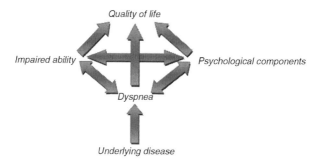

3.3   Measurement

Instruments have been developed to provide a standardized method to measure health status and levels of impairment (discriminative) en to detect how much HRQOL has changed in response to therapy (evaluative).

The interest for HRQOL measurement in patients with dyspnea has grown in recent years. The fact that HRQOL is the result of the interaction of multiple physical, psychological and social factors, unique for each individual, can justify this interest from the scientific community. HRQOL is a measurement that can be identified and quantified, but is different from physiologic measures or survival risks. The HRQOL can be quantified through various health evaluation instruments, both general and disease specific (Carrasco Garrido et al., 2006). These instruments are designed to provide a standardized method by which health status or levels of health impairment could be measured and compared in individual patients as well as in groups of patients. Simply put, HRQOL assessment quantifies the impact of the disease on activities of daily living (ADLs) and the individual's sense of well-being. To meet this goal we can use three different types of instruments (Guyatt et al., 1993) which are shortly presented in ❷ *Table 159-5*.

There is no consensus definition or method of measuring the quality of an individual, other than it should be judged by him or herself. Regardless of the type of the instrument or combination of instruments used in a battery, a good questionnaire should include the following markers, to assess the effect of dyspnea and its underlying disease on daily life of patients:

◻ Table 159-5

Types of instruments to measure HRQOL

Type	Example
Utility scale	A continuum from perfect health to death; EuroQol
General or generic health measures	The Sickness Impact Profile(SIP), the Short-Form 36-item questionnaire (SF-36), the Nottingham Health Profile
Disease-specific measures	1. COPD: the Clinical COPD Questionnaire (CCQ), the Chronic Respiratory Questionnaire (CRQ), the St.George's Respiratory Questionnaire (SGRQ), the Seattle Obstructive Lung Disease Questionnaire (SOLQ); 2. HF: the Minnesota Living with Heart Failure (MLHF), the Chronic Heart Failure Questionnaire (CHQ) and Quality of Life Questionnaire in Severe Heart Failure (QLQ-SHF), the Kansas cardiomyopathy clinical questionnaire (KCCQ)

This table shows some frequent measurement tools to evaluate HRQOL. There are many other less used instruments with different validity and reliability

1. Level of dyspnea (frequency, duration, and severity, sleep disturbance)
2. Activity levels (ability to exercise, perform activities of daily living)
3. Fatigue (severity and frequency)
4. General feeling of well-being
5. Social functioning status (ability to engage in social functions in and out of the home)
6. Emotional functioning status (depression, attitudes toward coping)

As the severity of underlying disease increases, dyspnea begins to have an impact on ADLs; eventually, some ADLs become limited or are completely eliminated. Whether an ADL is eliminated or continued depends on the interaction between the need of the patient to do that activity and the intensity of associated symptoms. ADL such as leisure activities are usually the first to be eliminated, since they generally require greater effort and are not critical to daily life. There are many tools to use for evaluation ADL, such as the Katz ADL scale and the Lawton ADL scale. ADL can be divided in two distinct category; *basic* (primary) and *instrumental* (secondary). Basic ADLs are those required for daily life, such as eating, dressing, personal hygiene, toileting, and physical mobility (moving from one place to another). Elderly patients with dyspnea have difficulty to do some or all of these activities, but they are seldom eliminated or appreciably limited except in far-advanced disease or because of substantial comorbidity. Thus, basic ADLs are the last activities they can do in their life. Instrumental ADLs are necessary for adapting independently to the environment; they include activities such as cooking, shopping, home chores, housework, laundry and gardening. Many of these activities are optional in a person's life, depending on the level of social support and other resources (Spector et al., 1987).

4   Dyspnea Management and Rehabilitation

Treatment of the underlying disease is the most effective method of alleviating dyspnea.

Most of these diseases are progressive, frustrating and debilitating and their influence permeates every aspect of the patient's life. Unfortunately, medical science seems to be unable to devise a way to reverse the diseases process. In elderly patients, the specific cause of the dyspnea is usually elusive and a specific treatment is not available, so treatment should be aimed at symptom relief.

Patients who have chronic dyspnea can be taught a variety of methods to help them alleviate or cope with their breathlessness. For a long time, rest and the avoidance of stress were the main strategies, but now a progressive increase in the patient's level of activity, according to a scientific based multidisciplinary rehabilitation program, is the main approach to diminish the effect of dyspnea on quality of life.

Through activity modification, elderly patients may be better able to plan their days so that they are capable of doing the things that are most important to them. Physical inactivity in this group of patients is a major risk factor for multiple complications and is also a mediator in the dyspnea-inactivity-deconditioning circle. Clinicians need to be aware of the importance of helping patients with dyspnea to balance appropriate amounts of activity and inactivity so that patients may be better able to control their dyspnea and preserve quality of life.

Pharmacologic therapy of the underlying diseases is beyond the scope of this chapter. However, we want to focus on components of cardiac and pulmonary rehabilitation programs together with psychosocial supports especially in COPD and CHF, two most common causes of dyspnea.

Pulmonary and cardiac rehabilitations are medically supervised programs to help lung and heart patients recover quickly and improve their overall physical, mental and social functioning. The goal is to stabilize, slow or even reverse the progression of the underlying disease. These goals should be discussed with the patient and family. An individualized plan should be created in collaboration with other team members, taking into consideration the patient's general condition, the presence and severity of symptoms, the expected survival, and the preferred place of care. The long-term success of any program is directly related to patient compliance and participation.

4.1   Pulmonary Rehabilitation

According to The American Thoracic Society and the European Respiratory Society, Pulmonary rehabilitation is an evidence-based, multidisciplinary, and comprehensive intervention for patients with chronic respiratory diseases who are symptomatic and often have decreased daily life activities.

Pulmonary rehabilitation typically includes several different components, including exercise training, education, instruction in various respiratory and chest physiotherapy techniques, and psychosocial support.

Pulmonary rehabilitation has no substantial effect on the lung impairment, such as the FEV1, of patients with COPD or other chronic respiratory diseases. Despite this, pulmonary rehabilitation usually results in beneficial outcomes in several important aspects of health and well-being, including dyspnea, exercise performance, disability, and quality of life.

A number of factors in patients with physical deconditioning, such as muscle atrophy, reduced capillarization, decreased oxidative capacity, and early lactic acidemia, which contribute to exercise limitation and dyspnea, are potentially reversible. Exercise training is the best available means for improving muscle function and is widely considered to be a manda-tory component of pulmonary rehabilitation (Ries et al., 2007).

Traditionally, pulmonary rehabilitation exercise programs have been based essentially on lower-extremity training, by use of a treadmill or a stationary ergometer. The exercise program should involve upper-limb exercises too, because many activities of daily living require the upper extremities. Upper-extremity training with an arm ergometer, free weights or elastic bands may reduce dyspnea and ventilator requirements for arm elevation (Derom et al., 2007).

An attempt should be made to propose high-intensity training to achieve maximal physiologic effects (Vallet et al., 1997). This should be performed under strict supervision. Training intensities exceeding 60% of peak exercise capacity is empirically considered suffi-cient, although more beneficial effects may be obtained if higher percentages are tolerated. Borg score, heart rate or power output have been proposed as aids to target training intensity (Puente-Maestu et al., 2000). Occasionally, training intensities should be reduced because of symptom limitation, comorbidities or level of motivation.

Pulmonary rehabilitation and pharmacologic therapy should be considered complemen-tary to each other. If a patient with COPD remains symptomatic despite bronchodilators, pulmonary rehabilitation would likely provide additional benefit. On the other hand optimal bronchodilation allows for higher intensity exercise training during pulmonary rehabilitation, thereby enhancing its effects (Zuwallack, 2007). A recent study has shown that using oxygen supplementation during exercise training has no significant effect on maximal exercise outcome and HRQOL of the patients (Nonoyama et al., 2007).

The effect of the program should be evaluated at least in terms of exercise tolerance and health related quality of life in the individual patient and by pooling the data, obtained over a certain period of time.

4.2   Cardiac Rehabilitation

Cardiac rehabilitation program (CRP) aims to reverse the limitations that have developed following adverse pathophysiologic and psychological consequences of cardiac events. It consists of interventions that improve patient outcomes such as exercise, education, psycho-social counseling and lifestyle modification.

Elderly patients who are often under represented in clinical trials, are perhaps most likely to benefit from such a multidisciplinary approach because of polypharmacy, co-morbidity and poor health-related quality of life. These benefits are associated with a reduction in hospital admissions attributable to heart disease. Despite this, older adults are not likely to participate. Older men feared physical pain with exercise and older women expressed a need for emotional support. A tailored CRP for these patients with cardiac diseases, decreases admissions to hospital and improves exercise capacity (Austin et al., 2005). It has been suggested that in older adults, CRPs could be improved by including more socialization opportunities, offering varied forms of exercise, enhancing teaching about stress management, and adapting teaching strategies (Austin et al., 2005; Dolansky et al., 2006).

Patients older than 60 years who received 8 months CRP focusing on exercise, attained a significant improvement in health-related quality of life that is likely to be of clinical impor-tance. The strongest effect occurred in the first 8 weeks, when patients were receiving the most intense phase of the intervention. Exercise training, as an isolated intervention, may not be able to cause significant reduction in the morbidity and mortality of cardiac patients

(Austin et al., 2005). Nevertheless, exercise training has the potential to act as a catalyst for promoting other aspects of rehabilitation, including risk factor modification through therapeutic lifestyle changes and optimization of psychosocial support. The focus of education is mainly concerned with moderation of risk factors which, if adequately controlled, can assist in reducing patients' morbidity and mortality. These include smoking, hypertension, diabetes, elevated serum cholesterol, hypertension and obesity.

Similarly, better fulfillment of therapeutic guidelines to treat hypertension, diabetes and dyslipidemia can prevent the appearance or progression of atherosclerosis.

The intended outcome of education in the area of risk factor management is to produce observable sustainable changes in patients' behavior. Changes in lifestyle behavior are aimed at reducing their risk of worsening disease, and improving their overall quality of life (Austin et al., 2005).

Long-term follow-up studies in elderly patients are not conclusive because of sample erosion and presence of cross interventions. Several meta-analyses have studied the effect of CRP on mortality in randomized trials, producing inconclusive results. The last and perhaps the most thorough finding in these trials was a fall in mortality related to cardiovascular diseases (Jolliffe et al., 2004; O'Connor et al., 1989).

Although the benefits of exercise are difficult to distinguish from the concurrent effects of other parts of CRP, the association between regular physical activity and improved health is clear. Therefore, regular exercise is to be recommended for most patients who suffer from dyspnea.

4.3   Psychosocial Supports

As the underlying diseases progress, elderly patients may enter a downward cycle of dyspnea, inactivity and physical deconditioning, often accompanied by fear, anxiety and depression.

Clinicians are often not aware that panic disorder or depression can present mainly with somatic symptoms. For example, shortness of breath and choking, but also chest pain, are common somatic symptoms during panic attacks. It is therefore not surprisingly that patients present themselves in somatic settings, rather than in psychiatric ones. A chronic condition like heart failure is, however, not only a somatic burden to the patient, but is also a burden in a psychological way. Consequences of heart failure are often difficult to accept by patients (Lesman-Leegte et al., 2007). Over 40% of heart failure patients (especially women) have depressive or anxiety symptoms. It is important to detect depression or anxiety, like panic disorder, in patients because it decreases quality of life, deteriorates patient's prognosis and reduces compliance with treatment and healthy life style due to for example smoking. Patients with heart failure should therefore be screened for depression and anxiety (Kuijpers et al., 2000; Strik et al., 2003).

Exercise training in cardiac and pulmonary rehabilitation programs can be completed with psychosocial, behavioral and educational interventions depending on individual needs of the patient, degree of scientific evidence, and resources available. This includes ❷ self-management of dyspnea and related fear and anxiety, nutritional intervention, and Occupational therapy.

4.3.1   Self Management

Self-management is a term applied to educational programs consists of teaching skills needed to carry out medical regimens specific to the disease and provide emotional support for patients to control their disease and improve their quality of life.

In elderly patients, dyspnea not only leads to reduced effort but commonly associates with anxiety. Anxiety made the perception of dyspnea more acute, and some patients avoided any activity in a phobic manner as though the resulting shortness of breath meant that they would die.

Patients are often capable of successfully modifying their own symptom experiences. In elderly patients, these modifying methods rely heavily on knowledge and skills they already possess. These have been derived from allopathic health practices, alternative and traditional remedies and self-healing capabilities.

Strategies selected by more than 50% of COPD patients with dyspnea, are moving slower, keeping still, using extra oxygen, performing breathing exercises (pursed-lips breathing), decreasing activities and using cool air. Other less used methods are transferring ADLs to others, using extra inhaler therapy, changing dressing habits, changing eating habits and using assistive devices such as walker and cane (Christenbery, 2005).

A comprehensive rehabilitation program including self management, leads to a decrease in unrealistic fear of activity and improve patient's self esteem and autonomy in the control of dyspnea. Under good instructions, patients begin to see shortness of breath as a physiologic event rather than as a frightening and dangerous crisis. Repeated and increasing exercise in the presence of monitoring equipment and medical staff, gives the patients feeling that they can tolerate some shortness of breath and still continue effort without dangerous consequences. At the same time, the elderly patient should feel they are treated as though they are salvageable in some way and worth the effort.

So the anxiety or phobic element of their avoidance of activity can be desensitized, and eventually they will be able to continue physical effort without the reassuring presence of the others.

To achieve these goals, group participation may offer a setting for mutual encouragement and further education and can be an important aid to any rehabilitation effort.

Depending on individual needs and capacities of the patient we can add some other components to their self management program such as:

- Group sessions or private counseling on the anatomy and physiological basis of dyspnea, adaptation to underlying disease and advice on how to manage it in everyday life.
- Relaxation training.
- Bronchial hygiene instructions (to teach the patients the most effective way of coughing and how to remove secretions from their lungs using simple postures).
- Breathing retraining (to teach the patients how to breathe in the most effective way in different situations; breathing techniques such as pursed lip breathing, diaphragmatic breathing, segmental breathing and walking with a forward leaning posture).
- Smoking cessation counseling; smoking is an important risk factor for many respiratory and cardiac diseases. Smoking cessation must be the cornerstone of treatment and rehabilitation programs. Successful treatment of tobacco dependence requires repeated intensive interventions.

Using exercise together with these components in rehabilitation program has shown a benefit in anxiety and depressive symptoms in COPD patients. The benefit seems to be especially significant in anxiety symptoms than depressive symptoms. In addition to the improvement in psychological symptoms, the health status, exercise tolerance and dyspnea intensity are also significantly improved in COPD patients who underwent the rehabilitation program (Kayahan et al., 2006).

4.3.2 Nutritional Intervention

Malnutrition is associated with progressive muscle wasting and loss of fat mass, and can be observed in several different chronic disorders. Although the real cause of malnutrition in chronic patients is unclear, a multi-factorial mechanism by which increased energy expenditure is not balanced by an adequate dietary intake seems to be crucial. Some patients with COPD experience dyspnea during eating and may decrease their intake of food to avoid the unpleasant sensation. Also the entire process of preparing and eating a meal can be very tiring for some older patients, and can lead to a reduction in energy intake.

Because older patients are at increased risk for multiple nutritional deficiencies, it is important to begin nutritional management with a comprehensive nutritional assessment as an evaluation of nutritional status including medical history, dietary history, physical examination and laboratory data.

Nutritional counseling for elderly dyspnea patients must recognized specific nutrient requirements related to age and process of underlying disease plus additional demands related to increased physical activity and exercise during rehabilitation programs. Counseling should survey caloric and nutrient intake, dietary fat intake, eating habits and preferences in order to optimally individualize the dietary plan (Balady et al., 2007). Appropriate nutrition intervention considering multiple comorbidities and multiple medications of the patients, can reduce the risk of a variety of chronic health problems such as cardiac cachexia in CHF and sarcopenia (age related waste of muscle mass) in COPD.

Combination of nutritional supplementation and an appropriate exercise program improve respiratory and peripheral muscle strength and walking capacity in elderly COPD patients and should be part of a comprehensive rehabilitation program (Bunout et al., 2001).

4.3.3 Occupational Therapy

Occupational therapy (OT) can be defined as a task of rehabilitation for disabled patients, giving them independence and ability to maintain specific activities of daily living and to improve the ability to cope with their work and social challenges.

OT intervention during comprehensive pulmonary rehabilitation must be promoted to specifically evaluate and solve problems related with respiratory disability (i.e., walking, dressing, bathing, feeding and weight lifting). Occupational tasks should be related to symptoms occurring during specific activities.

A recent study has shown that the addition of OT to a standard comprehensive pulmonary rehabilitation is able to specifically improve the outcome of severely disabled COPD patients (Lorenzi et al., 2004).

Summary Points

- The mechanisms that underlie the sensation of dyspnea remain poorly understood. It seems clear that its mechanisms are multifactorial.
- Decrease in quality of life is a decisive factor for dyspnea patients to visit a physician. In general practices, dyspnea was found as chief complaint in 3.0–3.8% of patients who were older than 65 years.

- The differential diagnosis of dyspnea can be divided into four general categories: cardiac, respiratory, mixed cardiac and respiratory, and noncardiac/nonrespiratory.
- To optimally enhance quality of life, it is important to investigate how to assess dyspnea, how other symptoms and coping are related to dyspnea, and what the consequences of dyspnea are, especially on quality of life.
- As impairment, dyspnea reduces a patient's activity tolerance, which can lead to functional limitation and disability. Physicians and other care-givers must be able to examine the patient thoroughly, evaluate the cause of dyspnea, and use the information acquired to guide therapeutic interventions.
- There are several objective instruments available to measure dyspnea. Some instruments require patient subjective awareness and proper cognitive function, others are observations.
- Dyspnea has an especially strong relation with the quality of life measurements, which is an indication of the substantial impact dyspnea has on patients' daily life.
- As the severity of underlying disease increases, dyspnea begins to have an impact on ADLs; eventually, some ADLs become limited or are completely eliminated.
- Treatment of the underlying disease is the most effective method of alleviating dyspnea.
- Pulmonary and cardiac rehabilitations are medically supervised programs to help lung and heart patients recover quickly and improve their overall physical, mental and social functioning.
- Exercise training in cardiac and pulmonary rehabilitation programs can be completed with psychosocial/psychiatric, behavioral and educational interventions depending on individual objective and subjective needs of the patient, degree of scientific evidence, and resources available.

References

Albert US, Koller M, Lorenz W, Kopp I, Heitmann C, Stinner B, Rothmund M, Schulz KD. (2002). Breast. 11: 324–334.

American Thoracic Society. (1999). Am J Respir Crit Care Med. 159: 321–340.

Anderson KL, Burckhardt CS. (1999). J Adv Nurs. 29: 298–306.

Apostolakis E, Akinosoglou K. (2007). Am J Cardiol. 100: 911–912.

Austin J, Williams R, Ross L, Moseley L, Hutchison S. (2005). Eur J Heart Fail. 7: 411–417.

Balady GJ, Williams MA, Ades PA, Bittner V, Comoss P, Foody JA, Franklin B, Sanderson B, Southard D. (2007). J Cardiopulm Rehabil Prev. 27: 121–129.

Beitman BD, Basha I, Flaker G, DeRosear L, Mukerji V, Lamberti J. (1987). Behav Res Ther. 25: 487–492.

Bunout D, Barrera G, de la Maza P, Avendano M, Gattas V, Petermann M, Hirsch S. (2001). J Nutr. 131: 2441S–2446S.

Carrasco Garrido P, de Miguel Diez J, Rejas Gutierrez J, Centeno AM, Gobartt Vazquez E, Gil de Miguel A, Garcia Carballo M, Jimenez Garcia R. (2006). Health Qual Life Outcomes. 4: 31.

Christenbery TL. (2005). Heart Lung. 34: 406–414.

Ciccone AM, Meyers BF, Guthrie TJ, Davis GE, Yusen RD, Lefrak SS, Patterson GA, Cooper JD. (2003). J Thorac Cardiovasc Surg. 125: 513–525.

Covey MK, Larson JL, Wirtz SE, Berry JK, Pogue NJ, Alex CG, Patel M. (2001). J Cardiopulm Rehabil. 21: 231–240.

Curkendall SM, DeLuise C, Jones JK, Lanes S, Stang MR, Goehring E Jr, She D. (2006). Ann Epidemiol. 16: 63–70.

Derom E, Marchand E, Troosters T. (2007). Ann Readapt Med Phys. 50: 615–626, 602–614.

Dolansky MA, Moore SM, Visovsky C. (2006). J Gerontol Nurs. 32: 37–44.

Fleet RP, Martel JP, Lavoie KL, Dupuis G, Beitman BD. (2000). Psychosomatics. 41: 311–320.

Guyatt GH, Feeny DH, Patrick DL. (1993). Ann Intern Med. 118: 622–629.

Hanania NA, Darken P, Horstman D, Reisner C, Lee B, Davis S, Shah T. (2003). Chest. 124: 834–843.

Havranek EP, Masoudi FA, Westfall KA, Wolfe P, Ordin DL, Krumholz HM. (2002). Am Heart J. 143: 412–417.

Huijnen B, Horst van der F, van Amelsvoort L, Wesseling G, Lansbergen M, Aarts P, Nicolson N, Knottnerus JA. (2006). Fam Pract. 23: 34–39.

Jaarsma T, Halfens R, Abu-Saad HH, Dracup K, Stappers J, van Ree J. (1999). Eur J Heart Fail. 1: 151–160.

Jolliffe JA, Rees K, Taylor RS, Thompson D, Oldridge N, Ebrahim S. (2004). Cochrane Database Syst Rev. CD001800.

Kayahan B, Karapolat H, Atyntoprak E, Atasever A, Ozturk O. (2006). Respir Med. 100: 1050–1057.

Kroenke K, Mangelsdorff AD. (1989). Am J Med. 86: 262–266.

Kubo SH, Schulman S, Starling RC, Jessup M, Wentworth D, Burkhoff D. (2004). J Card Fail. 10: 228–235.

Kuijpers PM, Honig A, Griez EJ, Braat SH, Wellens HJ. (2000). Ned Tijdschr Geneeskd. 144: 745–749.

Lareau SC, Meek PM, Roos PJ. (1998). Heart Lung. 27: 159–168.

Lesman-Leegte I, Jaarsma T, Sanderman R, Hillege HL, van Veldhuisen DJ. (2008). Eur J Cardiovasc Nurs. 7: 121–126.

Lorenzi CM, Cilione C, Rizzardi R, Furino V, Bellantone T, Lugli D, Clini E. (2004). Respiration. 71: 246–251.

Mahler DA, Fierro-Carrion G, Baird JC. (2003). Clin Geriatr Med. 19: 19–33, v.

Mahler DA, Weinberg DH, Wells CK, Feinstein AR. (1984). Chest. 85: 751–758.

Meek PM. (2004). Chron Respir Dis. 1: 29–37.

Morgan WC, Hodge HL. (1998). Am Fam Physician. 57: 711–716.

Nonoyama ML, Brooks D, Lacasse Y, Guyatt GH, Goldstein RS. (2007). Cochrane Database Syst Rev. CD005372.

O'Connor GT, Buring JE, Yusuf S, Goldhaber SZ, Olmstead EM, Paffenbarger RS Jr, Hennekens CH. (1989). Circulation. 80: 234–244.

Peruzza S, Sergi G, Vianello A, Pisent C, Tiozzo F, Manzan A, Coin A, Inelmen EM, Enzi G. (2003). Respir Med. 97: 612–617.

Puente-Maestu L, Sanz ML, Sanz P, Ruiz de Ona JM, Rodriguez-Hermosa JL, Whipp BJ. (2000). Eur Respir J. 15: 1026–1032.

Rector TS. (2005). J Card Fail. 11: 173–176.

Ries AL, Bauldoff GS, Carlin BW, Casaburi R, Emery CF, Mahler DA, Make B, Rochester CL, Zuwallack R, Herrerias C. (2007). Chest. 131: 4S–42S.

Rutten FH, Cramer MJ, Lammers JW, Grobbee DE, Hoes AW. (2006). Eur J Heart Fail. 8: 706–711.

Schrier AC, Dekker FW, Kaptein AA, Dijkman JH. (1990). Chest. 98: 894–899.

Spector WD, Katz S, Murphy JB, Fulton JP. (1987). J Chronic Dis. 40: 481–489.

Spilker, B, Revicki, DA. (1999). In: Taxonomy of Quality of Life. Quality of Life and Pharmacoeconomics in Clinical Trials. Lippincott-Raven, Philadelphia, pp. 25–32.

Strik JJ, van Praag HM, Honig A. (2003). Tijdschr Gerontol Geriatr. 34: 104–112.

Tessier JF, Nejjari C, Letenneur L, Filleul L, Marty ML, Barberger Gateau P, Dartigues JF. (2001). Eur J Epidemiol. 17: 223–229.

Thoonen BPA, van Weel C. (2002). Huisarts Wet. 45: 414–419.

Vallet G, Ahmaidi S, Serres I, Fabre C, Bourgouin D, Desplan J, Varray A, Prefaut C. (1997). Eur Respir J. 10: 114–122.

Molen van der T, Willemse BW, Schokker S, ten Hacken NH, Postma DS, Juniper EF. (2003). Health Qual Life Outcomes. 1: 13.

Zuwallack R. (2007). Proc Am Thorac Soc. 4: 549–553.

160 Quality of Life and Age Urinary Incontinence Severity: Turkish Perspectives

T. M. Filiz · P. Topsever

1   Introduction 2746

2   Definition 2747

3   Diagnosing Female Urinary Incontinence with Questionnaires 2747

4   Prevalence 2747

5   Therapy of Urinary Incontinence 2747

6   Quality of Life in Urinary Incontinence 2748

7   Urinary Incontinence QOL Measures Used in Turkey 2750

8   Review of Turkish Literature 2750

9   Original Data 2751

    Summary Points 2755

Abstract: ❷ Urinary incontinence (UI) is being perceived as a stigmatized condition since ancient times. Not much has changed up to date – although, posing a considerable disease burden and impairing health related quality of life-urinary incontinence (HRQOL- UI) is not perceived as a medical entity by adult females in Turkey, and -due to lack of medical help seeking- probably is underreported. Overall prevalence in Turkey has been reported to be between 16.4 and 68.8%, depending on research setting and methodology. Because HRQOL is a new concept in medical research, there are only few urinary incontinence (UI) studies addressing quality of life (QOL), as well. The studies assessing QOL of individuals with UI are mostly cross-sectional and -except for the recent ones- do not use grade A International Consultation on Incontinence (ICI) recommended instruments. This chapter summarizes the available instruments used for diagnosis, classification and severity grading, as well HRQOL assessment. According to the results of studies on UI and related QOL, the disease burden and bothersomeness created by the condition is impairing QOL and mostly is the determinant for medical help seeking behavior, which is displaying a transcultural trend being in accordance with the world literature. There is a need for a clearinghouse for studies on UI and related QOL to plan and conduct such studies, manage and organize dissemination of evidence, and take action according to health policy needs in that matter.

List of Abbreviations: *BFLUTS*, Bristol female lower urinary tract symptoms questionnaire; *DIS*, Detrusor instability score; *HRQOL*, health related quality of life; *ICI*, International Consultation on Incontinence; *ICIQ-SF*, International Consultation on Incontinence Questionnaire Short Form; *ICS*, International continence society; *ICSmale-LUTS*, International Consultation on Incontinence Questionnaire lower urinary tract symptoms; *IIQ*, incontinence impact questionnaire; *I-QOL*, incontinence QOL instrument; *IQOLI*, incontinence QOL index; *ISI*, incontinence severity index; *KHQ*, King's Health Questionnaire; *LUTS*, ❷ lower urinary tract symptoms; *MUI*, ❷ mixed urinary incontinence; *OAB*, ❷ overactive bladder; *PRAFAB*, protection, amount, frequency, adjustment, body image; *QOL*, quality of life; *RCT*, randomized controlled trial; *SF-36*, medical outcomes study (MOS) 36-item short-form health survey (SF-36); *SII*, symptom impact index; *SSI*, symptom severity index; *SUI*, ❷ stress urinary incontinence; *SUIQQ*, stress urinary incontince quality of life questionnaire; *UDI*, urogenital distress inventory; *UI*, urinary incontinence; *UUI*, ❷ urge urinary incontinence; *WHO*, World Health Organization

1   Introduction

The diseases of the sexual organs in females, although so various, so distressing to those who labor under them, and not unfrequently so fatal in their consequences, are perhaps less generally known and understood by practitioners, than any other complaints to which the human body is subject. They are often neglected by women during the early stages of them, concealed from a sense of delicacy during their progress, and are often only made known to practitioners, when they have proceeded so far as to be beyond the reach of remedy. In these latter stages, a disease becomes complicated with many symptoms not originally belonging to it, which are the consequences of high irritation, or great debility, or of the general disturbance of the constitution. (Charles Mansfield Clarke, Member of the College of Surgeons, Surgeon to the Queen's Lying-In Hospital, and lecturer in Midwifery in London) (Wall, 2003).

Urinary incontinence (UI) is a widespread health problem affecting the physical, psychological, social, and economic well being of affected individuals and their families. However, despite its heavy disease burden, UI very often is not perceived as a medical entity which can be prevented and – once established – treated. Therefore, UI is assumed to be underreported worldwide and termed "the silent epidemic."

2   Definition

Lower urinary tract symptoms (LUTS) are defined from the individuals perspective and divided into three groups – storage, voiding, and post micturation symptoms. UI is one of the storage symptoms associated with increased day time frequency, nocturia, and urgency (Abrams et al., 2002a). International Continence Society (ICS) changed the 1979 definition of UI from "the involuntary loss of urine that is a social and hygienic problem and objectively demonstrable" to "the complaint of any involuntary leakage of urine," in 2002 (Abrams et al., 2002b).

3   Diagnosing Female Urinary Incontinence with Questionnaires

Female LUTS questionnaires are designed to perform at least one of three functions:

- Discriminate between SUI and UUI
- Quantify the amount of symptoms
- Assess the impact of symptoms on activity and quality of life.

4   Prevalence

UI can occur at any age, but is more common in older women, and is estimated to affect 20–40% of adult women or 11–80% of elderly, depending on age, the health-care setting where the study was performed, and the definition of UI used (Brocklehurst, 1993; Hannestad et al., 2000; Holst and Wilson, 1988; Moller et al., 2000; Sandvik et al., 1993; Sommer et al., 1990; Swithinbank et al., 1999; Yarnell et al., 1981). The prevalence of any UI shows a pattern of an early prevalence peak in the middle ages and then a steady incline among the elderly. The median prevalence of any UI shows two peaks, one at the fifth decade (33%) and another at the eighth decade of life (34%) (Hunskaar et al., 2003; Minassian et al.,2003). Turkish studies revealed the female UI prevalence to be between 16.4 and 68.8% (Ateskan et al., 2000; Biri et al., 2006; Cetinel et al., 2007; Ekin and Karayalcin, 2004; Filiz et al., 2006a, b; Kocak et al., 2005; Maral et al., 2001; Oskay et al., 2005; Ozerdogan et al., 2004; Turan et al., 1996) (Turan et al., 1996; Maral et al., 2001; Ekin and Karayalcin, 2004; Filiz et al., 2006a, b; Cetinel et al., 2007) (❷ *Table 160-1*).

5   Therapy of Urinary Incontinence

Contemporary therapeutic approaches to UI range from non-surgical, non-pharmacological treatment over pharmacotherapy to surgery. Evidence from randomized controlled trials

◘ Table 160-1

Prevalence studies of urinary incontinence in Turkey

Study	Sampling	Age	Definition	Survey type	Prevalence (%)
Turan et al. (1996)	Cross-sectional, gynecologic outpatient clinic patients with any gynecologic complaint other than UI	18+	Any UI, past or present	Questionnaire	24.5
Ateskan et al. (2000)	Cross-sectional, internal medicine and geriatrics outpatient clinics patients with any complaint	65+	Any UI in the last year	Face to face interview	44.2
Maral et al. (2001)	Cross-sectional, cluster sampling, household register	15+	Any UI, past or present	Face to face interview, questionnaire	20.8
Ozerdogan et al. (2004)	Cross-sectional, random sample, household registers	20+	Any UI, past or present	Questionnaire	25.8
Ekin and Karayalcin (2004)	Cross-sectional, gynecology outpatient clinic patients	20+	Any UI, past or present	Questionnaire	33.7
Kocak et al. (2005)	Cross-sectional, random sample, household registers	18+	Any UI, past or present	Questionnaire	23.9
Oskay et al. (2005)	Cross-sectional, health care centre patients with any complaint other than UI and accompanies of patients	50+	Any UI, past or present	Questionnaire	68.8
Filiz et al. (2006a,b)	Cross-sectional, primary health care centre patients with any complaint	18+	Any UI, past or present	Questionnaire	16.4
Biri et al. (2006)	Cross-sectional, primary health care centre patients with any complaint	15+	Any UI, past or present	Face to face interview, questionnaire	20.5
Cetinel et al. (2007)	Cross-sectional, multicentric	–	Any UI, past or present	Face to face interview, questionnaire	35.7

(RCT) has shown that pelvic floor muscle training, bio-feedback, behavioral modification, electrical stimulation, catheterization, and some drugs (tolterodine, trospium, oxybutynin, propiverine, desmopressine) are effective in treating UI.

6   Quality of Life in Urinary Incontinence

Since the World Health Organization (WHO) redefinition of health as "a state of complete physical, mental and social well-being and not merely the absence of disease or infirmity" the concept of health related quality of life (HRQOL) has increasingly gained importance in medicine. In terms of patient oriented outcomes, contemporary clinical research assessing the efficacy of the intervention(s) is supposed to focus on HRQOL in generic and/or disease specific terms as well.

UI has been assessed using symptom scores and objective investigations concentrating on its etiology, diagnosis, and treatment. For standardization and practical purposes, the former definition also included the psychosocial aspects, UI was simplified into "any urinary leakage," in 2002. Although several validated disease specific QOL instruments for UI are in use, some new questionnaires are being introduced to meet various other needs.

When more detailed insight into a disease specific subdomain of HRQOL is required, dimension-specific instruments should be used.

The most widely used UI specific QOL measures in clinical trials are described.

- *Bristol Female Lower Urinary Tract Symptom Questionnaire (BFLUTS)* is a 34-item instrument with 19 symptom, 4 sexual function, and 11 QOL questions developed for women with LUTS (Jackson et al., 1999).
- *CONTILIFE®* is a 28-item questionnaire with six dimensions (daily activities, effort activities, self-image, emotional consequences, sexuality, well-being) producing a global score, as well as one for each dimension, appropriated for women with SUI, MUI, and UUI (Amarenco et al., 2003).
- *International Consultation on Incontinence Questionnaire Short Form (ICIQ-SF)* was developed by Subcommittee of Symptom and QOL Assessment of the ICI. It contains six questions inquiring about severity and impairment due to UI in both genders (Gotoh, 2007).
- *Incontinence Impact Questionnaire (IIQ)* investigates the impact of UI on 30 different activities comprising four domains: physical activity, travel, social relationships, and emotional health (Shumaker et al., 1994). Short form of IIQ contains seven items for each domain of the original version. It is used in women with UI specific to lower urinary tract dysfunction and genital prolapse (Uebersax et al., 1995).
- *Incontinence QOL Instrument (I-QOL)* is a subjective QOL questionnaire used in clinical trials covering patients with varying types (SUI, MUI, UUI) and severity of UI. It has 22 items with three subscales: avoidance and limiting behaviors (eight items), psychosocial impacts (nine items), social embarrassment (five items) (Wagner et al., 1996).
- *Incontinence QOL Index (IQOLI)* is a 25-item questionnaire developed for women with UUI (Renck-Hooper et al., 1998).
- *King's Health Questionnaire (KHQ)* featuring 21 items with three major sections (general health perceptions, symptom bother, quality of life), and eight domains (general health, incontinence impact, role limitation, physical and social limitations, personal limitations, emotional problems, sleep/energy disturbance, and severity measures) can be used in women with general symptoms of UI and in both genders with OAB symptoms (Kelleher et al., 1997). A 6-item short form has been developed in Japan, with two domains (limitations of daily life and mental health) (Uemura and Homma, 2004).
- *Urogenital Distress Inventory (UDI)* inquires bother caused by 19 symptoms with three subscales (irritative symptoms, obstructive/discomfort symptoms, stress symptoms) and has a short form. It is used for women with UI specific to lower urinary tract dysfunction and genital prolapse (Shumaker et al., 1994; Uebersax et al., 1995).
- *York Incontinence Perception Scale (YIPS)* is a questionnaire with eight items referring to a single domain (psychosocial impact) (Lee et al., 1995).

- The questionnaires for the symptoms and QOL of urinary incontinence that have been recommended by the ICI Subcommittee of Symptom and QOL Assessment are shown in ❷ *Table 160-2.* There is no UI QOL instrument specifically developed for men.

■ Table 160-2

Recommended questionnaires for the evaluation of in urinary incontinence and urinary incontinence/lower urinary tract symptoms, and urinary incontinence related quality of life

Questionnaire	Gender		Recommendation grade	Lower urinary tract symptoms	Quality of life
	Female	Male			
ICIQ-SF	Yes	Yes	A	Yes	Yes
BFLUTS-Short Form	Yes		A	Yes	Yes
SUIQQ	Yes		A	Yes	Yes
ICSmale-SF		Yes	A	Yes	Yes
UDI, UDI-6	Yes		A	Yes	
ISI	Yes		A	Yes	
ICSmale-LUTS		Yes	A	Yes	
I-QOL	Yes	Yes	A		Yes
KHQ	Yes		A		Yes
IIQ	Yes		A		Yes
UISS	Yes		A		Yes
CONTILIFE	Yes		A		Yes

ICIQ-SF international consultation on incontinence questionnaire short form; *BFLUTS* Bristol female lower urinary tract symptoms questionnaire; *SUIQQ* stress urinary incontinence quality of life questionnaire; *ICSmale-SF* international consultation on incontinence questionnaire short form; *UDI* urogenital distress inventory; *ISI* incontinence severity index; *ICSmale-LUTS* international consultation on incontinence questionnaire lower urinary tract symptoms; *I-QOL* incontinence quality of life questionnaire; *KHQ* King's health questionnaire; *IIQ* incontinence impact questionnaire

7   Urinary Incontinence QOL Measures Used in Turkey

- IIQ-7 (Incontinence impact questionnaire 7-item short form) (Cam et al., 2007)
- UDI-6 (Urogenital distress inventory 6-item short form) (Cam et al., 2007)
- IQOL (Ozerdogan et al., 2004)
- ICIQ-SF (Cetinel et al., 2004)

8   Review of Turkish Literature

In Turkey many studies about UI were conducted ranging from epidemiological studies to clinical trials, but when evaluated in terms of QOL the literature search revealed only very few Turkish studies (❷ *Tables 160-3* and ❷ *160-4*). There may be some local studies published in journals of medical institutions that have been missed in the electronic literature search as they

◼ Table 160-3
Review of studies assessing QOL in Turkish women with UI

Study	N	Method	Questionnaire(s)
Karan et al. (2000)	53	Cross sectional, gynecologic outpatient clinic patients with any gynecologic complaint	Wagner's QOL scale
Aslan et al. (2003)	50	Cross-sectional	SSI, SII
Kocak et al. (2005)	1,012	Cross-sectional, random sample, household registers	ICIQ-SF
Imamoglu et al. (2005)	52	Prospective clinical trial	Raz Inventory Scale
Filiz et al. (2007)	650	Cross-sectional, primary health care centre patients with any complaint	Severity index, SF-36
Aksakal et al. (2006)	28	Prospective clinical trial	Severity Index, BFLUTS
van den Muijsenbergh and Lagro-Janssen (2006)	30	Qualitative	PRAFAB
Seckiner et al. (2007)	120	Prospective clinical trial	ICIQ-SF
Cetinel et al. (2007)	5,565	Cross-sectional, multicentric	ICIQ-SF
Onur et al. (2007)	49	Prospective clinical trial	UDI-6, IIQ-7

N: Total observation number, *SSI* the symptom severity index; *SII* symptom impact index; *ICIQ-SF* international consultation on incontinence questionnaire short form; *SF-36* medical outcomes study 36-item short form health survey, *BFLUTS* Bristol female lower urinary tract symptoms questionnaire; *PRAFAB* protection, amount, frequency, adjustment, body image; *UDI* urinary distress inventory; *IIQ-7* incontinence impact questionnaire

are not indexed. Almost all studies reveal that QOL/bother in UI is positively correlated with both, frequency and amount of leakage. Help seeking behavior was correlating with the degree of bother, which is a trans-cultural trend previously shown in many studies conducted similarly in different countries.

9 Original Data

A primary care study about UI prevalence and associated QOL in adult females (generic instrument SF-36, diseases specific instrument I-QOL) was carried out in the western Marmara region in 2005, where a representative sample of 650 women was composed by randomly enrolling attendees of six primary health care institutions in Sakarya after their informed consent. None of the women had a reason for encounter related to UI. In general, UI was shown to be adversely affecting quality of life. According to the generic HRQOL results of this study, women over 30 years reported more limited physical role functioning. Furthermore, HRQOL in adult incontinent females was associated with UI severity index, and advancing age and severity index were associated with impairment in all SF-36 domain subscales (except for the mental health domain) (Filiz et al., 2007).

◻ Table 160-4

Results of studies assessing QOL in Turkish women with UI

Study	Age[a] (years)	Mean score	Interpretation	Conclusion
Karan et al. (2000)	37 ± 19	23.37 ± 17.38	1–28: mild; 29–56: moderate; 57–84: severe impairment	The fact that QOL score is not correlated with the underlying organic disorder suggests that multiple factors affect psychosocial health
Aslan et al. (2003)	47.19 ± 10.35	SSI: 11.48 ± 4.86; over 20 points	NG	It was also observed that both SSI and SII scores increased with increasing age of the women.
		SII: 4.34 ± 3.97 over 16 points		..... the severity of incontinence makes no difference in the effects of incontinence on the life quality of women.
Kocak et al. (2005)	43.60 ± 16.47	8.92 ± 4.35	Higher scores representing greater impact on quality of life	. . . the majority of the participants with UI reported UI related complaints. . . . but only a few of them declared severe impact on their QOL. We also found little sexual activity impairment related to UI

☐ Table 160-4 (continued)

Study	Ageª (years)	Mean score			Interpretation	Conclusion
Imamoglu et al. (2005)	NG	First operation: Preoperation: 32.5 Postoperation: 13.75 Second operation: Preoperation: 22.45 postoperation: 13.18			NG	… When the cost of the material utilized is considered, the shortness of the procedure, its not requiring general anesthesia, and high rates of success and ease of application makes it an ideal choice for treatment in selected patient groups
Filiz et al. (2007)	32.2 ± 10.6	SF-36 domain subscales	Urinary incontinence symptomª		Each of the dimension scores was expressed as a value between 0 and 100, with higher scores representing better health	Neither age nor UI severity can explain the SF-36 quality of life changes; there are other potential risks to be determined. Generic quality of life questionnaire is not solely enough to determine the changes due to UI-though presents difference between incontinent women and controls- thus it is better be used along with an incontinence-related quality of life questionnaire
			Positive (n=106)	Negative (n=544)		
		Physical functioning	73.77 (22.92)	91.52 (16.02)		
		Role physical	66.67 (26.05)	89.41 (20.00)		
		Bodily pain	55.71 (26.82)	75.85 (23.23)		
		General health	46.20 (18.40)	57.17 (14.56)		
		Vitality	49.52 (17.52)	58.48 (14.22)		
		Social functioning	70.09 (24.06)	77.29 (19.50)		
		Role emotional	75.93 (22.64)	93.63 (15.49)		
		Mental health	64.11 (15.57)	66.51 (13.96)		

■ Table 160-4 (continued)

Study	Age[a] (years)	Mean score	Interpretation	Conclusion
Aksakal et al. (2006)	45 ± NA	NG	NG	Transobturator suburethral tape is a safe and effective technique in the treatment of stress incontinence in short-term. Nevertheless, long-term data is not available
van den Muijsenbergh and Lagro-Janssen (2006)	45 ± 9	NG (Incontinence was chiefly moderate (n = 10) to severe (n = 16) according to the PRAFAB scores)	mild (1–7 points); moderate (8–13 points) and severe (14–20 points)	
Seckiner et al. (2007)	49.8 ± NA	Pre-treatment: 13.9 ± 3.7 Post-treatment: 9.4 ± 2.9	Higher scores representing greater impact on quality of life	ICIQ-SF scoring is a practical and reliable method for baseline and post-treatment evaluation of patients with urge incontinence. Significant correlation exists between ICIQ-SF score and urodynamic parameters
Cetinel et al. (2007)	44.71 ± 12.12	The mean ICIQ-SF score in the whole incontinent patient group (n=1,893) was 7.7 ± 4.1, while patients with non-bothersome and bothersome UI had a mean ICIQ-SF scores of 5.3 ± 2.2, and 10.4 ± 4.1, respectively	Higher scores representing greater impact on quality of life	Frequency, severity, and mixed type of UI were found to be the determinants of bothersome UI for which the ICIQ-SF cutoff score of 8 was obtained

◼ Table 160-4 (continued)

Study	Age[a] (years)	Mean score	Interpretation	Conclusion
Onur et al. (2007)	59 ± NG	NG (Quality-of-life assessment revealed that postoperative urinary leakage had a minor (slight or not at all) effect on daily activities in both groups)	NG	Use of allograft dermis as an alternative to autologous rectus fascia for pubovaginal sling had comparable improvement in patient satisfaction and quality of life at intermediate term

[a]Age and questionnaire scores are given as mean ± standard deviation of the mean

NA not available; *NG* not given; *SSI* the symptom severity index; *SII* symptom impact index; *ICIQ-SF* international consultation on incontinence questionnaire short form; *SF-36* medical outcomes study 36-item short form health survey; *BFLUTS* Bristol female lower urinary tract symptoms questionnaire; *PRAFAB* protection, amount, frequency, adjustment, body image; *UDI* urinary distress inventory; *IIQ-7* incontinence impact questionnaire

In the same study, I-QOL scores were independently determined by BMI, RUTI, mode of delivery and frequency of incontinence, rather than severity, i.e., women with frequent incontinence experienced higher disease burden (unpublished data).

This study also revealed a high correlation between generic and disease specific QOL measures in incontinent women. All SF-36 subscales – "social functioning," "mental health," "physical functioning" – were correlating with I-QOL subdomains, the latter showing the most consistent and strongest correlation with all I-QOL sub-domains. And vice versa, among I-QOL sub-domains, "Psychosocial impact" and "Avoidance and limiting behavior" were mostly correlating with SF-36 subscales (unpublished data).

As preliminary prevalence data revealed a high association between diabetes mellitus and female urinary incontinence, the same study protocol was applied to an expanded data set with the aim of investigating the associations between DM, UI and HRQOL. The findings of this study showed a higher prevalence of UI in diabetic women independent of age (Topsever et al., 2007).

Generic HRQOL in incontinent diabetic women was adversely affected independent of age, as shown by lower scores in most SF-36 domains-with lowest scores in the "pain" subscale-, as compared to their continent counterparts (Cinar et al., 2006).

Urinary incontinence specific QOL, as measured by the I-QOL instrument, was also significantly affected in the presence of diabetes in comparison with non-diabetic incontinent women. UI seemed to further increase the significant psychosocial burden of type 2 Diabetes Mellitus and therefore, should be investigated in diabetic women (Filiz et al., 2006a, b).

Summary Points

• Prevalence of UI depends mainly on study population and UI definition.

- UI has been demonstrated to be associated with perceived bother and limited functional health status (especially in the social domain) and low HRQOL in Turkish adult females. Thus, it is a medical condition with a considerable disease burden.
- In Turkey, UI – similar to many other cultures – generally is not perceived as a medical condition by females, there is a need for health education and awareness campaigns about the fact the UI is a preventable condition and – once established- can be treated.
- As medical help seeking behavior of affected individuals is limited, it can be concluded that UI is highly underreported, there is need for a population based epidemiological study about UI including both genders in Turkey.
- The QOL questionnaires used in Turkish UI studies do not mostly comply with the ICI grade A evidence recommendations.
- Turkish studies about UI retrieved in the literature search were local and either of epidemiological nature or clinical trials about efficacy of surgical or pharmacological treatment methods for UI. The concept of QOL is relatively new in Turkish clinical research and therefore, was only scarcely included as an outcome in those studies.
- There is a need for a national clearinghouse, coordinating research, and administrating evidence (like registration of trials and indexing of studies) about UI and related QOL in Turkey.
- There is a need for studies on male incontinence and its impact on HRQOL.

References

Abrams P, Cardozo L, Fall M, Griffiths D, Rosier P, Ulmsten U, van Kerrebroeck P, Victor A, Wein A. (2002a). Neurourol Urodyn. 21: 167–178.

Abrams P, Cardozo L, Fall M, Griffiths D, Rosier P, Ulmsten U, van Kerrebroeck P, Victor A, Wein A. (2002b). Am J Obstet Gynecol. 187: 116–126.

Aksakal OS, Gungor T, Karaer A, Ugurlu EN, Aral AM, Bilge U. (2006). J Turkish-German Gynecol Assoc. 7: 210–214.

Amarenco G, Arnould B, Carita P, Haab F, Labat JJ, Richard F. (2003). Eur Urol. 43: 391–404.

Aslan E, Beji NK, Coskun A, Yalcin O. (2003). Int Urogynecol J Pelvic Floor Dysfunct. 14: 316–319; discussion 320.

Ateskan U, Mas MR, Doruk H, Kutlu M. (2000). Turkish J Geriatrics. 3: 45–50.

Biri A, Durukan E, Maral I, Korucuoglu U, Biri H, Tyras B, Bumin MA. (2006). Int Urogynecol J Pelvic Floor Dysfunct. 17: 604–610.

Brocklehurst JC .(1993). BMJ. 306: 832–834.

Cam C, Sakalli M, Ay P, Cam M, Karateke A. (2007). Neurourol Urodyn. 26: 129–133.

Cetinel B, Demirkesen O, Tarcan T, Yalcin O, Kocak T, Senocak M, Itil I. (2007). Int Urogynecol J Pelvic Floor Dysfunct. 18: 659–664.

Cetinel B, Ozkan B, Can G. (2004). Turkish J Urol. 30: 332–338.

Cinar N, Topsever P, Uludag C, Gorpelioglu S, Aydin N, Filiz T. (2006). Diabet Med. 23(Suppl. 4): 168.

Ekin M, Karayalcin R. (2004). J Ankara Med School. 26: 21–25.

Filiz M, Topsever P, Cinar N, Uludag C, Gorpelioglu S, Aydin N. (2006a). Diabet Med. 23(Suppl. 4): 404.

Filiz TM, Topsever P, Uludag C, Gorpelioglu S, Cinar N. (2007). Turkiye Klinikleri J Med Sci. 27: 189–194.

Filiz TM, Uludag C, Cinar N, Gorpelioglu S, Topsever P. (2006b). Saudi Med J. 27: 1688–1692.

Gotoh M. (2007). Nagoya J Med. 69: 123–131.

Hannestad YS, Rortveit G, Sandvik H, Hunskaar S. (2000). J Clin Epidemiol. 53: 1150–1107.

Holst K, Wilson PD. (1988). N Z Med J. 101: 756–758.

Hunskaar S, Burgio K, Diokno A, Herzog AR, Hjalmas K, Lapitan MC. (2003). Urology. 62 (Suppl. 1): 16–23.

Imamoglu A, Ozturk U, Eroglu M, Taygun C, Kiper A. (2005). Ankara Üniversitesi Tip Fakültesi Mecmuasi. 58: 1–4.

Jackson S, Shepherd A, Brookes S, Abrams P. (1999). Br J Obstet Gynaecol. 106: 711–718.

Karan A, Aksac B, Ayyildiz H, Isikoglu M, Yalcin O, Eskiyurt N. (2000). Turk J Geriatrics 3(3): 102–106.

Kelleher CJ, Cardozo LD, Khullar V, Salvatore S. (1997). Br J Obstet Gynaecol. 104: 1374–1379.

Kocak I, Okyay P, Dundar M, Erol H, Beser E. (2005). Eur Urol. 48: 634–641.

Lee PS, Reid DW, Saltmarche A, Linton L. (1995). J Am Geriatr Soc. 43: 1275–1278.

Maral I, Ozkardes H, Peskircioglu L, Bumin MA. (2001). J Urol. 165: 408–412.

Minassian VA, Drutz HP, Al-Badr A. (2003). Int J Gynaecol Obstet. 82: 327–338.

Moller LA, Lose G, Jorgensen T. (2000). Acta Obstet Gynecol Scand. 79: 298–305.

Onur R, Singla A, Kobashi KC. (2007). Int Urol Nephrol. 40(1): 45–49.

Oskay UY, Beji NK, Yalcin O. (2005). Acta Obstet Gynecol Scand. 84: 72–78.

Ozerdogan N, Beji NK, Yalcin O. (2004). Gynecol Obstet Invest. 58: 145–150.

Renck-Hooper U, McKenna SP, Whalley D. (1998). J Drug Assess. 1: 41–48.

Sandvik H, Hunskaar S, Seim A, Hermstad R, Vanvik A, Bratt H. (1993). J Epidemiol Community Health. 47: 497–499.

Seckiner I, Yesilli C, Mungan NA, Aykanat A, Akduman B. (2007). Neurourol Urodyn. 26: 492–494.

Shumaker SA, Wyman JF, Uebersax JS, McClish D, Fantl JA. (1994). Qual Life Res. 3: 291–306.

Sommer P, Bauer T, Nielsen KK, Kristensen ES, Hermann GG, Steven K, Nordling J. (1990). Br J Urol. 66: 12–15.

Swithinbank LV, Donovan JL, du Heaume JC, Rogers CA, James MC, Yang Q, Abrams P. (1999). Br J Gen Pract. 49: 897–900.

Topsever P, Filiz TM, Uludag C, Dede Cinar N. (2007). Diabetologia. 50(Suppl. 1): 470.

Turan C, Zorlu CG, Ekin M, Hancerliogullari N, Saracoglu F. (1996). Gynecol Obstet Invest. 41: 132–134.

Uebersax JS, Wyman JF, Shumaker SA, McClish DK, Fantl JA. (1995). Neurourol Urodyn. 14: 131–139.

Uemura S, Homma Y. (2004). Neurourol Urodyn. 23: 94–100.

van den Muijsenbergh ME, Lagro-Janssen TA. (2006). Br J Gen Pract. 56: 945–949.

Wagner TH, Patrick DL, Bavendam TG, Martin ML, Buesching DP. (1996). Urology. 47: 67–72.

Wall LL. (2003). Int Urogynecol J Pelvic Floor Dysfunct. 14: 67–69.

Yarnell JW, Voyle GJ, Richards CJ, Stephenson TP. (1981). J Epidemiol Community Health. 35: 71–74.

161 Quality of Life Measures in Elderly Patients with Chronic Obstructive Pulmonary Disease: Japanese Perspectives

K. Kida · T. Motegi · T. Ishii · K. Yamada

1	*Introduction*	**2760**
2	*Problems of Increase in Aged Population*	**2761**
2.1	Characteristics of Chronic Illness and Home Care	2761
2.2	COPD in the Elderly Population	2763
2.3	Problems in the Clinical Course of Elderly COPD	2763
2.4	Home Care in Elderly COPD	2765
3	*Problems in Aged COPD*	**2767**
3.1	Delayed Early Detection	2767
3.2	Comorbidity	2767
3.2.1	Pathological Observations	2767
3.2.2	Comorbidity of Osteoporosis	2768
4	*QOL in Elderly COPD*	**2769**
4.1	Disability in COPD	2769
4.2	QOL Measures for Elderly Patients	2769
4.2.1	QOL Measures for COPD	2769
4.2.2	QOL Measures for Elderly COPD	2770
4.3	Cultural Background in Elderly COPD	2772
5	*Perspectives Based on Experiences in Japan*	**2773**
5.1	Cooperation by Medical Teams	2773
5.2	Factors Associated with QOL in Elderly COPD	2775
6	*Conclusions*	**2775**
	Summary Points	**2776**

Abstract: ❷ Chronic obstructive pulmonary disease (COPD) is a common disease with increasing prevalence, which tends to show accelerated progression in patients over 65 years old, consequently becoming a major public health problem among elderly populations world-wide. Patients experience a progressive deterioration up to end-stage COPD, characterized by airflow limitation, a severely limited and declining performance status with ❷ chronic respiratory failure, advanced age, and various ❷ comorbidities due to systemic manifestations. These are mainly attributed to a delay in diagnosis, leading to additional and unexpected comorbidities during the clinical course. These comorbidities can be divided into three major groups: one is a COPD-specific group such as lung cancer; the second group comprises comorbidities generally observed at an advanced age, such as aspiration pneumonia or cognitive impairment; and the third group is made up of a mixture of these, such as osteoporosis, stroke, or ischemic heart disease.

The majority of elderly patients with COPD are managed by primary care physicians who still may not be aware of the recent clinical guidelines; thus, these patients are unlikely to receive proper management in the long term. The culmination of a delayed clinical diagnosis and poor management results in the reduction of activities of daily living (❷ ADL), repeated exacerbations, a poor ❷ quality of life (QOL), and high mortality rate in the elderly with COPD, leading to an increasing socio-economic burden. The management of COPD in elderly patients requires multidisciplinary holistic care with a comprehensive approach based on home respiratory care. In this regard, the role of primary care cannot be overestimated, and cooperation between specialist groups and primary care physicians, along with the support of local health care professionals, is critical. Therefore, treatment improvements and a team approach regarding COPD and its comorbidities are urgently needed in terms of health care for elderly COPD patients in our aging society.

We have described problems concerning elderly COPD patients through our experiences in Japan, particularly from the aspect of the health-related QOL and its perspectives.

List of Abbreviations: *6MWD*, 6-minute walking distance; *11-Q*, pre-interview questionnaire with 11 questions; *ADL*, activities of daily living; *AQ*, airways questionnaire; *ATS*, American Thoracic Society; *BPQ*, breathing problems questionnaire; *COPD*, chronic obstructive pulmonary disease; *CRQ*, chronic respiratory questionnaire; *FEV1*, forced expiratory volume in 1 s; *GERD*, gastroesophageal reflux disorders; *GOLD*, Global initiative for Chronic Obstructive Lung Disease; *HOT*, home oxygen therapy; *HMV*, ❷ home mechanical ventilation; *HRQOL*, health-related quality of life; *IADL*, instrumental activities of daily living; *ICF*, international classification of functioning, ❷ disability, and health; *ICIDH-I*, international classification of impairments, disabilities, and handicaps; *LTOT*, ❷ long-term oxygen therapy; *LVRS*, lung volume reduction surgery; *OCD*, oxygen cost diagram; *OSAS*, obstructive sleep apnea syndrome; *QOL*, quality of life; *QOL-RIQ*, quality of life for respiratory illness questionnaire; *QOL scale*, questionnaires for quality of life using a linear analog scale; *SAS*, self-administered standardized; *SF-36*, 36-item short-form health survey; *SGRQ*, St George's respiratory questionnaire; *SIP*, sickness impact profile; *URI*, upper respiratory infection; *VAS*, visual analogue scale; *WHO*, World Health Organization

1 Introduction

According to recent clinical guidelines (Global Initiative for Chronic Obstructive Lung Disease; GOLD, 2007), chronic obstructive pulmonary disease (COPD) is defined as "a preventable and treatable disease with some significant extra-pulmonary effects that may contribute to the severity in individual patients. Its pulmonary component is characterized by airflow limitation that is not fully reversible. The airflow limitation is usually progressive and associated with an abnormal inflammatory response of the lung to noxious particles or gases." COPD is the major cause of morbidity and mortality worldwide, and represents a substantial economic and social burden (GOLD, 2007). Patients with COPD experience progressive dyspnea during daily activities up to end-stage COPD, characterized by severe airflow limitation, and a severely limited and declining performance status, hence, showing deterioration of the health status both generally and in terms of the disease-specific quality of life (QOL). Patients with COPD of marked severity frequently experience exacerbations which require hospitalization, and the lung function declines accordingly. Further, COPD is characterized as a disease of advanced age, and by its comorbidities. These comorbidities are also causes of hospitalizations or contribute to deteriorate the QOL. However, so far, problems which arise in elderly patients with COPD have been little described.

This review sheds light on problems in COPD of elderly patients from a Japanese perspective, particularly regarding the health-related QOL.

2   Problems of Increase in Aged Population

2.1   Characteristics of Chronic Illness and Home Care

The elderly population aged 65 and older is increasing, and is currently at its highest ever level, 26.49 million and 21.0% of the total population (2006) (Ministry of Health, Labour and Welfare, Vital statistics, 2006) in Japan. This increase in the elderly population will be accelerated furthermore when so-called "baby boomers" reach retirement (Ministry of Health, Labour and Welfare, Vital statistics, 2006) (❷ *Figure 161-1*). ❷ *Figure 161-2* shows the cumulative probabilities that different world regions will reach one-third of their population being over 60 years old over the course of the twenty-first century. By mid-century, the chance of having passed this specific ageing threshold is 98% in Japan/Oceania, 82% in Western Europe and even 69% in the China region (Lutz et al., 2008). This increase in the size of the elderly population inevitably increases that of patients with chronic illness, which has been mostly managed by local and larger hospitals in Japan. However, it was found that there were many problems on both sides regarding patients and their families, and policy makers in terms of reimbursement; thus, a strategy was promoted to place home care as the core of the system.

The following are a summary of traditional (Ikegami and Campbell, 1995) and current problems:

1. Hospital care includes treatment of chronic illness for outpatients as well as inpatients, so that many elderly patients visit large hospitals frequently, being of the opinion that larger hospitals can facilitate better treatment and outcomes.
2. These patients may occasionally stay in large hospitals for several months, including receiving long-term rehabilitation while undergoing hospitalization.
3. The families of patients are not ready for the patient's return home, mostly because of a lack of caregivers and limited space at home.
4. A prolonged hospital stay reduces the QOL for both patients and families, and also demoralizes of young doctors. As a result, these young doctors might leave hospitals and

◻ Figure 161-1

Changing rate of the increasing elderly population in Japan. The increase in the elderly population will be accelerated when baby boomers reach to elderly (>65 years old). Data source from Vital Statistics, Ministry of Health, Labour and Welfare, 2006 (http://wwwdbtk.mhlw.go.jp/toukei/index.html; accessed at 28 November, 2008)

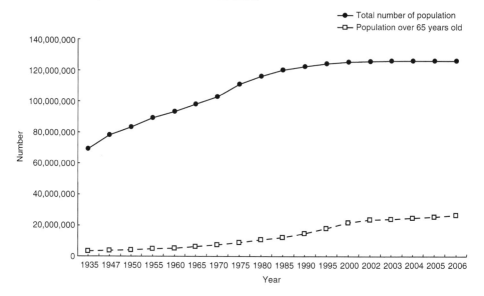

◻ Figure 161-2

Cumulative probabilities of reaching one-third of the population being over 60 years old or more for the world and selected world regions by calendar year. Reprint from Nature 2008; 451: 716–719 with permission

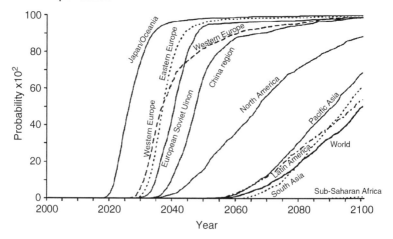

become primary care physicians at a small town clinic; thus, collapse of the current medical system is occurring in Japan.

5. Furthermore, health care costs and medical expenditure for the elderly sharply increase in this situation.

In this context, as a solution, home care for elderly patients in Japan has been established: the Medical Service Law was revised in 1992 and the health care insurance system was implemented in 1994; however, an increased cost in the future is not avoidable, and a new insurance system for the old-old elderly (>75 years old) starts in 2008. However, care systems in Japan for elderly patients still lead to problems, and urgently need improvements.

2.2   COPD in the Elderly Population

COPD is characterized by symptoms of cough, phlegm production, dyspnea, and exercise limitation. It is a common disease with an increasing prevalence, and currently is a major public health problem among elderly populations of developed countries (GOLD, 2007), including Japan (Japanese Respiratory Society; JRS, 2004). The number of COPD patients in Japan according to the Ministry of Health, Labour and Welfare in 2005 (Ministry of Health, Labour and Welfare, 2005) was estimated at only approximately 220,000. However, epidemiologic data on COPD (Fukuchi et al., 2004), performed in 2001, suggested that approximately 5.3 million Japanese aged 40 and older have COPD (Fukuchi et al., 2004), and 15.7% of those aged 60–69 and 24.4% of those aged 70 and older. Further, since they also showed that 1% of all COPD patients are in Stage IV, and long-term oxygen therapy is generally introduced in Stage IV of the GOLD guideline (GOLD, 2007), it is estimated that the total number of patients receiving or requiring long-term oxygen therapy in Japan could reach over 50,000. As 1–10% of all COPD patients are in Stage III-IV globally (the proportion varies among countries (Buist et al., 2007)), it is critical to prevent COPD and its progression, especially in the elderly population, by smoking cessation, education, early diagnosis, and treatment, and also by solving associated problems, for example, environmental pollution (GOLD, 2007).

2.3   Problems in the Clinical Course of Elderly COPD

Worldwide, smoking remains the main cause of COPD. The World Health Organization (WHO) estimates that in high-income countries, 73% of COPD mortality is related to smoking, with 40% related to smoking in nations of low and middle income (Lopez et al., 2006). In Japan, more than 95% of COPD patients have a smoking history (JRS, 2004) which is similar to other developed countries (American Thoracic Society; ATS/European Respiratory Society; ERS, 2005; GOLD, 2007), partly because, so far, been a very limited number of families with genetic α1 anti-trypsin deficiency have reported in Japan (Seyama et al., 1991). The number of patients with COPD in Japan is accordingly increasing, as it has done for approximately the last 20 years, following behind the increase in annual tobacco sales (❯ Figure 161-3).

The natural course of such COPD patients has not been precisely described since the landmark study of Fletcher and Peto (Fletcher and Peto, 1977). Persons who started smoking at the age of 20 show a have mild cough and phlegm production before age 40, approximately

◼ **Figure 161-3**

Correlation between tobacco sales and increasing COPD-related mortality in Japan. Number of deaths attributed to COPD in Japan follows approximately 20 years behind the annual sales of tobacco. Data source from (Curr Opin Pulm Med 2002; 8: 102–105 with permission)

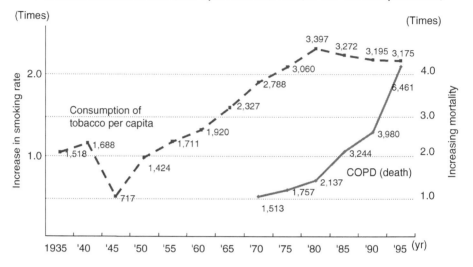

◼ **Figure 161-4**

Three typical clinical courses of elderly COPD patients regarding fatal cases. Reprinted from JAMA with permission. In the original manuscript, the figure explained the general trajectories of function and well-being over time in fatal cases of chronic illness, which is used to fit cases involving elderly COPD patients by authors' intuition. Type A = unexpected episode during the course which causes sudden death; Type B = gradual decline of lung function with multiple episodes of exacerbation; Type C = patients over 75 years old may exhibit fragility due to muscle weakness or malnutrition. Reprint from (JAMA, 2001; 285: 925–932) with permission

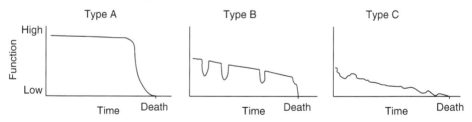

20 years from smoking onset. At around age 50, some complain of a frequent, common cold, particularly during winter, which may correspond to repeated mild exacerbations. The majority of patients complain of dyspnea on exertion before the age of 60, around the time of their retirement, then pharmacological therapy starts on their first visits to hospitals. At this stage, however, many patients have already reached beyond Stage II according to the ❷ GOLD guidelines (GOLD, 2007). In general, three typical clinical courses of chronic illness of elderly patients are proposed (Lynn, 2001) (❷ *Figure 161-4*). Elderly patients with COPD of type A may show comorbidity of the cardiovascular system. In fact, approximately one third of

COPD patient deaths were attributed to comorbidity of cardiovascular disease, and many sudden death cases were observed in this group (McGarvey et al., 2007). Although exacerbations have been clearly demonstrated to occur more frequently as COPD becomes more severe, the frequency of exacerbations varies widely among individuals with a similar degree of COPD severity. Mortality due to exacerbations is reported to be approximately 11–24% (Anzueto et al., 2007) which likely corresponds to type B, with a gradual decline of lung function. It should be noted that patients undergoing poor management require frequent hospitalizations due to exacerbations (Casas et al., 2006). However, type C patients are generally of an advanced age, such as over 75, called the old-old elderly. Such patients may have physical impairments due to stroke or severe muscle weakness in COPD per se, which is also one of the comorbidities of COPD (Agusti, 2005) and causes fragility. All these three types of COPD patient are seen at an advanced age and accordingly result in a deterioration of the activities of daily living (ADL) and profound impairment of both the generic and health related QOL. Further, patients with Stage IV COPD, the most severe stage, may require long term-oxygen therapy, which is called home oxygen therapy (HOT) in Japan.

2.4 Home Care in Elderly COPD

With an attempt to increase awareness of the huge burden of respiratory diseases among the public and policy makers, the JRS published a White Paper on a survey of home respiratory care in 2005 (JRS, 2006). A total of 2,237 patients who belong to the Japan Federation of Patient Organizations for Respiratory Diseases replied by post. Of these subjects who returned the questionnaire, 55% were receiving HOT and/or home mechanical ventilation (HMV), which is designated the HOT/HMV group in ❷ *Figure 161-5*. COPD was the leading cause of disease (39%) compared to the other two groups, namely, pulmonary tuberculosis sequalae (35%) and post-polio syndrome (15%). Reasons for joining the patient advocacy group were that "they could get information about their disease and treatment" (75%), and that they "could learn about their disease" (81%). It was found that the ADL of these subjects were restricted: 21% of those in the HOT/HMV group were home bound, although 87% overall were not home bound but their activities were severely restricted. The main reasons for restriction were inconvenience of ambulatory oxygen use (68%), fear of increasing dyspnea on leaving the home (63%), and solitude (50%). Regarding economic burden, personal expenditure of these subjects reached more than 12,000 yen per month (120 US$) in 26% of the cases, which was similar in 46% and 31% of the HOT/HMV and HOT only groups, respectively.

Then, a survey of institutions accredited by the Japanese Respiratory Society, the Japan Physicians Association (mainly general physicians), and randomly selected general hospitals conducted in 2004 also appeared in the White Paper (JRS, 2006). An itemized, clinical diagnosis of patients receiving HOT is shown in ❷ *Figure 161-6*. Among various diseases, COPD is the leading disease (48%), followed by pulmonary tuberculosis sequelae (18%), interstitial lung disease (15%), and lung cancer (5%).

From the survey on both patients and physicians who engaged in medical management, the following four areas were highlighted regarding the needs of patients: (1) improvement the education and support for self-management, (2) approach to welfare, (3) creating a system of safe and anxiety-free home respiratory care, and (4) increase public awareness of respiratory diseases and patients with respiratory disabilities. It should be noted that the above-mentioned are profoundly reflected by two factors: the nature of chronic respiratory illness, and advanced age.

◘ Figure 161-5
Surveys of subjects receiving respiratory care. Approximately half of the subjects receiving respiratory care were treated with LTOT or HMV or both. *LTOT* long-term oxygen therapy; *HMV* home mechanical ventilation. Reprint from Japanese White Paper on Home Respiratory Case, 2006 with permission

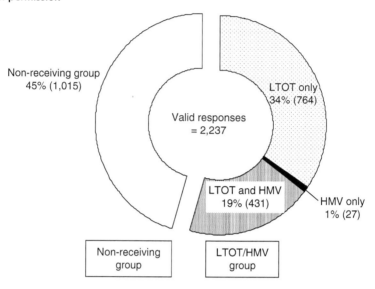

◘ Figure 161-6
Breakdown of patients receiving long-term oxygen therapy according to diseases. The total number of patients (n=20,860) seen by the responding physicians (n = 20,860) and each prevalence are shown. Reprint from Japanese White Paper on Home Respiratory Case, 2006 with permission

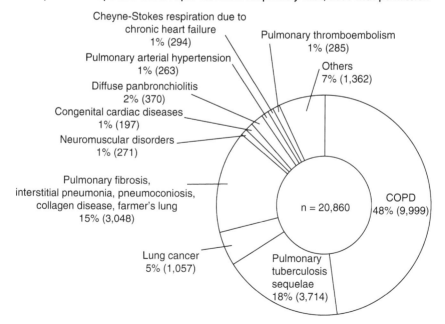

3 Problems in Aged COPD

3.1 Delayed Early Detection

In general, chronic illnesses of the elderly are characterized as showing poly-pathology, atypical clinical features, and fewer symptoms, and problems arising in COPD deeply reflect such clinical characteristics. Despite such complicated circumstances, early diagnosis is still central to the management of COPD. In time-constrained clinical situations, a pre-interview questionnaire can be a useful method for alerting both clinicians and patients regarding COPD, particularly in elderly patients. Currently, several questionnaires for detection are available (Price et al., 2006). However, those specifically targeting the elderly population are limited. To screen for subjects who might have COPD, we have developed an efficient pre-interview questionnaire for elderly COPD (Kida et al., 2006). The pre-interview questionnaire comprising 11 questions (11-Q), was found to be an appropriate tool to alert primary care providers to subjects with COPD and could also be used to distinguish COPD with a more than moderate severity from bronchial asthma. The 11-Q can be used as a simple and inexpensive method of predicting COPD on combined use with the MMSE (the mini-mental state examination) (Folestein et al., 1975) for cognitive function; thus, 11-Q is a useful tool to alert primary care providers to patients with suspected COPD, particularly among the elderly. The current American College of Physicians' guidelines for COPD indicate that spirometry should not be used to screen for airflow obstruction in asymptomatic individuals (Qaseem et al., 2007). Because many elderly COPD patients tend to complain less of respiratory symptoms compared with younger patients, 11-Q may be useful for early detection in elderly patients.

3.2 Comorbidity

3.2.1 Pathological Observations

The clinical course of COPD is affected by the type and severity of comorbidities and recent studies have revealed that there are many comorbidities of COPD, including cardiovascular diseases, lung cancer, osteoporosis, muscle weakness and wasting, and depression (Agusti, 2005). We previously reported (Kida and Motegi, 2000) comorbidities of emphysema in a consecutive autopsy series of elderly patients comprised of 4,553 cases, consisting of men (n = 2,337) and women (n = 2,216), with a mean age of 79.3. Pathological emphysema of over-moderate severity was compared with cases of less than mild or without emphysema regarding aspects of comorbidity (❷ Figure 161-7). Cerebrovascular disorder is the leading comorbiditiy of elderly populations, being significantly more common than emphysema. Although the incidence of coronary heart disease has been increasing recently, Steg et al. (2007) reported that the incidence of cerebrovascular disease is still higher in Japan or Asia compared with North America, in which heart disease is more common. From the observational data (Kida and Motegi, 2000), we concluded that: (1) the prevalence of pathological emphysema with moderate or marked severity reached approximately 20%, (2) centrilobular, panacinar, and combined types comprised approximately 30% each, suggesting that these variations might be caused by different mechanisms or different pathological processes, (3) a greater prevalence of lung cancer was noted in cases of severe emphysema, (4) the clinical features of focal

□ **Figure 161-7**

Comorbidities of pathological emphysema in a series of autopsies at a geriatric hospital (n = 4,553). Comorbidities were compared between two groups: cases with over moderate emphysema and cases with less than moderate emphysema. (Reprinted from Kokyu 2000; 19: 1235–1247 with permission) Original figure is in Japanese

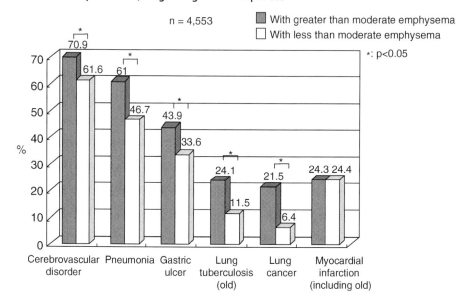

emphysema might differ from those of centrilobular emphysema, and (5) a smoking habit might be strongly correlated with the degree of pigmentation of the lung tissue and the severity of emphysema. It should be noted that there are various comorbidities with different severities in elderly COPD patients.

It has been reported that obstructive sleep apnea syndrome (OSAS) is also likely to be a comorbidity of COPD, called overlap syndrome. It was suspected that a high prevalence of overlap syndrome might be observed in COPD; however, more recent data indicate that this is not the case (Sanders et al., 2003) although precise data on overlap syndrome in elderly patients are still lacking.

3.2.2   Comorbidity of Osteoporosis

A recent study revealed that osteoporosis and vertebral fractures are quite common in patients with COPD, and that they showed a significant relationship with the mortality of these patients (Ionescu and Schoon, 2003). These results suggest that the management of osteoporosis in advanced COPD is important. Bodily pain, which frequently occurs in patients with osteoporosis, is considered to be similar to dyspnea regarding its difficulty of assessment, and patients experiencing this have an increased risk of exacerbations with COPD since suppression of the cough reflex occurs due to increased bodily pain. Thus, elderly patients with COPD require proper management for osteoporosis. Whether patients with COPD who have never received chronic systemic corticosteroids show a higher incidence of osteoporosis and whether these patients require treatment strategies to decrease osteoporotic fracture is not known. It is also unclear whether there are differences in terms of the degree of osteoporosis between patients with COPD and those with bronchial asthma. Previously, we reported (Katsura and Kida, 2002) data that compare the degree of osteoporosis and bone metabolism markers between elderly women with COPD and those with bronchial asthma who have never received chronic systemic corticosteroids, and determined factors influencing bone metabolism in these patients. In elderly female patients, osteoporosis is more common in cases of COPD than in bronchial asthma, even if these patients have never received systemic corticosteroids. A male predominance in COPD has been noted (Martinez et al., 2007), and the number of women with COPD is increasing, with an inevitable rise in problems concerning these patients, particularly in old age; preventive strategies to decrease osteoporotic fractures should be added to the management of elderly patients with COPD.

4 QOL in Elderly COPD

4.1 Disability in COPD

In 1980, the WHO published the International Classification of Impairments, Disabilities, and Handicaps (ICIDH-I). Over the 20 years since then, a new direction of promoting a new life with disability, rather than regarding the disability as negative, has been developed. The recent WHO concept of the International Classification of Functioning, Disability and Health (ICF: http://www.who.int/classifications/icf/site/icftemplate.cfm) is based on the idea that persons with disabilities resulting from chronic illness should be encouraged to participate actively in society and show higher levels of activity.

The time-course of the decrease in ADL after the onset of COPD and the corresponding new views on the management of these patients are shown in ❷ *Figure 161-8*. Formerly, the onset of COPD caused a gradual decrease in ADL, associated with marked limitations in the ability to participate in any occupation, daily activities, and pastimes. In contrast, in accordance with the new concept, the implementation of HOT, HMV, home respiratory rehabilitation, and appropriate drug therapy, the patient's life can be redefined so as to achieve the best possible QOL. ❷ *Table 161-1* shows the therapeutic and prophylactic aspects of home care in patients with COPD who are regarded as disabled persons. Impairment occurs according to the severity of the disease, leading to limitations in the ability of the patient to participate in any occupation and everyday activities.

4.2 QOL Measures for Elderly Patients

4.2.1 QOL Measures for COPD

The QOL can be defined as "the gap between that which is desired in life and that which is achieved" (Carr et al., 2001). According to Hyland (Hyland and Sodergren, 2005), there are three purposes of QOL assessment: resource allocation between diseases, treatment selection for a single disease, and clinical management. It is also stated that the management of a patient's QOL requires an individualized approach to treatment (Hyland and Sodergren, 2005). This approach can be assisted by a questionnaire, of which there are many types

◼ Figure 161-8

Decrease in forced expiratory volume in 1 s (FEV1) over the course of COPD and corresponding treatment. The possible course of illness from the onset to the terminal stage according to GOLD is shown. In general, COPD patients with FEV1 1.0 L need long-term oxygen therapy. *LTOT* long-term oxygen therapy; *LVRS* lung volume reduction surgery

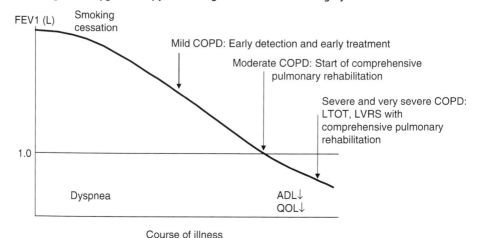

Course of illness

(see below). It is known that the disease-specific QOL is affected by various background factors, including gender, education, and cultural differences. However, assessing the effects of age on the disease-specific QOL is still controversial.

Health status measurement provides a standardized method of assessing the impact of disease on patients' daily lives, activity, and well-being. Health-related QOL (HRQOL) is a more specific term. Several questionnaires, including the Short-Form Health Survey (SF-36), are designed to assess health irrespective of disease. Whereas questionnaires to assess the long-term disease-specific health status and HRQOL are known, which include St George's Respiratory Questionnaire (SGRQ) (Jones et al., 1992). Questionnaires to assess the health status and QOL were summarized and described further in a recent review (Cazzola et al., 2008).

4.2.2 QOL Measures for Elderly COPD

Also, the simple visual analogue scale (VAS) is used (Schünemann et al., 2006). We previously examined the validity, discriminatory ability, and responsiveness of HRQOL questionnaires for QOL assessment using a linear analog scale (QOL scale) for COPD (Hiratuka and Kida, 1993; Katsura et al., 2003). In this study, elderly subjects with mild to severe COPD were recruited and scores on the QOL scale, SGRQ, and SF-36 and various clinical parameters were recorded. The correlations between these QOL questionnaires and various clinical parameters were then examined. The responses of elderly COPD patients to the QOL scale and the SGRQ before and 3 months after the completion of a comprehensive pulmonary rehabilitation program were compared longitudinally. The total score of the QOL scale was closely correlated with that of SGRQ. On cross-sectional study, the QOL scale showed a significant correlation with the total score and three components of the SGRQ. The QOL scale was correlated

◻ Table 161-1

Treatment and prophylaxis in home care of chronic respiratory diseases

Changing process	Measures	
	Treatment	Prophylaxis
Disease state	Comprehensive care by medical team collaboration	Health awareness, promotion
		Nutrition improvement
		Vaccination
↓		
Development of impairment	Early pulmonary rehabilitation	Prevention of activity limitation
↓		
Limited activities	LTOT/HMV	Prophylactic rehabilitation
	Visiting care, involvement of helpers	Prevention of limitations regarding social participation
	Pulmonary rehabilitation	
↓		
Limited participation	Improvement of residential environment	Change to better living environment
	Enlightenment of the public to promote acceptance	Consideration to avoid disadvantages concerning employment and social participation
	Prevention of discriminating against people with illness	Ensuring easily accessible services

Treatments and prophylaxis to prevent the reduction of daily activities in each changing process are shown. *LTOT* long-term oxygen therapy; *HMV* home mechanical ventilation

significantly with all components of the SF-36, but the total SGRQ score was correlated with only six components of the SF-36, excluding vitality and the mental health index (❷ *Table 161-2*). Both the QOL scale and total score of the SGRQ were correlated significantly with the oxygen cost diagram (OCD) (McGavin et al., 1978), morale scale (Liang et al., 1987), 6-minute walking distance (❷ 6MWD), forced expiratory volume in 1 s, and instrumental activities of daily living (IADL) score. When subjects were divided into three groups according to disease severity (mild, moderate, and severe) using the American Thoracic Society guidelines (ATS, 1997), the total SGRQ score discriminated between the three groups. However, the QOL scale could not discriminate between mild and moderate or moderate and severe. On longitudinal study, 3 months after finishing the comprehensive pulmonary rehabilitation program, the QOL scale, SGRQ, 6MWD, and OCD all showed significant improvements. The difference in the QOL scale after the comprehensive pulmonary rehabilitation program showed a significant correlation with changes in the SGRQ total score and the OCD but not with the 6MWD. The QOL scale is similar to more complex questionnaires such as the SGRQ in terms of its validity and responsiveness for evaluating the disease-specific HRQOL in elderly COPD patients. In clinical settings, the QOL scale, as a simple questionnaire, may be useful for disease-specific HRQOL assessments in elderly COPD patients (Katsura et al., 2003).

◻ Table 161-2

Correlations between each component of the 36-Item Short-Form Health Survey Questionnaire (SF-36) and the quality of life (QOL) scale and St. George's Respiratory Questionnaire (SGRQ) in the cross-sectional study. Reprint from J Am Geriatr Soc 2003; 51: 1131–1135 with permission

SF-36 scale	QOL scale	SGRQ			
		Total	Symptoms	Activity	Impact
Physical functioning	0.40*	0.30*	0.20*	0.23*	0.36*
Role-physical	0.42*	0.44*	0.37*	0.30*	0.46*
Bodily pain	0.35*	0.34*	0.15	0.32*	0.34*
General health	0.46*	0.24*	0.18	0.26*	0.24*
Vitality	0.37*	0.11	0.14	0.05	0.17
Social functioning	0.37*	0.29*	0.20*	0.22*	0.30*
Role-emotional	0.39*	0.36*	0.31*	0.23*	0.39*
Mental health	0.40*	0.10	0.16	0.02	0.17
Physical component summary	0.47*	0.47*	0.27*	0.42*	0.48*
Mental component summary	0.44*	0.19	0.23*	0.08	0.24*

The QOL scale correlated well with all eight components of SF-36. The total SGRQ score was correlated with all six components of the SF-36 except for vitality and the mental health index (Katsura et al., 2003)
*P <0.05

Since COPD is now thought to be a systemic disease, as described above, comorbidities could also affect QOL in COPD patients. The Charlson index is well-known as a general assessment of comorbidities (Charlson et al., 1987). However, the disease category included in the Charlson index is not specialized for comorbidity in COPD per se, and some comorbidities in COPD, e.g., osteoporosis and depression, are not included in this index. Comorbidity with COPD should be investigated in detail, and a weighted score other than the Charlson index should be determined to examine the association between comorbidities and QOL in COPD.

4.3   Cultural Background in Elderly COPD

It is interesting to assess primary outcome effects by types of caregiver in long-term home care in elderly patients with COPD. This may be affected by various cultural or religious factors, since, in some Asian countries, such as Korea or Japan, which are historically under Confucianism, family and relatives respect their elders and live together in a large house. We previously explored the problems that have arisen in elderly COPD in terms of types of caregivers in Japan (Wakabayashi et al., 2003). Patients with mild to moderate airflow obstruction were included. The types of in-home care were classified into the following three groups: live alone (Group A), with an elderly spouse or a single child (Group B), and with more than three persons (Group C). There were no significant changes among the three groups in basic ADL; however, Group A showed the highest instrumental ADL score, followed by Groups B and C. The 6MWD was shortest in Group A, followed by Groups B and C. Differences in the QOL scale among these three groups indicated that the QOL was highest in

Group C, followed that in Groups A and B. The frequency of hospitalization did not significantly differ among the groups, but emergency visits were required more frequently in Group A compared with Group B or C, with significance. We concluded that the types of in-home caregiver(s) profoundly affect outcomes in elderly COPD, although there was no significant difference observed in the QOL of patients. However, currently the Asian style of caregiver is rapidly changing and being modified to the Western style due to difficulties in maintaining enough space to live together as a whole family (❷ *Figure 161-9a, b*). It is expected that home care will play a central role in medical care of the elderly in the twenty-first century in Japan. Highly specialized medical care in university hospitals or core hospitals in the community has been developed, founded in evidence-based medicine or nursing. However, information is still lacking, and so further study is urgently needed. For the steady development of home care as a new, efficient form of medical care, it is also necessary to incorporate scientific elements into home care. From this viewpoint, the role of physicians would seem to be critical.

5   Perspectives Based on Experiences in Japan

5.1   Cooperation by Medical Teams

Primary care is becoming increasingly focused on the management of chronic disease in a health care system that is more suited to episodic care of acute illness. Seventy-eight percent of Medicare beneficiaries have one or more chronic health conditions, and 46% have three or more chronic conditions (Babbott et al., 2006). The 23% of Medicare beneficiaries with five or more chronic conditions account for 68% of all Medicare spending (Anderson, 2005). Patients with chronic disease take more medications, see more specialists, and receive more formal and informal care. This is the nature of elderly patients. For medical care of the elderly, information about the disease collected from younger adult patients is not always applicable to those elderly patients, and a wide range of information, extending from the changes associated with aging to the status of diseases of old age and health/well-being, must be sought. Medical care of the elderly should be holistic and comprehensive. Focusing only on the disease is to treat the disease, but not the patient, particularly when the patient is elderly. Such treatment is far from providing proper medical care. COPD is a progressive disease, with the reversibility of airway limitation being reduced with increasing severity. In this process, exacerbation may occur due to respiratory infection or other events or with complicated comorbidities. When pharmacological therapy or long-term oxygen therapy (LTOT) is administered, the presence/absence of cognitive impairment and the role of the family members (caregivers) that the patient is living with are extremely important. Physicians should take the central role in coordination with health care, medical care, and welfare services. The important prerequisite in medical care for the elderly is this coordination of health care, medical care, and welfare services. To maintain and prevent a decrease in the ADL as effectively as possible, holistic and comprehensive care of the patient involving medical care and welfare services is required, including early detection, early treatment, rehabilitation, and nursing care. Comprehensive respiratory rehabilitation is consistent with this concept, for which the United Nations designated the year of 1999 as the International Year of Older Persons, and promoted the Active Aging Initiative to facilitate active aging, devoid of diseases, and with only slight impairment, if any (Voelker, 1999). In this process, five goals, i.e., independence, participation,

◘ Figure 161-9

(a) The residential status of elderly subjects was compared among Asian (Japan and Korea) and Western (U.S.A., Germany, and France) countries. Residential types of the elderly population are different between Asian and Western countries: numbers of elderly who live together with their sons or daughters are greater in Asian than in Western countries. Data source from Cabinet Office, Government of Japan, 2005 (http://www8.cao.go.jp/kourei/ishiki/kenkyu1.htm).

(b) Number of elderly living with family members in five countries. The number of elderly living with family members is sharply decreasing in Asian countries (Japan and Korea) compared with USA, West Germany, and Sweden. Data source from White Paper on the National Lifestyle, Prime Minister's Office in Japan, 1994 (http://www5.cao.go.jp/seikatsu/whitepaper/; accessed at 28 November, 2008)

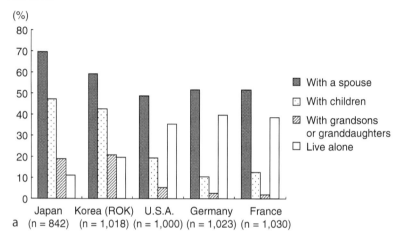

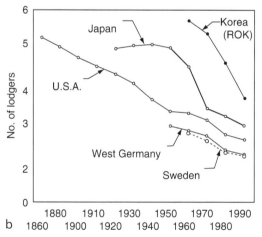

care, self-actualization, and dignity, are specified. Medical care is closely involved in attaining each of these five goals. Physicians should take the central role in maintaining orderly coordination between health care, medical care, and welfare work. However, there are still unresolved problems in elderly COPD that should be overcome in the future.

■ Figure 161-10

Impairment of QOL in elderly COPD. *URI* upper respiratory infection; *GERD* gastroesophageal reflux disorders. Complex factors related to pathophysiology of elderly COPD

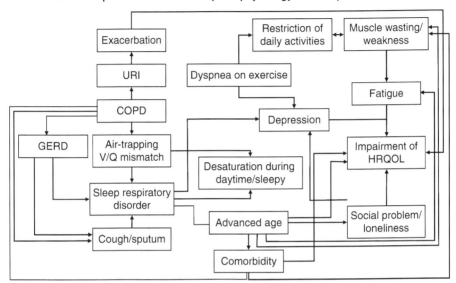

5.2   Factors Associated with QOL in Elderly COPD

Depression impairs the health status of people with chronic diseases, including COPD (Moussavi et al., 2007). Hence, the consideration and treatment of depression is clearly related to the outcome of chronic disease, such as COPD (Yohannes, 2005). It could be also speculated that cormobidity with depression significantly worsens the health of people with COPD. The need for the timely diagnosis and treatment of depressive disorders to reduce the burden on public health is imperative. In primary care settings, patients presenting with multiple disorders that include depression often fail to get diagnosed, particularly in COPD, and, if so, treatment is often focused on the other chronic diseases including COPD (Cassano and Fava, 2002). Depression can be treated in primary care or community settings with locally available, cost-effective interventions (Patel et al., 2004).

In fact, it is suspected that there are many factors which may be related to elderly COPD. ❯ *Figure 161-10* indicates factors associated with elderly COPD, although various comorbidities differently contribute during the clinical course. Further, these also differ between young-old (<75 years old) and old-old (>75 years old) groups of patients, by gender, and local network medical services. Both the generic and health-related QOL are deeply reflected and easily changed by the factors described above; thus, it should be noted that individual QOL is closely connected with the socio-economic burden of society as a whole.

6   Conclusions

The recently modified GOLD guidelines (GOLD, 2007) add brief recommendations for primary care in the last chapter, as follows: "older patients frequently have multiple chronic health conditions. Comorbidities can magnify the impact of COPD on a patient's health status, and can complicate the management of COPD." Problems covered by this thesis are extensive, very complicated, and will require much effort to overcome. To solve the problems, further research and the cooperation of medical teams, including primary care physicians, are clearly needed.

Summary Points

- An increase in the aged population inevitably increases patients with chronic illness.
- COPD is a typical chronic illness in aged people, characterized by not only a pulmonary component, but also some significant extra-pulmonary comorbidities.
- These comorbidities are also causes of hospitalization or contribute to a declining QOL.
- The natural course of elderly COPD is divided into three types, which lead to comorbidity and/or progression of the severity.
- A QOL measure for elderly COPD has not been established because it is affected by many external and internal factors, including severity, comorbidity, age, gender, and cultural background.
- Early detection should be stressed in primary care; however, this is still unresolved.
- Regarding the current status of COPD in Japan, major problem areas indicated by patients and medical staff are as follows: (1) improvement of education and support for self-management, (2) approach to welfare, (3) creating a system of safe and anxiety-free home respiratory care, and (4) increase public awareness of respiratory diseases and patients with respiratory disabilities.

References

Agusti AGN. (2005). Proc Am Thorac Soc. 2: 367–370.

American Thoracic Society. (1997). Am J Respir Crit Care Med. 152 (Suppl.): S77–S121.

American Thoracic Society/European Respiratory Society Task Force. Standards for the Diagnosis and Management of Patients with COPD [Internet]. Version 1.2. American Thoracic Society; 2004 [updated 2005 September 8], New York. Available at: http://www.thoracic.org/go/copd.

Anderson GF. (2005). N Engl J Med. 353: 305–309.

Anzueto A, Sethi S, Martinez FJ. (2007). Proc ATS. 4: 554–564.

Babbott SF, Bigby JA, Day SC, Dugdale DC, Fihn SD, Kapoor WN, McMahon LF Jr, Rosenthal GE, Sinsky CA. (2006). Available at: www.sgim.org/pdf/SGIMReports/BRPFinalReport71106.pdf/ Accessed on 14 Mar 2008.

Buist AS, McBurnie MA, Vollmer WM, Gillespie S, Burney P, Mannino DM, Menezes AM, Sullivan SD, Lee TA, Weiss KB, Jensen RL, Marks GB, Gulsvik A, Nizankowska-Mogilnicka E; BOLD Collaborative Research Group. (2007). Lancet. 370: 741–750.

Carr AJ, Gibson B, Robinson PG. (2001). BMJ. 322: 1240–1243.

Casas, A, Troosters T, Garcia-Aymerich J, Roca J, Hernandez C, Alonso A, del Pozo F, de Toledo P, Anto JM, Rodriguez-Roisin R, Decramer M. (2006). Eur Respir J. 28: 123–130.

Cassano P, Fava M. (2002). J Psychosom Res. 53: 849–857.

Cazzola M, MacNee W, Martinez FJ, Rabe KF, Franciosi LG, Barnes PJ, Brusasco V, Burge PS, Calverley PM, Celli BR, Jones PW, Mahler DA, Make B, Miravitlles M, Page CP, Palange P, Parr D, Pistolesi M, Rennard SI, Rutten-van Mölken MP, Stockley R, Sullivan SD, Wedzicha JA, Wouters EF. (2008). American Thoracic Society; European Respiratory Society Task Force on outcomes of COPD Eur Respir J. 31: 416–469.

Charlson ME, Pompei P, Ales KL, MacKenzie CR. (1987). J Chronic Dis. 40: 373–383.

Fletcher C, Peto R. (1977). Br Med J. 1: 1645–1648.

Folestein MF, Folestein SE, McHugh PR. (1975). J Psychiatr Res. 12: 189–198.

Fukuchi Y, Nishimura M, Ichinose M, Adachi M, Nagai A, Kuriyama T, Takahashi K, Nishimura K, Ishioka S, Aizawa H, Zaher C. (2004). Respirology. 9: 458–465.

Global Initiative for Chronic Obstructive Lung Disease. (GOLD). Global Strategy for Diagnosis, Management, and Prevention of COPD Updated 2007. Available at: http://www.goldcopd.org/

Hiratuka T, Kida K. (1993). Int Med. 32: 836–836.

Hyland ME, Sodergren SC. (2005). In: Ahmedzai SH, Muers MF (ed.) Supportive Care in Respiratory Disease. Oxford University Press, New York, pp. 57–66.

Ikegami N, Campbell JC. (1995). N Engl J Med. 333: 1295–1299.

Ionescu AA, Schoon E. (2003). Eur Respir J. 22: 64S–75S.

Jones PW, Quirk FH, Baveystock CM, Littlejohns P. (1992). Am Rev Respir Dis. 145: 1321–1327.

Katsura H, Kida K. (2002). Chest. 122: 1949–1955.

Katsura H, Yamada K, Kida K. (2003). J Am Geriatr Soc. 51: 1131–1135.

Kida K, Motegi T. (2000). Kokyu. 19: 1235–1247 (in Japanese).

Kida K, Wakabayashi R, Mizuuchi T, Murata A. (2006). Intern Med. 45: 1201–1207.

Liang J, Asano H, Bollen KA, Kahana EF, Maeda D. (1987). J Gerontol. 42: 37–43.

Lopez AD, Mathers CD, Ezzati M, Jamison DT, Murray CJL. (2006). Global Burden of Disease and Risk Factors. The World Bank, Washington.

Lutz W, Sanderson W, Scherbov S. (2008). Nature. 451: 716–719.

Lynn J. (2001). JAMA. 285: 925–932.

Martinez FJ, Curtis JL, Sciurba F, Mumford J, Giardino ND, Weinmann G, Kazerooni E, Murray S, Criner GJ, Sin DD, Hogg J, Ries AL, Han M, Fishman AP, Make B, Hoffman EA, Mohsenifar Z, Wise R; National Emphysema Treatment Trial Research Group. (2007). Am J Respir Crit Care Med. 176: 243–252.

McGarvey LP, John M, Anderson JA, Zvarich M, Wise RA; TORCH Clinical Endpoint Committee. (2007). Thorax. 62: 411–415.

McGavin CR, Artvinli M, Naoe H, McHardy GJ. (1978). Br Med J. 2: 241–243.

Ministry of Health, Labour and Welfare. (2005). Patient Survey.

Ministry of Health, Labour and Welfare. (2006). Vital statistics.

Moussavi S, Chatterji S, Verdes E, Tandon A, Patel V, Ustun B. (2007). Lancet. 370: 851–858.

Patel V, Araya R, Bolton P. (2004). Trop Med Int Health. 9: 539–541.

Price DB, Tinkelman DG, Nordyke RJ, Isonaka S, Halbert RJ; COPD Questionnaire Study Group. (2006). Chest. 129: 1531–1539.

Qaseem A, Snow V, Shekelle P, Sherif K, Wilt TJ, Weinberger S, Owens DK; Clinical Efficacy Assessment Subcommittee of the American College of Physicians. (2007). Ann Intern Med. 147: 633–638.

Sanders MH, Newman AB, Haggerty CL, Redline S, Lebowitz M, Samet J, O'Connor GT, Punjabi NM, Shahar E. (2003). Am J Respir Crit Care Med. 167: 7–14.

Schünemann HJ, Goldstein R, Mador MJ, McKim D, Stahl E, Griffith LE, Bayoumi AM, Austin P, Guyatt GH. (2006). Qual Life Res. 15: 1–14.

Seyama K, Nukiwa T, Takabe K, Takahashi H, Miyake K, Kira S. (1991). J Biol Chem. 266: 12627–12632.

Steg PG, Bhatt DL, Wilson PW, D'Agostino R Sr, Ohman EM, Röther J, Liau CS, Hirsch AT, Mas JL, Ikeda Y, Pencina MJ, Goto S; REACH Registry Investigators. (2007). JAMA 297: 1197–1206.

The Japanese Respiratory Society. (2004). Guidelines for the Diagnosis and Treatment of COPD (Chronic Obstructive Pulmonary Disease), 2nd ed. Available at: http://www.jrs.or.jp/home/modules/english/index.php?content_id = 15.

The Japanese Respiratory Society. (2006). Japanese White Paper on Home Respiratory Care. Available at: http://www.jrs.or.jp/home/modules/english/index.php?content_id = 15.

Voelker R. (1999). JAMA. 281: 1262.

Wakabayashi R, Katsura H, Yamada K, Motegi T, Omata M, Nishimura N, Goto R, Kida K. (2003). Eur Respir J. 22: 169s.

Yohannes AM. (2005). Br J Community Nurs. 10: 42–46.

3   Quality of Life Measures and
     Indices
3.4 Cancer

162 Chemotherapy for Brain Metastasis and Quality of Life

R. Addeo · G. Cimmino · S. D. Prete

1   *Introduction* 2782

2   *Chemotherapy: The Role of Temozolomide* 2784
2.1   TMZ Single Agent 2784
2.2   TMZ in Combination with Other Chemotherapeutic Drugs 2787

3   *Other Cytotoxic Agents and Combination Chemotherapy for the Treatment*
      of Brain Metastases 2788
3.1   Platinum-Based Regimen 2788
3.2   Other Drugs 2788

4   *Quality of Life* 2789
4.1   Review of Literature 2790
4.2   Original Data 2791

5   *Conclusions* 2791

      Summary Points 2793

Abstract: Brain ❷ metastases incidence is increasing among patients with ❷ solid tumors. Treatment options are limited and frequently the ❷ palliative approaches remain the standard treatment to relieve neurologic symptoms with a decrease in survival and ❷ quality of life. Therapeutic approaches to ❷ brain metastases include surgery, ❷ whole brain radiotherapy (WBRT), ❷ stereotactic radiosurgery (SRS), and ❷ chemotherapy.

For patients with multiple brain metastases, improvement in quality of life and neuralgic function remain important objectives. In this chapter the current role of chemotherapy and the impact on the Quality of life in these patients is summarized.

❷ Temozolomide, an oral imidazotetrazinone methylating agent, is highly bio-available after oral administration, has excellent central nervous system penetration, and reaches the brain in therapeutic concentrations. Tolerability of this agent has been confirmed by clinical trials in patients with BM.

Several combination chemotherapy in first-line treatment for brain metastases was investigated, and in newly diagnosed brain metastases, the tumors are responsive as the primary systemic cancer, as demonstrated by several phase II studies.

The results of recent trials support the efficacy and safety of WBRT and chemotherapy in the treatment of patients with BM from a variety of solid tumors. The data show that this choice can also offer significant palliation for BM, improving global Quality of Life.

List of Abbreviations: *BBB*, ❷ blood brain barrier; *BM*, brain metastases; *CNS*, central nervous system; *CR*, complete response; *EGFR*, epidermal growth factor receptor; *FACT*, functional assessment of cancer therapy; *5-FU*, 5-fluoruracil; *KPS*, Karnofsky performance status; *MRI*, magnetic resonance imaging; *NSCLC*, non small cell lung cancer; *PR*, partial response; *QOL*, quality of life; ❷ *RPA*, recursive partitioning analysis; *RTOG*, radiation therapy oncology group; *SRS*, stereotactic radiosurgery; *TMZ*, temozolomide; *WBRT*, whole brain radiotherapy

1 Introduction

Central Nervous system metastasis develops in 15–30% of patients with systemic malignancies and represent an important cause of morbidity and mortality. The incidence of brain metastases (BM) has increased in the last recent years, probably due to the longer survival of cancer patients given aggressive treatments for primary tumors (Hutter et al., 2003).The risk of developing BM varies according to primary tumor type, with lung cancer accounting for approximately half of all BM. Recent data evidenced that among patients with lung cancer and breast cancer, the incidence of BM is 40–50% and 15–25%, respectively, and there is an evident correlation between stage of disease and incidence of CNS metastases (Eichler and Loeffler, 2007).

In the era of magnetic resonance imaging (MRI), the majority of patients have multiple brain metastases at diagnosis. Common clinical features include headache, neurological deficit, and seizures. Detailed neuropsychological testing demonstrates cognitive impairment in 65% of patients with brain metastases, usually across multiple domains being favorable.

Despite the advances in the management of BM during the past 20 years the prognosis of patients remains generally poor; the median survival time of untreated patients is approximately 1 month (Zimm et al., 1981). Several studies in patients with BM have identified a number of patient characteristics that are associated with survival, the most notable of which is the recursive partitioning analysis (RPA) described by Gaspar and colleagues (❷ *Table 162-1*)

◘ Table 162-1

RPA prognostic classification according to RTOG recommendations

RPA class	Description	Median survival	Recommended
1st	KPS ≥ 70	7.1 months	Definite treatments
	Ages < 65		
	Controlled primary		
	No systemic metastases		
2nd	KPS ≥ 70	4.2 months	WBRT
	Ages > 65		
	Uncontrolled primary		
	Systemic metastases		
3rd	KPS < 70	2.3 months	WBRT o/e symptomatic cures

RPA prognostic classification identifies three prognostic classes for patients with brain metastases. *WBRT* whole brain radiotherapy; *KPS* Karnofsky performance status

◘ Table 162-2

Treatment modalities

Supportive care		Definitive
Medical		Surgery
Corticosteroids		Radio surgery
Anticonvulsants		Radiotherapy
		Chemotherapy
		Others

Management consists of symptomatic care and definitive treatment. Symptomatic management can result in a significant improvement in quality of life for patients with brain metastasis

The RTOG trial described three groups of patients according to prognostic factors related to tumor based on Karnofsky performance score, primary tumor status, presence of extra-cranial metastases and age. Patients with KPS≥70, age<65 years, no extra-cranial metastases and controlled primary tumor are considered Class I and have a median survival of 7.1 months; patients with KPS < 70 are class III with a median survival of 2.3 months. All other patients belong to class II with a median survival of 4.2 months (Gaspar et al., 1997).

The current standard of care for BM involves surgical resection, stereotactic radiosurgery (SRS), whole-brain radiation therapy (WBRT) and control of symptoms with steroids and anticonvulsants (◉ *Table 162-2*) (Jeyapalan and Batchelor, 2004).

Many patients are treated with a combination of these, and treatment decisions must take into account factors such as patient age, functional status, primary tumor type, extent of extracranial disease, prior therapies, and number of intracranial lesions (Langer and Mehta, 2005).

Chemotherapy has traditionally not played a major role in the treatment of patients with BM. The blood- brain-barrier (BBB) penetration is a limiting factor for the crossing of both chemotherapy and target-based agents. However contrast enhancement on computerized tomography scans suggests that the BBB may be partially disrupted in metastases (Davey, 2002). Another crucial factor is that steroids used to treat edema partially restore the disrupted BBB; reducing the ability of the drug to achieve adequate tumor concentrations. In addition, the intrinsic chemosensitivity of a cancer to a peculiar drug or regimen of agents is important. In patients who are chemotherapy naïve, responses of BM to chemotherapy have generally been comparable to response rates of extracranial disease. BM from germ cell tumors, small cell lung cancer, and lymphoid malignancies are the most sensitive to chemotherapy, whereas BM from non small cell lung cancer and breast cancer are somewhat less sensitive to these agents (Drappatz and Wen, 2006).

Currently only for exquisitely chemosensitive tumors, such as germ cell tumors, is chemotherapy accepted as first-line therapy of brain metastases; on the other hand for most cancer type the chemotherapy has a limited role in treating BM. and has been reserved for patients who have failed other treatment modalities.

As suggested in primary CNS cancer patients treated with concurrent TMZ and WBRT, the combination of traditional cytotoxic agents or targeted molecular drugs with radiation may hold promise for improving upon control rates of WBRT alone.

Data supporting the use of chemotherapy BM are limited. Only few number of prospective phase II and III trials have investigated the role of systemic chemotherapy in the treatment of BM. Frequently, the heterogeneous inclusion criteria, represent another limitation; in fact, most clinical trials incorporate patients with a variety of histologies, prior treatments and stages of systemic disease.

Maintenance and improvement of patients' quality of life (QOL) is regarded as an important goal for medical intervention in addition to tumor control and survival.

Despite the advances in the management of BM have provided patients with longer survival, long-Term survival after development of BM is rare. For these reasons, the control of neurocognitive function and the improvement of quality of life remain an end-point with high priority.

In this chapter we will analyze the chemotherapeutic regime used for the treatment of BM from breast and lung cancer, and discuss as these treatment can impact on the quality of life of theses patients.

2   Chemotherapy: The Role of Temozolomide

2.1   TMZ Single Agent

Despite the theoretic difficulties with delivering chemotherapy to intracranial targets, including the presence of the BBB, the poor efficacy of Whole Brain Radiotherapy alone, especially in Terms of controlling extra cranial disease, has led to a number of investigations that have sought to evaluate a role for these agents. The limited ability of most chemotherapeutic agents to cross the BBB is believed to be one of the principal reasons these agents are less active against disease in the CNS than extra cranial disease.

Recently, there as been much interest in the drug Temozolomide (TMZ), that is a second-generation alkylating agent that has shown a promising activity in primary brain tumors with

◻ Table 162-3

Phase II study of cytotoxic agents in BM from breast cancer

Author	Patients	Treatment	Response rate	Survival time	QOL/NCF assessment
Rosner	100	Various	50	6	No
Cocconi	22	CDDP + VP-16	55	13	No
Franciosi	56	CDDP + VP-16	38	8	No
Friedman	15	TMZ	0	NR	No
Addeo	21	WBRT + TMZ→ TMZ	70	13	Yes
Caraglia	8	TMZ + liposomal doxorubicin	62	10	Yes
Christodoulou	15	TMZ + CDDP	40	5.5	Yes
Abrey	10	TMZ	0	7	No
Rivera	24	TMZ + Capecitabine	18	4	Yes
Trudeau	19	TMZ	0	NR	No
Kouvaris	7	WBRT + TMZ → TMZ	28	12	No
Verger	6	WBRT + TMZ	NR	4.5	No

Responses and survival seen with chemotherapy treatments for NSCLC patients with brain metastases. *CDDP* cisplatin; *VP-16* vepesid; *TMZ* temozolomide; *WBRT* whole brain radiotherapy; *NR* not reported; *QOL* quality of life; *NCF* neurocognitive function

a low incidence of adverse hematological events. TMZ has the interesting qualities of near 100% bioavailability when administered orally and the ability to cross the BBB (Baker et al., 1999), achieving effective concentrations in cerebrospinal fluid (Plowman et al., 1994). TMZ has been investigated as a treatment for BM in four different scenarios: alone for newly diagnosed brain metastases; alone for recurrent/progressive disease; TMZ in combination with WBRT for newly diagnosed lesions; and more recently TMZ in combination with other chemotherapeutic agents (Langer and Mehta, 2005), both for breast and NSCLC (❯ *Table 162-3* and ❯ *162-4*).

Several trials have been investigated TMZ as single agent for the treatment of recurrent/progressive BM. The largest of these, reported by Friedman reported, among 52 patients enrolled, 3 partial responses and 33 stable diseases (Friedman et al., 2003). Other trials obtained similar results and suggest that TMZ, as single agent, has modest activity in patients with recurrent BM. In a phase II study, among the 41 patients with recurrent or progressive BM from a variety of primary malignancies, the authors achieved a disease control in 41% of patients, confirming that single agent TMZ has a definite activity for some patients with recurrent brain metastases, with minimal toxicity (Abrey et al., 2001).

Recently, in a study on 19 patients with breast cancer and BM, that had been received up to two prior chemotherapy regimens for metastatic disease, Trudeau and colleagues used TMZ as single agent. No objective responses to TMZ were achieved in those heavily pre treated women (Trudeau et al., 2006). For newly diagnosed BM, two different studies showed an interesting overall response rate for BM of 24%, but varied by primary cancer. Conversely, the efficacy and safety of using TMZ concurrently with WBRT for patients with newly diagnosed BM was evaluated in several recent phase II studies. Dardoufas et al. (2001) demonstrated radiographic

◘ Table 162-4

Phase II study of cytotoxic agents in BM from NSCLC

Author	Patients	Treatment	Response rate	Survival time	QOL/NCF assessment
Bernardo	22	VNR + GEM + CBDCA	45	7	No
Robinet	76	CDDP + VNR	21	5	No
Antonodou	16	WBRT + TMZ → TMZ	NA	8.5	Yes
Addeo	22	WBRT + TMZ → TMZ	45	13	Yes
Caraglia	6	TMZ + liposomal doxorubicin	0	NR	Yes
Kouvaris	11	WBRT + TMZ → TMZ	80	12	No
Franciosi	43	CDDP + VP-16	30	8	No
Friedman	29	TMZ	7	NR	No
Dardoufas	11	WBRT + TMZ → TMZ	82	NR	Yes
Christodoulou	12	TMZ + CDDP	18	5.5	No
Abrey	22	TMZ	9	7	No
Omuro	10	TMZ + VNR	NR	6	No
Cortot	50	TMZ + Cisplatin	16	5	No
Hedde	45	Topotecan	NR	4.5	No
Verger	20	WBRT + TMZ	NR	4.5	No

Responses and survival seen with chemotherapy treatment for breast cancer patients with brain metastases. *VNR* vinorelbine; *CBDCA* carboplatin; *TMZ* temozolomide; *GEM* gemcitabine; *WBRT* whole brain radiotherapy; *CDDP* cisplatin; *VP-16* vepesid; *NR* not reported; *QOL* quality of life; *NCF* neurocognitive function

complete or partial responses in 14 of 20 patients after six cycles of TMZ, with any unacceptable toxicities.

More recently, Antonadou performed a randomized phase II and a confirmatory phase III study. In both trials the authors found a significantly greater complete or partial response rate in patients receiving TMZ plus WBRT (96% objective response rate, vs. 66%), although the median survival time did not differ (8.6 months vs. 7.0 months; p _.447) (Antonadou et al., 2002).

In another randomized study, enrolling 82 patients with the same study design, failed to replicate the high objective response rate found by the previous authors. The authors demonstrated that the patients receiving TMZ in addition to WBRT had non significant improvements in survival, although they did find a significantly higher neurological progression-free survival rate in the TMZ arm (72 vs. 54%; $p < 0.03$) (Verger et al., 2005).

In the last year, other two different studies confirm the efficacy of this combination in Terms of objective responses. In the first study, developed by an Italian group on 59 patients with BM from different tumor histotypes, reported five complete responses, 21 partial response (❷ *Figure 162-1*) and 18 stable diseases, with an encouraging overall response rate (45%)with an encouraging median overall survival of 13 months (Addeo et al., 2007). Kouvaris and colleagues, in a trial that enrolled 33 patients with BM, found an objective response rate of 54%. The median overall survival was 12 months with an acceptable mild side effects (Kouvaris et al., 2007).

▣ Figure 162-1

Radiological responses to TMZ therapy in brain metastases. (a–b) Complete response to TMZ, after six cycles of TMZ in a patient with BM from breast cancer. (c–d) Partial response to TMZ, after six cycles of TMZ in a patient with BM from NSCLC

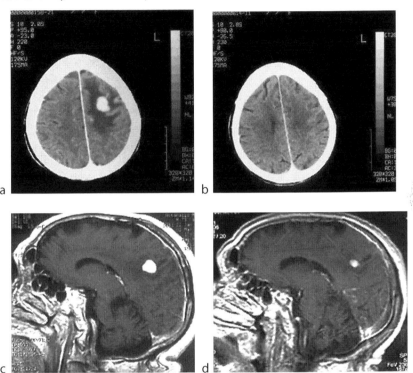

2.2 TMZ in Combination with Other Chemotherapeutic Drugs

More recently, there as been interest in improving the activity of TMZ using dose-intensive regimen, or by combining it with other therapeutic agents. The efficacy of the combination of TMZ with pegylated liposomal doxorubicin has been investigated in the treatment of brain metastases from solid tumors (Caraglia et al., 2006), as well as the combination if TMZ and Cisplatin (Christodoulou et al., 2005). The reported objective responses are 36.8% and 31.2%, respectively, with acceptable toxicity. However also this issue is controversial, and data against it has recently been demonstrated by Cortot in a phase II trials. Among 50 patients with BM from NSCLC received TMZ with Cisplatin, the authors reported eight objective responses (16%) (Cortot et al., 2006).

Omuro used an intensified regimen of TMZ in patients with brain metastasis. The combination had a favorable toxicity profile and at least stable disease was seen in eight out 18 assessable patients (44%) in a phase I study (Omuro et al., 2006). Recently, in the next phase II study, among 38 patients with BM from different types of primary cancer, they achieved an objective radiographic response rate of 5%, with a median overall survival of 5 months (Iwamoto et al., 2007).

In an other study, Rivera utilized a combination of TMZ with Capecitabine to treat breast cancer patients with BM. Among 24 patients, one complete response and three partial responses were achieved. The median response duration was 8 weeks. The combination is an active and well-tolerate regimen (Rivera et al., 2006).

3   Other Cytotoxic Agents and Combination Chemotherapy for the Treatment of Brain Metastases

3.1   Platinum-Based Regimen

Platinum-based chemotherapy has been evaluated in combination with other active agents. The Italian Oncology Group for Clinical Research treated chemotherapy and radiotherapy-naïve NSCLC patients who were not surgical candidates with etoposide and cisplatin and reported comparable response rate of 30%. Median time to progression was 4 months and median survival was 8 months. In other study paclitaxel in combination with cisplatin and either vinorelbine or gemcitabine as an up-front therapy in 38 BM patients from NSCLC achieved intracranial response rates of 38% (Cortes et al., 2003). Bernardo and colleagues treated 22 chemotherapy-naïve NSCLC patients with BM with a combination of vinorelbine, gemcitabine and carboplatin; this treatment yielded high response rates of 45%. These data suggest that the responsiveness of BM might be deTermined more by the chemo-sensitivity of the primary cancer than the ability of the cytotoxic agents to penetrate the BBB (Bernardo et al., 2002).

Two randomized phase III studies have showed the efficacy of chemotherapy in BM. One, of concurrent chemotherapy plus radiotherapy in BM from non-small-cell lung cancer, suggested that the timing of WBRT, with respect to chemotherapy with cisplatin and vinor-elbine did not influence survival (Robinet et al., 2001). The other, evaluating effect of adding WBRT to teniposide in small cell lung cancer, resulted in a better response rate and longer time to BM progression but had no impact on survival (Postmus et al., 2000).

The combination of cisplatin and etoposide has shown activity in two phase II studies totaling 78 patients with new brain metastases from breast cancer, with 12 CRs, 21 PRs, and a median overall survival time in the range of 31–58 weeks (Cocconi et al., 1990; Franciosi et al., 1999).

3.2   Other Drugs

Paclitaxel activity was evaluated in a phase III study in which 86 patients (56% lung cancer, 12% melanoma, 10% breast cancer) were randomized to receive WBRT alone or placlitaxel (250 mg/mq/week for 3 weeks).In the group of paclitaxel median survival was not improved, instead grade 3/4toxicity was higher (Glantz et al., 1999).

Recently, combination of topotecan and WBRT was checked in a phase I study, followed by a phase II study. Treatment was completed in 57 patients out the 80 brain metastases patients treated. Median survival was 25 weeks overall and 34 weeks in those with objective responses. The authors indicated that this combination was a tolerable regimen with high response rate of BM, but response rates for BM were not reported (Hedde et al., 2007; Korfel et al., 2002).

Rosner and colleagues treated 100 women with BM from breast cancer with several different regimens. A total of 50 patients demonstrated an objective response. The median duration of remission was10 months for complete responses and 7 months for partial responses. Primary chemotherapy achieved responses in 27 out 52 patients treated with cyclophosphamide, 5-FU and prednisone; 19 out 35 patients receiving cyclophosphamide, 5-FU, prednisone, vincristine andmethotrexate; in three out seven patients treated with prednisone, methotrexate and vincristine. The median survival for complete responders and partial responders was 39 and10 months, respectively, in contrast with non responders with a median survival of 1.5 months. naive patients treated with up-front chemotherapy (Rosner et al., 1986).

The activity of Gefinitib, an orally active inhibitor of the epidermal growth factor receptor-associated tyrosine kynase, in BM patients has been suggested in several case reports. Huang and colleagues, in a preclinical study, showed that Gefinitib enhances the antitumor activity of radiation (Huang et al., 2002). In a phase II study, Gefinitib was administered to 27 patients with BM. The authors described six partial responses (30%) and five stable diseases (25%). In Terms of BM, two patients had responses, including a complete remission. In the largest prospective series reported, Ceresoli et al. found a 27% disease control rate (4 of 41 patients [10%] with PRs, 7 of 41 patients [17%] with stable disease) in 41 patients with measurable brain metastases, 18 of whom had received WBRT _3 months prior to study entry (Ceresoli et al., 2004).

Finally, there is interest in the role of oral targeted agents, particularly in women with human epidermal growth factor receptor (HER)-2–positive tumors, who are known to be at high risk for brain metastases. The dual EGFR and HER-2 tyrosine kinase inhibitor lapatinib showed modest activity in a recent phase II study of lapatinib for recurrent brain metastases in women treated with trastuzumab for HER- 2–positive breast cancer. Lin et al. reported two PRs, six minor responses, and five patients with stable disease for _16 weeks in 34 patients treated, and a larger multinational phase II trial has recently completed enrolment (Lin et al., 2006).

4   Quality of Life

When assessing the value of a particular anticancer treatment it is important to consider the impact it may have not only on length of survival but also on health related quality of life.

Over the last few decades assessments of patients' QOL have been established as part of cancer clinical trials. Sometimes QOL variables are used as a primary endpoint, but more often they are used as subsidiary endpoints or descriptive data. Both medical and QOL results from clinical studies should influence how patients are treated in clinical practice (Bottomley, 2002).

QOL measurement scales and outcome concerns have become increasingly important as part of outcomes research programs in recent years, all in an effort to assess whether new therapeutic strategies are justified in Term of efficacy, cost, and net QOL benefits.

Although the induction of the remission of the disease and the improvement in overall survival remain central to cancer clinical research, it is now widely accepted that relief from symptoms and protection against brain complications should not be overlooked as therapeutic goals to be achieved in cancer patients with brain metastases. Therefore, the improvement in the quality of life may be as important as the increase in survival rates in these patients.

A phase II study revealed that Temozolomide has single-agent activity in patients with WHO grade II cerebral glioma, with an improvement in quality of life and improvement in epilepsy control (Brada et al., 2003). The efficacy of TMZ on QOL of patients with brain tumors was confirmed in an other study conducted by Pace and colleagues. The clinical benefit was significantly higher in patients with non-enhancing lesions than in those with enhancing lesions, ($P < 0.05$). Patients with a radiological response showed a relevant clinical benefit during TMZ treatment, with 41% gaining seizure control and QOL improvement (Pace et al., 2003).

4.1   Review of Literature

The evaluation of the clinical benefits, in Terms of seizure control, neurocognitive function, and improvement in quality of life (QOL), represents an important goal to establish the efficacy and usefulness of chemotherapy for patients with BM usually with a poor and prognosis. Moreover, only few trials developed in the last years, assessed these parameters (❷ Table 162-3 and ❷ 162-4).

Caraglia and colleagues observed a highly statistically significant improvement in the quality of life as measured by ❷ FACT-G, suggesting a clinically relevant impact of PLD/TMZ combination therapy in patients with brain metastases. The maximal percentage increase in mean FACT-G values from baseline was after 9 months of therapy. Interestingly, also in pts. who did not achieved an objective response a statistically significant amelioration of their QOL was recorded (Caraglia et al., 2006).

Recently we evidenced an interesting positive impact of the combination of TMZ and WBRT therapy in patients with brain metastases after 3 and 6 months from the beginning of the treatment with TMZ. The results speculate that TMZ has superior palliative effects despite the presence of toxicity; the improvement in the quality of life would have been greater if our study had been restricted to symptomatic patients. The aspects of the quality of life that are assessed with the FACT-G and ❷ FACT-Br questionnaires were maintained or improved during treatment, with the greatest benefit occurring for BM–specific concerns. We investigate the impact of TMZ and WBRT treatment combination on the quality of life of 59 patients enrolled in the study, measured using subject-completed Functional Assessment of Cancer Therapy (FACT) and FACT- brain metastases questionnaires (FACT-Br) developed to assess quality of life and symptom response at baseline and 1 month after whole-brain radiotherapy for BM (Bezjak et al., 2002). Baseline FACT-G questionnaires were completed by 59 patients (100%). The authors found a statistically significant improvement measured by the questionnaire, also in patients that not achieved any objective response. The FACT-Br questionnaire confirmed these encouraging results as they found an amelioration of quality of their life after 3 months of treatment. The analysis of the respondents, 34 patients, reported that they were "quite a bit" or "very much" content with the quality of their life after 3 months of treatment (79% positive respondents to 21% negative respondent), on the other and, the baseline value were following: positive respondents 51%, 21 patients, and negative respondents 49% (those patients who responded "not at all"/"a little bit"), 20 patients (Addeo et al., 2007).

Rivera evaluated the neurocognitive function in 24 patients with multiple BM treated with capecitabine and TMZ. After 1 months of treatment, the patients achieved a significant improvement in attention span and emotional function. These results suggest that this combination was not neurotoxic and may have a beneficial effect that can influences the QOL of these patients. Similar results was obtained by Antonadou in another trial, the percentage of patients that showed an improvement of neurological functional status after TMZ and WBRT treatment was higher than that of patients with BM treated with WBRT alone.

4.2 Original Data

We conducted a single-institution phase II clinical trial to deTermine the efficacy and the safety profile of new regimen based on dose-intensified, protracted course of TMZ, after WBRT in patients with multiple brain metastases from breast cancer and NSCLC. They were treated with 30 Gy WBRT with concomitant TMZ ($75mg/m^2$/day) for 10 days, and subsequently TMZ at $75mg/m^2$/day, for 21 days every 4 weeks, for up to 12 cycles. We also assessed whether there was an improvement in quality of life for patients with brain metastases as measured after three and six courses of TMZ therapy, using FACT-BR questionnaire. A two-tailed t test for paired samples was used to detect a statistically significant difference in global scores between pre-chemotherapy and post-chemotherapy quality-of-life assessments.

Thirty-two patients with BM from either breast cancer or NSCLC were enrolled and evaluated from November 2005 to March 2007. All patients who answered the questionnaire at baseline were included in the evaluation, and the FACT-G and FACT-BR scores ware compared with the baseline value for each of these patients.

We detect a difference in general quality of life score, FACT-G ($p = 0.022$) and brain subscale score, FACT-BR ($p = 0.012$) after three cycles of treatment. After 6 months of treatment, There was a statistical improvement toward worsening FACT-G scores, and FACT-BR, compared to baseline score (❷ *Table 162-5*).

The QOL analysis showed a high level of satisfaction among patients who have undergone TMZ plus WBRT treatment for brain metastases and provides excellent support for its acceptability. These data propose that TMZ has superior palliative effects despite the presence of toxicity.

5 Conclusions

Metastatic brain tumors are the most common intracranial neoplasm in adults, and although the exact incidence is unknown. The frequency of metastatic brain tumors appears to be rising as a result of superior imaging modalities and earlier detection as well as longer survival after a primary cancer diagnosis because of more effective treatment of systemic disease.

❏ Table 162-5
Quality of life scores compared to baseline scores, original results of our group

Total QOL score	t statistic	P value
FACT- G after three cycles of TMZ	2,320	0,022
FACT- G after six cycles of TMZ	2,880	0,012
FACT-BR after three cycles of TMZ	2.248	0,042
FACT-BR after three cycles of TMZ	3,107	0,009

Twenty-nine patients completed the FACT-BR and FACT-G questionnaires at baseline. poor agreement and values in between, moderate Twenty-one patients (72%) completed the questionnaires at third month of treatment, and 18 patients after six cycles of TMZ. A pair-wise t test of global score (FACT-G) as well as the brain subscale score (FACT-BR) as ranked by the patient was analyzed. A t statistic greater than 0 represents a higher absolute quality-of-life score at baseline. *QOL* quality of life; *FACT-G* functional assessment of cancer therapy-general; *FACT-BR* functional assessment of cancer therapy-brain

The management of brain metastases can be divided into symptomatic and therapeutic strategies. Symptomatic therapy (❷ Symptomatic Treatment of Brain Metastases) often includes corticosteroids to reduce peritumoral edema and anticonvulsants to prevent recurrent seizures.

Chemotherapy has traditionally played a limited role in the treatment of brain metastases and has been reserved for patients who have failed other treatment modalities or for diseases known to be "chemosensitive". Clinical data supporting the utility of chemotherapy for brain metastases in various solid tumors are limited primarily to small phase II studies, often in heavily pre treated patient populations.

For these patients, treatment strategies that prolong survival remain lacking; however, for this population intracranial disease control, time to neurologic progression, neurologic function, and quality of life may be more relevant endpoints because of the competing risk for death from systemic disease.

QOL especially is important for patients suffering from BM from solid tumors, whose life expectancy may be very short.

The results of QOL analysis shows a high level of satisfaction among patients who have undergone TMZ plus WBRT treatment for brain metastases and provides excellent support for its acceptability. Chemotherapy combined with radiotherapy appears to be promising in the treatment of patients with BM. Chemotherapy should also be considered in the treatment of progressive brain disease after radiotherapy.

The results support the efficacy and safety of chemotherapeutic agents in the treatment of patients with BM from a variety of solid tumors and confirm that this drug can also offer significant palliation for BM, improving global QOL. Moreover, in patients with brain metastases, the prospective evaluation of neurocognitive function or quality of life during and after treatment remain often problematic because of high dropout rates and the potential introduction of bias.

Recent results suggested that a more frequent or dose dense schedule of TMZ may obtain better cytotoxic activity, and the latter consideration is confirmed by initial encouraging results in patients with glioblastoma.

A possibility to combine TMZ with other agents, to allow the control of extra-brain disease sites that are poorly susceptible to TMZ, is given by lowering TMZ dosages reducing the occurrence of its side effects. In this view, metronomic chemotherapy may represent an alternative to conventional chemotherapy providing a number of favorable effects: (1) delay of the onset of acquired drug resistance; (2) reduction of host toxicity; (3) lack of prolonged drug-free break; (4) anti-angiogenic effects (Gasperini, 2001).

Although the role of chemotherapy for brain metastases has been limited in the past, it is likely that this will change significantly in the next future. The recent progress that has been obtained in the cure of systemic cancers with cytotoxic and targeted molecular agents can be checked for the treatment of brain metastases. The utilization, for the initial treatment of systemic malignancy, of drugs with a favorable profile of CNS penetration, will reduce the incidence of subsequent brain metastases.

In the future, patients will benefit from a multidisciplinary approach focused on the integration of multiple therapeutic options as surgery, radiation therapy, and chemotherapy focusing on neurologic and neurocognitive function and quality of life.

Summary Points

- Brain metastases occur in up to 40% of all cancer patients with metastatic disease and, are associated with poor prognosis.
- WBRT is the treatment of choice for patients with multiple brain metastases or lesions that are not amenable to surgical resection.
- The role of systemic chemotherapy in patients with brain metastases remains controversial.
- Temozolomide, an orally bioavailable alkylating agent that crosses the blood brain barrier, has activity against brain metastases when used as a single agent in combination with Whole brain radiotherapy.
- In patients with newly untreated BM, responses to several chemotherapeutic combinations have been similar to primary tumors.
- For patients with BM from solid tumors with a short life expectance, Quality of Life and control of neurologic functional status represent and important endpoint.
- Chemotherapy, in addition to whole brain radiotherapy, may represent an promising treatment choice for patients with BM to control the brain disease and improve the Quality of life.

References

Abrey LE, Olson JD, Raizer JJ, Mack M, Rodavitch A, Boutros DY, Malkin MG. (2001). J Neurooncol. 53: 259–265.

Addeo R, Caraglia M, Faiola V, Capasso E, Vincenzi B, Montella L, Guarrasi R, Caserta L, Del Prete S. (2007). BMC Cancer. 7: 18.

Antonadou D, Paraskevaidis M, Sarris M, Coliarakis N, Economou I, Karageorgis P, Throuvalas N. (2002). J Clin Oncol. 20: 3644–3650.

Baker SD, Wirth M, Statkevich P, Reidenberg P, Alton K, Sartorius SE, Dugan M, Cutler D, Batra V, Grochow LB, Donehower RC, Rowinsky EK. (1999). Clin Cancer Res. 5: 309–317.

Bernardo G, Cuzzoni Q, Strada MR, Bernardo A, Brunetti G, Jedrychowska I, Pozzi U, Palumbo R. (2002). Cancer Invest. 20: 293–302.

Bezjak A, Adam J, Barton R, Panzarella T, Lapierre N, Wong CS, Mason W, Buckley C, Levin W, McLean M, Wu JSY, Sia M, Kirkbride P. (2002). Eur J Cancer. 38: 487–496.

Bottomley A. (2002). Oncologist. 7: 120–125.

Brada M, Viviers L, Abson C, Hines F, Britton J, Ashley S, Sardell S, Traish D, Gonsalves A, Wilkins P, Westbury C. (2003). Ann Oncol. 14: 1715–1721.

Caraglia M, Addeo R, Costanzo R, Montella L, Faiola V, Marra M, Abbruzzese A, Palmieri G, Budillon A, Grillone F, Venuta S, Tagliaferri P, Del Prete S. (2006). Cancer Chemother Pharmacol. 57: 34–39.

Ceresoli GL, Cappuzzo F, Gregorc V, Bartolini S, Crinò L, Villa E. (2004). Ann Oncol. 15: 1042–1047.

Christodoulou C, Bafaloukos D, Linardou H, Aravantinos G, Bamias A, Carina M, Klouvas G, Skarlos D. (2005). J Neurooncol. 71: 61–65.

Cocconi G, Lottici R, Bisagni G, Bacchi M, Tonato M, Passalacqua R, Boni C, Belsanti V, Bassi P. (1990). Cancer Invest. 8: 327–334.

Cortes J, Rodriguez J, Aramendia JM, Salgado E, Gurpide A, Garcia-Foncillas J, Aristu JJ, Claver A, Bosch A, Lopez-Picazo JM, Martin-Algarra S, Brugarolas A, Calvo E. (2003). Oncology. 64: 28–35.

Cortot AB, Gerinière L, Robinet G, Breton JL, Corre R, Falchero L, Berard H, Gimenez C, Chavaillon JM, Perol M, Bombaron P, Mercier C, Souquet PJ, Groupe Lyon-Saint-Etienne d'Oncologie Thoracique, Groupe Français de Pneumo-Cancérologie. (2006). Ann Oncol. 17: 1412–1417.

Dardoufas C, Miliadou A, Skarleas C, Kouloulias V, Mavroidi P, Couvaris J, Gennatas K, Vassilaki M,

Gogas H, Polyzos A, Couvoussis E, Vlachos L. (2001). Proc Am Soc Clin Oncol. 20: 75 (Abs 2048).

Davey P. (2002). CNS Drugs. 16(5): 325 –338.

Drappatz J, Wen PY. (2006). Expert Rev Neurother. 6 (10): 1465–1479.

Eichler AF, Loeffler JS. (2007). Oncologist. 12: 884–898.

Franciosi V, Cocconi G, Michiara M, Di Costanzo F, Fosser V, Tonato M, Carlini P, Boni C, Di Sarra S. (1999). Cancer. 85: 1599–1605.

Friedman HS, Evans B, Reardon D, Quinn J, Rich J, Gururangan S, Stafford-Fox V, Chen C, Pati A, Schmidt W. (2003). Proc Am Soc Clin Oncol. 22: 102 (Abs. 408).

Gaspar L, Scott C, Rotman M, Asbell S, Phillips T, Wasserman T, McKenna WG, Byhardt R. (1997). Int J Radiat Oncol Biol Phys. 37: 745–751.

Gasperini G. (2001). Lancet Oncol. 2(12): 733–740.

Glantz M, Choy H, Chakravarthy A. (1999). Proc Am Soc Clin Oncol. 18: 140a, (Abstract 535).

Hedde JP, Neuhaus T, Schüller H, Metzler U, Schmidt-Wolf IG, Kleinschmidt R, Losem C, Lange O, Grohe C, Stier S, Ko YD. (2007). Int J Radiat Oncol Biol Phys. 68: 839–844.

Huang SM, Li J, Armstrong EA, Harari PM. (2002). Cancer Res. 62(15): 4300–4306.

Hutter A, Schwetye K, Bierhals A, McKinstry R. (2003). Neuroimaging Clin Am N. 2: 237–250.

Iwamoto FM, Omuro AM, Raizer JJ, Nolan CP, Hormigo A, Lassman AB, Gavrilovic IT, Abrey LE. (2008). J Neurooncol. 87(1): 85–90.

Jeyapalan SA, Batchelor T. (2004). Curr Treat Options Neurol. 6(4): 273–284.

Korfel A, Oehm C, von Pawel J, Keppler U, Deppermann M, Kaubitsch S, Thiel E. (2002). Eur J Cancer. 38: 1724–1729.

Kouvaris JR, Miliadou A, Kouloulias VE, Kolokouris D, Balafouta MJ, Papacharalampous XN, Vlahos LJ. (2007). Onkologie. 30(7): 361–366.

Lin NU, Carey LA, Liu MC, Younger J, Come SE, Bullitt E, Van Den Abbeele AD, Li X, Hochberg FH, Winer EP. (2006). J Clin Oncol. 24(Suppl 18): 503a.

Langer CJ, Mehta MP. (2005). J Clin Oncol. 23:6207–6219.

Omuro AM, Raizer JJ, Demopoulos D, Malkin MG, Abrey LE. (2006). J Neurooncol. 78: 277–280.

Pace A, Vidiri A, Galiè E, Carosi M, Telera S, Cianciulli AM, Canalini P, Giannarelli D, JandoloB, Carapella CM. (2003). Ann Oncol. 14: 1722–1726.

Plowman J, Waud WR, Koutsoukos AD, Rubinstein LV, Moore TD, Grever MR. (1994). Cancer Res. 54(14): 3793–3799.

Postmus PE, Haaxma-Reiche H, Smit EF, Smit EF, Groen HJ, Karnicka H, Lewinski T, van Meerbeeck J, Clerico M, Gregor A, Curran D, Sahmoud T, Kirkpatrick A, Giaccone G. (2000). J Clin Oncol. 18: 3400–3408.

Rivera E, Meyers C, Groves M, Valero V, Francis D, Arun B, Broglio K, Yin G, Hortobagyi GN, Buchholz T. (2006). Cancer. 107: 1348–1354.

Robinet G, Thomas P, Breton Jl, Léna, HGouva S, Dabouis G, Bennouna J, Souquet PJ, Balmes P, Thiberville L, Fournel P, Quoix E, Riou R, Rebattu P, Pérol M, Paillotin D, Mornex F. (2001). Ann Oncol. 12: 59–67.

Rosner D, Nemoto T, Lane WW. (1986). Cancer. 58(4): 832–839.

Trudeau ME, Crump M, Charpentier D, Yelle L, Bordeleau L, Matthews S, Eisenhauer E. (2006). Ann Oncol. 17: 952–956.

Verger E, Gil M, Yaya R, Viñolas N, Villà S, Pujol T, Quintó L, Graus F. (2005). Int J Radiat Oncol Biol Phys. 61: 185–191.

Zimm S, Wampler GL, Stablein D, Hazra T, Young HF. (1981). Cancer. 48: 384–394.

163 Quality of Life Measures in Patients with Esophageal Cancer

R. Parameswaran · J. C. Clifton · J. M. Blazeby

	Key Summary	2796
1	*Introduction*	2797
2	*Methods*	2798
3	*Questionnaires*	2798
3.1	The EORTC QLQ-OES18	2798
3.2	The FACT-E	2799
3.3	The EORTC QLQ-OG25	2799
3.4	The EQOL	2800
3.5	Questionnaire Development and Item Reduction	2800
3.6	Psychometric Properties	2802
3.7	Questionnaire Content	2802
3.8	Scoring Systems	2802
3.9	Cross Cultural Application	2804
4	*Discussion*	2805
	Summary Points	2806
	Appendices	2806

Abstract: Assessment of ❷ health-related quality of life in patients undergoing treatment for esophageal cancer is important as the disease is debilitating, treatments frequently toxic, and often life expectancy is poor. Measures need to be accurate, reliable, valid, and patient centred in order to be of clinical value. The aim of this chapter is to identify, summarise and evaluate ❷ patient reported outcome measures for this population. Literature reviews were undertaken and English language instruments that were multi-dimensional with reported psychometric properties were evaluated. Four questionnaires fulfilled these criteria (EORTC QLQ-OES18, FACT-E, EORTC QLQ-OG25, EQOL). Of these, one was developed from a questionnaire designed for patients with head and neck cancer (FACT-E) and one targeted patients undergoing potentially curative treatment alone (EQOL). ❷ Item reduction was generally performed with patient survey and expert opinion. The EORTC questionnaires formally tested scaling assumptions. Detailed ❷ validity testing was reported for all instruments, although the new EORTC module for oesophageal and gastric tumours lacks data supporting responsiveness. One questionnaire, the EORTC QLQ-OES18, fulfilled guidelines for instrument development and evaluation as outlined by the Medical Outcomes Trust and has been developed and most thoroughly tested in all appropriate patient groups. Rigorous instrument development is important for creating tools that can be used to inform clinical decision-making. More work is needed in evaluating current tools for esophageal cancer, with head to head comparisons and qualitative research to understand patients' experiences of treatment and patient reported outcomes.

List of Abbreviations: *ACA*, adenocarcinoma; *EORTC*, European Organization for Research and Treatment of Cancer; *ECS*, Esophageal Cancer Subscale; *EQOL*, Esophageal Quality of Life Questionnaire; *FACIT*, Functional Assessment of Chronic Illness and Therapy; *FACT-E*, Esophageal Cancer Quality of Life Questionnaire; *HRQL*, Health-related quality of life; *IRT*, ❷ Item Response Theory; *MOS-SF36*, Medical Outcomes Study Quality of Life Questionnaire; *PRO*, Patient reported outcome; *PROM*, Patient reported outcome measure; *QLQ-OES18*, Quality of Life Questionnaire – Esophageal Cancer; *QLQ-OG25*, Quality of Life Questionnaire – Esophageal & Stomach Cancer; *QLQ-STO22*, Quality of Life Questionnaire – Stomach Cancer; *SCC*, squamous cell carcinoma

Key Summary

- There are four validated self-reported multi-dimensional questionnaires for patients with esophageal cancer, EORTC QLQ-OES18, FACT-E, EORTC QLQ-OG25, and EQOL. Psychometric properties supporting clinical sensitivity and validity are growing.
- The quality of the questionnaires is variable with respect to their development, validation and psychometric properties. The EORTC QLQ-OES18 meets more of the criteria for questionnaire development as outlined by the Medical Outcomes Trust. Deficits in item development (FACT-E) or clinical responsiveness (EORTC QLQ-OG25) or scaling properties (EQOL) were identified.
- Both the EORTC and the FACT systems are available in several languages and therefore may be used in international clinical trials.
- Currently the EORTC QLQ-OES18 is the most widely used site-specific tool, and it accompanies the core questionnaire, the EORTC QLQ-C30.
- Further work determining relative merits of these tools is required.

1   Introduction

Esophageal cancer is a serious condition with an overall poor prognosis. The epidemiology of this disease is changing and in western parts of the world there has been a significant increase in adenocarcinoma of the esophagus and esophago-gastric junction. In other parts of the world (e.g. parts of China, Iraq and South Africa), esophageal squamous cell cancer prevails. Although it is likely that these two cell subtypes have different aetiologies, the treatment and outcomes are generally similar. Treatments aimed at cure involve major surgery or combination chemotherapy and radiotherapy and are associated with significant morbidity and five-year survival of approximately 20 to 30% survival. However, there doesn't appear to be any statistically significant difference in survival time between the various treatment modalities that are currently available.

When treatment is palliative in intent, the main aim is to relieve dysphagia (swallowing difficulties) and the median survival is approximately four to six months. There are a host of single or combination treatments for esophageal cancer and although some high quality evidence about outcomes is accruing, there is a lack of detailed information about the impact of specific treatments on patients' health-related quality of life (HRQL). Accurate assessment of HRQL is important for patients with esophageal cancer because of the poor prognosis and associated treatment risks.

Health-related quality of life is defined as a multi-dimensional concept that includes measures of physical, social and emotional function and self-reported symptoms. Historically the phrase 'quality of life' was used to assess these outcomes, but more recently it is becoming accepted that within the medical context HRQL is a more precise term. Another key phrase that requires definition is 'Patient reported outcome' (PRO). A PRO is an assessment of any symptom or function that is reported by the patient themselves and not by an observer. A PRO may be single or multi-dimensional. A multi-dimensional PRO measure is therefore similar to an assessment of HRQL.

Patient reported outcomes compliment standard clinical outcomes by providing insight into patients' experiences of treatment and the disease. There is evidence that patients' views differ from those of health professionals and therefore the information may be used to inform patients of likely treatment outcomes and it may influence clinical decision-making. There is also evidence that self-reported assessment of HRQL is predictive of survival. This finding has been observed particularly in patients with advanced disease and several studies demonstrate the independent predictive value of physical function for survival in esophageal cancer (Blazeby et al., 2001, Chau et al., 2004). Due to the clinical importance of HRQL assessment, it is critical that measurement be accurate, valid, reliable and clinically relevant. Standard generic HRQL measures (e.g. MOS-SF36) may be used, but they lack specific and common symptoms that patients experience. Such measures may also suffer ❷ floor effects and therefore not be sensitive to deteriorations in HRQL. Tools designed for patients with any diagnosis of cancer (e.g. EORTC QLQ-C30 or FACIT) are very valuable and these two tools are both designed to be supplemented by disease specific tools that will capture problems related specifically to esophageal cancer (e.g. dysphagia and eating restrictions) (Cella et al., 1993, Aaronson et al., 1993). The aim of this chapter is to review the published measures available for assessment of HRQL specifically for cancer of the esophagus and esophago-gastric junction.

The chapter will include a synopsis of the development and validation process, psychometric properties of the questionnaires and a concise summary of content. Finally, this chapter will review the clinical literature and will report on outcomes using these questionnaires in order to identify their strengths, weaknesses and areas for future research.

2　Methods

A review of the literature was performed to find questionnaires that were specifically developed and validated to use in patients with esophageal and/or esophagogastric cancer. If an article contained no information about instrument development or validation it was not included in the review. Two or more authors examined each article. Questionnaires were appraised for their adherence to international guidelines for the development and validation of health outcomes questionnaires as outlined by the Scientific Advisory Committee of the Medical Outcomes Trust (Aaronson et al., 2002). Psychometric properties were examined, content domains included in each questionnaire were summarised.

3　Questionnaires

The review revealed that there are four PROMs (patient reported outcome measures) that have been formally developed and validated in an esophageal cancer population (Blazeby et al., 2003, Blazeby et al., 1996, Clifton et al., 2007, Darling et al., 2006, Lagergren et al., 2007). Two of these were developed by the Quality of Life Group of the European Organization for Research and Treatment of Cancer (EORTC), one by the Functional Assessment of Chronic Illness and Therapy (FACIT) group and the fourth by a thoracic surgical department in North America – the EQOL. This instrument was developed for patients only undergoing potentially curative treatment (including surgery alone, adjuvant chemoradiotheray plus surgery, or definitive chemoradiotherapy) and the other three measures were designed for all other types of patients with esophageal cancer, whether undergoing treatment aimed at cure or palliation.

3.1　The EORTC QLQ-OES18

The EORTC site-specific module for esophageal cancer was developed in a total of 164 patients from the UK, Sweden and Spain. Initial literature searches, interviews with patients and health professionals generated 46 potential HRQL issues. Item reduction after further patient interviews to a provisional 32-item questionnaire was undertaken and pre-testing in the three European countries (n = 132) produced the EORTC QLQ-OES24. This was conceptualised as containing six scales, dysphagia, deglutition, eating restrictions, reflux, pain, and emotional items and five single items. During development the wording was modified to be consistent with other EORTC questionnaires and the response categories used a four-point Likert type scale, from 'not at all' to 'very much' (Blazeby et al., 1996). The international validation study was separately undertaken in 491 patients and eight different countries (Blazeby et al., 2003). This reduced the module to 18 items in four scales: dysphagia, eating restrictions, reflux and pain. Internal consistency of the scales was moderate to high, the module assessed clinically distinct domains to the QLQ-C30 and it was sensitive to changes over time. Indeed four distinct groups of patients completed questionnaires at two times points: surgery (n = 95), definitive chemoradiation (n = 172), endoscopic palliation (n = 96) and palliative chemoradiotherapy (n = 126). This study, therefore, was a large and very detailed psychometric and clinical study. The questionnaire, however, was not tested for stability (test retest).

A literature search was undertaken to identify randomised clinical trials and prospective longitudinal studies that have used the QLQ-OES18 or its original version the QLQ-OES24 in evaluation of the treatment of esophageal cancer. This search has shown that the EORTC esophageal module is currently the most widely used esophageal cancer site-specific questionnaire (Power et al., 2007, Reynolds et al., 2006, Dallal et al., 2001, Homs et al., 2004, Homs et al., 2004, 2004, Bergquist et al., 2005, 2005, Avery et al., 2007, Lagergren et al., 2007, McLarty et al., 1997, Schmidt et al., 2004, Viklund et al., 2006). One large randomised trial compared self-expanding metal stents with brachytherapy for the palliation of esophageal cancer and found that relief of dysphagia (reported by the OES18 scale) was significantly prolonged after brachytherapy (Homs et al., 2004). In a prospective study of patients surviving three or more years after surgery for oesophageal cancer, persistent significant problems with reflux (OES18), physical function, diarrhoea and dyspnoea (QLQ-C30) were identified (Lagergren et al., 2007). Articles using the newer instruments are likely to be published in the next few years. But currently the EORTC modules are the most widely used in clinical trials and research into PROs in esophageal cancer.

3.2   The FACT-E

The FACT esophageal cancer subscale (ECS) was developed using an iterative process of item generation, item reduction, scale construction and initial psychometric evaluation (Darling et al., 2006). Items were initially generated from a disease specific instrument for patients with head and neck cancer. Further qualitative interviews with 11 patients with esophageal cancer reduced this and added new items producing a 17-item esophageal cancer specific scale. Seven patients evaluated the new questionnaire and confirmed the appropriateness of the changes and ease of completion of the questionnaire. An expert panel revised the module to be consistent with existing FACT subscales and 38 patients confirmed that questions were easy to understand and answer (no clinical details of these patients provided, including whether they had a diagnosis of cancer or indeed esophageal cancer). Cronbach's alpha for this scale was 0.86. The validation included testing convergent and divergent validity with the EORTC QLQ-OES24 (the earlier version of the QLQ-OES18), establishing internal consistency and stability, concurrent validity in clinical groups and responsiveness to change of the FACT-E over time with clinical changes. This was performed in two patient cohorts. Cohort A was surgical patients (n = 54) and cohort B, patients undergoing definitive chemoradiotherapy (n = 29). These patients therefore were all fit and none had distant metastatic disease. The total score of the ECS may be combined with the FACT-G score to create the total FACT-E score. The ECS contains two major domains that were created a priori, eating (3 items) and swallowing (5 items) indices. All FACT-E items are rated on a five-point Likert type scale. Items change between positively and negatively worded phrasing (similar to the FACT-G) and the scoring system accounts for this reverse wording. One study has been identified reporting clinical outcomes with the FACT-E (Brooks et al., 2002).

3.3   The EORTC QLQ-OG25

The QLQ-OG25 is the result of a study to combine the QLQ-OES18 (esophageal cancer) and the QLQ-STO22 (stomach cancer) questionnaires into one instrument for assessment of

HRQL of both curative and palliative treatment of tumors of the esophagus, esophagogastric junction and the stomach. The new OG25 combined items from the two previous questionnaires. Semi-structured interviews then took place to record patients' opinions of the items. New items were added to improve wording of existing items, as deemed necessary. Multi-trait scaling analysis was performed in the aggregation process and exploratory analysis with item response theory (IRT) was used to confirm that the most useful items were retained. The resulting OG25 is comprised of 25 items with six scales: dysphagia; eating restrictions; reflux; odynophagia; pain and discomfort; anxiety; and 10 single item questions. Three hundred patients from seven institutions in four countries participated in the validation study. Seventy-two percent had local or locally advanced disease. Median age was 63, 69% were male and 148 (49%) had esophageal cancer, 66 (22%) had cancer of the esophagogastric junction, and 86 (29%) had cancer of the stomach.

Validity was assessed using Pearson's product moment correlation between the core questionnaire (QLQ-C30) and the new combined questionnaire (QLQ-OG25). Most items had low correlation with the core questionnaire suggesting that the new module was assessing clinically distinct HRQL issues. In addition, statistically significant differences were noted between the patient tumor groups in three of the scales of the QLQ-OG25: pain and discomfort; problems with saliva; problems with speech. This new module is now available for use in eight major European languages.

3.4   The EQOL

The Esophageal Quality of Life questionnaire (EQOL), is a 15-item, seven-point Likert questionnaire that covers five major domains: physical function, activities of daily living, emotional function, social function and symptoms. Developed and validated in two phases, it uses standard methodology. The first phase generated 195 items (divided into five domains) based on patient interviews (n = 20), existing literature, and expert opinion (n = 5). Item reduction was undertaken with further patient interviews (n = 38) and impact scores were calculated. The provisional 15-item module was pre-tested for patient understanding (n = 5). The second phase of the questionnaire – validation – enrolled 65 patients and examined ❯ reliability, responsiveness, criterion and construct validity. The Global Ratings Questionnaire was used to determine if change had occurred (Juniper et al., 1996). Of this patient sample, 49 (75%) had esophageal adenocarcinoma, 88% (n = 57) were male, 7 were undergoing palliative treatment and 9 (14%) were undergoing definitive chemoradiotherapy. The remaining 49 underwent surgical treatment. All patients in the validation study were interviewed and completed the questionnaires before and after treatment. The final questionnaire was found to have test-retest reliability, be responsive to change over time (physical, social and symptom domains) and had four a priori clinical predictions confirmed. External criterion validation was established using the MOS SF20. Minimally important clinical differences were calculated for the five major domains. Currently there are no published literature reporting further outcomes using this questionnaire.

3.5   Questionnaire Development and Item Reduction

❯ *Table 163-1* summarises the development and validation of the questionnaires. Three of the measures described item generation based upon standard interviews with patients, health

◘ Table 163-1

Health-related quality of life instruments for esophageal cancer: development and validation criteria

Evaluation	EORTC QLQ-OES18	FACT-E	EORTC QLQ-OG25	EQOL
Item generation				
Patient interviews	Yes	Yes*	Yes	Yes
Literature search	Yes	No	Yes	Yes
Expert opinion	Yes	Yes*	Yes	Yes
Develop conceptual model	Yes	Yes	Yes	Yes
Item reduction				
Expert opinion	Yes	No	Yes	Yes
Item redundancy	Yes	Yes	Yes	Yes
Endorsement frequencies	Yes	No	Yes	Yes
Missing data	Yes	No	No	No
Factor analysis	No	No	No	No
Testing of scaling assumptions	Yes	No	Yes	No
Psychometric analyses				
Acceptability	Yes	No	Yes	Yes
Internal consistency reliability	Yes	Yes	Yes	No
Item total correlations	N/A	Yes	N/A	N/A
Inter-rater reliability	No	No	No	No
Test-retest reliability	No	Yes	No	Yes
Face validity	Yes	Yes	Yes	Yes
Validity: construct	Yes	Yes	Yes	Yes
Validity: comparison with other measures	Yes	Yes	Yes	Yes
Validity: within scale	Yes	Yes	Yes	No
Validity: Hypothesis testing	Yes	Yes	Yes	Yes
Responsiveness to clinical changes	Yes	Yes	No	Yes

• initial items in the FACT-E were derived from interviews with patients with head and neck cancer

• N/A not applicable

This table summarizes whether the HRQL instruments used in esophageal cancer adhered to the standard psychometric properties commonly utilised in the development and validation of questionnaires

professionals and literature review. The FACT-E was developed from the questionnaire originally designed for patients with head and neck cancer and from early developmental work with the FACT-G. To supplement this, a further 17 patients with esophageal cancer were interviewed about item content. The clinical and demographic details of this group of patients are not reported. The original lengthy list of items considered in all four measures were reduced by checking for redundancy and overlap and the EORTC questionnaires and the

EQOL were also shortened by asking expert opinion and surveying patients' views. The scaling in the EORTC questionnaires was tested with multi-trait scaling techniques and none of the questionnaires were scaled using factor analyses.

3.6 Psychometric Properties

Different approaches to the psychometric testing of each of the instruments have been reported (❯ *Table 163-1*). No inter-rater reliability testing was performed for any of the questionnaires. Both the FACT-E and the EQOL underwent test retesting. Validity was carefully examined and reported for all four measures, although the EORTC QLQ-OG25 questionnaire was not examined for responsiveness of change over time and the EQOL was only tested for patients undergoing potentially curative treatments.

3.7 Questionnaire Content

A detailed evaluation of the domains in each questionnaire is presented in ❯ *Table 163-2*. Assessment of dysphagia (trouble swallowing) is covered with several items in each questionnaire except for the EQOL which asks only a single item about solid food sticking. All questionnaires contain a variety of items assessing eating restrictions, but the FACT-E does not specifically address issues related to reflux disease and the EQOL does not assess pain. The EQOL has some generic HRQL items under physical and social well-being, however, these items are assessed specifically due to esophageal cancer. For example: *How limited have you been in the past two weeks because you are unable to participate in activities that require physical exertion, because of your esophageal cancer or its treatment?* It also contains two items related to anxiety about cancer recurrence and treatment. The EORTC QLQ-OG25 contains items addressing body image and hair loss that were not included in the QLQ-OES18. It should be noted that the EORTC questionnaires and the FACT-E are specifically designed to supplement the core instrument. The QLQ-C30 has some single symptom items that are common in patients with esophageal cancer including, appetite loss, diarrhoea and trouble breathing, therefore they are not repeated within either of these modules. Although the EQOL is not an official EORTC module, it was developed for use with the EORTC QLQ-C30. It is currently only available in one language.

3.8 Scoring Systems

Each of the questionnaire modules produce several scales and single item scores. These are summarised in ❯ *Table 163-3*. Both the FACT-E and EQOL yield total scale scores, whereas the EORTC scales are designed only to be reported in multi-dimensional scales and single items. The QLQ-OES18 has four scales and six single times and the FACT-E has two scales (dysphagia and eating) or it can be scored separately or as a summary score. The updated EORTC questionnaire has six scales and 10 single items and the EQOL has four scales. Because the EORTC and FACT-E modules are designed for use with the core questionnaire, the scales and single items in these modules reflect very specific problems associated with esophageal cancer, whereas the EQOL uses generic scales (physical, social, activities of daily living and symptoms) but designed specifically for esophageal cancer.

◘ Table 163-2

Health-related quality of life instruments for esophageal cancer: content analysis

Domains	EORTC QLQ-OES18	FACT-E	EORTC QLQ-OG25	EQOL
Dysphagia				
Eating solid food	Yes	Yes	Yes	Yes
Eating soft foods	Yes	Yes	Yes	No
Drinking liquids	Yes	Yes	Yes	No
Swallow easily	No	Yes	No	No
Deglutition				
Being able to swallow saliva	Yes	No	Yes	No
Choking when swallowing	Yes	Yes	Yes	No
Eating related items				
Enjoying meals	Yes	Yes	Yes	No
Troublesome eating	Yes	No	Yes	No
Trouble eating in front of others/ with family	Yes	Yes	Yes	Yes
Trouble with taste	Yes	No	Yes	No
Feeling full up too quickly	Yes	No	Yes	Yes
Having to eat smaller meals	No	Yes	No	Yes
Good appetite	No	Yes	No	No
Eating slowly	No	No	Yes	No
Eating foods that they like	No	Yes	No	No
Avoiding foods/drinks	No	No	No	Yes
Unable to eat sufficient food	No	No	No	Yes
Indigestion				
Trouble with indigestion	Yes	No	Yes	No
Trouble with acid or bile/ regurgitation	Yes	No	Yes	Yes
Burping	No	No	No	Yes
Elevate the head end of the bed	No	No	No	Yes
Pain				
Pain when eating	Yes	Yes	Yes	No
Chest pain	Yes	Yes	Yes	No
Abdominal pain	Yes	Yes	Yes	No
Other symptoms				
Having a dry mouth	Yes	Yes	Yes	No
Troublesome coughing	Yes	Yes	Yes	No
Loss of weight	No	Yes	Yes	No
Increased sensitivity to cold	No	No	No	Yes
Troublesome talking	Yes	Yes	Yes	No

◘ Table 163-2 (continued)

Domains	EORTC QLQ-OES18	FACT-E	EORTC QLQ-OG25	EQOL
Problems with voice quality	No	Yes	No	No
Trouble breathing	No	Yes	No	No
General HRQL				
Physical well being	No	No	No	Yes
Emotional well being	No	No	Yes	No
Fearful of unpleasant treatment	No	No	No	Yes
Social well being	No	No	No	Yes
Fearful of cancer recurrence	No	No	No	Yes
Body image				
Physical appearance	No	No	Yes	No
Anxiety due to hair loss	No	No	Yes	No

This table describes in detail the various content domains of the four questionnaires in esophageal cancer

◘ Table 163-3

Scales and summary scores in validated HRQL measures for esophageal cancer

Scales	EORTC QLQ-OES18	FACT-E	EORTC QLQ-OG25	EQOL
Dysphagia	Yes	Yes	Yes	No
Eating	Yes	Yes	Yes	Yes
Pain	Yes	No	Yes	No
Reflux	Yes	No	Yes	No
Pain swallowing (odynophagia)	No	No	Yes	No
Anxiety	No	No	Yes	No
Symptoms	No	No	No	Yes
Physical	No	No	No	Yes
Social	No	No	No	Yes
Activities of daily living	No	No	No	Yes
Overall score	No	Yes	No	Yes

This table is a summary of the scales and single item scores produced by each of the questionnaire modules

3.9 Cross Cultural Application

Both the EORTC and the FACT systems are available in several languages and therefore may be used in international clinical trials. Details of current language availability may be obtained from the respective websites (www.eortc.be, www.facit.org).

4   Discussion

This review has identified four multi-dimensional HRQL questionnaires for use in patients with esophageal cancer. The quality of the questionnaires is variable with respect to their development, validation and psychometric properties. The EORTC QLQ-OES18 meets more of the necessary criteria for questionnaire development. Deficits in item development (FACT-E) or clinical responsiveness (EORTC QLQ-OG25) or scaling properties (EQOL) were identified.

Questionnaire content is particularly important in site-specific modules, where disease or treatment symptoms are unique, may be very distressing, or are not by definition included in core instruments. The EORTC QLQ-OG25 covers more key content than the other modules and it is very similar to the EORTC QLQ-OES18. Key domains of reflux, difficulties talking (recurrent laryngeal nerve palsy), respiratory morbidity of eosphagectomy are covered and the new module has items assessing body image. Both the EORTC questionnaires were developed and tested in very large numbers of patients undergoing a wide variety of curative and palliative treatments. They have also been developed for international trials, with the original questionnaire being developed in parallel in three language groups (English, Spanish and Swedish). None, however, have been tested in patients undergoing minimal access surgery and it is possible that specific side effects of this treatment need further items.

One of the reasons why the EORTC Quality of Life Group proceeded to update the QLQ-OES18 questionnaire was because of the changing epidemiology of esophageal cancer. In western parts of the world, this is becoming predominantly adenocarcinoma and tumors of the esophago-gastric junction are increasing in incidence. This type of esophageal cancer has a marked male predominance, and different aetiological risk factors compared to esophageal squamous cell cancer. The FACT-E which originated from a questionnaire designed for patients with head and neck cancer (entirely of squamous cell origin), was subsequently further developed and validated in patients with esophageal cancer. Unfortunately the proportions of patients with the more common cell type are not described in the main validation data.

One of the important features of a questionnaire is its ability to detect changes over time. Questionnaires therefore need development and validation in patients receiving palliative as well as curative treatment. Even after potentially curative treatment, about 50% of patients develop recurrent disease within two years and there are currently no effective second line treatments. The lack of palliative patients is a potential disadvantage of the FACT-E and the EQOL, which were both developed and tested in relatively fit patients undergoing potentially curative – treatments (surgery or definitive chemoradiotheray, with maximum M1a disease). In the case of the EQOL, the objective was to develop an instrument which could be used to determine the quality of life associated with available curative treatment modalities in Canada.

They may therefore fail to detect important HRQL domains in patients deteriorating with disease recurrence and possibly suffer from floor effects. Likewise, there are currently no data demonstrating the responsiveness of the EORTC QLQ-OG25 to changes over time, although the majority of the scales and items in this questionnaire have been derived from the EORTC QLQ-OES18 and the QLQ-STO22, which have been shown to be responsive and sensitive to clinically significant changes in the validation papers and subsequently clinical trials (Blazeby et al., 2004).

Although the questionnaires identified in this review have been carefully developed, tested and some widely used, little is known about their role and value in everyday clinical practice. Clinicians interested in PROs are generally unfamiliar with the science behind their construction and may be confused by the multi-dimensionality of HRQL assessment, as well as the supporting tests that are used for psychometric analyses. The use of summary scores, or Trial Index scores is particularly attractive for clinicians and further work with Rasch models and Item Response Theory models may increase the clinical utility of questionnaires for individual patients. Although this has intuitive attractiveness, in clinical practice many treatments are designed to specifically improve one or maybe two HRQL domains (e.g. endoscopic palliation of malignant dysphagia) Overcoming barriers to using HRQL tools in clinical practice, may therefore be achieved by collaborations between clinicians, psychometricians, statisticians and social scientists so that appropriate valid tools can be chosen to address specific clinical hypotheses.

Summary Points

- Esophageal cancer is the seventh leading cause of cancer deaths worldwide.
- Esophageal cancer is composed of two main histological subtypes: adenocarcinoma (ACA) and squamous cell carcinoma (SCC). It is much more common in men than in women.
- Adenocarcinoma of the esophagus has the fastest growing incidence rate of all cancers in the United States. Unlike in the United States, squamous cell carcinoma is responsible for 95% of all esophageal cancer worldwide.
- Patients with esophageal cancer commonly present with dysphagia (difficulty swallowing), weight loss, pain in the epigastric or retrosternal area, hoarseness of voice and respiratory symptoms caused by aspiration of undigested food.
- The diagnosis of esophageal cancer is confirmed with upper gastrointestinal endoscopy and biopsy. Pre-treatment staging is performed with a combination of endoscopic ultrasonography (EUS), and thoracic and abdominal computed tomographic (CT) scanning.
- Treatments aimed at cure involve major surgery or combination chemotherapy and radiotherapy and are associated with significant morbidity and five-year survival of approximately 20 to 30%.
- Palliative treatment is reserved for those who are unsuitable for surgery. It comprises of a variety of treatments like chemotherapy, radiation therapy, laser therapy, photodynamic therapy and intubation of the esophagus using expandable stents. The median survival is approximately four to six months.

Appendices

1. EORTC-QLQ OES18*
2. EORTC-QLQ OG25*
3. EORTC-QLQ STO22*
4. EQOL
5. FACT-E**

 *Permission to use EORTC questionnaires must be obtained from the EORTC Quality of life Unit prior to using either questionnaire.

 **Permission to reprint the FACT-E questionnaire was provided by Dr. David Cella and www.facit.org. Use of the questionnaire must be cleared through the website directly.

 The appendix for this chapter is available as electronic supplementary material at 10.1007/978-0-387-39940-9_163 and accessible for authorised users.

References

Aaronson N, Alonso J, Burnam A, et al. (2002). Qual Life Res. 11: 193–205.

Aaronson NK, Ahmedzai S, Bergman B, et al. (1993). J Natl Cancer Inst. 85: 365–376.

Avery KN, Metcalfe C, Barham CP, Alderson D, Falk SJ, Blazeby JM. (2007). Br J Surg. 94: 1369–1376.

Bergquist H, Wenger U, Johnsson E, et al. (2005). Dis Esophagus. 18: 131–139.

Blazeby JM, Alderson D, Winstone K, et al. (1996). Euro J Cancer. 32: 1912–1917.

Blazeby JM, Brookes ST, Alderson D. (2001). Gut. 49: 227–230.

Blazeby JM, Conroy T, Bottomley A, et al. (2004). Eur J Cancer. 40: 2260–2268.

Blazeby JM, Conroy T, Hammerlid E, et al. (2003). Euro J Cancer. 39: 1384–1394.

Brooks JA, Kesler KA, Johnson CS, Ciaccia D, Brown JW. (2002). J Surg Oncol. 81: 185–194.

Cella DF, Tulsky DS, Gray G, et al. (1993). J Clin Oncol. 11: 570–579.

Chau I, Norman AR, Cunningham D, Waters JS, Oates J, Ross PJ. (2004). J Clin Oncol. 22: 2395–2403.

Clifton JC, Finley RJ, Gelfand G, et al. (2007). Dis Esophagus. 20: 191–201.

Dallal HJ, Smith GD, Grieve DC, Ghosh S, Penman ID, Palmer KR. (2001). Gastrointest. Endosc. 54: 549–557.

Darling G, Eton DT, Sulman J, Casson AG, Celia D. (2006). Cancer. 107: 854–863.

Homs MY, Essink-Bot ML, Borsboom GJ, Steyerberg EW, Siersema PD. (2004). Eur J Cancer. 40: 1862–1871.

Homs MY, Steyerberg EW, Eijkenboom WM, et al. (2004). Lancet. 364(9444): 1497–1504.

Homs MY, Wahab PJ, Kuipers EJ, et al. (2004). Gastrointest Endosc. 60: 695–702.

Juniper EF, Guyatt GH, Jaeschke R. (1996). How to develop and validate a new health-related quality of life instrument. In: Quality of Life and Pharmacoeconomics in Clinical Trials. Edited by Spilker. Lippincott-Raven Publishers, Philadelphia, 49–56.

Lagergren P, Avery KN, Hughes R, et al. (2007). Cancer. 110: 686–693.

Lagergren P, Fayers P, Conroy T, et al. (2007). Eur J Cancer. 43: 2066–2073.

McLarty AJ, Deschamps C, Trastek VF, Allen MS, Pairolero PC, Harmsen WS. (1997). Ann Thoracic Surg. 63: 1568–1572.

Power C, Byrne PJ, Lim K, et al. (2007). Dis Esophagus. 20: 466–470.

Reynolds JV, McLaughlin R, Moore J, Rowley S, Ravi N, Byrne PJ. (2006). Br J Surg. 93: 1084–1090.

Schmidt CE, Bestmann B, Kuchler T, Schmid A, Kremer B. (2004). World J Surg. 28: 355–360.

Viklund P, Wengstrom Y, Rouvelas I, Lindblad M, Lagergren J. (2006). Eur J Cancer. 42: 1407–1414.

164 Quality of Life Measures in Head and Neck Cancer

C. D. Llewellyn

1	*Introduction*	*2810*
1.1	Head and Neck Cancer (HNC)	2810
2	*Definitions of "Quality of Life" in the Head and Neck Literature*	*2811*
3	*Health-Related Quality of Life Measures*	*2813*
3.1	HNC Specific HR-QOL Measures	2813
4	*The Impact of HNC and Treatment on HR-QOL*	*2816*
4.1	Study Design	2816
4.2	Short-term Impact on HR-QOL (≤12 Months Post-treatment)	2817
4.2.1	Prospective Studies	2817
4.3	Long-term Impact on HR-QOL (>12 Months Post-treatment)	2817
4.3.1	Prospective Studies	2817
4.3.2	Cross-sectional Studies	2818
5	*HNC Patient's Priorities Regarding Treatment Outcomes and QOL*	*2819*
6	*Specific Factors to Impact on HR-QOL*	*2820*
6.1	Disease or Treatment Related Factors	2820
6.1.1	Cancer Site and Stage	2820
6.1.2	Treatment Modality	2821
6.1.3	Radiotherapy	2821
6.1.4	Radiotherapy Versus Surgery	2822
6.1.5	The Impact of Neck Dissection on HR-QOL	2822
6.2	Demographic Factors	2823
6.2.1	Gender	2823
6.2.2	Age	2823
6.2.3	Ethnicity/Cultural Factors	2824
6.2.4	Employment and Educational Level	2824
6.2.5	Marital Status	2824
7	*Limitations of QOL Research in HNC*	*2825*
8	*Conclusions*	*2825*
	Summary Points	*2826*

Abstract: Quality of life (QOL) is an important patient reported outcome (PRO) in head and neck cancer (HNC) where survival rates remain at approximately 50% overall. HNC specific ❷ Health Related Quality of Life (HR-QOL) instruments typically measure aspects of communication, swallowing, chewing, nutrition and cosmesis. Nine disease specific HR-QOL instruments have been published for patients with HNC focusing on a range of treatments and outcomes. Treatment for HNC results in medium term morbidity and depression, much of which has been shown to improve within 1 year. There is no clear evidence for the impact of disease and treatment on PROs such as QOL. The emotional sequelae and perception of physical limitations may be more important to the patient than the actual limitations resulting from HNC and treatment. This chapter highlights the insensitivity of general measures of HR-QOL to accurately illustrate HNC specific problems or treatment related effects. The majority of published studies do not interpret HR-QOL scores in terms of clinical relevance. Using a global or total score for examining effects of treatment induced change may not be appropriate for this patient group. Further research is needed into the potentially modifiable aspects of QOL or modifiable factors related to PROs in order to design appropriate interventions.

List of Abbreviations: *CARES-SF,* cancer rehabilitation evaluation system – short form; *CES-D,* the center for epidemiologic studies depression scale; *EORTC,* The European Organisation for Research into Treatment of Cancer; *EORTC QLQ-C30 & HN35,* The European Organisation for Research into Treatment of Cancer Quality of Life Questionnaire & Head and Neck Cancer specific module; *FACT-G,* the functional assessment of cancer therapy general scale; *FACT-HNS,* the functional assessment of cancer therapy head and neck scale; *GHQ,* general health questionnaire; *H&N,* head and neck; *HNC,* head and neck cancer; *HNRQ,* the head and neck radiotherapy questionnaire; *HNQOL,* The University of Michigan head and neck quality of life questionnaire; *HR-QOL,* health related quality of life; *ICD,* International Classification of Diseases; *N-status,* nodal status; *ND,* ❷ neck dissection; *PGI,* patient generated index; *PRO,* patient reported outcome; *PSSHN,* performance status scale for head & neck cancer; *QL-H&N,* the quality of life instrument for head and neck cancer; *QLQ,* the quality of life questionnaire for advanced head and neck cancer; *QOL,* quality of life; *QOL-RTI/H&N,* the quality of life – radiation therapy instrument/head and neck module; *RT,* radiotherapy; *SF-12,* short form health survey (12-item); *SF-36,* short form health survey (36-item); *T-stage,* tumor stage; *UW-QOL,* The University of Washington quality of life questionnaire; *WHO,* World Health Organisation

1 Introduction

1.1 Head and Neck Cancer (HNC)

Head and neck cancer (HNC) encompasses cancers arising in any part of the mouth, tongue, lips, throat, salivary glands, pharynx, larynx, sinus, and other sites located in the head and neck area (❷ *Table 164-1*). Approximately 7,500 new cases of HNC were diagnosed in the UK between 2002 and 2004 (Cancer Statistics, 2004; National Statistics Online, 2007; Welsh Cancer Intelligence and Surveillance Unit, 2005). There have been minimal improvements seen in survival rates for HNC, with 5 year relative survival rates at approximately 50% (Carvalho et al., 2005). Consequently, quality of life (QOL) has become an increasingly important patient reported outcome (PRO).

◘ Table 164-1

Anatomical sites (ICD-9/10 codes) commonly included as "head and neck cancer"

Group of anatomical sites	Specific cancer site	ICD-10 code	ICD-9 group codes
Mouth, lip and oral cavity	Lip	C00	140–141, 143–145
	Base of tongue	C01	
	Other and unspecified parts of tongue	C02	
	Gum	C03	
	Floor of mouth	C04	
	Palate	C05	
	Other and unspecified parts of mouth	C06	
Salivary glands	Parotid gland	C07	142
	Other and unspecified major salivary glands	C08	
Pharynx (throat)	Tonsil	C09	146–149
	Oropharynx	C10	
	Nasopharynx	C11	
	Piriform sinus	C12	
	Hypopharynx	C13	
	Other and ill-defined sites in the lip, oral cavity and pharynx	C14	
Nasal cavity, ear and sinuses	Nasal cavity and middle ear	C30	160
	Accessory sinuses	C31	
Larynx (voice box)	Larynx	C32	161
Thyroid	Thymus	C73	193

ICD-9 International Classification of Disease (9th Revision); *ICD-10* International Classification of Disease (10th Revision); *HNC* head and neck cancer
Head and neck cancer (HNC) is not a single entity. HNC commonly refers to a heterogenous group that includes many different types of disease. There are over 30 specific sub-sites (ICD-10 codes) encompassing HNC and cancer at each site is relatively uncommon

The main objectives of this chapter are to present to researchers and practitioners in the field of head and neck oncology the current state of QOL literature in HNC and to discuss some of the issues surrounding its definition, measurement and interpretation.

It is beyond the scope of this chapter to include details of every primary study, editorial, letter and commentary published to date in this vastly expanding field, however, a comprehensive list of review articles has been provided in ❯ *Table 164-2* which should help those requiring further information to orientate themselves through this overwhelming body of literature.

2 Definitions of "Quality of Life" in the Head and Neck Literature

There is wide variation in what is meant by QOL. The World Health Organisation (WHO) has defined a high QOL as a "state of complete physical, mental and social well-being and not

◻ Table 164-2

Summary of articles reviewing primary literature on quality of life in head and neck cancer (1980–2007)

Author and year	Inclusion period	Patient population	Number of studies reviewed in article	Aim of review
Gotay and Moore (1992)	1980–1990	Head and neck cancer	N = 29. Only N = 18 documented QOL in specific patient population	A review of the definitions of QOL used in HNC studies, how QOL has been measured and how QOL data has been used in treatment
Dropkin (1998)	1996–1997	Head and neck cancer	N = 4	A review of four studies in relation to purpose, QOL definition and measurement, findings and implications to otorhinolaryngology nursing
De Boer et al. (1999)	1984–1996	Head and neck cancer	N = 50	A review of the physical and psychosocial correlates of HNC
Terrell (1999)	–	Head and neck cancer	N = 25	Reviews definitions and principles of QOL assessment, identifies QOL instruments and summarizes a selection of studies
Rogers et al. (1999a)	1980–1997	Oral and oropharyngeal cancer	N = 65	Comprehensive summary of the concepts of QOL evaluation, review of studies and outline of QOL measures
List and Stracks (2000)	1998–1999	Head and neck cancer	N = 34	Brief review of QOL in HNC with a focus on research and methodological developments
Ringash and Bezjak (2001)	1966–1999	Head and neck cancer	N = 8 HNC specific QOL instruments	A critical review of HNC specific HR-QOL instruments. Not a literature review as such
Schwartz et al. (2001)	1989–1999	Head and neck cancer	N = 61	A review of quality of life outcomes in the evaluation of HNC treatments. Includes comments on the use of terminology and study designs
Llewellyn et al. (2005)	1980–2003	Head and neck cancer	N = 16	Systematic review of studies investigating psycho-social or behavioral factors associated with QOL

◘ Table 164-2 (continued)

Author and year	Inclusion period	Patient population	Number of studies reviewed in article	Aim of review
Ledeboer et al. (2005)	1996–2003	Head and neck cancer	N = 87	A literature review of effects of disease and treatment, patient related factors and psychosocial interventions on QOL
Rogers et al. (2007)	2000–2005	Head and neck cancer	N = 154	The identification of papers reporting self-completed QOL outcomes

QOL quality of life; HNC head and neck cancer; HR-QOL health related quality of life
Articles published between 1980 and 2007 that describe and appraise peer-reviewed primary studies on quality of life in head and neck cancer patients, but do not present original data themselves

merely the absence of disease or infirmity." Assessing global QOL generally provides a broader picture of the impact of disease on an individual's life. In clinical practice, however, QOL generally refers to health-related quality-of-life (HR-QOL) which seeks to examine aspects of QOL thought to be impacted by a health or medical concern. Assessment of HR-QOL typically includes physical, psychological and social domains. Each domain may include measures that assess the patient's perception of symptoms, ability to function and disability, therefore, measures of purely functional status are not considered here.

3 Health-Related Quality of Life Measures

As it is accepted that "HR-QOL" is a broad, multi-dimensional concept, a number of questionnaires have been developed that reflect this complex conceptual framework. There are four main categories of questionnaire that are commonly applied to assess the HR-QOL of HNC patients, performance questionnaires aside: generic, cancer specific, HNC specific or individualized. Examples of studies using such measures are shown in ❷ Table 164-3.

Global or generic questionnaires can be applied to patients with any disease or a "normal" population and assess physical, psychological and social functioning. General cancer questionnaires focus on common symptoms and side-effects of cancer treatments. A review of general and cancer specific QOL measures is not within the scope of this chapter. HNC specific HR-QOL questionnaires are intended to assess the specific impact of HNC and its treatment on an individual's HR-QOL, which may include aspects of communication, swallowing, chewing, nutrition and cosmesis.

3.1 HNC Specific HR-QOL Measures

Nine *disease specific* HR-QOL instruments have been published for patients with HNC (❷ Table 164-4), with varying strengths and weaknesses. Studies assessing the ❷ psychometric properties of some of these instruments are still ongoing. The measures are discussed in chronological order.

◻ Table 164-3

Quality of life instruments used in research with head and neck cancer patients

Type of instrument	Example of instrument	Example of studies using instrument
Generic HR-QOL	Short Form Health Survey (SF-36/12) (Ware and Sherbourne, 1992; Ware et al., 1996)	Hammerlid and Taft (2001); Hjermstad and Fayers (1998a, b); Llewellyn et al. (2006)
	General Health Questionnaire (GHQ) (Goldberg and Williams, 1988)	Bjordal and Kaasa (1995); Morton and Witterick (1995)
Cancer Specific HR-QOL	The European Organisation for Research and Treatment of Cancer (EORTC) core questionnaire (Aaronson et al., 1993)	Allison et al. (1998); Pourel et al. (2002)
	The Functional Assessment of Cancer Therapy Scale (FACT-G) (Cella et al., 1993)	Long et al. (1996); Sehlen et al. (2002)
Head and neck cancer specific	The University of Washington Quality of Life Questionnaire (UW-QOL) (Hassan and Weymuller, 1993)	Deleyiannis et al. (1999); Lloyd et al. (2003); Rogers et al. (1999b)
	The European Organisation for Research into Treatment of Cancer Quality of Life Questionnaire for Head and Neck Cancer (EORTC QLQ-C30/HN35) (Bjordal et al., 1994a)	Bjordal et al. (2001); de Graeff et al. (2000); Hammerlid and Taft (2001)
Individualized	Patient Generated Index (PGI) (Ruta et al., 1999)	Llewellyn et al. (2006)

HR-QOL health related quality of life
Examples of commonly used instruments to measure quality of life in head and neck cancer. Generic health related quality of life instruments assess general aspects of HR-QOL that are applicable to any disease or health conditions, whereas, disease specific instruments assess the particular concerns and conditions related to that particular disease or health state. Individualized measures are also generic, however, they allow for the individual to state which areas of life they are impaired in and to rate accordingly

The *Quality of Life Questionnaire for Advanced Head and Neck Cancer* (QLQ), (Rathmell et al., 1991) was designed to ❷ discriminate between advanced stage HNC patients who have both surgery and radiotherapy and those who undergo radiation treatment only. Nineteen items cover four domains of physical, functional/mood, psychological and attitude to treatment. No reliability data and minimal validity has been established for this instrument and some of the item wording and general instructions may introduce bias.

The *Head and Neck Radiotherapy Questionnaire* (HNRQ), (Browman et al., 1993) was developed to measure radiation induced acute morbidity and HR-QOL in patients with locally advanced HNC. The interviewer administered scale consists of 22 items from six domains – skin, throat, oral stomatitis, digestion, energy and psychosocial aspects. An unspecified number of oncologists, nurses and patients generated the items and reduction was judged by health care workers. Content and face validity are lacking and the content of the questionnaire is mainly focused on physical symptoms rather than the patient's HR-QOL.

The *University of Washington Quality of Life Questionnaire* (UW-QOL), (Hassan and Weymuller, 1993) was developed to discriminate between a variety of HNC sites and stages.

◻ Table 164-4
List of head and neck cancer specific quality of life instruments developed in chronological order

References	Instrument
Rathmell et al. (1991)	The *Quality of Life Questionnaire for Advanced Head and Neck Cancer* (QLQ)
Browman et al. (1993)	The *Head and Neck Radiotherapy Questionnaire* (HNRQ)
Hassan and Weymuller (1993)	The *University of Washington Quality of Life Questionnaire* (UW-QOL)
Bjordal et al. (1994a)	The *European Organisation for Research into Treatment of Cancer Quality of Life Questionnaire for Head and Neck Cancer* (EORTC QLQ-C30/H&N35)
Morton and Witterick (1995)	The *Quality of Life Instrument for Head and Neck Cancer* (QL-H&N)
Lish et al. (1996)	The *Functional Assessment of Cancer Therapy- Head and Neck* (FACT-H&N)
Terrell et al. (1997)	The *University of Michigan Head and Neck Quality of Life* (HNQOL)
Trotti et al. (1998)	*Quality of Life – Radiation Therapy Instrument Head and Neck Module* (QOL-RTI/H&N)
Taylor et al. (2002)	The *Neck Dissection Impairment Index (NDII)*

List of measures developed to specifically assess quality of life amongst head and neck cancer patients with author details

The original self-administered questionnaire consists of 12 items: nine disease-specific items (pain, chewing, swallowing, speech, shoulder disability, appearance, activity, recreation and employment) in addition to three items measuring, global HR-QOL, change in HR-QOL since diagnosis and overall QOL. It is not known whether patients were involved with the item generation. ❯ Test-retest reliability is reported as very high with an acceptable ❯ internal consistency (Hassan and Weymuller, 1993). ❯ Responsiveness to change has also been reported (Deleyiannis et al., 1997). Since the original publication, this well used measure has seen several modifications and updated versions have been subsequently reported.

The *European Organisation for Research into Treatment of Cancer Quality of Life Questionnaire for Head and Neck Cancer* (EORTC QLQ-C30/H&N35), (Bjordal et al., 1994a), is a patient based, self-administered and multidimensional core and specific HR-QOL instrument developed across many cultural and language groups. The H&N module (H&N35) consists of 35 items from seven domains: pain; swallowing; senses; speech; social eating; social contact; and sexuality, in addition to 11 single items (e.g., problems with teeth and mouth, sticky saliva, weight and use of painkillers). This extensive questionnaire demonstrated reliability, validity and internal consistency in a trial of 500 patients (Bjordal et al., 1999), however, the social eating and speech domains did not show adequate reliability in this study. Responsiveness to change over time was seen in most domains, except for domains of social contact and single items assessing dry mouth, mouth opening, sticky saliva and feeling ill. Issues such as shoulder functioning and acute skin reactions to radiotherapy are not included.

The *Quality of Life Instrument for Head and Neck Cancer* (QL-H&N), (Morton and Witterick, 1995) is a short self-administered 29-item questionnaire with physical, social and psychological domains, however, a number of key issues for HNC patients have been overlooked. The psychometric properties of this instrument are difficult to establish since the entire version has not been published.

The *Functional Assessment of Cancer Therapy-Head and Neck* (FACT-H&N) version 3 (Cella, 1994) is a multidimensional, self-administered instrument consisting of 27 items from four core domains – physical, social/family, emotional and functional (FACT-G), plus a 12 item HNC symptom subscale. Original item generation was based on 15 HNC patients and five "experts." Item importance was determined by clinicians. Reliability and ❷ concurrent validity were found to be acceptable in this short questionnaire (D'Antonio et al., 1996; List et al., 1996) and responsiveness to change has also been demonstrated (D'Antonio et al., 1996).

The *University of Michigan Head and Neck Quality of Life* questionnaire (HNQOL), (Terrell et al., 1997) is an interviewer administered questionnaire consisting of 21 items from four domains – pain, emotion, communication and eating. Patients and health care workers generated the items. Face and content validity have been found to be moderate (Ringash and Bezjak, 2001) although the authors of the instrument advise that it is used in conjunction with a general HR-QOL instrument. Test-retest reliability and internal consistency were reported to be high (Terrell et al, 1997). ❷ Construct validity and ❷ convergent validity were also adequate. The newer 20-item version is undergoing testing.

The *Quality of Life – Radiation Therapy Instrument Head and Neck Module* (QOL-RTI/H&N), (Trotti et al., 1998) is intended to evaluate HR-QOL specifically in HNC patients undergoing radiotherapy. The self-administered questionnaire contains 25 items from four domains – functional, emotional, family/socio-economic and general, plus 14 items in the H&N module. Patients were not involved with item generation. Good internal consistency and test-retest reliability have been established (Trotti et al, 1998).

The *Neck Dissection Impairment Index* (NDII) (Taylor et al., 2002) is a 10-item self-report instrument to identify factors that affect HR-QOL in HNC patients following neck dissections. The measure was derived from a ❷ convenience sample of 54 patients who had undergone neck dissections 11–120 months previously and essentially measures degree of shoulder functioning. The measure demonstrated test-retest, internal consistency and convergent validity within this sample.

4 The Impact of HNC and Treatment on HR-QOL

4.1 Study Design

In clinical research, HR-QOL is recognized as an important endpoint, as changes in treatment policy are aimed not only at maximizing chances of survival, but also maintaining QOL (and possibly improving it) during treatment and long-term. Three basic types of study have been employed in HNC HR-QOL research: cross-sectional, prospective and case-control. ❷ Cross-sectional studies provide a snapshot evaluation from a specific time period but may have reduced sensitivity due to patient under-reporting. More importantly, without pre-treatment data, specific HR-QOL cannot be directly attributed to the effects of disease and treatment. Longitudinal (prospective) studies allow for the analyses of the impact of treatment, although selection bias is created due to loss of patients over the study period because of recurrent illness and death. ❷ Case-control studies allow for a comparison between the HR-QOL of the sample under study and another population, for example, another clinical sample or normative data.

In the past, the majority of published studies in this field were cross-sectional in design, but in the last few years the majority are now prospective. However, there have been very few studies published that have used control groups or ❷ randomized treatment groups.

4.2 Short-term Impact on HR-QOL ($\leqslant$ 12 Months Post-treatment)

4.2.1 Prospective Studies

Unsurprisingly, the majority of studies have found a temporary deterioration in HR-QOL in the first 3 months after treatment (de Graeff et al., 1999; Deleyiannis et al., 1997; Hammerlid and Taft, 2001; Kohda et al., 2005; List et al., 1999; Lloyd et al., 2003; Rogers et al., 1998, 2000), particularly in domains of physical and role functioning, probably caused by treatment itself. However, in the 12 months following treatment, the results are less consistent. In a study of 105 HNC patients, despite improvements in some physical functioning domains 1 month into recovery from treatment, patients still reported a decline from 1 month to 12 months in the domain of marital and sexual functioning and no significant improvement in other HR-QOL domains (as measured by the Cancer Rehabilitation Evaluation System- Short Form (CARES-SF)) (Gritz et al., 1999). These results highlight that, even with functional improvement, HR-QOL is impacted in other ways and for a significant time period after treatment. However, baseline (pre-treatment) levels of HR-QOL were not presented and it is unknown whether there were any significant differences between baseline HR-QOL and scores at 1 and 12 months. Functional status reflecting normal activity (as measured by the Karnofsky Performance Scale) was reached within 12 months (Gritz et al, 1999). The findings of this particular study contrast with several previous reports that indicate a gradual improvement in HR-QOL within the same time frame, in primary radiotherapy patients and with surgically treated patients (De Boer et al., 1995).

Paradoxically, despite the initial decline in *physical* aspects of HR-QOL, pain, mood and anxiety scores (UW-QOL) have been shown to significantly improve with surgical patients, at all post-operative time points (up to 12 months) compared to pre-operative scores (Lloyd et al., 2003) and similarly, with emotional functioning (EORTC QLQ-C30 & HN35) (Bjordal et al., 2001).

4.3 Long-term Impact on HR-QOL (>12 Months Post-treatment)

4.3.1 Prospective Studies

Until relatively recently, no prospective studies had been published with a follow-up of more than 1 year. However, several studies have now been reported with follow-up data of 2 and 3 years. For example, de Graeff et al. (2000) conducted a 3-year prospective study of 107 patients with mixed site HNC treated with surgery and/or radiotherapy. It was found that the majority of HR-QOL domains, (as measured by the EORTC QLQ-C30 & HN35), had returned to pre-treatment levels after 12 months with little change afterwards. However, at 36 months, domains of: physical functioning, taste/smell, dry mouth and sticky saliva were still significantly worse compared with baseline. The authors conclude that the magnitude of these differences was indicative of minor/moderate clinically relevant changes. Despite the longer-term deterioration of several physical symptoms and functioning scales, a gradual improvement of emotional functioning and depression (as measured with the CES-D) was reported.

A similar pattern was also reported in a 2 year ❯ longitudinal study of 201 HNC patients (Morton, 2003). Overall QOL (as measured by a modified 10 item version of the Life Satisfaction scale (Morton and Witterick, 1995) improved significantly from time of diagnosis to 24 months, although there was no significant difference between 12 and 24 months. Psychological distress (as measured by the GHQ-12) was significantly increased at 3 months but returned to at least pre-treatment levels by 12 and 24 months. However, all 201 patients at baseline were included in analyses when only 91 had completed questionnaires at 2 years. An analysis of these 91 patients demonstrated that only global QOL (life-satisfaction) was significantly better at 2 years and psychological distress was not. Amongst patients with cancer of the supraglottis and glottis, there was more difficulty speaking at 2 years post-diagnosis but not amongst patients with oral/oropharyngeal cancer. Many other mean scores of single item measures of somatic and physical dysfunction were found to increase over the 24 months follow-up.

4.3.2   Cross-sectional Studies

Cross-sectional studies have allowed the exploration of HR-QOL over longer time periods since treatment. Patients treated with primary surgery are considered to have poor physical and psychological outcomes as a result of surgery, however, advances in microvascular free tissue transfer has reduced the extent of physical deformity. Rogers et al. (1999b) conducted a cross-sectional study comparing 38 patients (out of an original cohort of 220 patients) treated 5–10 years after primary surgery for oral and oro-pharyngeal cancer, with 25 patients treated a year previously (Rogers et al., 1999b). The results at 1 year were similar to longer-term (5–10 year) survivors, suggesting that most of the longer term gain is achievable within 1 year. Indeed, UW-QOL scores in the longer-term group were better than at 1 year in all domains except shoulder function. This may have been due to the tendency towards radical neck dissection as compared to the function preserving neck dissections favored more recently. Despite the overall good level of functioning, it was found that a significant number of patients continued to experience severe problems, particularly in domains of: disfigurement, emotional and cognitive functions and chewing related functions (e.g., dry mouth, sticky saliva and trouble eating). Half of the longer-term survivors reported the use of painkillers in the last week. However it is not known whether this was specifically related to head and neck pain or not.

Several other survivor studies have demonstrated the long-term emotional effects of cancer and treatment. A European radiation therapy trial conducted between 1979 and 1984 randomly assigned 845 HNC patients into two radiotherapy schedules. The trial demonstrated no difference in survival or ❯ late effects of treatment between the study arms. However, 7–11 years later, a cross-sectional study of the HR-QOL of more than 200 of the trial survivors showed that emotional and social function were both adversely affected long-term if surgery was conducted as part of treatment (Bjordal et al., 1994b). Long-term psychological distress (using the GHQ) was also reported in 30% of the same cohort (Bjordal and Kaasa, 1995). This distress was found to be more pronounced in those with impaired cognitive function, impaired social function and pain. Pourel et al. (2002) reported similar results in a study of 113 patients at 2–9 years post-treatment (Pourel et al., 2002). Compared with the general population, the three scores indicating the most impaired HR-QOL (EORTC-QLQ-C30) were emotional and social functioning and fatigue. In addition, the physical functioning, role functioning and pain scores did not significantly differ from the general population.

One cross-sectional study compared the results from HNC patients 2 and 3 years post-diagnosis with general population norms (Hammerlid and Taft, 2001). The Swedish version of the SF-36 Health Survey and the EORTC QLQ-C30 & HN35 were used to examine how long term survivors of HNC 3 years after diagnosis ($n = 151$) compared with age and gender matched or adjusted norms of Swedish and Norwegian populations (Hjermstad and Fayers, 1998a, b). Comparison of the SF-36 demonstrated that only the role-physical functioning domain was significantly worse in the HNC patients compared to the population sample, although clinically worse for domains of role physical functioning and role-emotional functioning. A gender difference was noticed, whereby female HNC patients ($n = 42$) scored the same or better than the female reference group on all eight SF-36 domains. However, for males, an opposite pattern was found whereby the population sample scored better than the HNC patients ($n = 93$) on seven of the eight domains. A comparison of the EORTC QLQ-HN35 showed that HNC patients scored significantly worse compared to the population on all scales and single items except for coughing and feeling ill.

This study demonstrates that the general health status of long-term survivors is comparable or even better than age and gender matched normative populations. However, despite this, patients still report significant problems with more specific functions such as, social eating, pain and swallowing, 3 years after diagnosis. This highlights the importance of measuring HR-QOL with specific as well as generic questionnaires in order to elicit a more accurate picture of long standing problems. However, these results also illustrate that despite still having specific limitations; patients show functional adaptation both physically and emotionally over time.

Although these cross-sectional studies cannot provide any pre-treatment comparison data to test for causal relationships, they suggest that the emotional and social consequences of HNC to survivors remain even after a substantial time has elapsed since treatment.

5 HNC Patient's Priorities Regarding Treatment Outcomes and QOL

Despite the surfeit of publications measuring HR-QOL within this patient group, little has been published regarding patient priorities in terms of treatment outcomes or QOL. The crude effects of different treatment regimens on patients functioning is well recognized, therefore, patients can be more adequately informed as to the likely effects of treatment. Not much is known, however, as to how patients make treatment decisions when faced with the probabilities of survival versus likelihood of serious morbidity.

In an early innovative "trade-off" study involving healthy participants (McNeil et al., 1981), it was found that people were willing to "trade-off" years of life in order to retain normal vocal function, after being educated about the effects of having a laryngectomy. However, none were willing to trade off more than 5 years survival. Although this study was influential in suggesting that for some people quality of life was preferable to quantity of life, it is questionable whether one can extrapolate healthy patients priorities, using a standard gamble technique, to the priorities one would actually have when faced with laryngeal cancer.

More recently, a few studies have sought to examine patients' preferences among treatment effects. List et al. (2000), examined newly diagnosed, advanced stage HNC patients' pre-treatment preferences for a series of possible late stage effects of treatment (List et al., 2000). Results indicated that at this time point, survival was unsurprisingly top priority amongst patients. This data is consistent with newly diagnosed patients' willingness to accept highly toxic treatment with risk of chronic dysfunction for any chance of benefit (Slevin et al., 1990).

Studies of HR-QOL outcome typically focus on speech, swallowing and other functions that are affected, but the results by List et al. (2000) demonstrate that items relating to energy levels and normal activities were more frequently ranked in the top three considerations than items of appearance, chewing and being understood, irrespective of treatment. However, being newly diagnosed, patients had not yet experienced the morbidity in question and patient priorities may well change over time and with experience.

In a study reporting patients' importance ratings of HR-QOL longitudinally, Rogers et al. (2002) found that both pre- ($n = 48$) and post-treatment ($n = 35$) there was little correlation between importance rating and actual HR-QOL domain score (Rogers et al., 2002), thus indicating that patients do not necessarily rate their current functional limitation as being most important. This finding is supported by Deleyiannis et al. (1999), who reported that following laryngectomy the severity of functional disability did not correlate with its importance (Deleyiannis et al., 1999). At all time points (baseline, 6 and 12 months), patients tended to rate speech, chewing and swallowing as more important than other HR-QOL domains (as measured by the UW-QOL).

One recent study reported comparative data between individualized quality of life scores (as measured by the PGI) and standard measures of HR-QOL (EORTC QLQ-C30 and SF-12) (Llewellyn et al., 2006). The PGI allows for the assessment of an overall QOL score and also for the free expression of top priorities for the patient. Measures were found to be correlated as expected, however, the individualized measure tended to correlate with emotional, cognitive and mental health domains of the generalized HR-QOL and not physical, or pain related domains, indicating that these domains my be more important to the patient over more physical aspects. One limitation of this study is that it does not report the particular domains that were rated as most important to HNC patients.

Further prospective studies may help to identify whether particular functional problems associated with treatment are more amenable to adaptation than others and to what extent and why priorities change over time.

6   Specific Factors to Impact on HR-QOL

6.1   Disease or Treatment Related Factors

6.1.1   Cancer Site and Stage

Cancer site and stage are often interrelated, with patients with carcinoma of the hypopharynx, nasopharynx and oropharynx more likely to present with advanced stage of disease. Advanced disease in HNC has been reported as associated with poorer pre-treatment HR-QOL (Hammerlid et al., 2001) and a worse initial post-treatment decline in HR-QOL (Bjordal et al., 2001; Weymuller et al., 2000) with no return to baseline HR-QOL after 24 months (Weymuller et al., 2000). Similarly, a cross-sectional study of 60 patients with oropharyngeal cancer (Allal et al., 2003) found that tumor size was important when examining the effects of treatment. In patients with smaller tumors (T1-T2), there was no significant difference in HR-QOL between RT and surgical/RT treatment groups, whereas with larger tumor sizes (T3-T4) patients having undergone surgery/RT had significantly worse HR-QOL. In addition, the time since treatment for the surgical patients was much longer than that of the RT group. However, no multivariate analyses were conducted on these data and it was not known whether stage corresponded with tumor size in these patients as nodal involvement was not reported. Other studies also provide support for the finding that patients with later stage tumors have significantly worse HR-QOL than those with smaller tumors (Hammerlid et al., 2001; Rogers et al., 2000). However, similar to Allal et al. (2003), significant treatment effects were also reported and not controlled for. In contrast, the results from a cross-sectional study of 135 HNC patients showed that stage at presentation did not differentiate HR-QOL 3 years after treatment (Hammerlid and Taft, 2001). It is worth noting that tumor staging used in studies may differ, with respect to whether details of nodal involvement is known, which may influence the treatment and therefore resulting HR-QOL. Indeed, results from a longitudinal study of 91 HNC patients Morton (2003), found that nodal status (N-status) was significantly associated with a single-item measure of overall QOL and several single HR-QOL items such as head and neck pain and difficulty swallowing, whereas tumor size (T-stage) was not. T-stage, however, was positively correlated with a measure of psychiatric distress (GHQ). The inconsistency in the literature regarding the role of cancer stage or tumor size is further confounded by the results from a 3-year prospective study (de Graeff et al., 2000). In a multivariate analyses of 107 HNC patients, subgroup (oral/ oropharynx vs. larynx), stage of cancer and treatment were found to have significant effects on HR-QOL, particularly head and neck symptoms (EORTC HN35). Interestingly, these clinical factors were associated with physical symptoms but not with any psycho-social functioning or depressive symptoms.

The differences in HR-QOL due to tumor site are well reported in the literature with different tumor sites affecting different aspects of HR-QOL. Patients with pharyngeal cancer tend to have the most functional problems, followed by oral cancer then laryngeal cancer (Bjordal et al., 2001; Hammerlid et al., 2001). This is in line with the tendency for these cancers to be diagnosed at different stages. At 1 year post-treatment, patients with pharyngeal cancer reported clinically worse scores compared with patients with laryngeal or oral cancer on many HR-QOL domains, most of which related to swallowing and nutrition (Bjordal et al., 2001).

6.1.2 Treatment Modality

Choice of treatment is often dependent on the site and stage of disease, therefore, it is often not possible to disentangle treatment effects from disease related effects. However, studies have shown that there are specific consequences to HR-QOL as a result of different types of treatment.

6.1.3 Radiotherapy

Radiotherapy (RT) patients mainly report xerostomia (dry mouth) and related difficulties, namely problems with chewing and swallowing food, recurrent infections, mucositis, increased incidence of dental caries and sometimes problems with speech (Epstein et al., 1999). The majority of RT patients note a decrease in the amount of saliva or a change in its consistency. Studies have shown that long-term xerostomia has a more detrimental effect on QOL than voice function, which is often considered worse (Stoeckli et al., 2001).

Henson et al. (2001) and Lin et al. (2003) both conducted prospective, 12-month longitudinal studies examining whether the preservation of saliva post RT to the neck region resulted in better xerostomia-related QOL. Results were similar between the two studies (Henson et al., 2001; Lin et al., 2003). Key findings were the strong relationships demonstrated between all HNQOL domains and patient reported xerostomia, and the effect of time on xerostomia-related QOL.

The findings suggest that despite parotid sparing RT, salivary flow rates and HR-QOL decrease at the completion of RT but both improve over the following 12 months.

6.1.4   Radiotherapy Versus Surgery

Many of the major functional deficits commonly resulting from surgery have been alleviated by microsurgical reconstructive techniques. However, patients still face a certain amount of morbidity following surgery. Some of the issues more pertinent to surgical treatment are; difficulties with appearance, speech, swallowing, chewing, oral rehabilitation, nutrition and shoulder function.

Compared to surgery with or without post-operative RT, it has been suggested that non-surgical treatments are associated with superior functional outcomes in oral cancer. A recent cross-sectional study of 60 patients treated for oropharyngeal cancer with either RT (with or without chemotherapy) ($n = 40$) or surgery and post-operative RT ($n = 20$) provides support for this assertion (Allal et al., 2003). Using the Performance Status Scale for Head & Neck Cancer (PSSHN) (List et al., 1996), Allal et al. (2003) found significant group differences for the understandability of speech domain but not for other PSSHN domains or any functional domains of the EORTC QLQ-C30. However, when the patients were divided into two groups based on tumor size (T1/2 vs. T3/4), significant differences emerged. Patients with larger tumors (T3/4) who had undergone surgery, showed significantly worse scores on the PSSHN for; eating in public, understandability of speech and normalcy of diet than those with larger tumors who had non-surgical treatment. In addition, the T3/4 surgical group reported significantly more pain than the T3/4 RT group. However, patients with smaller tumors treated surgically, had significantly better scores for social functioning (EORTC QLQ-C30) than RT patients.

As before, it is also interesting to note that the time since treatment for these surgical patients was much longer than that of the RT group. Although multivariate analyses were not conducted, these results suggest there may also be important time considerations when comparing the HR-QOL between treatment groups. For example, high dose radiotherapy is associated with late toxic effects, therefore, depending on the timing of HR-QOL measurements, RT patients may still be experiencing serious side-effects of treatment. At a similar time point, surgical patients may be entering their recovery phase. Evidence suggests, however, that after 1 year, RT alone produces functionally superior results and better HR-QOL.

6.1.5   The Impact of Neck Dissection on HR-QOL

Neck dissection (ND) is often needed in the management of the HNC patient. Known complications and morbidities after ND often include numbness and/or pain in the neck or ear, shoulder and neck discomfort, functional problems with the arm and shoulder and lower lip weakness. Preservation of the spinal accessory nerve (i.e., selective ND) has been found to be associated with better HR-QOL in the few studies that have reported the impact of ND on HR-QOL.

In a cross-sectional study, Terrell et al. (2000) found that the spinal accessory nerve status (type of ND), HR-QOL emotion score, as measured by the HNQOL (Terrell et al., 1999), and time since treatment, were all independent predictors of HNQOL "shoulder or neck" pain score in 175 HNC patients (Terrell et al., 2000). This indicated that those who had a selective

ND, better HR-QOL emotion scores and surgery over 2 years previously, were less likely to score highly for "shoulder/neck" pain. Kuntz and Weymuller (1999), analyzed data from 84 HNC patients who had undergone ND and had completed a pre-treatment and 6 and 12 month post-treatment UW-QOL "shoulder domain." They also found that radical ND was associated with worse pain scores after treatment. There was a significant improvement in pain over time with selective ND only. However, it was also found that improvement in pain was also associated with T1–T3 tumors. Multivariate analysis was not performed.

6.2   Demographic Factors

6.2.1   Gender

Data from studies investigating the influence of gender on HR-QOL are conflicting. Some studies report no gender differences at any stage of assessment (Morton, 2003; Rogers et al. 1998) whereas others suggest females report worse symptoms and physical functioning (De Boer et al., 1995; de Graeff et al., 2000) and worse emotional functioning over time than males (Hammerlid et al., 2001).

Conversely, results from a longitudinal study using a normative population sample ($n = 871$) for comparison purposes, found that females 3 years after diagnosis scored the same or better than males on all domains of the SF-36 compared to an age and gender matched sample (Hammerlid and Taft, 2001). Comparisons between HNC patients only ($n = 135$) showed that females scored better than males on all scales except mental health. Although many of the gender differences in domains were clinically significant (physical, role physical, general health, vitality and role emotional), none proved statistically significant. Moreover, regression analyses with gender, age, disease stage, tumor site, treatment modality and number of co-morbidities as predictor variables, indicated that gender did not explain a significant proportion of the variance in any SF-36 domain (Hammerlid and Taft, 2001).

6.2.2   Age

Similarly to gender, the influence of age on HR-QOL is also not consistent in the literature. Studies have reported that age has no influence on HR-QOL except on physical functioning (de Graeff et al., 2000). A recent study comparing the HR-QOL of 54 elderly (≥ 70 years) and 75 younger patients (45–60 years) with HNC after surgery, supports this finding (Derks et al., 2003). The groups proved significantly different for gender, site, co-morbidities, Karnofsky performance status, radiotherapy and alcohol and tobacco use, with older patients scoring worse for co-morbidity and performance status. There was no age difference in tumor stage. Despite this, no significant differences were found in HR-QOL (EORTC QLQ-C30 & HN35) or depression (CES-D) between the younger and older samples both before and 3 months after surgery, controlling for tumor site.

Paradoxically, older patients (>75 years) have been reported at diagnosis as having clinically better HR-QOL scores on emotional functioning than younger patients despite having worse scores for domains reflecting physical functioning and symptoms. Significant correlations between increasing age and better social and emotional functioning have also been reported by (Hammerlid et al., 2001). However, these were all based on univariate analyses.

6.2.3 Ethnicity/Cultural Factors

Few studies have reported the effects of ethnicity on the HR-QOL of HNC patients. A recent cross-sectional study by Morton (2003) attempted to compare the HR-QOL in two geographically separate and culturally distinct populations. The 45 pairs of patients recruited from Canada and New Zealand were largely Caucasian and matched for age, gender, primary site, T and N stage and overall cancer stage. Psychological distress (GHQ-12) and country of residence were found to account for more than 40% of the variance in global QOL (life satisfaction) Morton (2003). Although there were treatment differences between the groups, these did not appear to contribute to overall QOL on multivariate analysis, with patients from Canada having worse HR-QOL than patients from New Zealand. The only other cross-cultural data on the HR-QOL of HNC patients was supplied from Europe as a result of a large-scale validation study of the EORTC QLQ-HN35 (Bjordal et al., 1999, 2000). Although baseline differences in HR-QOL were found between patients from Norway, Sweden and The Netherlands, any variation was attributed to differences between patients (site, stage and performance status). Further research is required in this area.

6.2.4 Employment and Educational Level

Employment status and educational level of the patient are rarely analyzed in relation to HR-QOL in this patient group but in the few papers that have, results are conflicting. No relationship was found between educational level (high school diploma or less vs. higher level) and HR-QOL (FACT-G & HNS, UW-QOL and PSS subscales of eating in public, speech and normalcy of diet) with multivariate analyses of a cross-sectional sample of 50 HNC patients up to 6 years post-surgery (Long et al., 1996). However, a prospective study (Sehlen et al., 2002) of 83 HNC patients 6 weeks after radiotherapy, found that five socio-demographic variables (having no children, a low secondary education, being unemployed, male, and abusing ethanol) could predict a quarter of the variance in HR-QOL (FACT-G). It was also emphasized that only socio-demographic variables could predict HR-QOL and not the various clinical and treatment related factors that were also analyzed.

Four studies highlight the relationship between poorer HR-QOL and unemployment. Allison et al. (1998) demonstrated that a range of clinical and socio-demographic factors could explain global HR-QOL (EORTC QLQ-C30) in a cross-sectional study of 188 post-treatment HNC patients. A multivariate model including clinical (dentate, stage and site) and socio-demographic factors (unemployment, age and gender) was found to explain a fifth of the variance in HR-QOL. The three strongest predictors of HR-QOL were unemployment, age and gender.

6.2.5 Marital Status

Long et al. (1996) found that married patients and those living with someone else had higher HR-QOL (using the FACT-G but not with the FACT-HNS or UW-QOL). However, Allison et al. (1998) failed to find a significant relationship between living arrangements (living alone vs. living with others) and HR-QOL, although the mean global QOL score was higher for those living with someone rather than living alone.

7 Limitations of QOL Research in HNC

Great variability in HR-QOL has been demonstrated with HNC patients. The minority of research studies to date have been longitudinal in design and very few have explicitly tested hypotheses. Potential biases within the data are likely to have been uniform across studies, namely, unavoidable selection bias for treatment decisions, since randomization is rarely feasible or ethical. In addition, variation in HR-QOL may be accounted for by the heterogeneous samples often included in analyses, in terms of site, stage and treatment modality. Although many studies do not have the statistical power for sub-analyses by site, stage or treatment modality, multivariate analyses have rarely been attempted in order to control for the effect of other variables on HR-QOL. When stratification by site, stage and treatment is carried out, the resultant small sample numbers do not achieve enough statistical power to allow for accurate between-groups comparisons. This is especially problematic for the longitudinal analyses of advanced stage tumors, where 40–50% of patients do not survive for 2-year follow-up (Weymuller et al., 2000). The small number of survivors after several years makes Type 2 statistical errors more likely when comparing groups. In addition, it is likely that those who drop-out are more at risk of poor HR-QOL.

Although particular types of HNC have been grouped together for analyses because they have been considered sufficiently homogenous, the question of whether they are homogenous in terms of HR-QOL has never been explored.

This review highlights the insensitivity of general measures of HR-QOL (for example, the EORTC-QLQ-C30 or SF-36) to accurately illustrate long-term H&N specific problems or treatment related effects. Many studies that have failed to find differences between treatment groups or site/stage of cancer have frequently used general measures of HR-QOL. Many studies have also not interpreted HR-QOL scores in terms of clinical relevance.

Weymuller et al. (2000) have reported the problems when examining global HR-QOL scores only, particularly when assessing the impact of treatment. The functional changes created by different treatment modalities affect different domains and this causes a cancellation effect when examining total scores only. Therefore, using a global or total score for examining effects of treatment induced change in HR-QOL may not be appropriate.

8 Conclusions

Treatment for HNC results in medium term morbidity and depression, much of which has been shown to improve within 1 year. In the long-term, despite an initially high level of depression, there is a gradual improvement in psychological functioning and global QOL over the next few years. However, there is subgroup of patients who continue to experience high levels of psychological morbidity years after treatment and it is important to note that this has been shown not to be wholly related to physical functioning.

Although a patient's characteristics are clearly important, there is no clear evidence for the impact of disease and treatment on outcomes such as QOL and many studies have reported that somatic symptoms and scores of dysfunction are not associated with emotional distress or QOL either.

Authors in the field are beginning to acknowledge that an individual's QOL is probably determined more by their perceptions of the disease than the disease itself and adaptational processes may be responsible for distorted interpretations of changes in QOL over time.

To date there has been little attempt to explain these discrepancies in QOL and although factors such as stage, site of disease and type of treatment, have some impact on HR-QOL, it is unclear what additional factors account for the large variation evidenced in ❷ patient-reported outcomes (PROs).

More recently, interest has been generated in the area of psychological factors (although most commonly the influence of depressive symptoms) to account for variation in HR-QOL. By understanding the relationship between HR-QOL and potentially modifiable patient factors, such as psychological factors, interventions could be designed with the aim of maximizing a patient's long-term QOL.

Summary Points

- QOL is an important patient reported outcome (PRO) in head and neck cancer (HNC) where survival rates remain at approximately 50% overall.
- HNC specific HR-QOL instruments typically measure aspects of communication, swallowing, chewing, nutrition and cosmesis.
- Nine disease specific HR-QOL instruments have been published for patients with HNC focusing on a range of treatments and outcomes.
- Treatment for HNC results in medium term morbidity and depression, much of which has been shown to improve within 1 year.
- There is no clear evidence for the impact of disease and treatment on PROs such as QOL.
- The emotional sequelae and perception of physical limitations may be more important to the patient than the actual limitations resulting from HNC and treatment.
- The review highlights the insensitivity of general measures of HR-QOL to accurately illustrate HNC specific problems or treatment related effects.
- The majority of studies do not interpret HR-QOL scores in terms of clinical relevance.
- Using a global or total score for examining effects of treatment induced change may not be appropriate for this patient group.
- Further research is needed into the potentially modifiable aspects of QOL or modifiable factors related to PROs in order to design appropriate interventions.

References

Aaronson NK, Ahmedzai S, Bergman B, Bullinger M, Cull A, Duez NJ, Filiberti A, Flechtner H, Fleishman SB, de Haes JCJM, Kaasa S, Klee M, Osaba D, Razavi D, Rofe PB, Schraub S, Sneeuw K, Sullivan M, Takeda F. (1993). J Natl Cancer Inst. 85: 365–376.

Allal AS, Nicoucar K, Mach N, Dulguerov P. (2003). Head Neck. 25: 833–840.

Allison PJ, Locker D, Wood-Dauphinee S, Black M, Feine JS. (1998). Qual Life Res. 7:713–722.

Bjordal K, Ahlner-Elmqvist M, Hammerlid E, Boysen M, Evensen JF, Biorklund A, Jannert M, Westin T, Kaasa S. (2001). Laryngoscope. 111: 1440–1452.

Bjordal K, Ahlner-Elmqvist M, Tollesson E, Jensen AB, Razavi D, Maher EJ, Kaasa S. (1994a). Acta Oncol. 33: 879–885.

Bjordal K, de Graeff A, Fayers PM, Hammerlid E, van Pottelsberghe C, Curran D, Ahlner-Elmqvist M, Maher EJ, Meyza JW, Brédart A, Söderholm AL, Arraras JJ, Feine JS, Abendstein H, Morton RP, Pignon T, Huguenin P, Bottomly A, Kaasa S. (2000). Eur J Cancer. 36: 1796–1807.

Bjordal K, Hammerlid E, Ahlner-Elmqvist M, de Graeff A, Boysen M, Evensen JF, Biorklund A, de Leeuw RJ, Fayers PM, Jannert M, Westin T, Kaasa S. (1999). J Clin Oncol. 17: 1008–1019.

Bjordal K, Kaasa S. (1995). Brit J Cancer. 71: 592–597.

Bjordal K, Kaasa S, Mastekaasa A. (1994b). Int J Radiat Oncol. 28: 847–856.

Browman GP, Levine MN, Hodson DI, Sathya J, Russell R, Skingley P, Cripps C, Eapen L, Girard A. (1993). J Clin Oncol. 11: 863–872.

Cancer Statistics. (2004). Registrations of cancer diagnosed in 2004, England. Series MB1, (Rep. No. 35). HMSO, London.

Carvalho AL, Nishimoto IN, Califano JA, Kowalski LP. (2005). Int J Cancer. 114: 806–816.

Cella DF. (1994). Manual for the Functional Assessment of Cancer Therapy (FACT) Measurement system Rush Medical Center, Chicago.

Cella DF, Tulsky DS, Gray G, Sarafian B, Linn E, Bonomi A, Silberman M, Yellen SB, Winicour P, Brannon J. (1993). J Clin Oncol. 11: 570–579.

D'Antonio LL, Zimmerman GJ, Cella DF, Long SA. (1996). Arch Otolaryngol. 122: 482–487.

De Boer MF, McCormick LK, Pruyn JF, Ryckman RM, van den Borne BW. (1999). Otolaryng Head Neck. 120: 427–436.

De Boer MF, Pruyn JFA, Van den BB, Knegt PP, Ryckman RM, Verwoerd CDA. (1995). Head Neck. 17: 503–515.

de Graeff A, de Leeuw JR, Ros WJ, Hordijk GJ, Blijham GH, Winnubst JA. (1999). Oral Oncol. 35: 27–32.

de Graeff A, de Leeuw JR, Ros WJ, Hordijk GJ, Blijham GH, Winnubst JA. (2000). Laryngoscope. 110: 98–106.

Deleyiannis FW, Weymuller EA Jr, Coltrera MD, Futran N. (1999). Head Neck. 21: 319–324.

Deleyiannis FWB, Weymuller EA, Coltrera MD. (1997). Head Neck. 19: 466–473.

Derks W, de Leeuw JR, Hordijk G, Winnubst JA. (2003). Clin Otolaryngol All. 28: 399–405.

Dropkin MJ. (1998). ORL Head Neck Nurs. 16: 22–23.

Epstein JB, Emerton S, Kolbinson DA, Le ND, Phillips N, Stevenson-Moore P, Osoba D. (1999). Head Neck. 21: 1–11.

Goldberg D, Williams P. (1988). A user's guide to the General Health Questionnaire. NFER-NELSON Publishing Company Ltd, Windsor, Berkshire.

Gotay CC, Moore TD. (1992). Qual Life Res. 1: 5–17.

Gritz E, Carmack C, de Moor C, Coscarelli A, Schacherer C, Meyers E, Abemayor E. (1999). J Clin Oncol. 17: 352–360.

Hammerlid E, Bjordal K, Ahlner-Elmqvist M, Boysen M, Evensen JF, Biorklund A, Jannert M, Kaasa S, Sullivan M, Westin T. (2001). Laryngoscope. 111: 669–680.

Hammerlid E, Taft C. (2001). Br J Cancer. 84: 149–156.

Hassan SJ, Weymuller EA Jr. (1993). Head Neck. 15: 485–496.

Henson BS, Inglehart MR, Eisbruch A, Ship JA. (2001). Oral Oncol. 37: 84–93.

Hjermstad M, Fayers P. (1998a). J Clin Oncol. 16: 1188–1196.

Hjermstad M, Fayers P. (1998b). Eur J Cancer. 34: 1381–1389.

Kohda R, Otsubo T, Kuwakado Y, Tanaka K, Kitahara T, Yoshimura K, Mimura M. (2005). Psychooncol. 14: 331–336.

Kuntz AL, Weymuller EA Jr. (1999) Larynygoscope. 109:1334–1338.

Ledeboer QCP, van der Velden LA, De Boer MF, Feenstra L, Pruyn JFA. (2005). Clin Otolaryngol. 30: 303–319.

Lin A, Hyungjin MK, Terrell JE, Dawson LA, Ship JA, Eisbruch A. (2003). Int J Radiat Oncol. 57: 61–70.

List MA, D'Antonio LL, Cella DF, Siston A, Mumby P, Haraf D, Vokes E. (1996). Cancer. 77: 2294–2301.

List MA, Siston A, Haraf D, Schumm P, Kies M, Stenson K, Vokes EE. (1999). J Clin Oncol. 17: 1020–1028.

List MA, Stracks J. (2000). Curr Opin Oncol. 12: 215–220.

List MA, Stracks J, Colangelo L, Butler P, Ganzenko N, Lundy D, Sullivan P, Haraf D, Kies M, Goodwin W, Vokes EE. (2000). J Clin Oncol. 18: 877–884.

Llewellyn CD, McGurk M, Weinman J. (2005). Oral Oncol. 41: 440–454.

Llewellyn CD, McGurk M, Weinman J. (2006). Brit J Oral Max Surg. 44: 351–357.

Lloyd S, Devesa-Martinez P, Howard DJ, Lund VJ. (2003). Clin Otolaryngol. 28: 524–532.

Long SA, D'Antonio LL, Robinson EB, Zimmerman G, Petti G, Chonkich G. (1996). Laryngoscope. 106: t-8.

McNeil BJ, Weichselbaum R, Pauker SG. (1981). New Engl J Med. 305: 982–987.

Morton RP. (2003). Laryngoscope. 113: 1091–1103.

Morton RP, Witterick IJ. (1995). Am J Otolaryngol. 16: 284–293.

National Statistics Online. (2007). Cancer Incidence and mortality in the UK 2002–2004, office for National Statistics (ONS), United Kingdom.

Pourel N, Peiffert D, Lartigau E, Desandes E, Luporsi E, Conroy T. (2002). Int J Radiat Oncol. 54: 742–751.

Rathmell AJ, Ash DV, Howes M, Nicholls J. (1991). Clin Oncol. 3: 10–16.

Ringash J, Bezjak A. (2001). Head Neck. 23: 201–213.

Rogers SN, Ahad SA, Murphy AP. (2007). Oral Oncol. 43: 843–868.

Rogers SN, Fisher SE, Woolgar JA. (1999a). Int J Oral Max Surg. 28: 99–117.

Rogers SN, Hannah L, Lowe D, Magennis P. (1999b). J Cranio Maxillofac Surg. 27: 187–191.

Rogers SN, Laher SH, Overend L, Lowe D. (2002). J Cranio Maxillofac Surg. 30: 125–132.

Rogers SN, Lowe D, Brown JS, Vaughan ED. (1998). Oral Oncol. 34: 361–372.

Rogers SN, Lowe D, Humphris G. (2000). Oral Oncol. 36: 529–538.

Ruta D, Garratt A, Russell I. (1999). Qual Health Care. 8: 22–29.

Schwartz S, Patrick DL, Yueh B. (2001). Arch Otolaryngol. 127: 673–678.

Sehlen S, Hollenhorst H, Lenk M, Schymura B, Herschbach P, Aydemir U, Duhmke E. (2002). Int J Radiat Oncol. 52: 779–783.

Slevin ML, Stubbs L, Plant HJ. (1990). BMJ. 300: 1458–1460.

Stoeckli SJ, Guidicelli M, Schneider A, Huber A, Schmid S. (2001). Eur Arch Oto-Rhino-Laryngol. 258: 96–99.

Taylor RJ, Chepeha JC, Teknos TN, Bradford CR, Sharma PK, Terrell JE, Hogikyan ND, Wolf GT, Chepeha DB. (2002). Arch Otolaryngol. 128: 44–49.

Terrell JE. (1999). Hematol Oncol Clin North Am. 13: 849–865.

Terrell JE, Nanavati K, Esclamado RM, Bradford CR, Wolf GT. (1999). Otolaryngol Head Neck. 120: 852–859.

Terrell JE, Nanavati KA, Esclamado RM, Bishop JK, Bradford CR, Wolf GT. (1997). Arch Otolaryngol. 123: 1125–1132.

Terrell JE, Welsh DE, Bradford CR, Chepeha DB, Esclamado RM, Hogikyan ND, Wolf GT. (2000). Laryngoscope. 110: 620–626.

Trotti A, Johnson DJ, Gwede C, Casey L, Sauder B, Cantor A, Pearlman J. (1998). Int J Radiat Oncol. 42: 257–261.

Ware JE, Kosinski M, Keller SD. (1996). Med Care. 34: 220–233.

Ware JE, Sherbourne DC. (1992). Med Care. 30: 473–483.

Welsh Cancer Intelligence and Surveillance Unit. (2005). Publication SA6/02 Cancer Incidence in Wales 2001–2005.

Weymuller EA Jr, Yueh B, Deleyiannis FW, Kuntz AL, Alsarraf R, Coltrera MD. (2000). Laryngoscope. 110: t-7.

165 Quality of Life in Breast Cancer Patients: An Overview of the Literature

A. Montazeri

1	*Introduction*	*2830*
2	*The Past*	*2831*
2.1	Two Historical Papers	2831
2.2	Reviews	2831
3	*Measurement*	*2834*
3.1	Instruments Used	2834
3.2	Validation Studies	2834
4	*Treatments*	*2836*
4.1	Surgical Treatment	2836
4.2	Systemic Therapies	2838
4.2.1	Examples from Early Studies	2838
4.2.2	Recent Studies	2838
5	*Quality of Life as Predictor of Survival*	*2842*
5.1	In Early-Stage Disease	2842
5.2	In Metastatic Patients	2842
5.3	Partial Relationship	2842
6	*Distress*	*2842*
6.1	Psychological Distress	2842
6.2	Symptoms	2846
6.3	Sexual Functioning	2849
7	*The Future*	*2849*
	Summary Points	*2849*
	Appendix	*2850*
	Some Key Facts About Breast Cancer	*2850*
	Breast Cancer Treatment Options	*2851*

Abstract: Quality of life in patients with breast cancer is an important outcome. This chapter presents an overview of the literature on the topic ranging from descriptive findings to clinical trials. There is quite an extensive body of the literature on quality of life in breast cancer patients. Studies on quality of life in breast cancer have made a considerable contribution in improving breast cancer care, although their exact benefit is hard to define. Quality of life data in breast cancer patients provided scientific evidence for clinical decision-making and conveyed helpful information concerning breast cancer patients' experiences during the course of the disease diagnosis, treatment, disease-free survival time, and recurrences; otherwise finding solutions for evidence-based selection of optimal treatments, psychosocial interventions, patient–physician communications, allocation of resources, and indicating research priorities were impossible. More qualitative research is needed for a better understanding of the topic. In addition, issues related to the disease, its treatment side effects and symptoms, and sexual functioning should receive more attention when studying quality of life in breast cancer patients.

List of Abbreviations: *A*, doxorubcin; *ALND*, axillary lymph node dissection; *ANA*, anastrozole; *BCPT-BESS*, breast cancer prevention trial eight symptom scale; *BCPT-SCL*, BCPT symptom checklist; *BCQ*, breast cancer chemotherapy questionnaire; *BCS*, breast conservation surgery; *BI*, body image; *BIBCQ*, body image after breast cancer questionnaire; *C*, cyclophosphamide; *CTCb*, cyclophosphamide, thiotepa, and carboplatin; *DPPE*, tesmilifene; *E*, epirubcin; *EORTC QLQ-BR23*, European Organization for Research and Treatment of Cancer breast cancer specific quality of life questionnaire; *EXE*, exemestane; *F*, 5-fluorouracil; *FACT-B*, functional assessment of cancer therapy breast cancer specific questionnaire; *FACT-B+4*, impact of arm morbidity subscale for FACT-B; *FACT-B-plus ES*, an endocrine symptom subscale for the FACT-B; *FACT-G*, functional assessment of cancer therapy-general; *FSAQ*, Fallowfield's sexual activity questionnaire; *FU*, future perspective; *G-CSF*, granulocyte colony stimulating factor; *HADS*, hospital anxiety and depression scale; *LASA*, linear analogue self-assessment; *LSQ-32*, life satisfaction questionnaire; *M*, methotrexate; *MAS*, mastectomy; *MRM*, modified radical mastectomy; *PTSD*, post-traumatic distress disorder; *QLACS*, quality of life in adult cancer survivors; *QOL*, quality of life; *RSC*, Rotterdam symptom checklist; *SEE*, sexual enjoyment; *SEF*, sexual functioning; *SF-36*, medical outcomes study short form survey; *SLDS-BC*, satisfaction with life domains scale for breast cancer; *SNLB*, sentinel lymph node biopsy; *T*, docetaxel; *TAM*, tamoxifen

1   Introduction

Health-related quality of life is now considered an important endpoint in cancer clinical trials. It has been shown that assessing quality of life in cancer patients could contribute to improved treatment and could even be as prognostic as medical factors (Montazeri et al., 1996a; 1996b; Montazeri et al., 2001). Among the quality of life studies in cancer patients, breast cancer has received most attention for several reasons. First, the number of women with breast cancer is increasing. It has been reported that each year over 1.1 million women worldwide are diagnosed with breast cancer and 410,000 die from the disease (Stewart and Paul Kleihues, 2003). Secondly, early detection and treatment of breast cancer have improved and survivors now live longer, so studying quality of life in this context is important. Thirdly, breast cancer affects women's identities and therefore studying quality of life for those who lose their breasts is vital. In addition, it is believed that females play important roles as partners, wives, and mothers within any family. Thus, when a woman develops breast cancer, all members of family might develop some sort of illnesses. In fact, breast cancer is a family disease. Other reasons could be added, but overall it is crucial to recognize that with increasing improvements in medicine and medical practice during recent years, studying quality of life for any cancer, for any anatomical site, and for either gender is considered highly relevant. A descriptive study of the published papers (230 articles) on non-biomedical outcomes (quality of life, preferences, satisfaction, and economics) in breast cancer patients, covering the literature from 1990–2000, found that the most frequently reported outcomes were health-related quality of life (54%), followed by economic analyses (38%), and patient satisfaction (14%). Only 9% measured patient preferences (Mandelblatt et al., 2004).

Over the past 10 years, much clinical effort has been expended in the treatment of breast cancer in order to improve survival. So the question is: to what extent have quality of life studies in breast cancer patients added to our information or contributed to improved outcomes in breast cancer care? This is very difficult to answer, but it is possible to try to investigate the contribution of quality of life studies to breast cancer care as a whole. The aim of this review is to give an outline of the most important findings, since the topic first appeared in English language biomedical journals. It is hoped that this may contribute to existing knowledge, help both researchers, and clinicians to have a better profile of the topic, and consequently aid in improving quality of life in breast cancer patients.

2 The Past

2.1 Two Historical Papers

The first paper on quality of life in breast cancer patients was published in 1974. In this historical paper, advanced breast cancer patients receiving adrenalectomy with chemotherapy were assessed for objective and subjective response rates, survival, and quality of life. The results showed that in 64% of the patients the subjective palliation involved a return to essentially normal living during the period of improvement (Moore et al., 1974). The second historical paper on the topic appeared 2 years later. Priestman and Baum (1976) used a linear analogue self-assessment (LASA) to measure the subjective effects of treatment in women with advanced breast cancer. The results showed that this technique might be used to monitor the subjective benefit of treatment and to compare the subjective toxicities of different therapeutic regimens. The results also suggested that the subjective toxicity of cytotoxic therapy was not related to the patient's age and diminished with successive courses of drugs. However, not until the late 1980s and early 1990s was the literature gradually supplemented with papers using relatively standard and established instruments to measure quality of life in breast cancer patients.

2.2 Reviews

There are a number of review papers about quality of life in breast cancer patients. However, a few systematic reviews with limited objectives exist on the topic. These are summarized in ❷ *Table 165-1*.

◻ Table 165-1

A list of systematic reviews on different aspects of quality of life in breast cancer patients

Author(s) (Year)	Main focus	Conclusion(s)
Irwig and Bennetts (1997)	A systematic review of quality of life after breast conservation or mastectomy	Apart body image it is unclear whether breast conservation or mastectomy results in better psychosocial outcomes
Bottomley and Therasse (2002)	Systemic therapy (chemotherapy, hormonal therapy, or biological therapy) in advanced breast cancer (1995–2001)	QOL data provide invaluable insights into the treatment and care of patients
Shimozuma et al. (2002)	Systematic overview of the literature (1982–1999)	To date there have been almost no appropriate systematic overviews or guidelines issued for QOL assessment studies related to breast cancer
Goodwin et al. (2003)	Randomized clinical trials of treatment (review of literature from 1980 to 2001)	Until results of ongoing trials in breast cancer are available, caution is recommended in initiating new QOL studies unless treatment equivalency is expected or unless unique or specific issues can be addressed
Rietman et al. (2003)	Late morbidity of breast cancer (review of literature from 1980 to 2000)	Significant relationship between late morbidity and restrictions of daily activities and poorer QOL was reported
Payne et al. (2003)	Racial disparities in the palliative care for African-American (review of literature from 1985 to 2000)	Differences in treatment patterns, pain management, and hospice care exist between African-American and other ethnic groups
Fossati et al. (2004)	Randomized clinical trials of cytotoxic or hormonal treatments in advanced breast cancer (review of published literature before Dec 2003)	QOL assessments added relatively little value to classical clinical endpoints
Mols et al. (2005)	Systematic review among long-term survivors	Focusing on the long-term effects of breast cancer is important when evaluating the full extent of cancer treatment
Grimison and Stockler (2007)	Adjuvant systemic therapy for early-stage breast cancer (review of literature from 1996 to Feb. 2007)	For the majority of breast cancer patients most aspects of health-related quality of life recover after adjuvant chemotherapy ends without long-term effects except vasomotor symptoms and sexual dysfunction
Perry et al. (2007)	Benefit, acceptability and utilization of quality of life assessment (review of literature from 1995 to 2005)	Implementation of quality of life assessments into clinical practice for breast cancer treatment has a high potential to benefit patients

◻ Table 165-1 (continued)

Author(s) (Year)	Main focus	Conclusion(s)
Lemieux et al. (2008)	Chemotherapy-induced alopecia	Hair loss consistently ranked amongst the most troublesome side effects, was described as distressing and may affect body image

This table summarizes the most recent systematic review papers on quality of life in breast cancer patients. *QOL* quality of life

Health-related quality of life in patients undergoing systemic therapy for advanced breast cancer was reviewed by Bottomley and Therasse (2002), covering the literature from 1995 to 2001. They indicated that there were 19 studies. Among these, there were 12 studies on chemotherapy, 6 on hormonal trials and 1 on biological therapy (Trastuzumab). They concluded that quality of life data provided invaluable insights into the treatment and care of patients.

To help selection of optimal treatment, Goodwin et al. (2003) conducted a review of measurements of health-related quality of life in randomized clinical trials in breast cancer patients, covering the literature from 1980 to 2000. They identified in breast cancer patients a total of 256 randomized trials that included health-related quality of life or psychosocial outcomes. Of these, 66 trials involved randomized different treatment options, 46 evaluated biomedical interventions, and 20 evaluated psychosocial interventions. They concluded that until results of ongoing trials on breast cancer are available, caution is recommended in initiating new quality of life studies unless treatment equivalence is expected or unless unique or specific issues can be addressed. Similarly, a critical review of published literature on randomized clinical trials of cytotoxic or hormonal treatments of advanced breast cancer indicated that quality of life assessments added relatively little value to classical clinical endpoints (Fossati et al., 2004).

Mols et al. (2005) reviewed the literature on quality of life among long-term survivors of breast cancer and found that although these patients experienced some specific problems such as a thick and painful arm and problems with sexual functioning, most reported good overall quality of life. The review also indicated that the current medical condition, amount of social support, and current income level were strong positive predictors of quality of life, and the use of adjuvant chemotherapy emerged as a negative predictor. The authors concluded that focusing on the long-term effects of breast cancer is important when evaluating the full extent of treatment.

A recent review of clinical randomized trials covering the literature from 1996 to 2007 described the effects of adjuvant chemotherapy and hormonal therapy on quality of life in women with early-stage breast cancer (Grimison and Stockler, 2007). The review concluded that adjuvant chemotherapy has acute detrimental effects on many physical and psychosocial aspects of health related quality of life, with longer and more aggressive therapies causing worse and persistent effects. Most aspects of health-related quality of life recover rapidly after the end of chemotherapy, without long-term effects for the majority of patients, except vasomotor symptoms and sexual dysfunction occurring as a result of chemotherapy-induced premature menopause.

3 Measurement

3.1 Instruments Used

Broadly, quality of life measures can be classified as: general, disease specific, and site-specific. Several valid instruments for measuring quality of life in breast cancer patients have been developed in recent years. The most commonly-used instruments are: the European Organization for Research and Treatment of Cancer (EORTC) Quality of Life Questionnaire and its Breast Cancer supplement (EORTC QLQ-C30 and QLQ-BR23); the Functional Assessment of Cancer Therapy General Questionnaire and its Breast Cancer Supplement (FACT-G and FACT-B); the Breast Cancer Chemotherapy Questionnaire (BCQ); the Hospital Anxiety and Depression Scale (HADS); and the Medical Outcomes Study Short Form Survey (SF-36). ❷ *Table 165-2* lists a number of most important instruments used in quality of life studies in breast cancer patients. Almost all these instruments proved to be valid and were found to be very popular among researchers and clinicians.

It seems that it is time to stop developing new instruments, since there are enough valid and comprehensive measures to assess quality of life in breast cancer patients. New instruments might cause confusion and may be regarded as a waste of resources, so any such developments would need robust justification. Depending on the objectives of any single study, one might use other existing valid measures such as the Satisfaction with Life Domains Scale for Breast Cancer (SLDS-BC), which can briefly and rapidly assess quality of life across the breast cancer continuum of care (Spagnola et al., 2003); the Body Image After Breast Cancer Questionnaire (BIBCQ), which is a valid measure for assessing the long-term impact of breast cancer on body image (Baxter et al., 2006); and the Fallowfield's Sexual Activity Questionnaire (FSAQ), which is a useful tool for measuring sexual activity in women with cancer (Atkins and Fallowfield, 2007).

3.2 Validation Studies

Developments of instruments for measuring quality of life in breast cancer patients, or cultural adaptation and validation studies of the existing instruments, are the major themes in a number of papers. These are presented in ❷ *Table 165-3*. A paper by Levine et al. in 1988 is the first validation study in this field. It reported a quality of life measure in breast cancer patients called the Breast Cancer Chemotherapy Questionnaire (BCQ). This is a 30-item questionnaire that focuses on loss of attractiveness, fatigue, physical symptoms, inconvenience, emotional distress, and feelings of hope and support from others (Levine et al., 1988). A few studies reported translation and validation findings for the instruments that are used to assess quality of life among breast cancer patients in different cultures (e.g., see Lee et al., 2004; Montazeri et al., 2000).

The latest development in this field relates to a new measure of symptoms for breast cancer patients. The Breast Cancer Prevention Trial Eight Symptom Scale (BCPT-BESS) derived from the BCPT Symptom Checklist (BCPT-SCL), is a 21-item questionnaire that measures eight clinically interpretable clusters of symptoms. These are: cognitive symptoms, musculoskeletal pain, vasomotor symptoms, nausea, sexual problems, bladder problems, body image, and vaginal symptoms (Cella et al., 2008).

◘ Table 165-2

A list of most important instruments used to measure quality of life in breast cancer patients

Types of measures	Measures full name	Abbreviation
General measures	Short Form Health Survey	SF-36
	Spitzer Quality of Life Index	QLI
	Sickness Impact Profile	SIP
	Ferrans and Powers Quality of Life Index	QLI
Cancer specific measures	European Organization for Research and Treatment of Cancer Core quality of Life questionnaire	EORTC QLQ-C30
	Functional Assessment of Chronic Illness Therapy General Questionnaire	FACIT-G (FACT-G)
	Functional Living Index-Cancer	FLI-C
	Ferrans and Powers Quality of Life Index-Cancer	QLI-C
Breast cancer specific measures	European Organization for Research and Treatment of Cancer Breast Cancer Quality of Life Questionnaire	EORTC QLQ-BR23
	Functional Assessment of Chronic Illness Therapy-Breast	FCIT-B (FACT-B)
	Breast Cancer Chemotherapy Questionnaire	BCQ
	The Satisfaction with Life Domains Scale for Breast Cancer	SLDS-BC
Psychological measures	General Health Questionnaire-28	GHQ-28
	Hospital Anxiety and Depression Scale	HADS
	Beck Depression Inventory	BDI
	Center for Epidemiologic Studies Depression Scale	CES-D
	State-Trait Anxiety Inventory	STAI
	Profile Mood State	PMS
	Mental Adjustment to Cancer Scale	MACS
	Psychosocial Adjustment to Illness Scale	PAIS
Symptom measures	Functional Assessment of Chronic Illness Therapy-Fatigue	FACIT-F (FACT-F)
	Piper Fatigue Scale	PFS
	Multidimensional Fatigue Inventory	MFI
	Functional Assessment of Chronic Illness Therapy-B plus Arm Morbidity Subscale	FACIT-B + 4 (FACT-B + 4)
	Hot Flash Related Interference Scale	HFRDIS
	Shoulder Disability Questionnaire	SDQ
	Brief Pain Inventory	BPI
	McGill Pain Questionnaire	MPQ
	Memorial Symptom Assessment Scale	MSAS
	Rotterdam Symptom Checklist	RSC

◻ Table 165-2 (continued)

Types of measures	Measures full name	Abbreviation
Other measures	Functional Assessment of Chronic Illness Therapy-Spiritual	FACIT-SP (FACT-SP)
	Body Image Scale	BIS
	Body Image After Breast Cancer Questionnaire	BIBCQ
	Watts Sexual Functioning Questionnaire	WSFQ
	Social Support Questionnaire	SSQ
	Life Satisfaction Questionnaire	LSQ
	Satisfaction With Life Scale	SWLS

These are among the most cited instruments used to measure quality of life in breast cancer patients

4 Treatments

4.1 Surgical Treatment

Breast cancer surgery including conservative surgery followed by irradiation, and modified radical mastectomy or radical mastectomy followed by immediate reconstruction is associated with different side-effects including pain, and fatigue and thus affecting quality of life in breast cancer patients. A list of recent studies on surgery and quality of life in breast cancer patients is given in ❷ *Table 165-4*.

The most important topic in studies of breast cancer surgery and quality of life relates to the type of surgery. Recent findings suggest that partial and total mastectomy appear to be equivalent treatments in terms of patients' long-term quality of life. However, both short-term and long-term distress levels after partial and total mastectomy may depend on patient's age at diagnosis (Dorval et al., 1998). A study of early breast cancer patients, 1 year after mastectomy or conservative surgery and radiation therapy found that the differences between treatment groups were mainly accounted for by adjuvant therapies. Those treated by breast conservation reported better body image but worse physical functions. The negative impact of breast cancer and its treatment was greater for younger women regardless of treatment type (Kenny et al., 2000).

In addition, one study found that aspects of quality of life other than body image were no better in women who underwent breast-conserving surgery or mastectomy with reconstruction than in women who had mastectomy alone. Furthermore, mastectomy with reconstruction was associated with greater mood disturbance and poorer health (Nissen et al., 2001). However, the results of a 5-year prospective study on quality of life following breast conserving surgery or mastectomy indicated that mastectomy patients had a significantly worse body image, role and sexual functioning, and their lives were more disrupted (Engel et al., 2004). A recent Japanese study performing multivariate analysis on the early effects of surgery in patients with breast cancer reported that there were no significant differences in quality of life before and after surgery, but quality of life was significantly better among women undergoing breast conservation than those undergoing mastectomy (Pandey et al., 2006).

◻ Table 165-3

A summary of validation studies of quality of life instruments in breast cancer patients

Author(s) (Year)	Instrument	Main focus
Levine et al. (1988)	The Breast Cancer Chemotherapy Questionnaire (BCQ)	Development an outcome measure in clinical trials of adjuvant chemotherapy
Carlsson and Hamrin (1996)	The Life Satisfaction Questionnaire (LSQ-32)	Development a tool to measure life satisfaction in breast cancer patients
Sprangers et al. (1996)	The European Organization for Research and Treatment of Cancer Breast Cancer Specific Quality of Life Questionnaire (EORTC QLQ-BR23)	Development of a breast cancer specific QOL measure
Brady et al. (1997)	The Functional Assessment of Cancer Therapy Breast Cancer Specific Questionnaire (FACT-B)	Development of a breast cancer specific QOL measure
de Haes and Olschewski (1998)	The Rotterdam Symptom Checklist (RSC)	Cross cultural validation
Fallowfield et al. (1999)	An Endocrine Symptom subscale for the FACT-B (FACT-B plus ES)	Validation in women undergoing hormonal therapy for breast cancer
Montazeri et al. (2000)	The EORTC QLQ-BR23	Validation of the Iranian version
Coster et al. (2001)	The Impact of Arm Morbidity (FACT-B+4)	Development a QOL scale to assess the impact of arm morbidity post-operatively
Carpenter (2001)	The Hot Flash Related Daily Interference Scale	Development of a tool for measuring the impact of hot flashes on QOL
Pandey et al. (2002)	The FACT Breast Cancer Specific Questionnaire (FACT-B)	Validation of the Malayalam version
Chie et al. (2003)	The EORTC QLQ-C30 and the EORTC QLQ-BR23	Validation of the Taiwan Chinese version
Lee et al. (2004)	The Functional Assessment of Cancer Therapy-General (FACT-G)	Validation of the Korean version
Yun et al. (2004)	The EORTC QLQ-BR23	Cross-cultural application in Korea
Avis and Foley (2006)	The Quality of life in Adult Cancer Survivors (QLACS)	Evaluation in long term breast cancer survivors
Wan et al. (2007a)	The FCT-B	Simplified Chinese version of the FACT-B
Wan et al. (2007b)	The EORTC QLQ-BR53	Simplified Chinese version of the EORTC QLQ-BR53

◻ Table 165-3 (continued)

Author(s) (Year)	Instrument	Main focus
Cella et al. (in press)	The Breast Cancer Prevention Trial Eight Symptom Scale (BCPT-BESS)	Psychometric properties of the BCPT-BESS

This table summarizes studies that report either about instruments that are validated for the first time or existing instruments that translated into other languages and validated in different populations of breast cancer patients. *BCQ* breast cancer chemotherapy questionnaire; *LSQ-32* life satisfaction questionnaire; *EORTC QLQ-BR23* European Organization for Research and Treatment of Cancer breast cancer specific quality of life questionnaire, *RSC* Rotterdam symptom checklist; *FACT-B* functional assessment of cancer therapy breast cancer specific question-naire; *FACT-B-plus ES* an endocrine symptom subscale for the FACT-B; *FACT-B+4* impact of arm morbidity subscale for FACT-B; *BCPT-BESS* breast cancer prevention trial eight symptom scale; *QLACS* quality of life in adult cancer survivors; *QOL* quality of life

4.2 Systemic Therapies

In order to reduce the risk of recurrence and death, breast cancer patients usually receive systemic therapies (chemotherapy, hormonal therapy, and biological treatments) after surgery. Several studies evaluated quality of life in breast cancer patients receiving systemic therapies. A list of studies reporting on the topic is given in ❷ *Table 165-5*.

4.2.1 Examples from Early Studies

In a study of postoperative adjuvant chemotherapy in primary node positive breast cancer patients (one or more axillary node), women receiving a single agent or a multi-drug regimen indicated that the treatment was *"unbearable"* (Palmer et al., 1980) or in a study of patients with early breast cancer receiving preoperative chemotherapy, almost all patients considered chemotherapy the most *"burdensome"* aspect of the treatment (Kiebert et al., 1990).

4.2.2 Recent Studies

To improve clinical outcomes, an international randomized controlled trial compared dose-intensive chemotherapy with standard systemic chemotherapy in patients with locally advanced breast cancer and showed that a dose-intensive regimen only has a temporary effect on health-related quality of life, thus enabling more research on intensive treatment for patients with locally advanced breast cancer, as it might also offer a survival benefit (Bottomley et al., 2005).

Recent studies focusing on adjuvant hormonal therapies (tamoxifen or aromatase inhibitors such as anastrozole, letrozole, exemestane) and quality of life in postmenopausal early-stage breast cancer patients reported more encouraging results. Most studies found that overall quality of life was improved in patients receiving either anstrozole or tamoxifen but patients reported different side effects (Fallowfield et al., 2004; Cella et al., 2006). A trial comparing tamoxifen with exemestane showed that quality of life did not change significantly in either groups, but there were improvements in endocrine-related symptoms (Fallowfield et al., 2006).

◼ Table 165-4

A list of recent studies of surgical treatment and quality of life in breast cancer patients

Author(s) (Year)	Treatment (assessment time)	Conclusion(s)
King et al. (2000)	MAS or BCS (3 months and 1 year after)	Most symptoms declined over time but arm and menopausal symptoms persisted; worse QOL in younger patients
Kenny et al. (2000)	MAS or BCS + irradiation (1 year after)	Better body image and physical function in BCS; more impact on younger women regardless of treatment type
Nissen et al. (2001)	MAS or MAS + reconstruction or BCS (6 times assessment up to 2 years after)	QOL other than body image were not better in BCS or MAS + reconstruction than in who had MAS alone; MAS + reconstruction was associated with greater mood disturbance and poorer QOL
Janni et al. (2001)	MAS or BCS (median 46 months follow-up)	Surgical modalities had no long-term impact on overall QOL, but certain body image related problems in MAS was observed
Girotto et al. (2003)	MAS + reconstruction in older women	Improved QOL in older patients especially improved mental health
Engel et al. (2004)	MAS or BCS (5 years follow-up)	MAS patients had lower body image, role and sexual functioning; BCS should be encouraged in all ages
Ganz et al. (2004)	Lumpectomy + chemotherapy or MAS + chemotherapy or Lumpectomy alone or MAS alone in non-metastatic breast cancer patients	At the end of primary treatment all treatment groups reported good emotional functioning but decreased physical health especially among women who had MAS or received chemotherapy
Elder et al. (2005)	MAS + immediate breast reconstruction (before and 12 months after)	After 12 months good QOL comparable with aged-matched women from the general population
Fleissig et al. (2006)	SLNB versus ALND	Regarding arm functioning and QOL the use of SLNB was recommended in patients with node negative breast cancer
Pandey et al. (2006)	MAS or BCS	No significant change in overall QOL after surgery; poorer QOL in MAS patients
Rietman et al. (2006)	SLNB or ALND (before and after 2 years)	Less treatment related upper limb morbidity, perceived disability in activities of daily life and worsening of QOL after SLNB compared with ALND

This table summarizes a number of studies that describe or compare quality of life in breast cancer patients who underwent breast conservation surgery or mastectomy. *MRM* modified radical mastectomy; *MAS* mastectomy; *BCS* breast conservation surgery; *SLNB* sentinel lymph node biopsy; *ALND* axillary lymph node dissection; *QOL* quality of life

However, as noted by Cella and Fallowfield (2008), recognition and management of treatment-related side-effects for breast cancer patients receiving adjuvant endocrine therapy is an important issue, since such side-effects negatively affect health-related quality of life and adherences to therapy. These authors argue that adverse events constitute the main reason for

■ Table 165-5

A list of recent studies on systemic therapies and quality of life in breast cancer patients

Author(s) (Year)	Treatment/patients	Conclusion(s)
Osoba et al. (2002)	Chemotherapy + Trastuzumab (Hercptin) vs. Chemotherapy alone in metastatic breast cancer	More improved global QOL with chemotherapy + Herceptin
de Haes et al. (2003)	Goserelin vs. CMF in peri-and pre-menopausal node-positive early breast cancer	Better QOL in favor of goserelin
Land et al. (2004)	CMF vs. AC in axillary node negative and estrogen receptor negative breast cancer	Overall QOL was equivalent between two groups
Fallowfield et al. (2004)	ANA vs. TAM alone or in combination in postmenopausal early breast cancer	Similar overall QOL impact but some small differences in side effects profiles
Bottomley et al. (2004)	AT vs. AC in metastatic breast cancer	No significant differences in QOL between two groups
Bernhard et al. (2004)	TAM for 5 years or three prior cycles of CMF followed by 57 months TAM in estrogen receptor-negative and estrogen receptor-positive breast cancer	At completion there were no differences by treatment groups
Galalae et al. (2005)	Radiotherapy and adjuvant chemotherapy vs. radiotherapy and hormonal therapy vs. radiotherapy alone after conserving surgery	Adjuvant chemotherapy lowered QOL vs. hormones or radiotherapy alone
Bottomley et al. (2005)	Dose-intensives chemotherapy (CE + filgrastim) vs. CEF in locally advanced breast cancer	Groups did not differ in progression free survival; lower QOL in intensified group at short term but no difference at long term
Ahles et al. (2005)	Standard-dose systemic chemotherapy vs. local therapy only in long-term breast cancer survivors	Lower overall QOL in chemotherapy group
Martin et al. (2006)	FAC vs. TAC or TAC + G-CSF in node negative breast cancer	Lower QOL in patients treated with TAC. Addition of G-CSF improves QOL
Fallowfield et al. (2006)	EXE vs. TAM after 2–3 years of TAM in postmenopausal primary breast cancer	Temporary decrease in overall QOL for EXE but no other differences
Cella et al. (2006)	ANA vs. TAM alone or in combination in postmenopausal breast cancer	ANA and TAM had similar impact on QOL
Karamouzis et al. (2007)	Chemotherapy vs. supportive care in metastatic patients	QOL was better in patients receiving chemotherapy than those under supportive care

◘ Table 165-5 (continued)

Author(s) (Year)	Treatment/patients	Conclusion(s)
Hopwood et al. (2007)	Adjuvant radiotherapy	QOL and mental health were favorable for most patients about to start radiotherapy but younger age and receiving chemotherapy were significant risk factors for poorer QOL

This table summarizes a number of studies that describe or compare quality of life in breast cancer patients who received different chemotherapy regimens, or hormonal therapies. *C* cyclophosphamide; *M* methotrexate; *F* 5-fluorouracil; *A* doxorubcin; *E* epirubcin; *T* docetaxel; *TAM* tamoxifen; *ANA* anastrozole; *EXE* exemestane; *QOL* quality of life; *DPPE* tesmilifene; *G-CSF* granulocyte colony stimulating factor; *CTCb* cyclophosphamide, thiotepa, and carboplatin; *QOL* quality of life

non-adherence to endocrine treatment, and across all adjuvant endocrine trials regardless of the treatment, vasomotor symptoms such as hot flushes are the most common side-effects. Other frequently reported side-effects such as vaginal discharge, vaginal dryness, dyspareunia, and arthralgia vary in prevalence between tamoxifen and aromatase inhibitors. A recent study reported that decline in health-related quality of life during therapy predicted treatment discontinuation even after adjusting for age and chemotherapy related side-effects (Richardson et al., 2007, also see ❷ *Figure 165-1*).

Finally, it has been recommended that currently in assessing quality of life in breast cancer patients receiving systemic therapies priorities should be given to cognitive functioning, menopausal symptoms, body image and long-term effects of new therapies that might cause musculoskeletal and neurological side-effects (Grimison and Stockler, 2007).

◘ Figure 165-1
Quality of life in a sample of 150 breast cancer patients at baseline and 3 months after treatment. This is an example of quality of life data in breast cancer patients as measured by the EORTC QLQ-BR23. The figure shows functioning scales and the higher scores indicate a better condition (scores ranging from 0 to 100). All measures decreased after treatment but future perspective increased indicating patients were hopeful that the treatment might cure their disease (From unpublished data by Montazeri et al., Iranian Centre for Breast Cancer). *BI* body image; *SEF* sexual functioning; *SEE* sexual enjoyment; *FU* future perspective

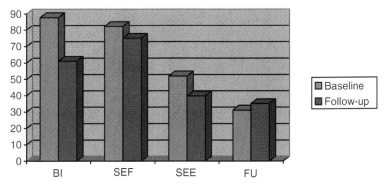

5 Quality of Life as Predictor of Survival

5.1 In Early-Stage Disease

Until recently, only a few studies had reported a relationship between quality of life and survival in breast cancer patients (Coates et al., 1987). Studies have shown that baseline quality of life predicts survival in advanced breast cancer but not in early stage of disease (Coates et al., 2000). Two recently published papers also confirmed that baseline quality of life is not a prognostic factor in non-metastatic breast cancer patients. One of these two studies, using Cox survival analysis, indicated that neither health-related quality of life nor psychological status at diagnosis or 1 year later was associated with medical outcome in women with early-stage breast cancer (Goodwin et al., 2004). The other study, on a sample of 448 locally advanced breast cancer patients, reported that baseline health-related quality of life parameters had no prognostic value in a non-metastatic breast cancer population (Efficace et al., 2004a).

5.2 In Metastatic Patients

A study using the Daily Diary Card to measure quality of life in advanced breast cancer showed that the instrument offered accurate prognostic data regarding subsequent response to treatment and survival duration (Fraser et al., 1993). Similarly, Seidman et al. (1995) evaluated quality of life in two phase II clinical trials of metastatic breast cancer and found that baseline scores of two validated quality of life instruments independently predicted the overall survival.

5.3 Partial Relationship

Studies have demonstrated that some aspects of quality of life data including physical health (Coates et al., 1992), pain (Kramer et al., 2000a,b; Luoma et al., 2003), and loss of appetite (Efficace et al., 2004b) are significant prognostic factors for survival in women with advanced breast cancer. In addition, one study demonstrated that baseline physical aspects of quality of life and its changes were related to survival, but psychological and social aspects were not (Shimozuma et al., 2000).

6 Distress

6.1 Psychological Distress

Women with breast cancer might develop psychological distress including anxiety and depression during diagnosis and treatment and after treatment. The psychological impact of breast cancer has received considerable attention. Since this is a separate topic, the focus here is on psychological distress as it relates to quality of life studies in breast cancer patients. ❍ *Table 165-6* summarizes the papers on the topic.

◻ Table 165-6

A list of studies on psychological distress and quality of life in breast cancer patients

Author(s) (Years)	Main focus	Results/conclusion(s)
Kissane et al. (1998)	Psychological morbidity in early-stage breast cancer	45% (135/303) had psychiatric disorder, 42% had depression, anxiety or both; QOL was substantially affected
Bloom et al. (1998)	Intrusiveness of illness in young women with newly-diagnosed breast cancer	Intrusiveness of illness mediated the effect of disease and treatment factors on QOL; neither time post-diagnosis nor type of treatment affected the psychological component of QOL
Longman et al. (1999)	Psychological adjustment over time	Over time depression burden and anxiety burden persist and each was negatively associated with overall and present QOL
Cotton et al. (1999)	Relationship among spiritual well-being, QOL, and psychological adjustment	Spiritual well-being was correlated with both QOL and psychological adjustment, but relationship was found to be more complex and indirect than previously considered
Ashing-Giwa (1999)	Psychological outcome in long-term survivors of breast cancer (focus on African-American)	Patients relied on spiritual faith and family support to cope; socio-cultural contexts of the women's lives need to be considered when studying QOL
Lewis et al. (2001)	Cancer-related intrusive thoughts and social support	In women with social support cancer-related intrusive thoughts had no significant negative impact on QOL, but in women with low social support there was negative effect on QOL
Amir and Ramati (2002)	Post-traumatic distress disorder (PTSD), QOL, and emotional distress in long term survivors of breast cancer and a control group	Higher PSTD, emotional distress and lower QOL in breast cancer mainly due to chemotherapy and disease stage
Ganz et al. (2003)	Psychosocial adjustment 15 months after diagnosis in older women with breast cancer	Psychosocial adjustment at 15 months was predicted by better mental health, emotional social support and better self-rated interaction with health care providers
Bordeleau et al. (2003)	Randomized trial of group psychological support vs. control in metastatic breast cancer	Supportive-expressive group therapy did not appear to influence QOL
Badger et al. (2004)	Depression burden and psychological adjustment	Depression burden had negative effect on psychological adjustment and QOL

◘ Table 165-6 (continued)

Author(s) (Years)	Main focus	Results/conclusion(s)
Schreier and Williams (2004)	Anxiety in women receiving either radiation or chemotherapy for breast cancer	No significant differences for total QOL or any subscales by treatment; trait anxiety was higher for chemotherapy patients; state anxiety was high and did not decrease over the course of the treatment for either group
Kershaw et al. (2004)	Coping strategies in advanced breast cancer patients and their family caregivers	Patients use more emotional support, religion and positive reframing strategies while family use more alcohol or drug. In both active coping was associated with higher QOL
Lehto et al. (2005)	Psychological stress factors as predictors of QOL in patients receiving surgery alone vs. adjuvant treatment	Psychosocial factors were strongest predictors of QOL but not cancer type or treatment; non-cancer related stresses showed strongest QOL decreasing influence
Roth et al. (2005)	Affective distress in women seeking immediate vs. delayed breast reconstruction after mastectomy	Women seeking immediate breast reconstruction showed relatively higher psychological impairment and physical disability
Okamura et al. (2005)	Psychiatric disorders and associated factors after first breast cancer recurrence	Patients' psychiatric disorders were associated with lower QOL
Golden-Kreutz et al. (2005)	Traumatic stress, perceived global stress, and life events	Initial stress at diagnosis predicted both psychological and physical health at follow-up
Deshields et al. (2005)	Emotional adjustment (at 4 points in time)	Primary psychological changes occur quickly after treatment conclusion and then it appeared to become stabled
Schou et al. (2005)	Dispositional optimism and QOL	Optimism was predictive for better emotional and social functioning 1 year after surgery; at time of diagnosis and throughout post-diagnosis dispositional optimism was associated with better QOL and fewer symptoms
Grabsch et al. (2006)	Psychological morbidity in advanced breast cancer	42% (97/277) had a psychiatric disorder, 36% depression or anxiety or both. QOL was substantially affected
Antoni et al. (2006)	Stress management after treatment for breast cancer	Stress management skill taught had beneficial effects on reduced social disruption, and increased emotional well-being, positive states of mind, benefit finding, positive lifestyle change, and positive affect

◘ Table 165-6 (continued)

Author(s) (Years)	Main focus	Results/conclusion(s)
Wonghongkul et al. (2006)	Uncertainty appraisal coping	Social support was used most to cope and confront-coping used the least; year of survival, uncertainty in illness and harm appraisal influenced QOL
Yen et al. (2006)	Depression and stress in breast cancer versus benign tumor	Stress from health problem was the most significant predictor for QOL among malignant group
Costanzo et al. (2007)	Distress and adjustment following treatment	Survivors demonstrated good adjustment on general distress indices following treatment. Some women were at risk for sustained distress; and cancer-related concerns were prevalent
Meneses et al. (2007)	Psycho-educational intervention and quality of life	Breast cancer education intervention is an effective intervention in improving quality of life during the first year of breast cancer survivorship
Parker et al. (2007)	Short-term and long-term psychosocial adjustment in patients undergoing different surgical procedure	Patients in stable condition and with psychosocial support can hope to enjoy good QOL with treatment

This table summarizes a number of studies that investigated psychological distress in breast cancer patients as relates to quality of life in this population. *PTSD* post-traumatic distress disorder; *QOL* quality of life

Psychological distress in breast cancer patients is mostly related to depression, anxiety, and low emotional functioning and almost all studies have shown that psychological distress contributed to impaired quality of life especially emotional functioning, social functioning, mental health and overall quality of life. It has been shown that the risk factors for depression (such as fatigue, past history of depression, job loss, etc.) impair quality of life in breast cancer patients (Golden-Kreutz et al., 2005).

The diagnosis of the disease, importance of fears and concerns regarding death and disease recurrence, impairment of body image, and alteration of femininity, sexuality and attractiveness are factors that can cause unexpected psychological distress even years after diagnosis and treatment (Baucom et al., 2006; Reich et al., 2008; Spiegel, 1997). Studies have shown that psychological factors predict subsequent quality of life (Deshield et al., 2005) or even overall survival in breast cancer patients (Groenvold et al., 2007). Furthermore, it has been shown that psychological adjustment such as the ability to cope with the disease, treatment and effects of treatment could improve outcome. A recent publication reported that the experience of distressing symptoms is predicted by coping capacity and the coping efforts experiences predict health related quality of life. In other words, patients with lower coping capacity report higher prevalence of symptoms, experience worse perceived health that in turn may decrease their quality of life (Kenne Sarenmalm et al., 2007). In addition, the relationship between positive thinking and longer survival and a better quality of life are well documented (Spiegel, 2001).

6.2 Symptoms

There are several studies on breast cancer symptoms and their relationship to quality of life. Most of these studies are related to fatigue, lymphedema, pain, and menopausal symptoms. The results are summarized in ❷ *Table 165-7*. It is argued that symptoms are important contributors to the distress experience and in turn distress has a severe impact on quality of life (Kenne Sarenmalm et al., 2008).

◘ Table 165-7

A list of studies of quality of life and common symptoms in breast cancer patients

Author(s) (Year)	Main focus	Results/conclusion(s)
Hann et al. (1998)	Fatigue following radiotherapy	Women experienced fatigue but not worse than expected
Carpenter et al. (1998)	Hot flushes	65% (n = 114) reported ht flushes, with 59% of women with hot flushes rating the symptom as severe; hot flushes were most severe in women with a higher body mass index, those who were younger at diagnosis, and those receiving tamoxifen
Hann et al. (1999)	Fatigue after high-dose therapy and autolougous stem cell rescue	Fatigue was related to medical and psychosocial factors
Velanovich and Szymanski (1999)	Lymphedema	Lymphedema occurred in a minority of patients and negatively affected QOL
Bower et al. (2000)	Fatigue, occurrence, and correlates	About one-third (n = 1,957) reported more severe fatigue which was associate with higher level of depression, pain, and sleep difficulties
Kuehn et al. (2000)	Surgery related symptoms following ALND	Shoulder-arm morbidity following ALND was found to be the most important long-term sources of distress
Stein et al. (2000)	Hot flushes	Hot flushes have a negative impact on QOL that may be due to fatigue and interference with sleep
Beaulac et al. (2002)	Lymphedema in survivors of early-stage breast cancer	MAS or BCS patients had similar lymphedema rates (28%-42/151) and had negative impact on long-term QOL in survivors
Kwan et al. (2002)	Arm morbidity after curative breast cancer treatment	Symptomatic patients and patients with lymphedema had impaired QOL compared to patients with no symptoms

◘ Table 165-7 (continued)

Author(s) (Year)	Main focus	Results/conclusion(s)
Fortner et al. (2002)	Sleep difficulties	Most patients had significant sleep problems that frequently being disturbed by pain, nocturia, feeling too hot, and coughing or snoring loudly; patients having significant sleep problems had greater deficits in QOL
Engel et al. (2003)	Arm morbidity	Up to 5 years after diagnosis 38% (n = 990) were still experienced arm problems and for these patients QOL was significantly lower than patients without arm morbidity; extent of axilla, younger age, and operating clinic significantly contributed to arm morbidity
Caffo et al. (2003)	Pain after surgery	Pain distressed 40% of patients (n = 529) regardless of treatment type and had negative effect on patients' QOL
Rietman et al. (2004)	Impairments and disabilities (2.7 years after surgery)	Pain was the most frequent assessed impairment after breast cancer treatment with strong relationship to perceived disability and QOL
Schults et al. (2005)	Menopausal symptoms	Menopausal signs and symptoms may not be different or the breast cancer survivors and they should not be confused with the QOL/psychosocial issues of the cancer survivors
Ridner (2005)	Lymphedema	Survivors with lymphedema reported poorer QOL; a symptom cluster including limb sensation, loss of confidence in body, decreased physical activity, fatigue and psychological distress was identified
Conde et al. (2005)	Menopausal symptoms	Prevalence of menopausal symptoms was similar in women with and without breast cancer; sexual activity was less frequent in breast cancer patients
Burckhardt et al. (2005)	Pain	Widespread pain significantly caused more experience of pain severity, pain impact and lower physical health than regional pain
Mills et al. (2005)	Fatigue	Pre-chemotherapy and chemotherapy induced inflammation were related to fatigue and QOL

◼ Table 165-7 (continued)

Author(s) (Year)	Main focus	Results/conclusion(s)
Massacesi (2006)	Effects of endocrine related symptoms in breast cancer who had switched from tamoxifen to anastrozole	Endocrine related symptoms improved but higher rate of mild arthritic and bone pain were reported
Land et al. (2006)	Tamoxifen or raloxifene related symptoms	No significant differences between groups; tamoxifen group reported better sexual function, more gynecological problems and vasomotor symptoms while raloxifene group reported more musculoskeletal problems and weight gain
Heidrich et al. (2006)	Symptoms, and symptom beliefs in older breast cancer patients vs. older women without breast cancer	Symptom experience and QOL of older breast cancer survivors were similar to those of older women with other chronic health problems
Gupta et al. (2006)	Menopausal symptoms	96% reported vasomotor, 83% psychological and 90% somatic symptoms (n = 200) which negatively correlated not only their own but also with their partners' QOL
Byar et al. (2006)	Fatigue	Fatigue was associated with other physical and psychological symptoms and higher fatigue compromised QOL
Arndt et al. (2006)	Fatigue	Fatigue emerged as the strongest predictor of QOL
Pyszel et al. (2006)	Disability, and psychological distress in breast cancer survivors with and without lymphedema	Patients with arm lymphedema were more disabled, experienced a poorer QOL and had increased psychological distress in comparison to those without lymphedema
Janz et al. (2007)	Relationship between symptoms and post-treatment QOL	Five most common symptoms were: systemic therapy side effects, fatigue, breast symptoms, sleep difficulties, and arm symptoms. Fatigue had the greatest impact on QOL
Mehnert et al. (2007)	Association between neuropsychological impairment, cognitive deficits, fatigue and QOL	The role of self-perceived cognitive deficits and fatigue should be considered in educational interventions and counseling

This table summarizes a number of studies that report on the relationship between quality of life and common symptoms in breast cancer patients. *ALND* axillary lymph node dissection; *ASCT* autologous stem cell transplantation; *QOL* quality of life; *MAS* mastectomy; *BCS* breast conservation surgery

Fatigue is the least definable symptom experienced by patients with breast cancer and its effect on impaired quality of life cannot be explained precisely. A recent publication studying 1,588 breast cancer patients showed that fatigue (as measured by the EORTC QLQ-C30 fatigue subscale) independently predicted longer recurrence-free survival when biological factors were controlled in the analysis. When combined with the biological model, fatigue still remained a significant predictor of recurrence-free survival (Groenvold et al., 2007).

6.3   Sexual Functioning

Breast cancer could be regarded as a disease that relates to women's identities. In this respect, sexual functioning is an important issue, especially in younger breast cancer patients. About 60% of women usually report disruption in their sexual quality of life (Beckjord and Campas, 2007). Among quality of life studies in breast cancer patients a few papers focused especially on sexual functioning (Knapp, 1997; Makar et al., 1997; Ganz et al., 1998; Marsden et al., 2001; Malinovszky et al., 2006; Beckjord and Campas, 2007). The findings indicated that disrupted sexual functioning or unsatisfactory sexual life is related to poorer quality of life at younger age, treatment with chemotherapy, emotional distress consequent on an unsatisfactory sexual life, and difficulties with partners because of sexual relationships. It is argued that younger survivors may need interventions that specifically target their needs related to menopausal symptoms and problems with relationships, sexual functioning and body image (Avis et al., 2005).

7   The Future

The literature reveals how much effort has been made in studying quality of life in breast cancer patients and shows the achievements of a journey that was started more than 30 years ago. If quality of life has now become an important part of breast cancer patients' care, it is due to all these efforts.

There are few qualitative studies. Since these could provide more insight into quality of life in breast cancer patients, we need more such studies to collect data and indicate how breast cancer patients interpret life after diagnosis and during and after treatment. Breast cancer survivors even might rate their quality of life more favorably than outpatients with other common medical conditions and identify many positive aspects from the cancer experience (Ganz et al., 1996). However, it is not only the study of quality of life in newly diagnosed breast cancer patients that is necessary; studying quality of life in long-term survivors is equally important. As suggested, when assessing quality of life in breast cancer patients, the stage of disease should also be considered. There are differences in quality of life between patients with non-invasive breast cancer, newly diagnosed breast cancer and advanced local breast cancer, and disease-free breast cancer survivors, women with recurrence breast cancer, and women with advanced metastatic breast cancer (Ganz and Goodwin, 2005).

Finally, issues related to the disease, its treatment side effects and symptoms, and sexual functioning should receive more attention when studying quality of life in breast cancer patients.

Summary Points

- There is quite an extensive body of the literature on quality of life in breast cancer patients. These papers have made a considerable contribution to improving breast cancer care, although their exact benefit is hard to define.
- Measuring quality of life in breast cancer patients is both crucial and scientific.

- Several valid instruments exist to measure quality of life in breast cancer patients. The European Organization for Research and Treatment of Cancer Core Cancer Quality of Life Questionnaire (EORTC QLQ-C30) and its breast cancer specific complementary measure (EORTC QLQ-BR23) and the Functional Assessment Chronic Illness Therapy General questionnaire (FACT-G) and its breast cancer module (FACT-B) are the most common and well developed instruments to measure quality of life in breast cancer patients.
- Similar to known medical factors, quality of life data in metastatic breast cancer patients is found to be prognostic and predictive of survival time.
- Different surgical procedures lead to relatively similar results in terms of quality of life assessments, although mastectomy patients compared to conserving surgery patients usually report a lower body image and sexual functioning.
- Breast cancer patients receiving chemotherapy might experience several side effects and symptoms that negatively affect their quality of life. Adjuvant hormonal therapies also have similar negative impact on quality of life, although in general they are associated with improved survival.
- Anxiety and depression are common among breast cancer patients even years after the disease diagnosis and treatment. Psychological factors might predict subsequent quality of life or even overall survival in breast cancer patients.
- Pain, fatigue, arm morbidity and postmenopausal symptoms are the most common symptoms among breast cancer patients. As recommended, recognition and management of these symptoms is an important issue since such symptoms impair health-related quality of life.
- Breast cancer patients especially younger patients suffer from poor sexual functioning that negatively affect quality of life.

Appendix

Some Key Facts About Breast Cancer

- The most common sign of breast cancer is a new lump or mass. A lump that is painless, hard, and has uneven edges is more likely to be cancer. Sometimes cancers can be tender, soft, and rounded. Other signs of breast cancer include a swelling of part of the breast; skin irritation or dimpling; nipple pain or the nipple turning inward; redness or scaliness of the nipple or breast skin; a nipple discharge (other than breast milk); and a lump in the under arm area.
- The cause of breast cancer is not known. Factors that can increase a woman's risk include heredity, early puberty, late childbearing, obesity, and lifestyle factors such as heavy alcohol consumption and smoking. The biggest risk factor for breast cancer is age that is growing older. Most breast cancers occur in women over the age of 50, and women over 60 are at the highest risk.
- A woman's risk for developing breast cancer increases if her mother, sister, daughter, or two or more other close relatives, such as cousins, have a history of breast cancer, especially at a young age. However, 85% of women who develop breast cancer have no known family history of the disease.
- Changes in certain genes (BRCA1, BRCA2, and others) make women more susceptible to breast cancer. Genetic testing can determine whether a woman has these abnormal genes.

- Based on involvement of breasts, breast cancer can be categorized as stage 0 (cancer cells remain in the breast duct), stage I (cancer is 2 cmentimeters or less), stage II (tumor is over 2 but not larger than 5 cm or is spread to the lymph nodes under the arm), stage III or locally advanced (tumor is more than 5 cm or is extensive in the under arm lymph nodes or spread to other lymph nodes or tissues near the breast) and stage IV (cancer has spread or metastasized to other parts of the body).
- 5-year survival time for breast cancer patients vary depending on stage and treatment received. However, there are differences between survival for the same breast cancer patients in developed and developing countries.

Source: adapted from www.breastcancer.org

Breast Cancer Treatment Options

- Surgery is the treatment of choice for breast cancer. There are different surgery options for breast cancer: breast conservation surgery and mastectomy.
- In breast conservation surgery we save the breast and it includes: lumpectomy (malignant tumor and a rim of normal tissue are removed) or quadrantectomy (malignant tumor and a large rim of normal tissue are removed) with axillary dissection.
- In mastectomy the whole breast is removed and it includes: total or simple mastectomy (whole breast is removed); or modified radical mastectomy (the whole breast is removed with under arm lymph nodes); or radical mastectomy (the whole breast, chest muscles, all lymph nodes under the arm, and some additional fat and skin are removed).
- Chemotherapy uses drugs to destroy cancer cells. It is given systemically (throughout the body) after surgery to kill cancer cells that may have been left behind (adjuvant therapy). Also it may be given before surgery to reduce the size of the cancer (neoadjuvant therapy).
- Hormonal therapy is a form of whole body (systemic) treatment for breast cancer. In hormonal therapy, drugs are used to reduce or block the effects of hormones (including estrogen and progesterone) that can promote the growth of breast cancer. Hormonal therapy protects the whole body from breast cancer cells that may have been left behind after surgery, radiation, or chemotherapy. It can also lower the risk of a new cancer developing in the other breast.

Source: adapted from www.breastcancer.org

References

Ahles TA, Saykin AJ, Furstenberg CT, Cole B, Mott LA, Ttius-Ernstoff L, Skalla K, Bakitas M, Silberfarb PM. (2005). J Clin Oncol. 23: 4399–4405.

Amir M, Ramati A. (2002). J Anxiety Disord. 16: 191–206.

Antoni MH, Lechner SC, Kazi A, Wimberly SR, Sifre T, Urcuyo KR, Phillips K, Gluck S, Carver CS. (2006). J Consult Clin Psychol. 74: 1143–1152.

Arndt V, Stegmaier C, Ziegler H, Brenner H. (2006). Cancer. 107: 2496–2503.

Ashing-Giwa K. (1999). J Psychosoc Oncol. 17: 47–62.

Atkins L, Fallowfield LJ. (2007). Menopause Int. 13: 103–109.

Avis NE, Crawford S, Manuel J. (2005). J Clin Oncol. 23: 3322–3330.

Avis NE, Foley KL. (2006). Health Qual Life Outcomes. 4: 92.

Badger TA, Braden CJ, Mishel MH, Longman A. (2004). Res Nurs Health. 27: 19–28.

Baucom DH, Porter LS, Kiby JS, Gremore TM, Keefe FJ. (2006). Breast Dis. 23: 103–113.

Baxter NN, Goodwin PJ, Mcleod RS, Dion R, Devins G, Bombardier C. (2006). Breast J. 12: 221–232.

Beaulac SM, McNair LA, Scott TE, LaMorte WW, Kavanah MT. (2002). Arch Surg. 137: 1253–1257.

Beckjord E, Campas BE. (2007). J Psychosoc Oncol. 25: 19–36.

Bernhard J, Zahrieh D, Coates AS, Gelber R, Castiglione-Gertsch M, Murray E, Forbes JF, Perey L, Collins J, Snyder R, Rudenstam CM, Crivellari D, Veronesi A, Thurlimann B, Fey MF, Price KN, Goldhirsch A, Hurny C. (2004). Br J Cancer. 91: 1893–1901.

Bloom JR, Stewart SL, Johnston M, Banks P. (1998). Psycho-Oncol. 7: 89–100.

Bordeleau L, Szalai JP, Ennis M, Leszcz M, Speca M, Sela R, Doll R, Chochinov HM, Navarro M, Arnold A, Pritchard KI, Bezjak A, Liewellyn-Thomas HA, Sawka CA, Goodwin PJ. (2003). J Clin Oncol. 21: 1944–1951.

Bottomley A, Biganzoli L, Cufer T, Coleman RE, Coens C, Efficace F, Calvert HA, Gamucci T, Twelves C, Fargeot P, Piccart M. (2004). J Clin Oncol. 22: 257–286.

Bottomley A, Therasse P. (2002). Lancet Oncol. 3: 620–628.

Bottomley A, Therasse P, Piccart M, Efficace F, Coens C, Gotay C, Welnicka-Jaskiewicz M, Mauriac L, Dyczka J, Cufer T, Lichinitser MR, Schornagel JH, Bonnefoi H, Shepherd L. (2005). Lancet Oncol. 6: 287–294.

Bower JE, Ganz PA, Desmond KA, Rowland JH, Meyetowitz BE, Belin TR. (2000). J Clin Oncol. 18: 743–753.

Brady MJ, Cella DF, Mo F, Bonomi AE, Tulsky DS, Lloyd SR, Deasy S, Cobleigh M, Shiomoto G. (1997). J Clin Oncol. 15: 974–986.

Burckhardt CS, Carol S, Jones KD. (2005). Health Qual Life Outcomes. 3: 30.

Byar KL, Berger AM, Bakken SL, Cetak MA. (2006). Oncol Nurs Forum. 33: E18–E26.

Caffo O, Amichetti M, Ferro A, Lucenti A, Valduga F, Galligioni E. (2003). Breast Cancer Res Treat. 80: 39–48.

Carlsson M, Hamrin E. (1996). Qual Life Res. 5: 265–274.

Carpenter JS. (2001). J Pain Symptom Manag. 22: 979–989.

Carpenter JS, Andrykowski MA, Cordova M, Cunningham L, Studts J, McGrath P, Kenady D, Sloan D, Munn R. (1998). Cancer. 82: 1682–1691.

Cella D, Fallowfield L, Barker P, Cuzick J, Locker G, Howell A. (2006). Breast Cancer Res Treat. 100: 273–284.

Cella D, Fallowfield LJ. (2008). Breast Cancer Res Treat. 107: 167–180.

Cella D, Land SR, Chang CH, Day R, Costantino JP, Wolmark N, Ganz PA. (2008). Breast Cancer Research Treat. 109: 515–526.

Chie WC, Chang KJ, Huang CS, Kuo WH. (2003). Psychooncology. 12: 729–735.

Coates A, Gebski V, Bishop JF, Jeal PN, Woods RL, Snyder R, Tattersall MH, Byrne M, Harvey V, Gill G. (1987). N Engl J Med. 317: 1490–1495.

Coates A, Gebski V, Signorini D, Murray P, McNeil D, Byne M, Forbes JF. (1992). J Clin Oncol. 10: 1833–1838.

Coates AS, Hurny C, Peterson HF, Bernhard J, Castinglione-Gertsch M, Gelberg D, Goldhirsch A. (2000). J Clin Oncol. 18: 3768–3774.

Conde DM, Pinto-Neto AM, Cabello C, Santos-Sa D, Costa-Paiva L, Martinze EZ. (2005). Menopause. 12: 436–443.

Costanzo ES, Lutgendorf SK, Mattes ML, Trehan S, Robinson CB, Tewfik F, Roman SL. (2007). Br J Cancer. 97: 1625–1631.

Coster S, Poole K, Fallowfield LJ. (2001). Breast Cancer Res Treat. 68: 273–282.

Cotton SP, Levine EG, Fitzpatrick CM, Dold KH, Targ E. (1999). Psychooncology. 8: 429–438.

de Haes H, Olschewski M, Kaufmann M, Schumacher M, Jonat W, Sauerbrei W. (2003). J Clin Oncol. 21: 4510–4516.

de Haes JC, Olschewski M. (1998). Ann Oncol. 9: 745–750.

Deshields T, Tibbs T, Fan MY, Bayer L, Taylor M, Fisher E. (2005). Support Care Cancer. 13: 1018–1026.

Dorval M, Maunsell E, Deschenes L, Brisson J, Masse B. (1998). J Clin Oncol. 16: 487–494.

Efficace F, Biganzoli L, Piccart M, Coens C, van Steen K, Cufer T, Coleman RE, Calvert HA, Gamucci T, Twelves C, Fargeot P, Bottomley A. (2004a). Eur J Cancer. 40: 1021–1030.

Efficace F, Therasse P, Piccart MJ, Coens C, van Steen K, Welnicka-Jaskiewicz M, Cufer T, Dyczka J, Lichinitser M, Shepherd L, de Haes H, Srangers MA, Bottomley A. (2004b). J Clin Oncol. 22: 3381–3388.

Elder EE, Brandberg Y, Bjorklund T, Rylander R, Lagergren J, Jurell G, Wickman M, Sandelin K. (2005). Breast. 14: 201–208.

Engel J, Kerr J, Schlesinger-Raab A, Sauer H, Halzel D. (2004). Breast J. 10: 223–231.

Engel J, Kerr J, Schlesinger-Raab A, Sauer H, Holzel D. (2003). Breast Cancer Res Treat. 79: 47–57.

Fallowfield L, Cella D, Cuzick J, Francis S, Locker G, Howll A. (2004). J Clin Oncol. 22: 4261–4271.

Fallowfield LJ, Bliss JM, Porter LS, Price MH, Snowdon CF, Jones SE, Coobes RC, Hall E. (2006). J Clin Oncol. 24: 910–917.

Fallowfield LJ, Leaity SK, Howell A, Benson S, Cella D. (1999). Breast Cancer Res Treat. 55: 189–199.

Fleissig A, Fallowfield LJ, Langridge CI, Johnson L, Newcombe RG, Dixon JM, Kissin M, Mansel RE. (2006). Breast Cancer Res Treat. 95: 279–293.

Fortner BV, Stepanski EJ, Wang SC, Kasprowicz S, Durrence H. (2002). J Pain Symptom Manag. 24: 471–480.

Fossati R, Confalonieri C, Mosconi P, Pistotti V, Apolone G. (2004). Breast Cancer Res Treat. 87: 233–243.

Fraser SCA, Ramirez AJ, Ebbes SR, Fallowfield LJ, Dobbs HJ, Richards MA, Bates T, Baum M. (1993). Br J Cancer. 67: 341–346.

Galalae RM, Michel J, Siebmann JU, Kuchler T, Eilf K, Kimmig B. (2005). Strahlenther Onkol (Strahlentherapie und Onkologie). 181: 645–651.

Ganz PA, coscarelli A, Fred C, Kahn B, Polinsky ML, Petersen L. (1996). Breast Cancer Res Treat. 38: 183–199.

Ganz PA, Goodwin PJ. (2005). In: Lipscomb J, Gotay CC, Snyder C (ed.) Outcomes Assessment in Cancer: Measures, Methods, and Applications. Cambridge University Press, Cambridge, UK, pp. 93–125.

Ganz PA, Guadagnoli E, Landdrum MB, Lash TL, Rakowski W, Silliman RA. (2003). J Clin Oncol. 21: 4027–4033.

Ganz PA, Kwan L, Stanton AL, Krupnick JL, Rowland JH, Meyerowitz BE, Bower JE, Belin TR. (2004). J Natl Cancer Inst. 96: 376–387.

Ganz PA, Rowland JH, Desmond K, Meyerowitz BE, Wyatt GE. (1998). J Clin Oncol. 16: 501–514.

Girotto JA, Schreiber J, Nahabedian MY. (2003). Ann Plast Surg. 50: 572–578.

Golden-Kreutz DM, Thornton LM, Wells-Di GS, Frierson GM, Jim HS, Carpenter KM, Shelby RA, Andersen BL. (2005). Health Psychol. 24: 288–296.

Goodwin PJ, Black JT, Bordeleau LJ, Ganz PA. (2003). J Natl Cancer Inst. 95: 263–281.

Goodwin PJ, Ennis M, Bordeleau LJ, Pritchard KT, Trudeau Me, Koo J, Hood N. (2004). J Clin Oncol. 22: 4184–4192.

Grabsch B, Clarke DM, Love A, McKenzie DP, Snyder RD, Bloch S, Smith G, Kissane DW. (2006). Palliat Support Care. 4: 47–56.

Grimison PS, Stockler M. (2007). Expert Rev Anticancer Ther. 7: 1123–1134.

Groenvold M, Petersen MA, Idler E, Bjorner JB, Fayers PM, Mouridsen HT. (2007). Breast Cancer Res Treat. 105: 209–219.

Gupta P, Sturdee DW, Pallin SL, Majumder K, Fear R, Marshall T, Paterson I. (2006). Climacteric. 9: 49–58.

Hann DM, Garovoy N, Finkelstein B, Jacobsen PB, Azzarello LM, Fields KK. (1999). J Pain Symptom Manage. 17: 313–319.

Hann DM, Jacobson P, Martin S. (1998). J Clin Psychol Med S. 5: 19–33.

Heidrich SM, Egan JJ, Hengudomsub P, Randolph SM. (2006). Oncol Nurs Forum. 33: 315–322.

Hopwood P, Haviland J, Mills J, Sumo G, Bliss MJ. (2007). Breast. 16: 241–251.

Irwig L, Bennetts A. (1997). Aust N Z J Surg. 67: 750–754.

Janni W, Rjosk D, Dimpfl T, Haertl K, Strobl B, Hepp F, Hanke A, Bergauer F, Sommer H. (2001). Ann Surg Oncol. 8: 542–548.

Janz NK, Mujahid M, Chung LK, Lantz PM, Hawley ST, Morrow M, Schwartz K, Katz SJ. (2007). J Women's Health. 16: 1348–1361.

Karamouzis MV, Ioannidis G, Rigatos G. (2007). Eur J Cancer Care. 16: 433–438.

Kenne Sarenmalm E, Ohlen J, Oden A, Gaston-Johansson F. (2007). J Pain Symptom Manage. 34: 24–39.

Kenne Sarenmalm E, Ohlen J, Oden A, Gaston-Johansson F. (2008). Psychooncology. 17: 497–505.

Kenny P, King MT, Sheill A, Seymour J, Hall J, Langlsnds A, Boyages J. (2000). Breast. 9: 37–44.

Kershaw T, Northouse L, kritpracha C, Schafenacker A, Mood D. (2004). Psychol Health. 19: 139–155.

Kiebert GM, Hanneke J, de Haes CJ, Kievit J, van de Velde CJ. (1990). Eur J Cancer. 26: 1038–1042.

King MT, Kenny P, Shiell A, Hall J, Boyages J. (2000). Qual Life Res. 9: 789–800.

Kissane DW, Clarke DM, Ikin J, Bloch S, Smith GC, Vietta L, McKenzie DP. (1998). Med J Aust. 169: 192–196.

Knapp J. (1997). J Gynecol Oncol Nurs. 7: 37–40.

Kramer JA, Curran D, Piccart M, de Haes JC, Bruning PF, Klijn JG, Bontenbal M, van Pottelsberghe C, Groenvold M, Paridaens R. (2000a). Eur J Cancer. 36: 1488–1497.

Kramer JA, Curran D, Piccart M, de Haes JC, Bruning PF, Klijn JG, van Hoorebeeck I, Paridaens R. (2000b). Eur J Cancer. 36: 1498–1506.

Kuehn T, Klauss W, Darsow M, Regele S, Flock F, Maiterth C, Dahlbender R, Wendt I, Kreienberg R. (2000). Breast Cancer Res Treat. 64: 275–286.

Kwan W, Jackson J, Weir LM, Dingee C, McGregor G, Olivotto IA. (2002). J Clin Oncol. 20: 4242–4248.

Land SR, Kopec JA, Yothers G, Anderson S, Day R, Tang G, Ganz PA, Fisher B, Wolmark N. (2004). Breast Cancer Res Treat. 86: 153–164.

Land SR, Wickerham DL, Costantino JP, Ritter MW, Vogel VG, Lee MK, Pajon ER, Wade JL III, Dakhil S, Lockhart JB, Wolmark N, Ganz PA. (2006). JAMA. 295: 2742–2751.

Lee EH, Chun M, Kang S, Lee HJ. (2004). Jap J Clin Oncol. 34: 393–399.

Lehto US, Ojanen M, Kellokumpu-Lehtinen P. (2005). Annal Oncol. 16: 805–816.

Lemieux J, Maunsell E, Provencher L. (2008). Psychooncology. 17: 317–328.

Levine MN, Guyatt GH, Gent M, De Pauw S, Goodyear MD, Hryniuk WM, Arnold A, Findlay B,

Skillings JR, Bramwell VH. (1988). J Clin Oncol. 6: 1798–1810.

Lewis JA, Manne SL, DuHamel KN, Vickburg SMJ, Bovjerg DH, Currie V, Winkel G, Redd WH. (2001). J Behav Med. 24: 231–245.

Longman AJ, Braden CJ, Mishel MH. (1999). Oncol Nurs Forum. 26: 909–915.

Luoma ML, Hakamies-Blomqvist L, Sjostrom J, Pluzanska A, Ottoson S, Mouridsen H, Bengtsson NO, Bergh J, Malmstrom P, Valvere V, Tennvall L, Blomqvist C. (2003). Eur J Cancer. 39: 1370–1376.

Makar K, Cumming CE, Lees AW, Hundleby M, Nabholtz J, Kieren DK, Jenkins H, Wentzel C, Handman M, Cumming DC. (1997). Can J Hum Sex. 6: 1–8.

Malinovszky KM, Gould A, Foster E, Cameron D, Humphreys A, Crown J, Leonard RC. (2006). Br J Cancer. 95: 1626–1631.

Mandelblatt J, Armetta C, Yabroff KR, Liang W, Lawreence W. (2004). J Natl Cancer Inst Monographs. 33: 8–44.

Marsden J, Baum M, A'Hern R, West A, Fallowfield L, Whitehead M, Sacks N. (2001). Br J Menopause Soc. 7: 85–87.

Martin M, Lluch A, Segui MA, Ruzi A, Ramos M, adrover E, Rodriguez-Lescure A, Grosse R, Calvo L, Fernandez-Chacon C, Roset M, Anton A, Isla D, del Prado PM, Iglesias L, Zaluski J, Arcusa A, Lopez-Vega JM, Munoz M, Mel JR. (2006). Annal Oncol. 17: 1205–1212.

Massacesi C, Sabbatini E, Rocchi MB, Zepponi L, Rossini S, Pilone A, Burattini L, Pezzoli M. (2006). Am J Cancer. 5: 433–440.

Mehnert A, Scherwatch A, Schirmer L, Schleimer B, Petersen C, Schulz-Kindermann F, Zander AR, Koch U. (2007). Patient Educ Couns. 66: 108–118.

Meneses KD, McNees P, Loerzel VW, Su X, Zhang Y, Hassey LA. (2007). Oncol Nurs Forum. 34: 1007–1016.

Mills PJ, Parker B, Dimsdale JE, Sadler GR, Ancoli-Israel S. (2005). Biol Psychol. 69: 85–96.

Mols F, Vingerhoets AJ, Coebergh JW, van de Poll-Franse LV. (2005). Eur J Cancer. 41: 2613–2619.

Montazeri A, Gillis CR, McEwen J. (1996a). Eur J Cancer Care. 5: 159–167.

Montazeri A, Gillis CR, McEwen J. (1996b). Eur J Cancer Care. 5: 168–175.

Montazeri A, Harirchi I, Vahdani M, Khaleghi F, Jarvandi S, Ebrahimi M, Haji-Mahmoodi M. (2000). Qual Life Res. 9: 177–184.

Montazeri A, Milroy R, Hole D, McEwen J, Gillis CR. (2001). Lung Cancer. 31: 233–240.

Moore FD, van de Vanter SB, Boyden CM, Lokich J, Wilson RE. (1974). Surgery. 76: 376–390.

Nissen MJ, Swenson KK, Ritz LJ, Farrell JB, Sladek ML, Lally RM. (2001). Cancer. 91: 1238–1246.

Okamura M, Yamavaki S, Akechi T, Taniguchi K, Uchitomi Y. (2005). Jpn J Clin Oncol. 35: 302–309.

Osoba D, Slamon DJ, Burchmore M, Murphy M. (2002). J Clin Oncol. 20: 3106–3113.

Palmer BV, Walsh GA, McKinna JA, Greening WP. (1980). Br Med J. 281: 1594–1597.

Pandey M, Thomas BC, Ramdas K, Eremenco S, Nair K. (2002). Qual Life Res. 11: 87–90.

Pandey M, Thomas BC, Ramdas K, Ratheesan K. (2006). Jpn J Clin Oncol. 36: 468–472.

Parker PA, Youssef A, Walker S, Basen-Engguist K, Cohen L, Gritz ER, Wei QX, Robb SL. (2007). Ann Surg Oncol. 14: 3035–3036.

Payne R, Medina E, Hampton JW. (2003). Cancer. 97 (Suppl. 1): 311–317.

Perry S, Kowalski TL, Chang CH. (2007). Health Qual Life Outcomes. 5: 24.

Priestman TJ, Baum M. (1976). Lancet. i: 899–900.

Pyszel A, Malyszezak K, Pyszel K, Andrzejak R, Szuba A. (2006). Lymphology. 39: 185–192.

Reich M, Lesur A, Perdrizet-Chevallier C. (2008). Breast Cancer Res Treat. 110: 9–17.

Richardson LC, Wang W, Hartzema AG, Wanger S. (2007). Breast J. 13: 581–587.

Ridner SH. (2005). Support Care Cancer. 13: 904–911.

Rietman J, Dijkstra P, Debreczeni R, Geertzen J, Robinson D, de Vries J. (2004). Disabil Rehabil. 26: 78–84.

Rietman JS, Dijkstra PU, Hoekstra HJ, Eisma WH, Szabo BG, Groothoff JW, Geertzen JH. (2003). Eur J Surg Oncol. 29: 229–238.

Rietman JS, Geertzen JH, Hoekstra HJ, Baas P, Dolsma WV, de Vries J, Groothoff JW, Eisma WH, Dijkstra PU. (2006). Eur J Surg Oncol. 32: 148–152.

Roth RS, Lowery JC, Davis J, Wilkins E. (2005). Plast Reconstr Surg. 116: 993–1002.

Schou I, Ekeberg O, Sandvik L, Hjermstad MJ, Ruland CM. (2005). Qual Life Res. 14: 1813–1823.

Schreier AM, Williams SA. (2004). Oncol Nurs Forum. 31: 127–130.

Schults PN, Klein MJ, Beck ML, Stava C, Sellin RV. (2005). J Clin Nurs. 14: 204–211.

Seidman AD, Portenoy R, Yao TJ, Lepore J, Mont EK, Kortmansky J, Onetto N, Ren L, Grechko J, Beltangady M. (1995). J Natl Cancer Inst. 187: 1316–1322.

Shimozuma K, Okamoto T, Katsumata N, Koike M, Tanaka K, Osumi S, Saito M, Shikama N, Watanabe T, Mitsumori M, Yamauchi C, Hisashige A. (2002). Breast Cancer. 9: 196–202.

Shimozuma K, Sonoo H, Ichihara K, Tanaka K. (2000). Surg Today. 30: 255–261.

Spagnola S, Zabora J, BrintzenhofeSzoc K, Hooker C, Cohen G, Baker F. (2003). Breast J. 9: 463–471.

Spiegel D. (1997). Semin Oncol. 24 (Suppl. 1): S36–S47.

Spiegel D. (2001). J Psychosom Res. 50: 287–290.

Sprangers MAG, Groenvold M, Arraras JI, Franklin J, te Velde A, Muller M, Franzini L, Williams A, de Haes HC, Hopwood P, Cull A, Aaronson NK. (1996). J Clin Oncol. 14: 2756–2768.

Stein KD, Jacobsen PB, Hann DM, Greenberg H, Lyman G. (2000). J Pain Symptom Manage. 19: 436–445.

Stewart BW, Paul Kleihues P. (2003). World Cancer Report. International Agency Research on Cancer, Lyon, France.

Velanovich V, Szymanski W. (1999). Am J Surg. 177: 184–187.

Wan C, Tang X, Tu XM, Feng C, Messing S, Meng Q, Zhang X. (2007b). Breast Cancer Res Treat. 105: 187–193.

Wan C, Zhang D, Yang Z, Tu X, Tang W, Feng C, Wang H, Tang X. (2007a). Breast Cancer Res Treat. 106: 413–418.

Wonghongkul T, Dechaprom N, Phumivichuvate L, Losawatkul S. (2006). Cancer Nurs. 29: 250–257.

Yen JY, Ko CH, Yen CF, Yang MJ, Wu CY, Juan CH, Hou MF. (2006). Psychiatry Clin Neurosci. 60: 147–153.

Yun YH, Bae SH, Kang IO, Shin KH, Lee R, Kwon SI, Park YS, Lee ES. (2004). Support Care Cancer. 12: 441–445.

166 Quality of Life with Localized Prostate Cancer: Japanese Perspectives

S. Namiki · L. Kwan · Y. Arai

1 *Introduction* *2858*

2 *Trends and Characteristics in Prostate Cancer Mortality in Japan* *2859*

3 *Methodology of HRQOL Research in Men with Localized Prostate Cancer* *2860*

4 *Prostate Cancer Specific HRQOL Instruments* *2860*

5 *Radical Prostatectomy* *2861*

6 *Radiation Therapy* *2866*

7 *Androgen Deprivation Therapy* *2867*

8 *Cross-Cultural Comparative Study* *2867*

9 *Future Directions* *2870*

   Summary Points *2871*

Abstract: With the established effectiveness of diverse treatments for localized prostate cancer, identification of the physical and psychological consequences of the disease and various treatments becomes critical. Race and ethnicity are important factors in health-related quality of life (HRQOL) because preferences and health system trust factors that are predominant in certain racial groups are likely to influence HRQOL and satisfaction with care. In Japan, increased screening for prostate cancer has lead to an increase in the apparent incidence of prostate cancer, and resulted in a shift to an earlier age and stage at diagnosis, a trend similar to that in US or European countries. The aim of this article is to selectively review the current research findings related to HRQOL for Japanese men with localized prostate cancer. Studies show that prostate cancer treatment affects both disease-specific HRQOL (i.e., urinary, sexual and bowel function and bother) as well as general HRQOL (i.e., energy/vitality, performance inn physical and social roles). In addition, race/ethnicity (Japanese vs. American men) independently predicted the patterns of urinary and sexual recovery up to 24 months after curative therapy for localized prostate cancer. More attention should be given to fully evaluating HRQOL in Asian populations including Japanese men with localized prostate cancer.

List of Abbreviations: *ADT,* androgen deprivation therapy; *EBRT,* external beam radiation therapy; *HRQOL,* health-related quality of life; *PSA,* prostate specific antigen; *RP,* radical prostatectomy; *WW,* watchful waiting

1   Introduction

Worldwide, prostate cancer is the third most common cancer and the cause of 6% of all cancer deaths in men (Parkin et al., 2001). The Incidence rate of localized prostate cancer in Japanese men is projected to increase by 2.8-fold from 1995 to 2015 with the wide-spread use of the prostate specific antigen (PSA) test and changing in dietary habits. For this subset of patients various treatment modalities including surgery, radiation therapy, androgen deprivation therapy and, in selected cases, watchful waiting are proposed. For the early stage, low risk patients, surgery and radiotherapy can equally provide excellent long-term survival (Potters et al., 2004). Decision-making therefore mostly depends on how the patient feels about morbidities associated with the treatment intervention. Under these circumstances, health-related quality of life (HRQOL) outcome in patients who are treated with each treatment modality has become a pivotal concern among both patients and physicians (Litwin et al., 1995). HRQOL encompassed a wide range of experience, including the daily necessities of life, such as intrapersonal and interpersonal responses to illness, and activities associated with professional fulfillment and personal happiness. HRQOL also includes the overall sense of satisfaction that an individual experiences with life and, most importantly, patient perceptions of personal health and ability to function. The concept of HRQOL includes not only the symptoms of a given disease or treatment and their impact on functional status, but also the degree of associated bother, typically defined as the degree of distress associated with functional limitations or symptoms (Gill and Feinstein, 1994). Importantly, HRQOL is a patient centered outcome. A prior study comparing patients and physician quality of life ratings in prostate cancer have shown significant disparities, typically with the physician underestimating the impact of the disease and its treatment on the patients (Litwin et al., 1998b).

Race and ethnicity are important factors in HRQOL because preferences and health system trust factors that are predominant in certain racial groups are likely to influence HRQOL and satisfaction with care (Rose et al., 2004). Another consideration is that there appear to be racial differences in HRQOL preferences even before treatment, which may potentially explain differences in the administration of initial treatment and subsequent HRQOL patients following treatment. In a large multi-center study Lubeck et al. studied baseline differences in HRQOL in patients of differing races with prostate cancer and found that African-American men had worse HRQOL at presentation even when controlling for a number of potential confounders (Lubeck et al., 2001). Most ethnic comparisons of HRQOL after prostate cancer treatment have been limited to studies of non-Hispanic whites, African-Americans, and Hispanics in the U.S. (Johnson et al., 2004). The HRQOL articles originated from 22 countries with the U.S producing the majority (47%), followed by the United Kingdom (8%), Canada (8%) and Japan (6%) (Ramsey et al., 2007). Thus, there is insufficient information regarding HRQOL for Japanese men diagnosed with prostate cancer with most HRQOL information coming from the experience of well educated white men. Because prostate cancer is so common and it is not confined to any particular racial or sociodemographic group, it is crucial that researchers should be particularly careful to collect information on race in their study. This review synthesized the findings of the fields of HRQOL for Japanese men with localized prostate cancer.

2   Trends and Characteristics in Prostate Cancer Mortality in Japan

In the U.S., the incidence rate of prostate cancer showed a rapid increase in the late 1980s because of widespread screening with PSA, which continued until the beginning of the 1990s. However, more recently, the reported incidence and mortality rates of prostate cancer have been declining, which suggested that early diagnosis and treatment of localized prostate cancer may improve patient survival (Shaw et al., 2004). Contrary to this trend in U.S., although the incidence of prostate cancer is not so high compared to that of Western countries, the prostate cancer death rate has been rapidly increasing in Japan, especially since the 1990s (Nakata et al., 1998). One reason for the difference in the trends may be the prevalence of PSA testing. In addition, Japanese eating habits in these past decades have rapidly become more westernized, characterized by high fat, which is considered to be a risk factor for prostate cancer. However, the age-adjusted death rate remained stable from 1996 to 2001. The Japanese Society of Urology survey, which was started in 2001 and performed at 173 facilities, enrolled 4,529 patients newly diagnosed with prostate cancer during 2000 (Cancer Registration Committee of the Japanese Urological Association, 2005). According to this survey, prostate cancer clinical T stage was T1c, T2a, T2b, T3a, T3b and T4 in 20.3, 21.8, 17.3, 15.8, 11 and 8% of the subjects, respectively. On the other hand, CaPSURE data reported that a majority presents with a biopsy Gleason score of seven or less (81%) and with clinical stage T1 or T2 disease (85%) in the U.S. radical prostatectomy (RP) is the most common primary treatment (41%), followed sequentially by androgen deprivation therapy (ADT) (16.9%), external beam radiation therapy (EBRT) (12%), brachytherapy (BT) (10%) and watchful waiting (6%) (Cooperberg et al., 2004). It is worth nothing that ADT was often selected with localized prostate cancer as well as advanced cancer (Akaza et al., 2006). In recent years, however, increased screening for prostate cancer, primarily with PSA testing, has lead to an increase in the apparent incidence of prostate cancer, and resulted in a shift to an earlier age and stage at diagnosis, a trend similar to that in the U.S. and European countries.

3 Methodology of HRQOL Research in Men with Localized Prostate Cancer

The vast majority of publications on HRQOL in prostate cancer focuses on men with localized disease. HRQOL is especially relevant to many individuals with localized prostate cancer who anticipate a long life expectancy following diagnosis and therapy, regardless of treatment choice. Given the well-known complications of sexual, urinary and bowel dysfunction associated with all forms of therapy for localized disease, patients and clinicians must seriously consider HRQOL when choosing primary therapy for localized prostate cancer. HRQOL is a patient centered variable, measured using questionnaires or surveys that are administered directly to patients in a standardized manner. HRQOL instruments typically contain questions, or items, that are organized into scales. Each scale measures a different aspect, or domain, of HRQOL, and domains may be generic or disease specific. Generic HRQOL domains address general aspects relevant to ill and well persons, and include the components of overall well-being that are common to all patients, regardless of their disease. Disease specific domains focus on the impact of particular organic dysfunctions that affect HRQOL, and involve symptoms and/or concerns directly relevant to the condition (Patrick and Deyo, 1989).

Many researchers consider the Medical Outcomes Study 36-Item Short Form (SF-36) as the "gold standard" for measuring general HRQOL. The 8 domains of the SF-36 address the health concepts of physical function, social function, bodily pain, emotional well-being, energy/fatigue, general health perceptions, role limitations due to physical problems and role limitations due to emotional problems (Ware and Sherbourne, 1992). Several HRQOL instruments have been developed to assess domains of significance to all patients with cancer, regardless of the site of the malignancy. The European Organization for Research and Treatment of Cancer (EORTC) Quality of life Core Questionnaire (QLQ-C30) is a 30-item survey that incorporates five function scales (physical, role, emotional, cognitive and social), a global health scale, three symptom scales concerning dyspnea, insomnia, appetite loss, consumption, diarrhea and financial difficulties due to disease (Aaronson et al., 1993). Another cancer specific HRQOL is the Functional Assessment of Cancer Therapy-General (FACT-G) (Cella et al., 1993). Each item of the FACT-G contains a statement with which a patient may agree or disagree across a 5-point range. The FACT-G has 4 domains – physical, social-family, emotional and functional well-being. All of the aforementioned questionnaires were translated to Japanese version.

4 Prostate Cancer Specific HRQOL Instruments

The most commonly used HRQOL instruments for prostate cancer patients are: (1) the European Organization for Research and Treatment of Cancer Core Quality of Life Questionnaire with a prostate-cancer-specific module (EORTC-P) (Aaronson et al., 1993), (2) the Functional Assessment of Cancer Therapy-Prostate (FACT-P) (Esper et al., 1997), (3) the University of California, Los Angeles Prostate Cancer Index (UCLA PCI) (Litwin et al., 1998), and (4) Expanded Prostate Cancer Index Composite (EPIC) (Wei et al., 2000). UCLA PCI and EPIC differs from EORTC-P and FACT-P in providing distinct, domain-specific summary scores for urinary, bowel, sexual, and hormonal symptoms. The UCLA PCI was developed by Litwin et al. (1998a) to evaluate the HRQOL of men who underwent surgery or radiotherapy for localized prostate cancer. The 20 prostate specific items address 6 domains – urinary function and bother, sexual function and bother, and bowel function and bother. The fact that the UCLA PCI generates separate scores to quantify the degree of symptoms (function) and perception of problem due to symptoms (bother) is important because the bother experienced by patients may not necessarily correlate highly with the level of dysfunction. The Japanese version demonstrated good psychometric properties (reliability and validity) and it was easy to answer and easily understandable by patients and physicians (Kakehi et al., 2002). Since then, the Japanese version of UCLA-PCI has been incorporated in many outcome studies of Japanese patients (❷ Table 166-1). The EPIC instrument (50 items) was constructed by modifying the UCLA PCI (20 items): items regarding irritative, obstructive urinary symptoms and irritative bowel symptoms, and symptoms intimately related to ADT, were added. Recently, Japanese version of the EPIC was available (Kakehi et al., 2007) and Namiki et al. (2007) evaluated the correspondence between UCLA PCI and EPIC using linking analysis method. In this study the urinary and sexual domains of the UCLA PCI and EPIC exhibited strong correlations. In contrast, the correlation for the bowel domain was relatively weak. Once investigators choose a survey, they will usually continue to use the same survey to achieve consistent comparisons. While it would be ideal for researchers to agree on using the same surveys, this study may be useful for translating one survey score into another as different surveys are being used across studies.

5   Radical Prostatectomy

Radical prostatectomy (RP) is a standard treatment for patients with localized prostate cancer and a life expectancy of more than 10 years who accept the risk of treatment-related complications (Bill-Axelson et al., 2005). Urinary incontinence and erectile dysfunction represent the principal sources of postoperative adverse events for patients who have undergone RP even with nerve-sparing techniques. Longitudinal studies have revealed that some physical function domains were lower than baseline score just after RP. However, these domains recovered to baseline scores 6 months post-operatively. Furthermore, mental health, classified as the emotional well-being domain of SF-36, revealed that some postoperative groups had higher scores than the preoperative group. Previous studies found that, following surgery, with the relief accompanying the perceived cure, the tension level was reduced which was correlated in turn with a reduction in feelings of confusion, depression and anger (Talcott et al., 1998).

Urinary incontinence is cited as a significant drawback of RP, and although the definition of continence is inconsistent across studies, urinary function and bother are often used as measures of QOL in this population (Krupski et al., 2003). But what is consistent is that incontinence causes significant decreases in HRQOL (Carlson and Nitti, 2001). Researchers have found that significant differences in QOL exist between men who wear one pad a day for control of leakage as compared with men who do not wear any protection at all (Cooperberg et al., 2003). According to UCLA PCI scores which represent disease specific HRQOL, the urinary function domain, which reflects leakage substantially declined at 3 months and continued to recover at 6, 12, 18, and 24 months after RP. However, scores were still lower at 24 months than at baseline. Urinary bother had a significantly worse score at 3 months than that at baseline. At 6 months postoperatively, however, it returned to baseline levels. When continence was defined as "leaked urine not at all," only 46% of the patients were continent at 24 months after RP. On the other hand, when continence was defined as "no pads," overall 50.5, 84.4, 87.6, 88.5 and 90.5% of men were continent at the 3, 6, 12, 18 and 24-month follow up points, respectively. Younger men tended to show more rapid recovery than older men

◻ Table 166-1

Selected studies comparing HRQOL following treatment for Japanese men with localized prostate cancer

Study	Design	No of pt.	Therapy	Summary of major findings
Akakura (1999)	Longitudinal	46	RP, EBRT	More surgery patients complained of urinary incontinence. Quality of life was less disturbed in the radiation group
Arai (1999)	Comparison group	60	RP	General HRQOL does not appear to be compromised following radical prostatectomy. Patients are willing to accept some morbidity for a perceived survival benefit. Although minimal urinary dysfunction was reported, most patients were dissatisfied with postoperative sexual function
Egawa et al. (2003)	Cross-sectional	85	EBRT	Study patients had statistically significant decreases in five SF-36 domains during the first month of treatment. All measures recovered by 12 months. Sexual function was not affected by irradiation
Kakehi et al. (2002)	Cross-sectional	125	RP, EBRT	Sexual function scores did not correlate highly with sexual bother scores. Furthermore, poor sexual function and bother had little association with the SF-36 scores
Hara et al. (2003)	Cross-sectional	106	RP	The general HRQOL survey revealed no significant differences in health before and after laparoscopic and open prostatectomy. However, sexual quality of life was markedly lower after surgery
Yoshimura et al. (2003)	Longitudinal	37	ADHT	The scores for sexual problem and sexual desire domains were significantly higher in the flutamide group than in the LHRH group
Yoshimura et al. (2004)	Longitudinal	135	RP, EBRT	Rapid decline of sexual function and increase in sexual bother were observed throughout follow-up in the RP group, and did not change thereafter in the XRT group. Overall satisfaction with urinary condition significantly improved after treatment
Namiki et al. (2004)	Cross-sectional	264	RP, EBRT	The patients who underwent RP had significantly worse urinary and better bowel function than those treated with EBRT. Both treatment groups had decrements in sexual function throughout the post-treatment period
Hashine et al. (2005)	Cross-sectional	57	EBRT	The combination of radiotherapy and hormone therapy had a good outcome and patients did not experience poor HRQOL, except for sexual problems. Moreover, the disease-specific QOL is good, especially for urinary bother

◻ Table 166-1 (continued)

Study	Design	No of pt.	Therapy	Summary of major findings
Matsubara (2005)	Longitudinal	41	RP	The majority of patients who undergo RPP rapidly regain urinary continence and QOL within 3–6 months. RPP has a favorable impact on LUTS
Namiki et al. (2005c)	Longitudinal	72	RP, ADHT	Neoadjuvant hormonal therapy may decrease not only sexual function, but also general HRQOL before surgery. The recovery of HRQOL appeared to be further prolonged in patients who received long-term neoadjuvant hormonal therapy
Namiki et al. (2005b)	Longitudinal	112	RP	Despite reports of problems with sexuality and urinary continence, general HRQOL was mostly unaffected by surgery after 6 months. Although urinary function did not completely return to the baseline level even at 2 years after surgery, Urinary bother returned to baseline at 6 months postoperatively
Ishihara et al. (2006)	Comparison group	141	Before treatment	Compared to age-gender adjusted population norms, patients demonstrated better physical function and worse mental health. Characteristic age-related changes were found in physical function and sexual function; however, disease stage exhibited no relevant
Namiki et al. (2006b)	Longitudinal	144	EBRT	The IMRT approach produced little impairment in bowel and sexual function compared with conventional radiation therapy
Namiki et al. (2006a)	Longitudinal	225	RP	Radical retropubic prostatectomy has a significant beneficial effect on lower urinary tract symptoms. The rate of improvement was lowest for nocturia among the seven symptoms of IPSS. Urinary continence after surgery and age can affect the recovery of voiding
Namiki et al. (2006c)	Longitudinal	137	RP, BT	The RRP group reported a lower post-treatment urinary function score, which reflected leakage, than the BT group. The data from the International Prostate Symptom Score showed adverse effects from BT on voiding symptoms for the initial 6 months after treatment
Mizokami (2007)	Cross-sectional	628	RP, EBHT	Only sexual function, and not other QOL variables, in men aged 50–59 years appeared to be reduced in men who had hormonal therapy, compared to age-matched controls

⬛ Table 166-1 (continued)

Study	Design	No of pt.	Therapy	Summary of major findings
Kakehi et al. (2007)	Cross-sectional	460	RP, EBRT, ADHT, BT	Known groups validity revealed significant improvement in urinary domain scores with time in patients treated with radical prostatectomy plus permanent (125) I seed implantation. Bowel domain scores were worse in patients treated with external beam radiation
Kato et al. (2007)	Comparison group	56	ADHT	General HRQOL was mostly unaffected by ADT in Japanese men. Disease-specific questions indicated an increase in urinary function. Although deterioration of sexual function was marked, most patients did not report sexual bother
Namiki et al. (2007a)	Longitudinal	113	RP	The bilateral nerve sparing group showed more rapid recovery than the unilateral nerve sparing plus sural nerve graft group after RP. The unilateral nerve sparing group reported lower urinary function and sexual function scores after RP compared to the other groups
Namiki et al. (2007c)	Cross-sectional	385	RP, RT, WW	The RP group had the worst urinary function of all the groups. Each group except for the WW group had poor sexual function
Namiki et al. (2008a)	Longitudinal	558	RP	Japanese and American men experience different patterns of recovery of their sexual function and bother after RP
Namiki et al. (2007b)	Cross-sectional	340	RP, EBRT	Most patients who underwent RP or EBRT for localized prostate cancer experienced low levels of psychological distress after treatment. However, men who were experiencing urinary and bowel symptoms tended to suffer from moderate to higher distress compared with men reporting no or fewer such symptoms
Okeneya (2007)	Longitudinal	100	BT	Urinary retention was rare, but voiding symptoms were persistent in Japanese patients

within 12 months after RP (Namiki et al., 2004a). Hoffman and colleagues showed that 75% of those who developed daily urinary incontinence still reported that the poor function was at most only a small problem (Hoffman et al., 2003).

Erectile dysfunction represents the principal sources of postoperative adverse events for patients who have undergone RP. Men who had RP seem to experience improvements in sexual functioning in the year after RP. Catalona et al. reported excellent results, with overall postoperative potency rates of 68% and postoperative continence rates of 92% (Catalona et al., 1999). However, this is affected by age, preoperative sexual function, and whether nerve-sparing surgery was performed (Litwin et al., 1999). The Japanese data on sexual function showed a substantially lower score just after RP and remained at a deteriorated level. Thirty-eight percent of patients stated at baseline that they had sexual intercourse once or more often during the last 4 weeks. However, this reduced to only 15% at 24 months after RP. In addition, 25 and 65% of the patients considered their ability to have erection as "poor" and "very poor," respectively at 24 months (Namiki et al., 2005b).

The majority of men who underwent RP were between 50 and 70 years old. It has been shown that 44% of men with localized prostate cancer who present for RP have moderate to severe lower urinary tract symptoms (LUTS) that may be due to benign prostatic enlargement (BPE) (Schwartz and Lepor, 1999). Accordingly, evaluation of lower tract function after RP is as important as that of urinary incontinence. A prospective, consecutive study which examined the impact of RP on LUTS revealed that mean total IPSS and IPSS QOL score showed significant improvement after RP. Especially, in men with moderate or severe urinary symptoms, RP significantly improved the total IPSS, as reported in another study (Namiki et al., 2006a). The positive effects of RP on LUTS had a greater beneficial impact than the negative effects of stress urinary incontinence. This improvement in the IPSS, however, was not noted in men with no or mild symptoms but rather in those with moderate to severe symptoms. Therefore, LUTS in men selected for RP may be attributable to underlying BPE rather than prostate cancer.

Laparoscopic radical prostatectomy, used as a minimally invasive approach to radical prostatectomy, has been developed as an alternative to retropubic radical prostatectomy. A multi-institutional longitudinal study in Japan revealed that the laparoscopy group reported delayed recovery of urinary and sexual function, which seemed to affect their general HRQOL. When performed by an experienced surgeon, however, the two approaches appeared to be equivalent in terms of HRQOL. Laparoscopic radical prostatectomy appears to be still an evolving procedure in Japan (Namiki et al., 2005a).

Nerve-sparing RP procedures appear to preserve erectile function in certain men. Nerve grafting is a surgical technique that has been used for decades. With low-volume and low-stage disease, nerve sparing dose not compromise surgical margins; however, nerve-sparing might not be appropriate in men with high-grade tumors or palpable disease extending toward neurovascular bundle. Interposition of sural nerve graft (SNG) to replace resected cavernous nerves during RP confers a greater chance of recovering erectile function than without grafts. The grafted nerve serves primarily as a channel or scaffold for regenerating axons to reestablish connection between the severed segments. Scardino reported that with nerve grafting for the side of neurovascular bundle resection, erectile function of the patients undergoing unilateral nerve-sparing has recovered to a level approximating bilateral nerve-sparing (Scardino and Kim, 2001). Namiki et al. (2007a) conducted a 3-year longitudinal study assessing the impact of unilateral SNG on recovery of potency and continence following RP They found that the bilateral nerve sparing group tended to show more rapid recovery than the unilateral nerve sparing plus SNG group within 12 months after RP. After 24 months, however, there were no significant differences observed between the bilateral nerve sparing group and the unilateral nerve sparing plus SNG group. The bilateral nerve sparing group maintained significantly better urinary function at 1 month after RP than the unilateral nerve-sparing plus SNG. After 3 months, both groups were almost continent. However, definitive conclusions about the SNG procedure are difficult to draw as men who elect it often constitute a highly selective sample of men. Without randomized studies, the superiority of this procedure over standard RP cannot be definitively determined.

As shown in previous studies, the Japanese RP group was older than the American RP group. The men most likely to benefit from RP are those with a life expectancy of more than 10 years and those with a few comorbidities (Andersson et al., 2004). Life expectancy calculations in the U.S. suggest an upper age limit of 70–72 years for offering RP. Currently, the life expectancy of a 75-year-old Japanese man is 11.2 years, (Tubaro and La Vecchia, 2004) while the life expectancy of a 75-year-old American man is 10.3 years (Blanker et al., 2000). The Japanese prostatectomy group was older than our American group in part because many Japanese urologists consider 75 years as an upper age limit for RP.

6   Radiation Therapy

External radiation therapy (EBRT) is often though of as having fewer and less debilitating side effects than surgery in the context of prostate cancer treatment. It is apparent, however, that transient irritative and obstructive urinary symptoms occur during and in the period immediately after EBRT. Questions about urgency as well as incontinence seem relevant to those experiencing urinary problems and for whom their daily activities were affected. These seem to be important symptoms to consider in evaluating side effects after EBRT or brachytherapy (BT) against prostate cancer.

Japanese men with localized prostate cancer who underwent EBRT appear to have similar general HRQOL to men who have received RP (Namiki et al., 2004b), which was similar to other groups (Frank et al., 2007). Among men treated with EBRT, fatigue appears to be the most common complication. EBRT has been associated with increased fatigue from pretreatment to 3 and 12-month follow-up (Talcott et al., 1998).

Findings from several studies appear to indicate that bowel problems are more likely to occur after treatment, especially after EBRT (Fowler et al., 1996; Potosky et al., 2004). Problems such as increased frequency, increased urgency, diarrhea, and bleeding with movements are reported more often by men with EBRT than by men treated with RP.

Intensity modulated radiation therapy (IMRT) has been shown to improve the local control and disease-free survival in patients with localized prostate cancer compared with conventional external beam or conformal radiation (Zelefsky et al., 2001). Zelefsky et al. reported that IMRT reduced acute and rectal toxicities compared with conventional radiotherapy techniques (Zelefsky et al., 2002). Namiki et al. demonstrated better HRQOL for Japanese men treated with IMRT compared with those who were treated with conventional or comformal radiotherapy (Namiki et al., 2006b; Yoshimura et al., 2007).

BT has been accepted as an option for the treatment of localized prostate cancer in selected patients and the 10-year survival data appear favorable (Downs et al., 2003). In Japan, the use of iodine-125 seed source was legally approved in June 2003. Eton et al. analyzed the immediate changes in general HRQOL in 256 men after treatment with BT, RP or external beam radiotherapy (Eton et al., 2001). HRQOL differences were noted in the domains of physical function, role physical, social function and bodily pain. In each domain, the patients who underwent BT had higher HRQOL scores than those treated with RP. On the other hand, mental health improved substantially and appeared to continue to improve for as long as 12 months after RP, while the BT patients consistently remained stable.

Although BT appeared to have a clear advantage over RP in terms of urinary function (urinary control), transient irritative and obstructive urinary symptoms occurred during and after BT (Litwin et al., 2002). The BT group experienced a significant increase in IPSS and this trend continued for more than 6 months after treatment. These symptoms were relatively apparent in our analysis using IPSS. Thus, the urinary bother curve shows more significant adverse treatment effects. In our experience, the IPSS had more than doubled at 3 months following BT. This sharp increase in urinary symptoms in a short period of time is clinically significant (Namiki et al., 2006c). By 1 year, however, the IPSS are indistinguishable from the baseline measures. This study revealed that continence is not a sole determining factor in urinary bother, and BT patients may be "dry" but suffer from urgency, frequency, and dysuria. The potency rates following BT have been encouraging, as high as 90%, although a decrease occurs from 3 to 6 years (Merrick et al., 2002). Additional long-term studies with a larger number of patients are necessary to fully understand the impact of each treatment on the HRQOL for Japanese men who undergo BT.

7 Androgen Deprivation Therapy

There are a few articles reporting the effects of Androgen deprivation therapy (ADT) on HRQOL. Heer and O'Sullivan (2000) compared patients receiving hormone therapy versus those observed for asymptomatic advanced cancer. They documented better HRQOL among patients who elected to defer treatment compared to those who opted for early interventions. Potosky et al. studied HRQOL in patients with localized prostate cancer treated initially with ADT or no therapy and reported that protracted ADT was associated with worse physical function and more fatigue compared with patients receiving no therapy (Potosky et al., 2002). On the other hand, Lubeck et al. stated that there were no noticeable decrements with the hormonal therapy in the first year scores of the general HRQOL (Lubeck et al., 1999). With regard to Japanese subjects, almost all HRQOL measures except for sexual function was mostly unaffected by ADT (Kato et al., 2007). Whereas there was a substantial decrease in sexual function, they did not complain sexual bother. Patients receiving ADT felt less bothered by sexual dysfunction presumably because they are well informed of the potential for deterioration of sexual function before treatment and thus have lowered expectations about post-treatment sexual function.

8 Cross-Cultural Comparative Study

Cross-cultural comparative studies using the same instrument will certainly contribute to the global advancement of outcome assessment. Namiki et al. conducted a cross-cultural comparison of the recovery of sexual and urinary function and bother during the first 2 years after radical prostatectomy (RP) between American and Japanese men (Namiki et al., 2008a). Using a self-reported questionnaire, Japanese men reported lower sexual function scores at baseline, even after adjusting for age, prostate-specific antigen (PSA) and comorbidity (38 vs. 61, p < 0.001). At 2 years postoperatively, 22% of Japanese men and 35% of American men had fully returned to baseline sexual function. In addition, American men were more likely than Japanese men to regain their baseline sexual function by 24 months after treatment. This finding is consistent with other reports in which ED and decreased libido were noted in a greater proportion of Japanese than American men (Masumori et al., 1999). Population-based data from Japan indicate that the proportion of ED is 20, 42 and 64% for ages 50–59, 60–69 and 70–79, respectively, all higher than in other countries (Marumo et al., 2001; Shabsigh et al., 2004). On the other hand, Japanese and American men did not differ in sexual bother score at baseline (70 vs. 68, p = 0.64). After RP, the Japanese men demonstrated significantly equivalent or better sexual bother scores (less distress) than did the American men at all postoperative time points. Whereas only 24 and 40% American men did at the same time points, 39 and 73% Japanese men returned to baseline sexual bother score at 1 and 6 months postoperatively. (❯ *Figures 166-1* and ❯ *166-2*) Multivariate modeling revealed that American men were less likely than Japanese men to return to their baseline sexual bother.

Even before treatment Japanese men with localized prostate cancer were more likely than American men to report poor sexual desire, poor erection ability, poor overall ability to function sexually, poor ability to attain orgasm, poor quality of erections, infrequency of sexual erections, infrequency of morning erections, and less intercourse in the previous 4 weeks. However, Japanese men were less likely than American men to be bothered by their sexual function (Namiki et al., 2008c). This suggests that cultural factors and deeply embedded health beliefs may play a decisive role in defining health-seeking behaviors for sexual problems. Even though Japanese beliefs regarding sexuality have changed considerably recently, Japanese men still hesitate in consulting physicians about their sexual issues. Thus, the deterioration of sexual activity did not appear to impact HRQOL in Japanese men as much as that in American men. This suggests that cultural factors and deeply embedded health beliefs may play a decisive role in defining health-seeking behaviors for sexual problems. Among those who do not seek treatment, younger men seem to believe that their ED would resolve spontaneously, while older men resisted seeking treatment because they felt ED was a natural part of aging. Moreover, while male erectile rigidity contributes to the frequency of sexual intercourse, it is not necessarily associated with a satisfactory sexual life in the Japanese men's partners (Hisasue et al., 2005). The discrepancy between Japanese males and their partners' responses might be explained by discordant views of what constitutes a satisfactory sexual life (e.g., non-coital intimate activities).

Japanese urologists' attitudes toward their patients' sexual problems may compound the hesitation to talk about sexual issues. They seem less proactive in dealing with ED in cancer patients, choosing to focus more on outcomes such as laboratory test results. This is consistent with previous study which was utilized a nationwide survey in Japan on the attitudes of breast cancer surgeons., One-third reported addressing "nothing in particular" about their patients' sexuality after surgery (Takahashi et al., 2006). Physical conditions in Japanese hospitals often limit confidentiality, perhaps decreasing motivation to discuss such sensitive issues. American

◻ **Figure 166-1**

Longitudinal changes in sexual function and bother over time in Japanese and American men

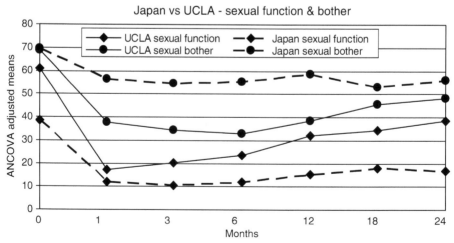

▣ Figure 166-2

Kaplan-Meier analysis of the proportion of subjects returning to baseline over time

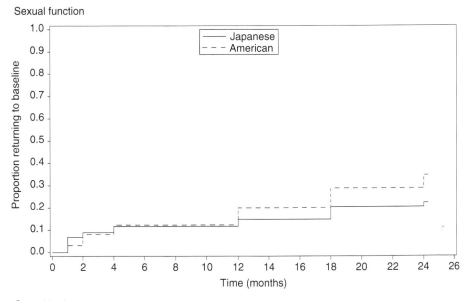

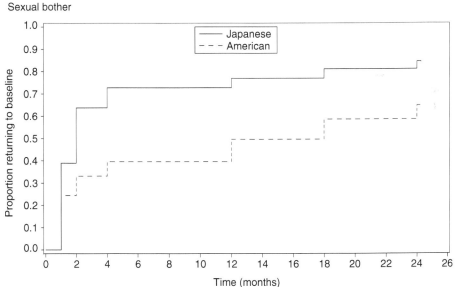

urologists tend to prescribe therapy for their patients with post-prostatectomy ED, in part because of theories that early sexual rehabilitation may promote post-surgical recovery of erectile function (Gontero et al., 2003).

The use of phosphodiesterase-5 (PDE-5) inhibitors (such as sildenafil, tadanafil, and vardenafil) has been widely touted as a solution for ED after prostate cancer treatment. Although PDE-5 inhibitors have been available since 1999 in Japan, it was striking that

Japanese men were much less likely than American men to use PDE-5 inhibitors (10% vs. 71%). In Japan, moreover, those who used PDE-5 inhibitors reported better sexual function than those who did not after RP as well as before RP. Contrary to Japanese men, the American men who took PDE-5 inhibitors reported lower sexual function than those who did not after RP (Namiki et al., 2008b). This finding mirrors differences between Japanese and American men in the motivations for sexuality. Even though Japanese beliefs regarding sexuality have changed considerably recently, Japanese men still hesitate in consulting physicians about their sexual issues. Conversely, American men are more assertive in seeking care for ED after prostate cancer treatment (Shabsigh et al., 2004). In Japan most men take no action, while in America men may seek help from their partners, family members or other sources of social support.

With regard to urinary HRQOL, there were no differences about urinary function or bother at baseline between Japanese men and American men. Japanese men reported a lower incidence of urinary dysfunction (urinary incontinence) and felt less distress than American men at 1 month after RP. For RP patients, urinary function and bother scores decreased from baseline to a nadir at 1 month after surgery and then continued to increase through 12 months post-operatively. Mean scores at 1 month differed significantly between the countries. Multivariate analyses revealed non-liner pattern of recovery and a significant difference in this pattern between countries with regard to urinary function (control) and bother after RP (both $p < 0.0001$) (❷ *Figure 166-3*). If Japanese men have historically not been screened as often, they would be expected to have presented with worse disease, making them more like the African-American men and reporting worse outcomes (Jayadevappa et al., 2007). In this analysis, however, the opposite was observed: Japanese men presented with worse disease but reported better outcomes than the American men. It is not clear whether the national variations we found in early urinary function recovery were attributable to intrinsic differences or the relative disease severity in our twosamples. The two cultures may simply have different concepts of health, well-being, and illness or disease with regard to urination. Even though we used validated survey instruments, we must remain aware that cross-cultural issues still significantly affect clinical assessment.

9   Future Directions

There is insufficient information regarding HRQOL for Asian men including Japanese men diagnosed with prostate cancer. In the absence of an underlying biological explanation for cross-national differences, however, we suspect that cultural differences in how the HRQOL surveys were interpreted may explain the differences in Japanese and American men with prostate cancer. Different cultures have different concepts of health, well-being, illness, and health insurance systems. A concept that is well developed in one country may not even exist in another one. Even if we use HRQOL study with validated survey instrument in English, we need to be aware that these multicultural issues may be introduced a significant bias in the collection of data and reflect not the men's preferences but the medical care they received.

Given that prostate cancer is one of the most common solid tumor in Japanese men, it is important to focus on the cancer and its various treatment have unique effects on quantity and quality of life. Further, while men with prostate cancer are being diagnosed at a younger age and living longer with the disease, it is critical that we obtain a better understanding of all the facts that could influence short-term and long-term functional states and HRQOL in prostate cancer patients.

□ Figure 166-3

Longitudinal changes in raw scores of urinary domains measured by UCLA Prostate Cancer Index over time

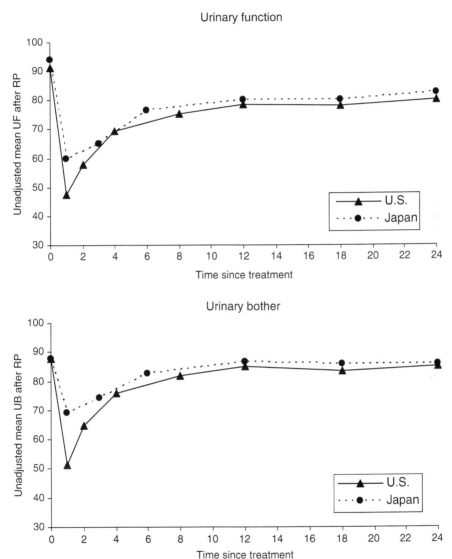

Summary Points

- In recent years, increased screening for prostate cancer, primarily with prostate specific antigen testing, has lead to an increase in the apparent incidence of prostate cancer, and resulted in a shift to an earlier age and stage at diagnosis, a trend similar to that in the U.S. and European countries.

- The Japanese version of UCLA Prostate Cancer Index demonstrated good psychometric properties (reliability and validity) and it was easy to answer and easily understandable by patients and physicians and it has been incorporated in many outcome studies of Japanese patients.
- Among the men who underwent radical prostatectomy, urinary function and bother scores decreased from baseline to a nadir at 1 month after surgery and then continued to increase through 12 months post-operatively.
- Although the majority of postoperative patients reported good general HRQOL, significant deteriorations of sexual function and sexual bother were observed.
- Japanese men with localized prostate cancer who underwent external beam radiation therapy appear to have similar general HRQOL to men who have received radical prostatectomy.
- The irritative and obstructive urinary symptoms occur during and in the period immediately after brachy therapy as well as external beam radiation therapy. These tend to improve over time but persist at the 12-month mark.
- Almost all HRQOL measures of Japanese men with prostate cancer except for sexual function was mostly unaffected by androgen deprivation therapy.
- Using a self-reported questionnaire, Japanese men reported lower sexual function scores at baseline. In addition, American men were more likely than Japanese men to regain their baseline sexual function by 24 months after treatment.
- Race and ethnicity are important factors in HRQOL because preferences and health system trust factors that are predominant in certain racial groups are likely to influence HRQOL and satisfaction with care.
- Multivariate analyses revealed a non-liner trend of recovery and an interaction between time and country with regard to urinary function (control) and bother after radical prostatectomy.

References

Aaronson NK, Ahmedzai S, Bergman B, Bullinger M, Cull A, Duez NJ, Filiberti A, Flechtner H, Fleishman SB, de Haes JC. (1993). J Natl Cancer Inst. 85: 365–376.

Akaza H, Hinotsu S, Usami M, Ogawa O, Kagawa S, Kitamura T, Tsukamoto T, Naito S, Hirao Y, Murai M, Yamanaka H, Namiki M. (2006). J Urol. 176: S47–49.

Akakura K, Isaka S, Akimoto S, Ito H, Okada K, Hachiya T, Yoshida O, Arai Y, Usami M, Kotake T, Tobisu K, Ohashi Y, Sumiyoshi Y, Kakizoe T, Shimazaki J. (1999). Urology. 54: 313–318.

Andersson SO, Rashidkhani B, Karlberg L, Wolk A, Johansson JE. (2004). BJU Int. 94: 323–331.

Arai Y, Okubo K, Aoki Y, Maekawa S, Okada T, Maeda H, Ogawa O, Kato T. (1999) Int J Urol. 6: 78–86.

Bill-Axelson A, Holmberg L, Ruutu M, Häggman M, Andersson SO, Bratell S, Spångberg A, Busch C, Nordling S, Garmo H, Palmgren J, Adami HO, Norlén BJ, Johansson JE, Scandinavian Prostate Cancer Group Study No. 4. (2005). N Engl J Med. 352: 1977–1984.

Blanker MH, Bohnen AM, Groeneveld FP, Bernsen RM, Prins A, Ruud Bosch JL. (2000). J Urol. 164: 1201–1205.

Cancer Registration Committee of the Japanese Urological Association. (2005). Int J Urol. 12: 46–49.

Carlson KV, Nitti VW. (2001). Urol Clin North Am. 28: 595–612.

Catalona WJ, Carvalhal GF, Mager DE, Smith DS. (1999). J Urol. 162: 433–438.

Cella DF, Tulsky DS, Gray G, Sarafian B, Linn E, Bonomi A, Silberman M, Yellen SB, Winicour P, Brannon J. (1993). J Clin Oncol. 11: 570–579.

Cooperberg MR, Broering JM, Litwin MS, Lubeck DP, Mehta SS, Henning JM, Carroll PR. (2004). CaPSURE Investigators J Urol. 171: 1393–1401.

Cooperberg MR, Master VA, Carroll PR. (2003). J Urol. 170: 512–515.

Downs TM, Sadetsky N, Pasta DJ, Grossfeld GD, Kane CJ, Mehta SS, Carroll PR, Lubeck DP. (2003). J Urol. 170: 1822–1827.

Egawa S, Shimura S, Irie A, Kitano M, Nishiguchi I, Kuwao S, Hayakawa K, Baba S. (2003). Int J Urol. 10: 207–212.

Esper P, Mo F, Chodak G, Sinner M, Cella D, Pienta KJ. (1997). Urology. 50: 920–928.

Eton DT, Lepore SJ, Helgeson VS. (2001). Cancer. 92: 1451–1459.

Frank SJ, Pisters LL, Davis J, Lee AK, Bassett R, Kuban DA. (2007). J Urol. 177: 2151–2156.

Fowler FJ Jr., Barry MJ, Lu-Yao G, Wasson JH, Bin L. (1996). J Clin Oncol. 14: 2258–2265.

Gill TM, Feinstein AR. (1994). JAMA. 272: 619–626.

Gontero P, Fontana F, Bagnasacco A, Panella M, Kocjancic E, Pretti G, Frea B. (2003). J Urol. 169: 2166–2169.

Hara I, Kawabata G, Miyake H, Nakamura I, Hara S, Okada H, Kamidono S. (2003). J Urol. 169: 2045–2048.

Hashine K, Azuma K, Koizumi T, Sumiyoshi Y. (2005). Int J Clin Oncol. 10: 45–50.

Heer HW, O'sullivan M. (2000). J Urol. 163: 1743–1746.

Hisasue S, Kumamoto Y, Sato Y, Masumori N, Horita H, Kato R, Kobayashi K, Hashimoto K, Yamashita N, Itoh N. (2005). Urology. 65: 143–148.

Hoffman RH, Hunt WC, Stephenson RA. (2003). Cancer. 97: 1653–1662.

Ishihara M, Suzuki H, Akakura K, Komiya A, Imamoto T, Tobe T, Ichikawa T. (2006). Int J Urol. 13: 920–92.

Jayadevappa R, Johnson JC, Chhatre S, Wein AJ, Malkowicz SB. (2007). Cancer. 109: 2229–2238.

Johnson TK, Gilliland FD, Hoffman RM, Deapen D, Penson DF, Stanford JL, Albertsen PC, Hamilton AS. (2004). J Clin Oncol. 22: 4193–4201.

Kakehi Y, Kamoto T, Ogawa O, Arai Y, Litwin MS, Suzukamo Y, Fukuhara S. (2002). Int J Clin Oncol. 7: 306–311.

Kakehi Y, Takegami M, Suzukamo Y, Namiki S, Arai Y, Kamoto T, Ogawa O, Fukuhara S. (2007). J Urol. 177: 1856–1861.

Kato T, Komiya A, Suzuki H, Imamoto T, Ueda T, Ichikawa T. (2007). Int J Urol. 14: 416–421.

Krupski TL, Saigal CS, Litwin MS. (2003). J Urol. 170: 1291–1294.

Litwin MS, Flanders SC, Pasta DJ, Stoddard ML, Lubeck DP, Henning JM. (1999). Urology. 54: 503–508.

Litwin MS, Hays RD, Fink A, Ganz PA, Leake B, Brook RH. (1998a). Med Care. 36: 1002–1012.

Litwin MS, Hays RD, Fink A, Ganz PA, Leak B, Leach GE, Brook RH. (1995). JAMA. 273: 129–135.

Litwin MS, Lubeck DP, Henning JM, Carroll PR. (1998b). J Urol. 159: 988–992.

Litwin MS, Lubeck DP, Spitalny GM, Henning JM, Carroll PR. (2002). Cancer. 95: 54–60.

Lubeck DP, Kim H, Grossfeld G, Ray P, Penson DF, Flanders SC, Carroll PR. (2001). J Urol. 166: 2281–2285.

Lubeck DP, Litwin MS, Henning JM, Stoddard ML, Flanders SC and Carroll PR. (1999). Urology. 53: 180–186.

Marumo K, Nakashima J, Murai M. (2001). Int J Urol. 8: 53–59.

Masumori N, Tsukamoto T, Kumamoto Y, Panser LA, Rhodes T, Girman CJ, Lieber MM, Jacobsen SJ. (1999). Urology. 54: 335–344.

Matsubara A, Yasumoto H, Mutaguchi K, Mita K, Teishima J, Seki M, Kajiwara M, Kato M, Shigeta M, Usui T. (2005). Int J Urol. 12: 953–958.

Merrick GS, Butler WM, Galbreath RW, Stipetich RL, Abel LJ, Lief JH. (2002). Int J Radiat Oncol Biol Phys. 52: 893–902.

Mizokami A, Ueno S, Fukagai T, Ito K, Ehara H, Kinbara H, Origasa H, Usami M, Namiki M, Akaza H. (2007) BJU Int. 99 Suppl 1: 6–9.

Nakata S, Ohtake N, Kubota Y, Imai K, Yamanaka H, Ito Y, Hirayama N, Hasegawa K. (1998). Int J Urol. 5: 364–369.

Namiki S, Egawa S, Baba S, Terachi T, Usui Y, Terai A, Tochigi T, Kuwahara M, Ioritani N, Arai Y. (2005a). Urology. 65: 517–523.

Namiki S, Ishidoya S, Saito S, Satoh M, Tochigi T, Ioritani N, Yoshimura K, Terai A, Arai Y. (2006a). Urology. 68: 142–147.

Namiki S, Ishidoya S, Tochigi T, Kawamura S, Kuwahara M, Terai A, Yoshimura K, Numata I, Satoh M, Saito S, Takai Y, Yamada S, Arai Y. (2006b). Jpn J Clin Oncol. 36: 224–230.

Namiki S, Kwan L, Kagawa-Singer M, Arai Y, Litwin MS. (2008b). Urology. 71: 901–905.

Namiki S, Kwan L, Kagawa-Singer M, Saito S, Terai A, Satoh T, Baba S, Arai Y, Litwin MS. (2008c). J Urol. 179: 245–249.

Namiki S, Kwan L, Kagawa-Singer M, Tochigi T, Ioritani N, Terai A, Arai Y, Litwin MS. (2008a). Prostate Cancer Prostatic Dis. 11: 298–302.

Namiki S, Saito S, Nakagawa H, Sanada T, Yamada A, Arai Y. (2007b). J Urol. 178: 212–216.

Namiki S, Saito S, Satoh M, Ishidoya S, Kawamura S, Tochigi T, Kuwahara M, Aizawa M, Ioritani N, Yoshimura K, Ichioka K, Terai A, Arai Y. (2005b). Jpn J Clin Oncol. 35: 551–558.

Namiki S, Saito S, Tochigi T, Kuwahara M, Ioritani N, Yoshimura K, Terai A, Koinuma N, Arai Y. (2005c). Int J Urol. 12: 173–181.

Namiki S, Saito S, Tochigi T, Numata I, Ioritani N, Arai Y. (2007c). Int J Urol. 14: 924–929.

Namiki S, Satoh T, Baba S, Ishiyama H, Hayakawa K, Saito S, Arai Y. (2006c). Urology. 68: 1230–1236.

Namiki S, Takegami M, Kakehi Y, Suzukamo Y, Fukuhara S, Arai Y. (2007d). J Urol. 178: 473–477.

Namiki S, Tochigi T, Kuwahara M, Ioritani N, Terai A, Numata I, Satoh M, Saito S, Koinuma N, Arai Y. (2004a). Int J Urol. 11: 619–627.

Namiki S, Tochigi T, Kuwahara M, Ioritani N, Yoshimura K, Terai A, Nakagawa H, Ishidoya S, Satoh M, Ito A, Saito S, Koinuma N, Arai Y. (2004b). Int J Urol. 11: 742–749.

Okaneya T, Nishizawa S, Nakayama T, Kamigaito T, Hashida I, Hosaka N. (2007). Int J Urol. 14: 602–606.

Parkin DM, Bray FI, Devesa SS. (2001). Eur J Cancer. 37 (Suppl. 8): S4–66.

Patrick DL, Deyo RA. (1989). Med Care. 27: S217–232.

Potosky AL, Davis WW, Hoffman RM, Stanford JL, Stephenson RA, Penson DF, Harlan LC. (2004). J Natl Cancer Inst. 96: 1358–1367.

Potosky AL, Reeve BB, Clegg LX, Hoffman RM, Stephenson RA, Albertsen PC, Gilliland FD, Stanford JL. (2002). J Natl Cancer Inst. 94: 430–437.

Potters L, Klein EA, Kattan MW, Reddy CA, Ciezki JP, Reuther AM, Kupelian PA. (2004). Radiother Oncol. 71: 29–33.

Ramsey SD, Zeliadt SB, Hall IJ, Ekwueme DU, Penson DF. (2007). J Urol. 177: 1992–1999.

Rose A, Peters N, Shea JA, Armstrong K. (2004). J Gen Intern Med. 19: 57–63.

Scardino PT, Kim ED. (2001). Urology. 57: 1016–1019.

Schwartz EJ, Lepor H. (1999). J Urol. 161: 1185–1188.

Shabsigh R, Perelman MA, Laumann EO, Lockhart DC. (2004). BJU Int. 94: 1055–1065.

Shaw PA, Etzioni R, Zeliadt SB, Mariotto A, Karnofski K, Penson DF, Weiss NS, Feuer EJ. (2004). Am J Epidemiol. 160: 1059–1069.

Takahashi M, Kai I, Hisata M, Higashi Y. (2006). J Clin Oncol. 24: 5763–5768.

Talcott JA, Rieker P, Clark JA, Propert KJ, Weeks JC, Beard CJ, Wishnow KI, Kaplan I, Loughlin KR, Richie JP, Kantoff PW. (1998). J Clin Oncol. 16: 275–283.

Tubaro A, La Vecchia C. (2004). Eur Urol. 45: 767–772.

Visser A, van Andel G, Willems P, Voogt E, Dijkstra A, Rovers P, Goodkin K, Kurth KH. (2003). Patient Educ Couns. 49: 225–232.

Ware JE and Sherbourne CD. (1992). Med Care. 30: 473–483.

Wei JT, Dunn RL, Litwin MS, Sandler HM, Sanda MG. (2000). Urology. 56: 899–905.

Yoshimura K, Arai Y, Ichioka K, Matsui Y, Ogura K, Terai A. (2004). Prostate Cancer Prostatic Dis. 7: 144–151.

Yoshimura K, Kamoto T, Nakamura E, Segawa T, Kamba T, Takahashi T, Nishiyama H, Ito N, Takayama K, Mizowaki T, Mitsumori M, Hiraoka M, Ogawa O. (2007). Prostate Cancer Prostatic Dis. 10: 288–292.

Yoshimura K, Sumiyoshi Y, Hashimura T, Ueda T, Kamiryo Y, Yamamoto A, Arai Y. (2003). Int J Urol. 10: 190–195.

Zelefsky MJ, Fuks Z, Hunt M, Lee HJ, Lombardi D, Ling CC, Reuter VE, Venkatraman ES, Leibel SA. (2001). J Urol. 166: 876–881.

Zelefsky MJ, Fuks Z, Hunt M, Yamada Y, Marion C, Ling CC, Amols H, Venkatraman ES, Leibel SA. (2002). Int J Radiat Oncol Biol Phys. 53: 1111–1116.

167 Quality of Life in Men Undergoing Radical Prostatectomy for Prostate Cancer

M. Pearson · E. M. Wallen · R. S. Pruthi

1   *Introduction* 2877

2   *Treatment Options* 2877

3   *Radical Prostatectomy as Treatment for Localized Prostate Cancer* 2878
3.1   Potential Advantages 2878
3.2   Potential Disadvantages 2880
3.3   Urinary Incontinence 2880
3.4   Erectile Dysfunction 2880

4   *Measures of Quality of Life* 2881

5   *Quality of Life Following Prostatectomy* 2882

6   *Relevance to Other Disease Sites* 2884

7   *Conclusion* 2885

Abstract: Prostate cancer is the most common noncutaneous cancer in men and the second-leading cause of death from cancer in men in the United States. Approximately one in six men will be diagnosed with the disease during his lifetime. When a man is diagnosed with clinically localized prostate cancer, he is immediately faced with a number of complex issues regarding the management of the disease. Options available to him include surgical management in the form of radical prostatectomy, radiotherapy including external beam radiation therapy and brachytherapy, hormone ablation, and expectant management or active surveillance (i.e., "watchful waiting").

Radical prostatectomy remains one of the most important tools for localized disease – a "gold-standard" for definitive treatment to which novel therapies are compared (❷ *Table 167-1*). It is estimated that in the United States that approximately 77,000 of the procedures are performed annually. To assist clinicians along these lines, several validated questionnaires have been developed and are commonly used to monitor quality of life changes in patients as they relate to treatment of localized prostate cancer. Providers who treat localized prostate cancer should be familiar with and utilize these instruments as part of their routine post-treatment evaluation of patients over time (❷ *Table 167-2*).

Improved understanding of the side effects of interventions and their impact of health-related quality of life (HRQOL) is an important part of understanding of the impact of the cancer as well as the modalities to treat the malignancy. To this end, HRQOL assessments have become and important area of interest with respect to radical prostatectomy. Researchers have evaluated many different aspects of this topic, including the impact of comorbidities, socioeconomic status, type of prostatectomy, as well as comparisons to other treatments for prostate cancer. However, despite the potential for side effects, overall satisfaction with the surgery remains high, and patients report little decrease in their overall quality of life. A thorough understanding of these issues is essential for clinicians who must assist their patients through complicated decision processes once they are diagnosed with localized prostate cancer.

List of Abbreviations: *EBRT,* external beam radiation therapy; *EORTC QLQ-C30,* the European organization for research and treatment of cancer core quality of life questionnaire with its prostate cancer specific module; *EPIC,* the expanded prostate cancer index-composite; *FACT-P,* The functional assessment of cancer therapy-prostate instrument; *HRQOL,* health-related quality of life; *RALRP,* robotic-assisted laparoscopic radical prostatectomy; *SES,* socioeconomic status; *UCLA PCI,* The UCLA prostate cancer index

◻ Table 167-1

Key facts about radical prostatectomy

Involves the surgical treatment for prostate cancer with curative intent
Estimated that over 100,000 procedures performed each year in the United States
Involves removal of entire prostate and seminal vesicles. On occasion, may include removal of pelvic lymph nodes
Common surgical techniques include retropubic, perineal, laparoscopic, and robotic-assisted laparoscopic approaches
Most common side effects which may impact quality of life include urinary leakage (< 10%) and erectile dysfunction (15–40%)

◘ Table 167-2

Commonly-used and validated measures of QOL after radical prostatectomy

1. *The UCLA Prostate Cancer Index (UCLA PCI)*: 20-item instrument that is prostate-specific in nature. Does not contain questions regarding general HRQOL, and therefore commonly administered along with general health instrument (e.g., RAND SF-36).
2. *The Expanded Prostate Cancer Index-Composite (EPIC)*: Expanded version of the UCLA PCI with 30 additional disease-specific items to more comprehensively define QOL outcomes following prostate cancer treatment. The EPIC includes additional 8 disease specific domains.
3. *The European Organization for Research and Treatment of Cancer Core Quality of Life Questionnaire with its prostate cancer specific module (EORTC QLQ-C30)*: Broad-based questionnaire was originally designed to measure cancer-specific QOL outcomes with various types of malignancies. Includes five general scales, a global health scale, three symptom scales, and 6 additional items. A prostate cancer module of 20 additional questions regarding bowel, urinary, and sexual function was added.
4. *The Functional Assessment of Cancer Therapy-Prostate Instrument (FACT-P)*: Questionnaire containing 38 items; 26 measure five general QOL domains with the remaining 12 measuring disease-specific issues. Perhaps better suited to assessing men with metastatic disease.

1   Introduction

Prostate cancer is the most common noncutaneous cancer in men and the second-leading cause of death from cancer in men in the United States. Approximately one in six men will be diagnosed with the disease during his lifetime. It was estimated that in January 2004, 2 million men living in the U.S. had either active prostate cancer or had been cured of the disease. In 2008, it is estimated that another 186,000 new cases of prostate cancer will be diagnosed and 28,000 men will die of the disease. (Website of the National Cancer Institute, 2008) Since the widespread implementation of PSA as a screening tool for prostate cancer in the early 1990s, prostate cancer is being diagnosed earlier. Approximately 90% of all prostate cancers are now diagnosed while the cancer is still confined to the primary site or to regional lymph nodes (Website of the National Cancer Institute, 2008).

2   Treatment Options

When a man is diagnosed with clinically localized prostate cancer, he is immediately faced with a number of complex issues regarding the management of the disease. Options available to him include surgical management in the form of radical prostatectomy, radiotherapy including external beam radiation therapy and brachytherapy, hormone ablation, and expectant management or active surveillance (i.e., "watchful waiting"). None of these modalities have shown definitive superiority compared to the others in terms of overall survival (Klein, 1998). However, each has a unique side-effect profile that impacts the quality of life of patients in different ways. Therefore, the choice of management of localized prostate cancer must be tailored to the individual patient based on his unique situation and preferences. The clinician has an important role in assisting the patient through this complicated decision process. In order to best advise the patient along these lines, the provider must looking beyond just disease-specific outcomes and have an understanding of how these modalities uniquely impact the quality of life of those who undergo them.

3   Radical Prostatectomy as Treatment for Localized Prostate Cancer

Radical prostatectomy involves complete removal of the prostate gland and seminal vesicles and sometimes includes a modified pelvic lymph node dissection (❷ *Figure 167-1*). Traditionally, prostatectomy is a formidable procedure. However refinement of the surgical technique over a century of experience has made the risk of operative mortality extremely low and has reduced the risks and complications of the operation. Indeed, recent advances in laparoscopic and robotic techniques have reduced the perioperative morbidity following prostatectomy to extremely low levels. Despite the advent of numerous other treatment modalities for localized prostate cancer, radical prostatectomy remains one of the most important tools for localized disease – a "gold-standard" for definitive treatment to which novel therapies are compared. It is estimated that in the United States that approximately 77,000 of the procedures are performed annually (Patel et al., 2007).

◻ Figure 167-1

Prostate and Relevant Pelvic Anatomy. Legend: Line drawing of lateral view of prostate and relevant pelvic anatomy. The figure reproduced from NCI website (www.cancer.gov)

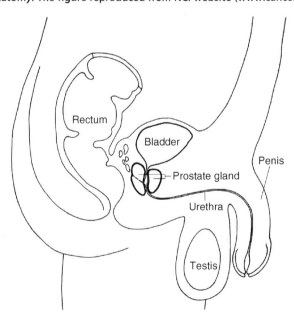

3.1   Potential Advantages

Compared to the other modalities used in the treatment of localized prostate cancer, radical prostatectomy offers several advantages. First, by providing specimens for pathologic evaluation, it offers more accurate staging than other therapies. Second, it significantly reduces local progression and distant metastases compared to watchful waiting (Bill-Axelson et al., 2005). Also, treatment failure is more readily identifiable after prostatectomy and may potentially be salvaged with postoperative radiotherapy (Stephenson et al., 2004b). However, the most important advantage of prostatectomy compared to other modalities is that it offers the possibility of complete eradication of the disease. This affords patients a relative peace-of-mind not afforded them by the other modalities used to treat localized prostate cancer. This may also be one reason why patient satisfaction after prostatectomy is generally high even in those who suffer side-effects of the surgery as discussed below (Clark et al., 2003) (❯ *Table 167-3*).

◻ Table 167-3

Studies on HRQOL after prostatectomy

Reference	HRQOL Measurement Tool	No. Pts	Main Outcome	Conclusion
Karakiewicz et al., 2008	UCLA-PCI	2,415	Association between comorbidity, SES, and HRQOL	Comorbidity and SES are strongly associated with sexual, urinary, and general HRQOL
Sadetsky et al., 2008	SF-36	2,258	Association between insurance status and HRQOL	Insurance associated with wide range of changes in HRQOL
Yang et al., 2005	EPIC	187	HRQOL after radical perineal prostatectomy (RPP)	HRQOL outcomes are favorable following RPP
Namiki et al., 2006	SF-36 UCLA-PCI	349	Comparison of HRQOL outcomes after retropubic, laparoscopic, and perineal, approaches	Similar HRQOL outcomes for each approach
Miller et al., 2007	SF-12	142	Impact of robotic assisted laparoscopic prostatectomy on short-term HRQOL	Faster return to baseline HRQOL after robotic prostatectomy vs. open
Litwan et al., 2007	SF-36 UCLA-PCI AUA-SI	580	Comparison of HRQOL outcomes after RRP, EBRT, and brachytherapy	Treatment modalities each of unique effect on HRQOL
Sanda et al., 2008	EPIC-26 SCA	1,201 patients; 625 partners	Comparison of HRQOL outcomes of patients and partners after RRP, EBRT, and brachytherapy	HRQOL of both patients and partners affected uniquely by each modality
Bacon et al., 2002	SF-36 CARES-SF, UCLA-PCI	783	Effect of treatment-related symptoms on overall HRQOL	Sexual, urinary, and bowel symptoms each associated with nearly all HRQOL outcomes examined

3.2   Potential Disadvantages

As noted previously, radical prostatectomy can be a morbid procedure relative to other, less invasive modalities used in the treatment of localized prostate cancer. Post-operative hospitalization is often required followed by a period of short-term disability and recovery (Miller et al., 2007). However, with the advent of laparoscopic and robotic techniques, the postoperative convalescent times have been substantially reduced (Miller et al., 2007). Many patients undergoing these minimally invasive techniques are able to leave the hospital on the first postoperative day and return to somewhat normal activity in a matter of days to weeks. The main disadvantage of prostatectomy concerning to patients contemplating surgery is the potential to develop two well-known side-effects postoperatively. These include urinary incontinence and erectile dysfunction, both of which result from disruptions of key anatomic structures during surgery due to their proximity to the prostate gland. It is the occurrence of one or both of these post-operative side effects that is most detrimental to a patient's quality of life after prostatectomy.

3.3   Urinary Incontinence

Urinary incontinence results from disruption of the external uretheral sphincter which lies at the apical end of the prostate and controls flow of urine out of the bladder. During prostatectomy meticulous dissection of the prostate from the external sphincter is required for maintenance of urinary continence. Contemporary series depicting post-prostatectomy incontinence rates have used varying definitions of the endpoint which has made comparisons between studies difficult. For instance, Stanford et al., reported that only 32% of men had total urinary control at 24 months following prostatectomy compared to 78% at baseline (Stanford et al., 2000). However, other single-center series utilizing more liberal definitions of continence have reported continence rates of greater than 90% at 18 months (Kundu et al., 2004; Walsh et al., 2000). In general, some percentage of men will suffer from incontinence immediately after prostatectomy. Most will regain urinary control by 6 months post-operatively (Burnett, 2005). Men who have not regained urinary control by 24 months should not anticipate any improvement thereafter (Penson et al., 2005). The main risk factor for failure to regain continence postoperatively is the age of the patient at the time of prostatectomy.

3.4   Erectile Dysfunction

Postoperative erectile dysfunction results from disruption of the cavernous nerves that innervate the penile erectile bodies and run along the posterolateral aspect of the prostate. Meticulous dissection of the neurovascular bundles from the surface of the prostate during resection is critical for maintenance of postoperative erectile function. This "nerve sparing" technique has been widely accepted and shown to have a significant impact on return of erectile function following prostatectomy (Quinlan et al., 1991). Again, methodological differences between studies make comparison of erectile dysfunction rates following prostatectomy difficult. However, contemporary estimates of recovery of erectile function in men with normal preoperative potency range from 60 to 85% (Donatucci and Greenfield, 2006). Unlike the recovery of continence following prostatectomy which normally occurs within the first 6 months, the return of erectile function is a slower process that may continue for up to 2 years after the surgery. This delayed recovery most likely coincides with the regeneration of the cavernous nerves injured during prostatectomy (Burnett, 2005). Return of erectile function has been correlated with the patient's age and preoperative potency status as well as the extent of the nerve sparing surgery performed.

4   Measures of Quality of Life

To assist clinicians along these lines, several validated questionnaires have been developed and are commonly used to monitor quality of life changes in patients as they relate to treatment of localized prostate cancer. Providers who treat localized prostate cancer should be familiar with and utilize these instruments as part of their routine post-treatment evaluation of patients over time. Research has shown that without such instruments, providers are not accurate in their assessment of the quality of life impact on patients due to the treatment modalities they provide (Penson and Litwin, 2003). Therefore, these patient-centered questionnaires are critical to a more complete awareness on the part of the clinician regarding how their patients are coping with the long-term effects of their disease and its treatment.

A brief summary of the four most commonly used questionnaires is provided below. Each of these instruments is patient-based and can be self-administered. Also, each attempts to break down overall health-related quality of life into domains to more precisely describe the patient experience. These domains may be general (common to all patients regardless of disease) or disease-specific (pertaining only to those with localized prostate cancer). Finally, each has been thoroughly validated for reproducibility (Borghede et al., 1997; Esper et al., 1997; Litwin et al., 1998; Wei et al., 2000).

1. *The UCLA Prostate Cancer Index (UCLA PCI)*: This is a 20-item instrument that is prostate-specific in nature and does not contain questions regarding general health-related quality of life (Litwin et al., 1998). Therefore, it is commonly administered along with the RAND 36-item General Health Survey (SF-36) (Ware and Sherbourne, 1992). The UCLA PCI divides prostate specific quality of life into six domains including urinary function and bother, sexual function and bother, and bowel function and bother.
2. *The Expanded Prostate Cancer Index-Composite (EPIC)*: This questionnaire is an expanded version of the UCLA PCI with 30 additional disease-specific items to more comprehensively define quality of life outcomes following prostate cancer treatment (Wei et al., 2000). The EPIC includes eight disease specific domains as it also queries hormonal function and bother in addition to the six included in the UCLA PCI. It also subdivides the urinary function domain into subscales of urinary incontinence and urinary irritation/obstruction. Because of its longer length, the EPIC is usually administered concurrently with the 12-item RAND SF-12 (Ware et al., 1996).
3. *The European Organization for Research and Treatment of Cancer Core Quality of Life Questionnaire with its prostate cancer specific module (EORTC QLQ-C30)*: This broad-based questionnaire was originally designed to measure cancer-specific quality of life outcomes with various types of malignancies (Aaronson et al., 1993). It includes five general scales (physical, role, emotional, cognitive, and social functioning), a global health scale, three symptom scales (fatigue, nausea/vomiting, and pain) and six additional items. As originally formulated, it was most suited to measure quality of life in men with

metastatic disease (Klein, 1998). However, a prostate cancer module of 20 additional questions regarding bowel, urinary, and sexual function was added and validated making it more specific for prostate cancer patients.

4. *The Functional Assessment of Cancer Therapy-Prostate Instrument (FACT-P)*: This questionnaire contains 38 items; 26 measure five general quality of life domains with the remaining 12 measuring disease-specific issues (Esper et al., 1997). However, because it uses only single items to assess the domains most affected by treatment of localized prostate cancer such as urinary difficulties and erectile dysfunction, the FACT-P is better suited to assessing men with metastatic disease (Klein, 1998).

5   Quality of Life Following Prostatectomy

Health-related quality of life (HRQOL) has become and important area of interest with respect to radical prostatectomy. Researchers have evaluated many different aspects of this topic. Several recent studies have evaluated the impact of population characteristics of patients on quality of life outcomes after prostatectomy. For example, using the UCLA PCI and the SF-36 as measures of prostate cancer-specific and overall health-related quality of life, Karakiewicz et al., evaluated associations between comorbidity and socioeconomic status (SES) with quality of life after prostatectomy. In general, the authors found a stronger effect on quality of life outcomes due to comorbidity. However, they also demonstrated an association with SES as well. For instance, 11 of the tested comorbidity and SES variables such as lower extremity circulation problems and education had a clinically significant impact on quality of life measures after prostatectomy (Karakiewicz et al., 2008). Another recent study by Sadetsky et al., found that the health insurance status of men undergoing prostatectomy had a strong association with HRQOL outcomes as measured by the SF-36 questionnaire as well (Sadetsky et al., 2008). Both of these studies correctly conclude that these demographic variables require consideration when interpreting HRQOL studies especially from heterogeneous patient populations.

Other studies have evaluated the effect of different forms of prostatectomy on HRQOL outcomes. As indicated above, several different surgical approaches are commonly used to accomplish prostatectomy including retropubic, perineal, pure laparoscopic, and robotic-assisted laparoscopic (❷ *Figure 167-2*). Most of the literature has focused on retropubic prostatectomy since this has been the most commonly performed technique historically. However, a recently published study by Yang et. al evaluated the HRQOL impact of prostatectomy performed via a perineal approach. The researchers conducting this study used the EPIC questionnaire and found that patients with at least 2 years follow-up after perineal prostatectomy had clinically similar HRQOL scores compared to a cohort of prostatectomy candidates prior to surgery (Yang et al., 2005). Another study from Japan directly compared the HRQOL impact of retropubic, perineal, and laparoscopic prostatectomies with 1 year of follow-up. Using the UCLA PCI and the SF-36, this study showed that each of the modalities resulted in the similar decrements in post-operative urinary and sexual dysfunction at 1 year. However, the perineal and laparoscopic groups showed decreased bodily pain immediately after surgery compared to the retropubic group. This difference was no longer detectable at 6 months post surgery (Namiki et al., 2006).

Recently, robotic-assisted laparoscopic radical prostatectomy (RALRP) has quickly gained wide-spread use in the urologic community as a method of performing prostatectomy with

◘ Figure 167-2

Commonly Used Approaches to Radical Prostatectomy. Legend: Diagram representing surgical incisions with retropubic (*left*) and robotic-assisted laparoscopic (*right*) prostatectomy

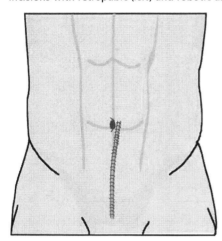 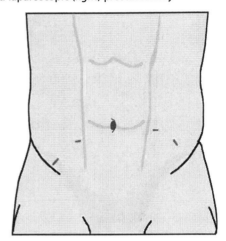

minimal perioperative morbidity while maintaining oncologic and functional outcomes. Due to the novelty of this procedure, research into its quality of life impact on patients is limited thus far. However, a study by Miller et al., compared the short-term impact of this modality versus retropubic prostatectomy using weekly SF-12 questionnaires for the first 6-weeks after surgery. This study demonstrated that patients undergoing RALRP had greater physical well-being and function compared those undergoing retropubic prostatectomy beginning the first week after surgery. It also demonstrated a swifter return to baseline for this component of quality of life (Miller et al., 2007). The combination of equivalent functional and oncologic outcomes with earlier return to baseline physical well-being as demonstrated by this article helps explain the current interest in RALRP.

The majority of research involving the quality of life impact due to treatment of localized prostate cancer has focused on comparing radical prostatectomy (RP) versus brachytherapy (BT) and external beam radiation therapy (EBRT). A number of studies have been conducted evaluating this, and the particular HRQOL impact of each has been convincingly discerned. A recently reported study by Litwin et al., exemplifies these findings. It used the SF-36 and the UCLA PCI to prospectively assess a cohort of 580 men at baseline and through 24 months after undergoing treatment for localized prostate cancer. It found that irritative urinary symptoms after RP were better than after BT but worse than after ERBT. In terms of urinary control, the RP group faired worse than both the BT and ERBT groups. In terms of sexual function, men potent at baseline who underwent bilateral nerve-sparing prostatectomy had equivalent outcomes compared to the BT group but worse outcomes compared to the ERBT group. Finally, bowel dysfunction was more common after ERBT than after BT and almost non-existant in the RP group (Litwan et al., 2007). This study corroborates previous findings along these lines and is useful to clinicians in clarifying to patients the risks and benefits of the various treatment modalities (Clark et al., 2003; Penson and Litwin, 2003; Sanda et al., 2008).

It is clear that a significant number of patients that undergo radical prostatectomy will suffer from incontinence, erectile dysfunction, or both. Studies have also shown that these side-effects will cause a significant amount of bother in the lives of these patients as well (Bacon et al., 2002; Sanda et al., 2008). However, paradoxically, these treatment-related side-effects do not seem to appreciably change the overall health status or health-related quality of life of these patients. For instance Clark et al., demonstrated that patients that underwent radical prostatectomy reported relatively high levels of confidence about cancer control as well as overall cancer-related outlook compared with those who underwent other treatment modalities for localized prostate cancer. This was despite the same cohort reporting relatively high levels of bother from erectile dysfunction and incontinence (Clark et al., 2003). It seems that men undergoing prostatectomy may "mentally exchange" the risk of treatment related side-effects for perceived better survival. Thus, satisfaction with prostatectomy and overall quality of life postoperatively remain high despite the occurrence of adverse treatment effects in many cases.

6   Relevance to Other Disease Sites

The study of HRQOL in men with prostate cancer provides a appropriate model for other benign and malignant disease states. Certainly, oncologic outcomes remain paramount prostatic carcinoma and other malignancies. However, as we have improved disease-specific outcomes in prostate cancer, attention to the impact of our treatments on HRQOL has become increasingly relevant. Perhaps because the natural history of prostate cancer progression is somewhat more protracted – at least for certain individuals – minimizing side effects have long been an important secondary goal of treatments. As such, development of prostate cancer-specific HRQOL instruments, such as those described in this chapter, have particular importance and relevance to the clinician caring for the prostate cancer patient. Development of such disease-specific measures – extending well beyond general QOL instruments – remains an important goal for many, if not all, cancer disease states. By defining, devising, and validating such measures of treatment success, we can ensure that we not only maximize oncologic efficacy, but also understand and minimize treated-related side effects. The experience in prostate cancer has this far been a sound model to this end.

◻ Table 167-4
Summary Points

• Prostate cancer is the most common non-cutaneous cancer among men in the United States
• Several validated self-assessment questionnaires exist and are routinely used in the evaluation of health-related quality of life as it relates to prostate cancer
• Radical prostatectomy is the most commonly performed therapeutic modality used in the treatment of localized prostate cancer
• Radical prostatectomy has a unique impact on the quality of life of those patients undergoing it relative to the other commonly used treatments for localized prostate cancer
• Two domains of health-related quality of life most commonly impacted by prostatectomy include urinary control and sexual function
• Overall health-related quality of life is typically maintained after prostatectomy even in cases in which specific domains of quality of life are diminished

7   Conclusion

Radical prostatectomy is the most frequently utilized modality in the treatment of localized prostate cancer. It has a unique side-effect profile relative to the other modalities with relatively high rates of post-operative incontinence and erectile dysfunction. Patients who experience these treatment-related effects do report increased bother because of them. However, despite this, overall satisfaction with the surgery remains high, and patients report little decrease in their overall quality of life. A thorough understanding of these issues is essential for clinicians who must assist their patients through complicated decision processes once they are diagnosed with localized prostate cancer (❷ *Table 167-4*).

References

Aaronson NK, Ahmedzai S, Bergman B, Bullinger M, Cull A, Duez NJ, Filiberti A, Flechtner H, Fleishman SB, deHaes JC, Kaasa S, Klee M, Osoba D, Razavi D, Rofe PB, Schraub S, Sneeuw K, Sullivan M, Takeda F. (1993). J Natl Cancer Inst. 85: 356–365.

Bacon CG, Giovannucci E, Testa M, Glass TA, Kawachi I. (2002). Cancer. 94: 862–871.

Bill-Axelson A, Holmberg L, Ruutu M, Häggman M, Andersson SO, Bratell S, Spångberg A, Busch C, Nordling S, Garmo H, Palmgren J, Adami HO, Norlén BJ, Johansson JE. (2005). Scandinavian Prostate Cancer Group Study No 4. N Engl J Med. 352: 1977–1984.

Borghede G, Karlsson J, Sullivan M. (1997). J Urol. 158: 1477–1485.

Burnett AL. (2005). JAMA. 293: 2648–2653.

Clark JA, Inui TS, Silliman RA, Bokhour BG, Krasnow SH, Robinson RA, Spaulding M, Talcott JA. (2003). J Clin Oncol. 21: 3777–3784.

Donatucci CF, Greenfield JM. (2006). Curr Opin Urol. 16: 444–448.

Esper P, Mo F, Chodak G, Sinner M, Cella D, Pienta KJ. (1997). Urology. 50: 920–928.

Karakiewicz PI, Bhojani N, Neugut A, Shariat SF, Jeldres C, Graefen M, Perrotte P, Peloquin F, Kattan MW. (2008). J Sex Med. 5: 919–927.

Klein EA. (1998). Semin Radiat Oncol. 8: 87–94.

Kundu SD, Roehl KA, Eggener SE, Antenor JA, Han M, Catalona WJ. (2004). J Urol. 172: 2227–2231.

Litwan MS, Gore JL, Kwan L, Brandeis JM, Lee SP, Withers HR, Reiter RE. (2007). Cancer. 109: 2239–2247.

Litwin MS, Hays RD, Fink A. (1998). Med Car. 36: 1002–1012.

Miller J, Smith A, Kouba E, Wallen E, Pruthi RS. (2007). J Urol. 178: 854–859.

Namiki S, Egawa S, Terachi T, Matsurbara A, Igawa M, Terai A, Tochigi T, Ioritani N, Saito S, Arai Y. (2006). J Urol. 67: 321–327.

Patel VR, Chammas MR Jr, Shah S. (2007). Int J Clin Pract. 61: 309–314.

Penson DF, Litwin MS. (2003). Curr Urol Reports. 4: 185–95.

Penson DF, McLerran D, Feng Z, Li L, Alertsen PC, Gilliland FD, Hamilton A, Hoffman RM, Stephenson RA, Potosky AL, Stanford JL. (2005). J Urol. 173: 1701–1705.

Quinlan DM, Epstein JI, Carter BS, Walsh PC. (1991). J Urol. 145: 998–1002.

Sadetsky N, Lubeck DP, Pasta DJ, Latini DM, DuChane J, Carroll PR. (2008). BJU Int. 101: 691–697.

Sanda MG, Dunn RL, Michalski J, Sandler HM, Northouse L, Hembroff L, Lin X, Greenfield TK, Litwin MS, Saigal CS, Mahadevan A, Lkein E, Kibel A, Pisters LL, Kuban D, Kaplan I, Wood D, Ciezki J, Shah N, Wei JT. (2008). N Engl J Med. 358: 1250–1261.

Stanford JL, Feng Z, Hamilton AS, Gilliland FD, Stephenson RA, Eley JW, Albertsen PC, Harlan LC, Potosky AL. (2000). JAMA. 283: 354–360.

Stephenson AJ, Shariat SF, Zelefsky MJ, Kattan MW, Butler EB, Teh BS, Klein EA, Kupelian PA, Roehrborn CG, Pistenmaa DA, Pacholke HD, Liau WSL, Katz MS, Leibel SA, Scardino PT, Slawin KM. (2004b). JAMA. 291: 1325–1332.

Walsh PC, Marschke P, Ricker D, Burnett AL. (2000). Urology. 55: 58–61.

Ware JE Jr, Kosinski M, Keller SD. (1996). Med Care. 34: 220–233.

Ware JE Jr, Sherbourne CD. (1992). Med Care. 30: 473–483.

Website of the National Cancer Institute. (2008). Cancer fact sheets: cancer of the prostate. Accessed March, 2008.

Wei JT, Dunn RL, Litwin MS, Sandler HM, Sanda MG. (2000). Urology. 56: 899–905.

Yang BK, Crisci A, Young MD, Silverstein AD, Peterson BL, Dahm P. (2005). J Urol. 65: 120–125.

168 Myeloproliferative Disorders and the Chronic Leukemias: Symptom Burden and Impact in Quality of Life

R. A. Mesa · D. P. Steensma · T. Shanafelt

1	*Introduction: Background*	**2889**
1.1	The Chronic Leukemias: A Primer	2889
1.1.1	Myeloproliferative Disorders	2889
1.2	Current Status of Treatment Options	2890
1.2.1	Short Term Therapeutic Plan	2890
1.2.2	Long Term Therapeutic Plan	2891
1.3	Chronic Leukemias and Why QOL Matters	2891
1.3.1	So Why the Focus on the Chronic Leukemias When We Discuss QOL?	2892
2	*Defining Symptomatic Burden in Chronic Leukemias*	**2892**
2.1	Chronic Leukemias: Spectrum of Disease – Spectrum of Symptoms	2892
3	*Other Chronic Leukemias*	**2893**
4	*Measured Impact on Quality of Life*	**2894**
4.1	Measuring Impact on Quality of Life in Chronic Leukemias: A Survey Based Approach	2894
4.1.1	Survey Content	2894
4.2	MPDS: Symptom Burden and Impact on QOL	2894
4.2.1	Respondents Encompassed Full Range of MPD Clinical Characteristics	2894
4.2.2	Majority of MPD Respondents Described Significant Symptoms and Medical Disability Secondary to their MPD	2895
4.2.3	MPD Patients Suffer from Significant Fatigue Compared to Published Norms	2895
4.2.4	MPD Related Fatigue Correlates with Many Disease Related Features	2897
4.2.5	Patients with Minimal "Objective" Manifestations of their MPD Suffer from Mild to Severe Fatigue	2897
4.2.6	Fatigue Is a Major Problem in MPD Patients Despite Therapy and Normal Co-Morbidity Burden	2898
4.3	MDS: Symptom Burden and Impact on QOL	2899
4.3.1	Participant Demographics and Disease Characteristics	2899
4.4	CLL: Symptom Burden and Impact on QOL	2900

5   Discussion: Implications of QOL Observations on Caring for
        Chronic Leukemia Patients 2900
5.1   What Have We Learned from Our Patients? 2900
5.2   How Should Symptoms and QOL Influence Treatment Decisions
        in Patients with Chronic Leukemias? 2901

6   Conclusions 2902

        Summary Points 2903

        Appendix 2903

Abstract: Optimizing health-related quality of life (QOL) is an important goal for patients with any hematological malignancy, but for those who suffer from disorders that follow a relatively indolent yet refractory course, QOL is an especially prominent consideration. These latter conditions include the chronic myeloproliferative disorders (MPD), myelodysplastic syndromes (MDS), and chronic lymphocytic leukemia (CLL) – diseases that are rarely curable, but that are often associated with prolonged survival. The MPD include polycythemia vera, essential thrombocythemia, and myelofibrosis (which can be primary, or can arise during the course of polycythemia vera or essential thrombocythemia). MPD-associated symptoms that compromise QOL include pruritus, night sweats, unintentional weight loss, loss of lean muscle mass, and profound fatigue, while QOL-impairing complications include thrombosis, bleeding, and often-dramatic splenic enlargement. Likewise, MDS suffer symptoms related to cytopenias, and CLL patients must contend with cytopenias, complications related to adenopathy and splenomegaly, and "B symptoms" (night sweats, weight loss, and unexplained fevers). By directly surveying large cohorts of MPD, MDS, and CLL patients using validated QOL instruments, we demonstrated that the burden of symptoms in these patients is severe, and that excessive fatigue is the most common and troublesome symptom of all, far exceeding levels reported for matched disease-free controls in the general population. Management of patients with MPD, MDS, or CLL needs to take into consideration QOL issues, and clinical trials of therapeutic agents should include improved QOL as a valid treatment endpoint.

List of Abbreviations: *BFI*, Brief Fatigue Inventory; *CLL*, Chronic Lymphocytic Leukemia; *CMML*, Chronic Myelomomonocytic Leukemia; *ESA*, Erythropoietin Stimulating Agent; *ET*, Essential Thrombocythemia; *FACTG*, Functional Assessment of Cancer–General; *FDA*, Federal Drug Administration; *MDS*, Myelodysplastic Syndrome; *MPD*, Myeloproliferative Disorder; *PV*, Polycythemia Vera; *Post ETMF*, Post Essential Thrombocythemia Myelofibrosis; *Post PVMF*, Post Polycythemia Vera Myelofibrosis; *PMF*, Primary Myelofibrosis; *QOL*, Quality of Life; *RA*, Refractory Anemia; *RAEV*, Refractory Anemia with Excess Blasts; *RAEV-T*, Refractory Anemia with Excess Blasts in Transformation; *RARS*, Refractory Anemia with Ringed Sideroblasts; *RCMV*, Refractory Cytopenia with Multilineage dysplasia

1   Introduction: Background

1.1   The Chronic Leukemias: A Primer

1.1.1   Myeloproliferative Disorders

The Philadelphia Chromosome-negative chronic myeloproliferative disorders (MPD) are a pathophysiologically interrelated group of clonal hematopoietic stem cell disorders which include polycythemia vera (PV), essential thrombocythemia (ET) and primary myelofibrosis (PMF) (Adamson and Fialkow, 1978; Dameshek, 1951; Gilbert, 1973). The MPD have a cumulative incidence of approximately 6/100,000/year and have a median age of onset of approximately 60 years of age (however patients <50 years of age are still commonly seen) (Mesa et al., 1999). Clinically, early in the disease course MPD patients are at risk of thrombohemorrhagic complications, and with progression can develop profound cytopenias, hepatosplenomegaly, eventually culminating in leukemic transformation. MPD can lead to premature death, with the most aggressive entity, myelofibrosis, having a median survival of

3–5 years (Dupriez et al., 1996). Patients both may have primary myelofibrosis (PMF) or may develop a myelofibrosis in the advanced phases of PV and ET; the latter complication is known as post polycythemia vera myelofibrosis (Post PV MF) and post essential thrombocythemia myelofibrosis (Post ET MF), respectively. Even in the absence of myelofibrosis, patients with PV and ET also have compromised survivals compared to age matched controls (Passamonti et al., 2004). The sources of mortality in ET and PV are the short-term risk of thrombohemor-rhagic complication and long-term risk of leukemic transformation, as well as development of Post ET/PV MF with their attendant cytopenias (Passamonti et al., 2004).

1.2   Current Status of Treatment Options

Currently available therapies are rarely able to alter the natural history of disease in MPD, although they may offer symptom palliation or decrease the risk of vascular events. Given these limitations, how should MPD patients be optimally managed?

When a diagnosis of an MPD is established or suspected, patients need to be stabilized, and immediate coagulopathies from severe erythrocytosis, thrombocytosis, or thrombotic/bleed-ing events must be urgently addressed. Management decisions then will depend on the treating clinician's estimation of overall disease prognosis, and the separate estimation of the individ-ual patient's risk of vascular events. In patients with ET and PV, patients at high risk for vascular events are those who have had a prior vascular event or are older than 60 years of age; low risk patients lack either of these features (and also have a platelet count $<1,000 \times 10^9$/L). Intermediate risk ET and PV are less than 60 and have not had a prior event, but have cardiovascular risk factors. Potential newly identified vascular risk factors include leukocytosis at diagnosis in PV $>15 \times 10^9$/L (Landolfi et al., 2007) or high JAK2V617F mutation allele burden in all MPD (Vannucchi et al., 2007). How these new factors should be included in modeling MPD vascular risk is not yet known, and requires further study.

1.2.1   Short Term Therapeutic Plan

The immediate therapeutic concerns for MPD patients at presentation are both an adequate prophylaxis against vascular events, and palliation when possible of MPD symptoms. Man-agement of PV patients includes control of erythrocytosis (by phlebotomy), and when no contraindication exists the use of low dose aspirin (Landolfi et al., 2004). The degree to which a patient needs to be phlebotomized has been questioned, with traditional dogma suggesting a goal hematocrit of $<42\%$ for women and 45% for men. Recent retrospective analysis of vascular events of patients on the ECLAP trial (European Collaborative Low Dose Aspirin Trial) has suggested that modestly higher targets (perhaps up to hematocrits of 55%) may not increase the risk of vascular events (Di Nisio et al., 2007). Whether goal hematocrits should be changed for PV needs to be addressed by appropriately designed trials.

What about myelosuppressive therapy for managing the MPDs? Hydroxyurea was shown in a randomized fashion to aid in the prevention of thrombotic events in patients with high risk ET (Cortelazzo et al., 1995). The UK MRC (United Kingdom Medical Research Council) PT-1 (primary thrombocythemia-1) trial compared in a randomized fashion hydroxyurea and anagrelide (both along with low dose aspirin) for ET patients and found hydroxyurea plus aspirin to be superior in regards to preventing arterial events, hemorrhage, and transformation to post-ET MF (Harrison et al., 2005). Therefore, standard front-line therapy for high risk ET and PV patients who require platelet lowering therapy is hydroxyurea. Although concerns linger about whether hydroxyurea accelerates an MPD towards leukemic transformation, this has never been proven (Finazzi et al., 2005). Pegylated interferon-2 alpha has shown clinical activity, and and may be more tolerable than traditional interferon, for especially PV (Kiladjian et al., 2006). How interferon compares with hydroxyurea for control of vascular events has not yet been studied in a randomized fashion.

Current attempts at palliating symptoms in MPD patients can include therapies for pruritus (anti-histamines, and selective serotonin reuptake inhibitors), erythromelalgia (aspirin), and fatigue (exercise). Cytopenias have improved in subsets of patients with erythropoietin supplementation (Cervantes et al., 2004), androgens (Cervantes et al., 2000), and/or corticosteroids. Similarly, the use of non-specific myelosuppressive regimens such as oral hydroxyurea (Lofvenberg et al., 1990) and cladribine (Faoro et al., 2005) have all been reported to provide palliative reduction in painful splenomegaly. Early reports of Phase I trials of JAK2 inhibitors indicate that these may also provide medical therapy of splenomegaly.

1.2.2   Long Term Therapeutic Plan

Currently, no therapy has been shown to be curative, alter natural history, or prolong survival in MPD patients, with the exception of allogeneic stem cell transplantation, for which few patients are eligible due to age and comorbidity. The long-term therapeutic plan for MPD patients, and particularly those with PMF (and post ET/PV MF), can be divided into (1) observation (2) proceeding directly to a allogeneic stem cell transplant and (3) enrollment in an appropriate clinical trial. Observation as a medical plan implies continued vigilance and therapy for prevention of vascular events and appropriate therapy for palliation of MPD symptoms. Observation is most appropriate for those patients with low risk PMF, and controlled ET and PV. Additionally, observation requires continued vigilance of the patient's disease status for disease progression to a point where (1) a clinical trial would be appropriate or 2) a stem cell transplant would be considered.

1.3   Chronic Leukemias and Why QOL Matters

While the major focus of this chapter is the impact of the MPD on quality of life, many of the challenges that these patients face are not unique and are shared by the other chronic hematological malignancies. Patients with the myelodysplastic syndromes (MDS) – a group a clonal bone marrow failure syndromes formerly known as "preleukemia," also suffer from debilitating fatigue and complications of cytopenias. Chronic lymphocytic leukemia (CLL) is a B-cell lymhoproliferative disorder characterized by cytopenias, lymphadenopathy, and hepatosplenomegaly due to organ expansion by clonal cells. MDS and CLL share several common several features with MPD. First, all three disorders are increasingly common with age, and thus will be a growing problem with the aging of our current population. Second, MDS and CLL also have few curative options. Finally, these diseases are associated with reduced survival but a highly variable prognosis; patients may live with their disease from anywhere from weeks to months in the most extreme cases, to survivals measured in years and in some instances almost as long as aged-matched controls.

Patients with MDS are currently managed with supportive care measures to improve disease associated cytopenias, and allogeneic stem cell transplant for individuals with the most adverse prognostic features who are candidates for such an aggressive intervention. There are now three therapeutic FDA-approved drugs for patients with MDS–namely lenalidomide, azacytidine, and decitabine. Efficacy from these agents is mainly related to improving cytopenias, and potentially prolonging survival and delaying transformation to acute leukemia. None of the agents is curative, and they come with a high risk of myelosuppression.

The range of treatment options for CLL is more broad than for MDS or MPD. Therapies include alkylating agents, purine nucleoside analogues, and monoclonal antibody based treatments. These drugs are employed when cytopenias and symptoms become problematic during disease progression. However, none of these agents are curative.

1.3.1 So Why the Focus on the Chronic Leukemias When We Discuss QOL?

Chronic hematological malignancies such as CLL, MDS, and MPD are incurable and significantly affect the QOL in individuals afflicted. In the absence of curative therapy, a better understanding of the impact of these disorders on their QOL as well as the ability of current or future therapeutic options to either reduce symptoms or improve quality of life is essential in both assessing the utility of currently available therapeutic options and future options that will become available.

2 Defining Symptomatic Burden in Chronic Leukemias

2.1 Chronic Leukemias: Spectrum of Disease – Spectrum of Symptoms

MPD patients suffer from a full range of disease associated symptoms, some of which are shared with patients with other chronic leukemias and other malignancies and some which are unique to the disorders themselves. Symptoms which are particularly associated and sometimes uniquely so with the myeloproliferative disorders include a risk of both thrombosis and/or bleeding especially in patients with ET and PV. These symptoms have a range of manifestations. (1) In the setting of acute venous thrombosis, one can be left with deep venous thrombosis or post phlebitic symptoms of the legs including pain, chronic peripheral edema, and difficulties of that nature. Chronic pulmonary emboli which can arise in these patients can lead to both short term morbidity from arrhythmia; but over the long term, can lead to pulmonary hypertension, chronic dyspnea, and a range of significant impact on these patients from dyspnea and compromise cardiac or lung function. Vascular events can also be more subtle. Individuals with extremes of either erythrocytosis or thrombocytosis even in the absence of frank thrombosis can have compromise microvascular circulation and have periods that are self described by patients as confusion, lack of ability to concentrate, migraine headaches, and visual disturbances. Hemorrhagic symptoms can range from acute gastrointestinal bleeding to more chronic bleeding events from esophageal varices or gastrointestinal sources that can lead to or exacerbate chronic anemia and all of the challenges with dyspnea and fatigue that the anemia can bring.

The presence of itching or pruritus is very common across the spectrum of myeloproliferative disorders and particularly amongst those individuals with polycythemia vera. These individuals classically have aquagenic pruritus meaning that after exposure to water and drying, the itching in the skin is its most prominent. The itching can occur in the absence of exposure to water. It is felt that this is potentially associated with histamine release and other cytokine mediators in the skin. Other skin mass sensations can include painful microvascular circulation, difficulties known with erythromelalgia. Patients with MPDs can suffer from significant constitutional symptoms including a loss of lean muscle mass or a cachexia that we feel is potentially associated with underlying disease manifestations having a selective predisposition for the consumption of lean muscle mass. Additionally, they can have fevers and night sweats that are likely cytokine driven in association with the underlying myeloid process. The myeloproliferative disorders are characterized by increases in circulating white blood cells; and in the case of primary myelofibrosis, a variety of immature myeloid cells. This can lead to the development of sequestration of these cells or extramedullary hematopoiesis (EMH). This particularly can lead to significant splenomegaly and/or hepatomegaly. The splenomegaly can be sufficient to cause significant early satiety, pain, abdominal bloating, difficulty with finding a comfortable position, difficulties with bending over, portal hypertension, worsening of peripheral edema, and a whole constellation of symptoms including painful splenic infarcts. EMH can develop in a variety of organs, and we have found it everywhere from in the pericardium causing pericardial effusions and in the spinal canal causing cord compression, in the lungs causing pulmonary hypertension, all of which can lead to very significant symptomatic burden in these groups of patients.

The intramedullary manifestations of the disease can lead to compromises in the ability of the bone marrow to produce sufficient numbers of red cells causing anemia and the constellation of fatigue and problems with organ function that anemia can bring, as well as, a decrease in platelet count or white count especially with progressive disease that can lead to problems with risk of infection and bleeding. On occasion, bone pain from the significant intramedullary process occurring in these patients can occur. They can refractory to therapy.

Fatigue is a common feature particularly amongst patients with primary and post ET and PV myelofibrosis and to a lesser degree in individuals with ET and polycythemia vera and PV. This fatigue, we believe, is multifactorial not only related with anemia as we will discuss in our subsequent data from our internet based surveys, but is directly a cytokine driven process both in the MPDs and in the other chronic leukemias and is probably the single largest contributor of decreased quality of life in these patients and up to this point has not been significantly impacted by current therapeutic options.

3 Other Chronic Leukemias

So, how does the constellation of disease associated symptoms differ in the other chronic leukemias? Amongst patients with MDS, these individuals can share many of the features present in MPDs typically with the exception of the significant pruritus and symptoms with the organomegaly. The symptoms associated with cytopenias, fatigue, and the anemia are equally shared by both diseases. Individuals with CLL have inherently different disease. They share the features of MPDs with the potential for splenic enlargement, fevers, night sweats, weight loss, and cytopenia associated symptoms but also can experience more infectious complications related to intrinsic immunodeficiency associated with the disease (hypogammaglobulinemia, T-cell function) and the profound and prolonged T-cell immu-nosupression associated with some CLL therapies (e.g., purine nucleoside analogues, alemtu-zemab). In addition, however, they can develop significant bulky enlargement in their lymph nodes which depending upon the distribution of the lymph nodes can lead to significant local symptomatic effects including problems with edema, discomfort, drainage, and problems with organ function.

4   Measured Impact on Quality of Life

4.1   Measuring Impact on Quality of Life in Chronic Leukemias: A Survey Based Approach

The challenge, how to gather data from large numbers of patients from relatively uncommon disorders in an efficient manner? We decided to partner with our patients, and patient groups to utilize the internet to obtain anonymous, self reported information using a survey patients could access through a variety of webportals (patient groups sites, LIST-SERVEs). Patients were recruited principally through partnership with disease specific patient advocacy organizations around the world.

4.1.1   Survey Content

The surveys collected patient demographics, employment status, disease specific information (diagnosis, treatment, and complications), co-morbidities (through the Charlson Co-Mor-bidity Index (Charlson et al., 1987), results of validated instruments including the Brief Fatigue Inventory (BFI) (Mendoza, 1999) (This nine question survey allows the rating of specific fatigue items from 0 to 10), the Functional Assessment of Cancer Therapy – Anemia (FACT-An) (Cella, 1997) or Functional Assessment of Cancer Therapy – General (FACT-G) (Cella et al., 1993). Demographic and disease specific information were compiled and descrip-tive statistics were computed for describing the patient population. Our patient popula-tion mean scores for the BFI, FACT-An, and FACT-G were compared to published norms (Mendoza, 1999; Cella et al., 2003; Godin and Shephard, 1985).

4.2   MPDS: Symptom Burden and Impact on QOL

4.2.1   Respondents Encompassed Full Range of MPD Clinical Characteristics

There were 1,179 MPD patients who responded to the internet based survey over the study interval representing a balanced range of MPD diagnoses including PV (n = 405) 34.8%, ET (n = 304) 26.1%, and Myelofibrosis (n = 456) 39.1% from around the world (33 countries). Amongst those patients with Myelofibrosis the subset of their disease was most accurately categorized as PMF (71.6%), Post ET MF (13.9%), or Post PV MF (14.4%) respectively). A history of thrombosis (n = 261; 22.1%), and/or hemorrhage (n = 272; 23.1%) was reported in about a quarter of patients. Additionally, 42.8% (n = 478) of respondents reported splenomegaly with 21% (n = 231) reporting at least occasional pain or discomfort from the enlarged spleen. Anemia occurred in 39% of the patients, with 10.1% of these having hemoglobin <10 g/dL. The vast majority of respondents had undergone at least one form of therapy for controlling their MPD including phlebotomy (44.1%), splenectomy (3.7%), allogeneic stem cell transplant (1.2%), and some form of medical therapy (70.5%).

4.2.2   Majority of MPD Respondents Described Significant Symptoms and Medical Disability Secondary to their MPD

Characterization of subjective symptoms from respondents demonstrated MPD patients suffer from significant fatigue, with 81.1% (n = 945) self-reporting fatigue. Additional symptomatology included pruritus (52.2%), night sweats (49.2%), bone pain (43.9%), fevers (13.7%), and undesired weight loss (13.1%). Further symptomatic breakdown by specific MPD diagnosis, MDS, and CLL is provided in ❷ *Table 168-1*. MPDs also have a significant effect upon afflicted patient's ability to work (❷ *Table 168-2*). Although the majority of MPD patients work outside the home (n = 604; 52.1%), 14.2% (n = 163) report being medically disabled (❷ *Table 168-2*). The majority of this latter group (n = 130; 11.2% of all respondents) were disabled specifically due to their MPD. Additionally 25.3% (n = 293) are currently retired.

4.2.3   MPD Patients Suffer from Significant Fatigue Compared to Published Norms

Fatigue (self described as related to their underlying MPD diagnosis in 78.7% of patients (n = 928)) quantification through the BFI and FACT-An demonstrated MPD patients have increased fatigue compared to published norms (Mendoza, 1999; Cella et al., 2003) (see ❷ *Table 168-3*). Specifically, MPD respondents had a mean score of 47.3 (range of 3.8–79.2)

◻ Table 168-1

Self-reported constitutional symptoms in 1,179 patients with MPN patients

Symptom	PV (N = 405) (%)	ET (N = 304) (%)	MF (N = 456) (%)	Total (N = 1,179) (%)	P value
Fatigue	85	72	84	81	<0.0001
Bone pain	65	40	50	53	<0.0001
Fever	49	41	56	50	0.0002
Pruritus	43	41	47	44	0.2480
Night sweats	13	9	18	14	0.0013
Symptomatic Splenomegaly	10	7	20	13	<0.0001
Weight loss (>10%)	4	9	7	6	<0.0001

PMF (Primary Myelofibrosis)
Post PV MF (Post Polycythemia Vera Myelofibrosis)
Post ET MF (Post Essential Thrombocythemia Myelofibrosis)

◻ Table 168-2

Employment status of 1,179 myeloproliferative patients whom responded to an international internet based survey of fatigue and disease symptoms

	PV (N = 405)	ET (N = 304)	MF (N = 456)	Total (N = 1,179)	p value
Work outside the home?					
Yes	227 (56.6%)	183 (60.6%)	192 (42.7%)	602 (52.2%)	<0.0001
No					
Retired	99 (24.7%)	60 (19.9%)	131 (29.1%)	290 (25.2%)	
Medically disabled due to MPD	34 (8.5%)	15 (5%)	80 (17.8%)	129 (11.2%)	<0.0001
Medically disabled other cause	13 (3.2%)	12 (4%)	9 (2%)	34 (2.9%)	
Personal choice (non-medical)	25 (6.2%)	31 (10.3%)	36 (8%)	92 (8%)	
Unknown reason	3 (0.7%)	1 (0.3%)	2 (0.4%)	6 (0.5%)	

◻ Table 168-3

Comparison of self reported fatigue in patients with chronic leukemias compared to published norms

Disease	N	BFI mean (SD)	FACT-An mean (SD)	P value compared to controls	
				BFI	FACT-An
MPD patients (All)	1,158	4.9 (2.42)	47.3 (19.03)	<0.0001	<0.0001
Essential thrombocythemia	300	4.4 (2.28)	51.6 (17.64)	<0.0001	<0.0001
Polycythemia vera	397	5.1 (2.45)	46.5 (19.82)	<0.0001	<0.0001
Myelofibrosis	450	5.2 (2.42)	45.5 (18.79)	<0.0001	<0.0001
MDS (Steensma et al., 2007)	345	5.8 (2.58)	46.1 (24.6)	<0.0001	<0.0001
CLL (Shanafelt et al., 2007)	1,482				
Early stage	2.2		NA	NS	NA
Intermediate	2.6		NA	=0.017	NA
Advanced stage	3.6		NA	<0.001	NA
Controls (BFI)	275	2.2 (1.80)	–	–	–
Controls (FACT-An)	1,078	–	77.1 (19.9)	–	–

Brief Fatigue Inventory (BFI)) (Mendoza, 1999): The nine items in the BFI were all on a scale from 0 to 10 where 0=No Fatigue/Does not interfere with activity and 10=As bad as you can imagine/Completely interferes with activity. The BFI score is the mean of all nine questions

FACT-An) (Cella et al., 2003): The Fact-An questions are on a scale from 0 to 4 where 0=not at all and 4=very much. The Fatigue subscale consists of 13 questions and it is scored by calculating the sum of all questions and converting the result into a 0–100 scale where 0=poor QOL and 100=is high QOL. The Anemia subscale consists of the 13 fatigue questions plus 7 anemia specific questions. The Anemia scores are calculated in the same manner on the Fact-An Fatigue subscale out of a possible 100. This value demonstrates a level of fatigue far in excess of published norms (mean of 77.1, difference p < 0.0001) (Cella et al., 2003). These observations were further corroborated by the mean survey BFI score being 4.9 (with a range of 1–10.0, where the higher score indicates higher fatigue) out of a possible 10. The mean for the general population is 2.2 (difference p < 0.0001) (Mendoza, 1999). Fatigue score differed between MPD diagnosis where, the increased burden of fatigue was present across all MPD diagnoses, it was more pronounced in Myelofibrosis patients (p < 0.001) (❱ Table 168-3). All three MPD diagnoses fatigue burden were significantly different than published controls (p < 0.0001 for all). There was no significant difference in the distribution of these symptoms among the three MF subcategories (PMF, post-PV MF, and post-ET MF) with the exception of pruritus, which was more prevalent in post-PV MF, and weight loss and splenomegaly, which were more prevalent in PMF. Fatigue was by far the most frequently reported symptom being listed by over 80% of patients and was shown to be in excess of what is expected from age-matched norms for each MF subcategory.

4.2.4   MPD Related Fatigue Correlates with Many Disease Related Features

Fatigue is frequently a multi-factorial process whether in MPD patients or the general population. As might be anticipated, the degree of fatigue described by respondents correlated with advanced disease features, type of MPD therapy and known complications of their underlying disease. Not unexpectedly, fatigue is more common in patients with myelofibrosis. Post ET MF and Post PV MF patients had more significant fatigue than their ET and PV counterparts respectively. Additionally, and not unexpectedly, the presence of anemia led to a stepwise increase in fatigue from mild anemia (just below normal), to significant anemia (hemoglobin <10 g/dL), to erythrocyte transfusion dependence. Additionally, the presence of other symptoms (i.e., pruritus, fever, weight loss) or prior MPD related thrombohemorrhagic complications all correlated with increasing fatigue. Patients who currently smoke are also clearly more fatigued than their non-smoking counterparts.

4.2.5   Patients with Minimal "Objective" Manifestations of their MPD Suffer from Mild to Severe Fatigue

Fatigue is a problem even in the majority of patients with early stages of MPDs (asymptomatic). The survey included a group (n = 279 (23.6%)) of patients (PV (41.5%), ET (31%), Myelofibrosis (24.7%)) who denied any features typically felt to be signs of problematic MPD. Specifically these are a history of thrombo-hemorrhagic events, splenomegaly, or anemia. These individuals reported fatigue measured by the FACT-An (mean 51.6, SD 18.33) and BFI (mean 4.2, SD 2.4) scores which were significantly greater than published norms (p < 0.001 for both). They also reported the full range of other subjective symptomatology exhibited by patients with more advanced disease features including pruritus (43.4%), bone pain (35.5%), night sweats (35.1%), unexplained fevers (6.1%), and undesired weight loss (3.2%). Finally, 2.6% of these same patients reported being medically disabled from their constitutional symptoms arising from their MPD, and 115/279 were no longer working. The majority (52%) of this latter group being <65 years of age.

4.2.6 Fatigue Is a Major Problem in MPD Patients Despite Therapy and Normal Co-Morbidity Burden

Comparisons of means for the Fact-An, Fact-An fatigue subscale and BFI scores were performed between PV patients focusing on the effect of therapy (❯ *Table 168-4* and ❯ *168-5*). First, an analysis was performed regarding the results of the fatigue metric between patients according to their most recent main PV therapy employed (phlebotomy alone, hydroxyurea, anagrelide, or interferon alpha). A further analysis was performed amongst patients focusing on the impact of phlebotomy on fatigue. First, the patients current perception of fatigue, and fatigue in the prior calendar year. Additionally, we attempted to determine the impact of the intensity of phlebotomy (patients stratified according to number of units phlebotomized during past calendar year).

Therapy for the 405 PV patients was reported by 96% (n = 388) patients, with 89% (361) having been phlebotomized, 72% (n = 291) received aspirin, 64% (n = 261) having received one or more myelosuppressive agent (hydroxyurea 53% (n = 216), anagrelide 22% (n = 88),

■ Table 168-4

Impact of phlebotomy upon fatigue in 405 patients with polycythemia vera

	Instrument				P value (BFI/ FACT-An)
	Brief Fatigue Inventory (BFI)		FACT-Fatigue subscale		
Phlebotomy	% Yes median score (Q1:Q3)	% No median score (Q1:Q3)	% Yes median score (Q1:Q3)	% No median score (Q1:Q3)	
Ever required	89% 5.3 (2.9:6.9)	11% 6.3 (2.3:7.5)	89% 48.1 (30.8:61.5)	11% 44.2 (23.1:69.2)	0.29/0.34
Required past year	43% 5.1 (2.7:6.8)	57% 5.4 (3.1:7.0)	43% 48.1 (32.7:60.4)	57% 48.1 (28.8:63.5)	0.38/ 0.78
Comparing last 2 years	89% 5.3 (2.9:6.9)	11% 6.3 (2.3:7.5)	89% 48.1 (30.8:61.5)	11% 44.2 (23.1:69.2)	0.29/ 0.34
+/− MPD therapy	77% 5.6 (3.4:7.0)	23% 4.8 (2.7:6.4)	77% 48.1 (28.8:61.5)	23% 48.1 (30.8:68.3)	0.13/ 0.51
Control values	2.2 (STD DEVIATION 1.80)		77.1 (STD DEVIATION 19.9)		

■ Table 168-5

Impact of current upon fatigue in 405 patients with polycythemia vera

	Instrument	
Therapy	BFI median score (Q1:Q3)	Fact-An median score (Q1:Q3)
Phlebotomy alone (56%)	5.3 (2.7:6.8)	46.2 (30.8:61.5)
Hydroxyurea (31%)	5.6 (2.9:7.0)	48.1 (28.8:61.5)
Anagrelide (3.5%)	4.4 (2.9:5.9)	56.8 (42.3:71.2)
Interferon (9.5%)	5.2 (3.0:7.1)	51.9 (34.6:69.2)
Difference between treatments	P = 0.67	P = 0.41
Control values	2.2 (STD DEVIATION 1.80)	77.1 (STD DEVIATION 19.9)

interferon-alpha 16% (n = 63)). Amongst patients whom were phlebotomized over the past year (43%; n = 174: median 4 units (range 1–18)), 53% (n = 92) received concurrent myelosuppressive therapy. Amongst patients whom originally, but no longer required phlebotomy 35% (n = 142), 94% (n = 134) were receiving myelosuppressive treatments. QOL assessments indicated fatigue as measured by both instruments is clearly increased across the PV respondents compared to published controls for those instruments (p < 0.001). Additionally, although the burden of fatigue was not significantly higher in "high-risk" PV, fatigue levels were higher amongst those with prior thrombo-hemorrhagic events (p = 0.03, or both types of events p < 0.01). In regards to the impact of PV therapy upon fatigue, the burden of this symptom was not significantly diminished for those individuals on phlebotomy alone compared to those on cytoreductive therapy. Neither did fatigue levels correlate with the frequency or intensity of phlebotomy. Additionally, although fatigue burden was high (compared to controls) amongst patients on cytoreductive therapy, no agent had a clear advantage in alleviating (or disadvantage in exacerbating) fatigue.

In an attempt to quantify the possible contributing effect of co-morbid conditions on the respondents the survey included the Charlson Co-Morbidity Index questionnaire (Charlson et al., 1987). This validated measure showed that the vast majority of individuals (86.8%) had 0–2 positive responses on the 10 point co-morbidity score. These values are similar to age matched controls from the published literature (Charlson et al., 1987) and supports our hypothesis that the increased fatigue burden is related to their underlying disease and not a manifestation of co-morbidities due to age.

4.3   MDS: Symptom Burden and Impact on QOL

4.3.1   Participant Demographics and Disease Characteristics

A parallel study with similar design to the MPD trial was undertaken in MDS (Steensma et al., 2007) with, 359 patients. Diagnoses spanned the MDS spectrum: RA 14%; RARS 12%; RCMD 6%; RAEB 16%; 5q- syndrome 11%; CMML 3%; RAEB-t 4%, unclassifiable/subtype unknown, 33%. By far the most common symptom endorsed by patients with MDS was excessive fatigue (in 89% of surveys). Other troublesome symptoms included bruising/bleeding (55%), night sweats (43%), bone pain (39%), fevers (28%), skin rash (25%), undesired weight loss (25%), and recurrent infections (20%). With respect to the site of bleeding in those 28% of patients who reported hemorrhagic episodes, 20% of reported nosebleeds, 9% gingival bleeding, 5% intestinal hemorrhage, 3% vaginal bleeding, 1% bleeding into the brain or eye, and 8% "other site." MDS impaired patients' ability to work: only 28.5% of respondents were working outside the home, and among those who were not working, 30% blamed MDS-related disability, while 60% considered themselves "retired." Respondents' normalized scores on the FACT-An were markedly worse than the general population: 40.3 in MDS versus 77.1 for controls (100 is best QOL); p < 0.0001 (❷ Table 168-3). The same was true for fatigue measurement via the BFI: 5.8 in MDS versus 2.2 for controls, (0 is "no fatigue"); p < 0.0001(❷ Table 168-3).

Fevers were more common in advanced MDS (i.e., RAEB and RAEB-t) – these groups also reported a lower mean neutrophil count – whereas weight loss was more common in RA, CMML, RAEB and RAEB-t than in RARS, 5q-, and RCMD. Skin rashes correlated with transfusion dependency and ESA use, while infection and fevers were more common in patients with diabetes mellitus as a comorbidity.

The symptoms of bone pain, fatigue, and skin rash were each strongly associated with the use of ESAs. With respect to fatigue, 95% of patients with fatigue reported ESA use, compared to 82% who had not used these agents (p = 0.0001), suggesting that these agents are commonly used by clinicians for patients with fatigue. Likewise, 30% of patients using ESAs reported skin lesions versus 18% of patients without ESA use (p = 0.005), and 48% of ESA users reported bone pain versus 28% of ESA non-users (p = 0.001), consistent with the known adverse event profile of these agents. Additionally, two of the dichotomized FACT-An components, walking and enjoying life, were significantly improved in patients reporting ESA use (p = 0.04 for each), but other FACT-An items as well as the FACT-An composite score, BFI score, and Godin LAS score did not correlate with ESA use. Patients who had used azacitidine scored more poorly on the Fatigue Subscale Score of FACT-An; an increase in fatigue is a known adverse effect of nucleoside analogues including azacitidine. Other treatments were not used frequently enough for symptom correlations to achieve statistical significance. Logistic regression modeling revealed that fatigue and BFI/FACT-An scores did not correlate with Hb level, an observation also made in the MPD QOL survey, but in contrast to findings in a 50-patient QOL analysis of MDS patients (Mesa et al., 2007).

4.4   CLL: Symptom Burden and Impact on QOL

A parallel study was performed using an internet-based approach with patients with CLL (Shanafelt et al., 2007). Similar to our other studies in MDS and MPDs, the brief fatigue inventory was measured as well as the FACT-G. Overall, 1,482 patients participated in this internet-based survey, and it was found the physical, functional, and overall quality of life scored the CLL patients were similar to age-matched control. In contrast, the emotional well-being scores of patients with CLL were lower than the general population and other types of cancer. A subsequent analysis was undertaken and found that aspects of the physician patient relationship including patients comfort being able to talk to their physician about QOL (more comfortable associated better emotional QOL) and whether physicians used language that minimized its impact on patients (i.e., by being described as the "good" leukemia associated worse emotional QOL) significantly impacted patients emotional well being (Shanafelt et al., 2007). Ongoing efforts to try to best delineate the reason for more emotional impact on these patients is being analyzed as well as data trying to be collected in our myeloid disorders to assess this difficulty. In contrast to the MPD and MDS, the fatigue scores (BFI) of CLL patients were only modestly higher than age-matched controls with significant variation present based on disease stage (❷ Table 168-3). Disability secondary to CLL was also common with 911 employed (61.5%), retired 326 (26.7%), disabled 175 (11.8%). Among the 175 patients who reported being medically disabled, the majority (n = 137, 78.3%) attributed their disability to CLL.

5   Discussion: Implications of QOL Observations on Caring for Chronic Leukemia Patients

5.1   What Have We Learned from Our Patients?

Patients with MPDs have long been known to suffer from a series of objective problems related to their hematologic disorder. Specifically, it has long been demonstrated these patients are at risk of thrombotic events (both micro and macrovascular) in both venous and arterial sites.

Additionally, as patients have progressive or advanced disease (namely Myelofibrosis either *de novo* or secondary) patients experience progressive cytopenias, progressive hepatosplenomegaly and portal hypertension. These patients all have a risk of eventual transformation to acute leukemia and risk of premature death. In concert with these objective disease features, MPD patients have been noted to suffer from a range of "constitutional symptoms," but the burden and character of these symptoms have been not been well quantified in the literature. We have demonstrated using an international, geographically diverse group of unselected MPD patients that the majority of MPD patients suffer from the significant symptoms of fatigue, pruritus, night sweats, and bone pain.

Fatigue, although long recognized as occurring in MPD patients, has been in the past poorly quantified due to the subjective nature of the complaint. Using two distinct instruments we clearly demonstrated that all subsets of MPD patients suffer from significant fatigue compared to published norms. The interesting aspect of this observation is that the fatigue is present across the spectrum of severity of disease, and was not attributable to co-morbidity or age. Additionally, although fatigue was associated with features clearly contributory to fatigue (such as anemia), the vast majority of even "asymptomatic" MPD patients still have clearly definable fatigue they attribute to their disease. The presence of this latter finding suggests that there is an aspect of the underlying myeloproliferative process that may well directly cause fatigue even in the absence of a clear source.

The National Comprehensive Cancer Network (NCCN) defines fatigue as a persistent, subjective sense of tiredness related to cancer or cancer therapy that interferes with usual functioning. Although there is no direct data for mechanisms of fatigue in MPD patients, amongst cancer patients fatigue is felt to be related to multiple contributory factors including anemia, therapeutic toxicity, tumor burden, tumor related cachexia, and a variety of contributory cytokines (Ahlberg et al., 2003). MPDs share several of these potential mechanisms, and MPDs also exhibit other commonalities such as anorexia from disease, and hypermetabolism. Additionally, various key cytokines have been implicated in exacerbating fatigue, such as tumor necrosis factor alpha (TNF-a), interleukin 1 and 6 (Ahlberg et al., 2003). Indeed, recent reports demonstrate that fatigue in cancer patients correlates with functional alteration in pro-inflammatory cytokines (Collado-Hidalgo et al., 2006), and that the degree of functional alteration may explain the broad variability seen in cancer related fatigue not easily explainable by stage of disease. In regards to MPD patients TNF-a specifically has been shown to be increased in patients with Myelofibrosis, and blockade of this cytokine is one of the few agents demonstrated to help abrogate fatigue in MPDs (Steensma et al., 2002).

The vast majority of patients whom responded to the survey had significant fatigue despite therapy. This would suggest that the therapies these patients are undergoing do not abrogate their fatigue. Indeed, in many cases the therapy patients are utlilizing may well contribute to their fatigue. Our data would suggest that current therapeutic approaches to MPDs have largely not been successful in abrogating fatigue, and in many cases may augment the intrinsic fatigue of the disorders (❷ *Table 168-5*).

5.2 How Should Symptoms and QOL Influence Treatment Decisions in Patients with Chronic Leukemias?

We have clearly demonstrated that in patients with chronic leukemias have variable but potentially significant impact on their quality of life through fatigue, direct disease related symptoms, and even their emotional well being from their disease. The real question is; how do we deal with this information therapeutically. First, we think it is important to have a sensitivity to these issues to identify them with patients to help highlight them and work on multi-factorial ways of trying to improve these issues. (1) Validating patient's concerns, raising these issues, and knowing they are disease related will, we think, help patients deal with them in a better fashion and decrease the stress in emotional impact that these symptoms and the disease can occur. (2) It is fairly clear from all of our studies that the ability of current therapeutic options for each of the chronic leukemias have very limited efficacy in their ability to reverse some specific QOL related symptoms.

How do we begin to target fatigue and QOL as therapeutic endpoints in MPDs and chronic leukemia clinical trials? Traditional endpoints in MPD trials have included firmly objective endpoints of decreases in thrombo-hemorrhagic complications, improvement in cytopenias, reduction in splenomegaly, or reduction in bone marrow features of disease. Improvement in fatigue, or other constitutional symptoms has not been directly targeted because of the subjective (and hence difficult to quantify) nature of these complaints. Likewise, it has been assumed that if the hard endpoints of disease (i.e., anemia) improve, than fatigue would also automatically improve as well. The reality, as shown by the results of this trial, is that previously tested agents even when able to improve anemia do not necessarily resolve fatigue and future agents need to prove efficacy against disease associated symptoms.

How else might we decrease fatigue in chronic leukemia patients? Fatigue, as a morbidity from a host of malignant disorders is common, yet pharmacologic stimulants to abrogate this symptom have rarely been successful. Exercise has the ability to potentially improve fatigue in patients with malignancies, but published data remains limited in scope. In a recent analysis of 26 published trials (mainly breast cancer patients and survivors) (Galvao and Newton, 2005) of exercise interventions in patients with malignancies it was shown that (1) patients with compromised performance status from disease (and therapy) are able to undergo cardiovascular exercise safely and (2) positive benefits reported included increased lean tissue mass (Winningham et al., 1989), decreased fatigue (Winningham et al., 1994), decreased resting heart rate, and decreased stress. Amongst patients with hematologic malignancies (data limited to patients who are either undergoing systemic chemotherapy or allogeneic stem cell transplantation (Hayes et al., 2004) results were similarly encouraging. In a prospective trial of patients undergoing intensive chemotherapy (with or without stem cell transplant) daily exercise on a treadmill led to stabilization of physical performance even in the face of chemotherapy and a decrease in hemoglobin (Dimeo et al., 2003).

6   Conclusions

The myeloproliferative disorders and the chronic leukemias of MDS and CLL significantly impact on patients in many ways that extend beyond measurable disease in terms of peripheral blood counts, adenopathy, or abnormalities that are present radiographically. These issues need to be considered in terms of therapeutic intervention, as well as, the utilization of current supportive care options. We are hopeful that better target therapies will have an impact upon these disease associated symptoms, but expect that a better understanding, quantification, and tracking of these symptoms in response to current and future therapies will be important in trying to expand the quality of care provided to these patients.

Summary Points

- Patients with the chronic myeloproliferative disorders (MPDs), the myelodysplastic syndromes (MDS), and chronic lymphocytic leukemia (CLL) share both a variable (but frequently chronic) natural history characterized by significant burden of symptoms and fatigue.
- Utilizing standardized instruments of fatigue we have shown and published that patients with MPDS, MDS, and CLL typically have fatigue worse than published controls.
- Amongst chronic leukemia patients the severity of fatigue was worst amongst MDS patients. Amongst each subset of disease worsening fatigue indices correlated with more advanced stages of disease.
- Fatigue was shown not to be a mere surrogate of anemia in patients with MDS and MPDs.
- Impact of current therapeutic options upon disease associated fatigue, and ability to improve quality of life, is quite limited. Novel therapeutic trials need to measure objective impact on QOL in these patients by therapeutic intervention.

Appendix

Key Facts on Myeloproliferative Disorders (MPDs)

What Diseases are included in the MPDs?	• Essential Thrombocythemia (ET)
	• Polycythemia Vera (PV)
	• Primary Myelofibrosis (PMF)
	  • Post Polycythemia Vera Myelofibrosis (Post PV MF)
	  • Post Essential Thrombocythemia Myelofibrosis (Post ET MF)

Age at Presentation	Typically in mid 60's for all subtypes, but ages 18–? is possible
Survival	ET and PV: Can be as long as age matched controls, but dropoff after a decade of disease PMF (Post ET-PV MF): Variable but typically 3–5 years (except in patients <60 usually 10 years or more)
Predisposing Causes	Usually not known, there is an association with radiation or carcinogen exposure
Hereditary Implications	Familial Cases of MPDs do exist, there is an increased incidence amongst afflicted family members but still absent in most cases
Main Clinical Implications	ET/PV: Short Term risk of thrombohemorrhagic complications. Long term risk of myelofibrotic or leukemic transformation. PMF (Post ET-PV MF): Significant constitutional symptoms, anemia, splenomegaly, extramedullary hematopoiesis, risk of acute leukemia and death
Main Therapies Employed	ET/PV: Thrombohemorrhagic prophylaxis (aspirin, phlebotomy, targeted cytoreduction with hydroxyurea, anagrelide or interferon) PMF (Post ET-PV MF): Allogeneic stem cell transplant in high risk patients whom are candidates. Palliative options for anemia, splenomegaly, and constitutional symptom exist. Active novel therapy program ongoing

References

Adamson JW, Fialkow PJ. (1978). Br J Hematol. 38: 299–303.

Ahlberg K, Ekman T, Gaston-Johansson F, Mock V. (2003). The Lancet. 362(9384): 640–650.

Cella D. (1997). Semin Hematol. 34(3 Suppl 2): 13–19.

Cella D, Tulsky D, Gray G, Sarafian B, Bonomi A, Silberman, et al. (1993). J Clin Oncol. 11: 570–579.

Cella D, Zagari MJ, Vandoros C, Gagnon DD, Hurtz H-J, Nortier JWR. (2003). J Clin Oncol. 21(2): 366–373.

Cervantes F, Alvarez-Larran A, Hernandez-Boluda JC, Sureda A, Torrebadell M, Montserrat E. (2004). Br J Haematol. 127(4): 399–403.

Cervantes F, Hernandez-Boluda JC, Alvarez A, Nadal E, Montserrat E. (2000). Haematologica. 85(6): 595–599.

Charlson ME, Pompei P, Ales KL, MacKenzie CR (1987). J Chronic Dis. 40(5): 373–383.

Collado-Hidalgo A, Bower JE, Ganz PA, Cole SW, Irwin MR. (2006). Clin Cancer Res. 12(9): 2759–2766.

Cortelazzo S, Finazzi G, Ruggeri M, Vestri O, Galli M, Rodeghiero F, et al. (1995). N Engl J Med. 332(17): 1132–1136.

Dameshek W. (1951). Blood. 6: 372–375.

Dimeo F, Schwartz S, Fietz T, Wanjura T, Boning D, Thiel E. (2003). Support Care Cancer. 11(10): 623–628.

Di Nisio M, Barbui T, Di Gennaro L, Borrelli G, Finazzi G, Landolfi R, et al. (2007). Br J Haematol. 136(2): 249–259.

Dupriez B, Morel P, Demory JL, Lai JL, Simon M, Plantier I, et al. (1996). Blood. 88(3): 1013–1018.

Faoro LN, Tefferi A, Mesa RA. (2005). Eur J Haematol. 74(2): 117–120.

Finazzi G, Caruso V, Marchioli R, Capnist G, Chisesi T, Finelli C, et al. (2005). Blood. 105(7): 2664–2670.

Galvao DA, Newton RU. (2005). J Clin Oncol. 23(4): 899–909.

Gilbert. (1973). Med Clin North Am. 57: 355–393.

Godin G, Shephard RJ. (1985). Can J Appl Sport Sci. 10(3): 141–146.

Harrison CN, Campbell PJ, Buck G, Wheatley K, East CL, Bareford D, et al. (2005). N Engl J Med. 353(1): 33–45.

Hayes S, Davies PS, Parker T, Bashford J, Newman B. (2004). Bone Marrow Transplant. 33(5): 553–558.

Kiladjian JJ, Cassinat B, Turlure P, Cambier N, Roussel M, Bellucci S, et al. (2006). Blood. 108(6): 2037–2040.

Landolfi R, Di Gennaro L, Barbui T, De Stefano V, Finazzi G, Marfisi R, et al. (2007). Blood. 109(6): 2446–2452.

Landolfi R, Marchioli R, Kutti J, Gisslinger H, Tognoni G, Patrono C, et al. (2004). N Engl J Med. 350(2): 114–124.

Lofvenberg E, Wahlin A, Roos G, Ost A. (1990). Eur J Haematol. 44(1): 33–38.

Mendoza TR, et al. (1999). Cancer. 85(5): 1186–1196.

Mesa RA, Niblack J, Wadleigh M, Verstovsek S, Camoriano J, Barnes S, et al. (2007). Cancer. 109 (1): 68–76.

Mesa RA, Silverstein MN, Jacobsen SJ, Wollan PC, Tefferi A. (1999). Am J Hematol. 61(1): 10–15.

Passamonti F, Rumi E, Pungolino E, Malabarba L, Bertazzoni P, Valentini M, et al. (2004). Am J Med. 117(10): 755–761.

Shanafelt TD, Bowen D, Venkat C, Slager SL, Zent CS, Kay NE, et al. (2007). Br J Haematol. 139(2): 255–264.

Shanafelt TD, Bowen D, Venkat C, Slager SL, Zent CS, Kay NE, et al. (2007). ASH Annual Meeting Abstracts. 110(11): 2060.

Steensma DP, Heptinstall KV, Johnson VM, et al. (2008). Leuk Res. 32: 691–698.

Steensma DP, Mesa RA, Li CY, Gray L, Tefferi A. (2002). Blood. 99(6): 2252–2254.

Vannucchi AM, Antonioli E, Guglielmelli P, et al. Blood. 110: 840–846.

Winningham ML, MacVicar MG, Bondoc M, Anderson JI, Minton JP. (1989). Oncol Nurs Forum. 16(5): 683–689.

Winningham ML, Nail LM, Burke MB, Brophy L, Cimprich B, Jones LS, et al. (1994). Oncol Nurs Forum. 21(1): 23–36.

169 Quality of Life in Advanced Renal Cell Carcinoma: Effect of Treatment with Cytokine Therapy and Targeted Agents

S. Shah · K. Gondek

1	*Introduction*	*2906*
2	*Treatment for Advanced RCC*	*2907*
2.1	Cytokine Therapy	2907
2.2	Targeted Agents	2910
2.2.1	Multikinase Inhibitors	2910
2.2.2	Anti-Vascular Endothelial Growth Factor Anti-Bodies	2911
2.2.3	Mammalian Target of Rapamycin Inhibitors (mTOR)	2911
3	*Quality of Life*	*2912*
3.1	Assessment of PRO Using Validated Questionnaires	2912
3.2	Evaluation of Change in Symptom Response/QoL	2912
4	*Quality of Life in Advanced RCC Patient*	*2914*
4.1	Effects of Cytokine Therapy and Other Non-Targeted Agents on Quality of Life	2914
4.2	Effect of Targeted Therapy on Quality of Life	2917
4.2.1	Mutikinase Inhibitors	2917
4.2.2	Mammalian Target of Rapamycin (mTOR) Inhibitors	2919
5	*Conclusions*	*2919*
	Summary Points	*2920*
	Appendix	*2920*

Abstract: Renal Cell Carcinoma (RCC) is the most common type of kidney cancer and its' incidence is increasing steadily worldwide. Due to the asymptomatic nature of the disease it is often diagnosed in advanced stages and treatment options have been limited. Symptoms of the advanced disease along with side-effects of available treatment options can greatly affect a patients' everyday living. The goal of therapeutic interventions in such advanced diseases is not only to increase survival but maintain or improve ❷ quality of life and functioning.

Cytokine therapy has been effective in only a select group of patients and has been associated with poor quality of life. A review of literature on quality of life in patients in advanced RCC treated with cytokine therapy revealed the use of cytokine therapy was associated with decrease in overall quality of life. Also a comparison of quality of life of patients treated with cytokine therapy with general population showed that patients treated with cytokine therapy had lower quality of life. Limited efficacy of cytokine therapies along with deterioration in QoL has led to use of these drugs in only select population.

❷ Targeted agents such as sorafenib and sunitinib have improved efficacy. In addition these agents have an overall better QoL and improved kidney-cancer symptoms and concerns as compared to interferon. Another targeted agent temsirolimus had significantly greater quality-adjusted survival than interferon.

The current trend in the management of advanced renal cell carcinoma is the utilization of these targeted agents either alone or in combination with other agents. Targeted agents have shown efficacy and safety, and maintenance or improvement of quality of life in patients with advanced renal cell carcinoma.

List of Abbreviations: *CR,* ❷ complete response; *EORTC-QLQ 30,* European Organization for Research and Treatment of Cancer Quality of Life Questionnaire Core 30; *EQ-5D,* Euro-QoL-5 Dimensions; *FACT,* functional assessment of cancer therapy; *FACT-BRM,* functional assessment of cancer therapy – biologic response modifier; *FACT-G,* functional assessment of cancer therapy –, general; *FKSI,* functional assessment of cancer therapy – kidney symptom index; *HRQoL,* health related quality of life; *IFN-α,* interferon-alpha; *IL-2,* interleukin-2; *mTOR,* ❷ mammalian target of rapamycin; *ORR,* ❷ overall response rate; *OS,* ❷ overall survival; *PDGF,* platelet driven ❷ growth factor; *PFS,* ❷ progression free survival; *PR,* ❷ partial response; *PRO,* patient reported outcomes; *QoL,* quality of life; *QTWiST,* quality-adjusted time without symptoms and toxicity; *RCC,* renal cell carcinoma; *RR,* response rate; *SF-12,* Short Form-12 Health Survey; *SF-36,* Short Form-36 Health Survey; *TWiST,* time without symptoms and toxicity; *US,* United States; *VEGF,* vascular endothelial growth factor; *VHL,* von Hippel-Lindau gene

1 Introduction

Renal cell carcinoma (RCC) is the most common type of kidney cancer and comprises 90–95% of kidney neoplasms (Jemal et al., 2006; Lam et al., 2005). In 2006, there were greater than 200,000 newly diagnosed cases of RCC and greater than 100,000 deaths worldwide (Albers, 2008; American Cancer Society, 2006). Even though RCC is relatively rare as compared to other cancer types, the incidence of RCC has been steadily increasing over the past 30 years and represents a significant clinical burden.

RCC is characterized by lack of early warning signs and presentation of diverse clinical manifestations. Small localized tumors rarely produce symptoms and therefore RCC is often diagnosed at advanced stages. This makes it a difficult malignancy to treat (Motzer et al., 1996). Until recently systemic treatments for advanced RCC had been proven to be ineffective.

Historically advanced RCC had been treated with chemotherapy, radiotherapy, hormonal therapy and cytokine therapy but advanced RCC is generally resistant to these therapies. Objective response rates (ORR) of less than 10% has been observed with frequently used chemotherapeutic agents such as gemcitabine, fluorouracil, capecitabine, etc (Costa and Drabkin, 2007; Waters et al., 2004). Response rates of patients treated with cytokine therapies (Interleukin -2 (IL-2) and Interferon-alpha (IFN-alpha)) have also been relatively low in the range of 10–20% (Costa and Drabkin, 2007). In addition both IL-2 and IFN-α are associated with significant toxicity.

Recent advances in the understanding of the molecular biology of RCC, specifically the von Hippel-Lindau (VHL) gene mutation leading to overexpression of vascular endothelial growth factor (VEGF) and platelet derived growth factor (PDGF), have led to development of targeted therapies for the treatment of advanced RCC (van Spronsen et al., 2005). Targeted therapies such as sorafenib, sunitinib, and temsirolimus have received regulatory approval and many more are in clinical trials. The availability of multiple drugs represents a significant improvement in management of RCC. In choosing the most appropriate therapy for an individual the benefits have to be balanced with the toxicity profile and the potential impact on quality of life (QoL).

Quality of life assessments provides insight into positive impact of treatment on disease as well as capturing any negative impact from adverse events associated with the treatment (Lipscomb et al., 2007). Since RCC is often diagnosed late, patients commonly have metastases in the lung, liver, bone and other. The various sites of renal metastases in combination with a wide of treatment options from highly toxic cytokine therapy to newer targeted agents can affect a patients' health-related quality of life (HRQoL). For patients with metastatic disease which are incurable and associated with reduced life-expectancy, relief of disease-related symptoms and maintenance of function are primary objectives of medical intervention (Cella et al., 2006). Therefore in addition to measuring traditional outcomes such as survival and response rates it is important to assess quality of life of patients.

In this chapter we will review the cytokine therapy and targeted therapy used to treat advanced RCC and their impact on patients' quality of life.

2   Treatment for Advanced RCC

2.1   Cytokine Therapy

In 1980s, in prospective studies it was observed that patients with advanced RCC had spontaneous regression rates of about 7% (Parton et al., 2006; Snow and Schellhammer, 1982). This led to the idea that spontaneous remission may be immune mediated and search for therapeutic agents that improve immunologic response against RCC tumor cells was initiated. Since then both IL-2 and IFN-α, along or in combination with other agents have been tested in many clinical trials with no regimen revealed to be consistently superior.

Multiple clinical trials have investigated single agent IFN-α and IL-2 for treatment of advanced RCC with a wide range of response rates (❍ Table 169-1). A recent Cochrane review analyzed 53 studies involving 6,117 patients that utilized immunotherapy in at least one study arm and reported remission or survival (Coppin et al., 2005). The pooled analyses of this review showed that patients with advanced RCC receiving immunotherapy had 12% partial or complete remission rates versus 2% in non-immunotherapy arms. However improvement in remission rate did not correlate with improvement in survival.

□ Table 169-1
Selected randomized studies of IL-2 and IFN-α in the treatment of mRCC

Study	No. of patients	Regimen		CR/PR	RR (%)	Response duration	Survival	Comments
		IL-2 dose	IFN-α Schedule					
Atkins et al. (1993)	71	1.33 mg/m2 IV q8h; days 1–5, days 15–19		4/8	17	Nine patients with over 15 months	Median 15.5 months	Dose is equivalent to 600,000 U/kg; no survival difference
	28	0.8 mg/m2 IV q8h; days 1–5, days 15–19	3 MU/m2 IV q8h; days 1–5, days 15–19	0/3	11	No response duration >15 months	Median 16 months	
Negrier et al. (2006)	138	18 MIU/m2/day; CIV days 1–5		2/7	6.5	–	1-year event-free survival 15%	RR P < .01 in favor of combination treatment; crossover study therefore survival data difficult to interpret; no overall survival difference in 2000 update
	147		18 MIU/m2 once daily SC TIW	0/11	7.5		1-year event-free survival 12%	
	140	18 MIU/m2/day; CIV days 1–5	6 MIU once daily SC TIW	1/25	18.6		1-year event-free survival 20%	
Niedhart et al. (1991)	82	–	20 MU/m2 IM daily (14 d)	–	12	–	10 months	
MRC collaborators (1999)	167	–	10 MU SC TIW	–	14	–	8.5 months	

Study	N	Dose						Comments
Motzer et al. (2000)	145	—	3 MU SC daily	—	6	—	15 months (95% CI: 12–17)	
Flanigan et al. (2001)	120 (+nephrectomy)	—	5 MU/m2 SC TIW	—	3.3 (n = 92)	—	11.1 months (95% CI: 9.2–16.5)	
	121		5 MU/m2 SC TIW		3.6 (n = 83)		8.1 months (95% CI: 5.4–9.5)	
Aass et al. (2005)	144	—	3–9 MU SC daily	—	—	—	13.2 months (95% CI: 11–17.8)	
McDermott et al. (2005)	95	600,000 U/kg IV q8h; days 1–5, days 15–19		8/14	23	Median 14 months	Median 17.5 months	RR is greater with high-dose IL-2; P = .018; no difference in overall survival
	91	IL-2 5 MIU/m2 SC q8h day 1, once daily SC 5 days weeks 1–4	5 MIU/m2 SC TIW weeks 1–4	3/6	10	Median 7 months	Median 13.5 months	

Multiple clinical trials have shown that activity of interferon and interleukine in advanced renal cell carcinoma is modest in a selected group of patients

Source: Adapted from Parton M et al. Role of Cytokine Therapy in 2006 and Beyond for Metastatic Renal Cell Cancer. J Clin Oncol. 2006; 24(35): 5584–5592. Reprinted with permission.

IL-2 Interleukin 2; *mRCC* metastatic renal cell cancer; *IFN-α* interferon-alpha; *CR* complete response; *PR* partial response; *RR* response rate (CR + PR); *IM* intramuscular; *IV* intravenous; *d* days; *q8h* every 8 h; *MU* million units; *MIU* million international units; *CIV* continuous intravenous infusion; *SC* subcutanous; *TIW* three times per week; *q3w* every 3 weeks

(Parton et al., 2006) reviewed the historic use of IL-2 in advanced RCC patients (❷ *Table 169-1*). The landmark study by Fyfe and colleagues (n = 255) that led to FDA approval of IL-2 demonstrated ORR of 14% with 12 complete responses (CRs) and 24 partial response (PRs) (Fyfe et al., 1995). Despite these high response rates there is considerable systemic toxicity during treatment, an area of major concern. Since this landmark study, results of many trials show that the response rates remain low and most patients do not benefit from treatment.

In summary, cytokine therapy is suitable for a select group of patients with good risk profile and clear cell subtype histology. It is not recommended in patients with intermediate or poor prognosis.

2.2 Targeted Agents

Research into molecular basis of RCC and identification of VHL gene mutation and its pathway that is correlated to majority of clear-cell RCC has been led to the significant progress in development of new targeted agents. Targeted agents were developed to impact components in VHL pathway thereby reducing the effects of VEGF, PDGF and blocking angiogenesis (van Spronsen et al., 2005). ❷ *Figure 169-1* shows the different targeted agents and the multiple pathways they block. This section provides a brief review on efficacy and safety of multikinase inhibitors, anti-VEGF antibodies and mammalian target of rapamycin (mTOR) inhibitors.

2.2.1 Multikinase Inhibitors

Sorafenib and sunitinib are two currently approved multikinase inhibitors that directly inhibit the VEGF and PDGF receptors thus blocking their actions. Several other agents such as pazopanib and axitinib are under investigation. This section discusses only currently approved therapies.

Sorafenib in advanced RCC was evaluated in a phase III multinational clinical trial. A total of 903 patients with previously treated advanced RCC were randomized to receive sorafenib or placebo. An ❷ interim analysis showed the median progression free survival (PFS) was 5.5 months in sorafenib group and 2.8 months in the placebo group (p < 0.001) (Escudier et al., 2007). As a result the study was stopped and patients on the placebo arm were allowed to cross-over to receive sorafenib. The difference in overall survival (OS) was not statistically significant (p = 0.015) based on the pre-specified p value at the interim analysis of p < 0.0005. However, the impact of cross-over was evident from a pre-specified analysis that showed a statistically significant OS advantage of sorafenib over placebo (Bukowski et al., 2007a). Sorafenib was found to be tolerable in these patients.

The efficacy of sunitinib was first evaluated in two single arm phase II trials in cytokine-refractory advanced RCC patients. The regulatory approval was based on data from these two phase II trials. In the first phase II trial (n = 106) an ORR of 34% was observed while in the second trial (n = 63) an ORR of 36.5% was observed (Motzer et al., 2006a,b).

The efficacy of sunitinib was evaluated in 750 patients in a phase III trial against IFN-α. ORR of 31% in sunitinib arm versus 6% in interferon arm was observed. The PFS was 11 months in sunitinib arm versus 5 months in the interferon arm. OS was not significant in interim analysis. The side-effect profile of sunitinib was tolerable (Motzer et al., 2007).

■ **Figure 169-1**

Inhibition of angiogenesis pathway in renal cell carcinoma by Targeted AgentsPathways leading to angiogenesis in advanced RCC can be inhibited at several steps (i) Depletion of VEGF by monoclonal antibody (e.g., bevacizumab). (ii) Inhibition of receptor tyrosine kinases: VEGFR and PDGFR by PTK787, SU11248 (sunitinib) and BAY43–900 (sorafenib) (iii) Inhibition of the Ras/Raf pathway (by BAY 43–9006). (iv) Inhibition of mTOR (by CCI-779 or temsirolimus). Adapted from van Spronsen DJ et al. Novel treatment strategies in clear-cell metastatic renal cell carcinoma. Anticancer Drugs 2005; 16(7): 709–717

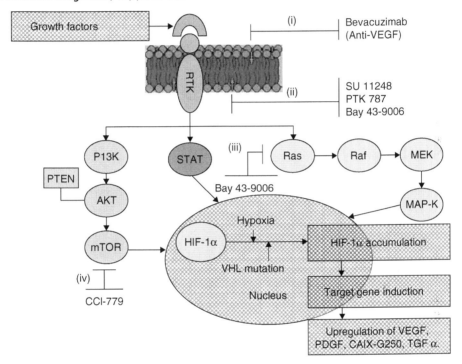

2.2.2   Anti-Vascular Endothelial Growth Factor Anti-Bodies

Bevacizumab is an anti-VEGF antibody that binds with VEGF receptors thereby inhibiting angiogenesis. The activity of bevacizumab in advanced RCC was recently evaluated in phase III trial involving 641 patients. Patients were randomized to receive IFN-α + bevacizumab or IFN-α + placebo. The PFS was 10.2 months for bevacizumab + IFN-α arm versus 5.4 months for IFN-α + placebo arm but no significant survival advantage was reported in an interim analysis (Melichar et al., 2008).

2.2.3   Mammalian Target of Rapamycin Inhibitors (mTOR)

mTOR inhibitors inhibit mTOR kinase, a molecule that up-regulates HIF gene transcription in response to hypoxia. One mTOR inhibitor temsirolimus has received regulatory approved in US and others agents are being currently developed.

In a phase III trial, 626 previously untreated RCC patients with poor prognostic features received IFN-α, temsirolimus or both in combination. It was shown that temsirolimus alone, but not in combination, was superior to single agent IFN-α with a PFS of 5.5 months versus 3.1 months (p < 0.001) and OS of 10.7 months versus 7.3 months (p = 0.008). However the response rates were low and no significant differences were found among the three arms. Among the three treatments temsirolimus had the lowest grade 3 or 4 adverse events (Hudes et al., 2007).

In Feb 2008 independent data committee stopped a phase III multinational trial of comparing everolimus against placebo in previously treated advanced RCC patients including multikinase inhibitors, anti-VEGF antibodies and IFN-α. The study was stopped as patients receiving everolimus showed a statistically significant better PFS as compared to placebo (4.0 months vs. 1.9 months). The safety profile was reported as manageable (Motzer et al., 2008). The regulatory approval has not yet achieved.

3 Quality of Life

For diseases such as cancer that are incurable and are treated with interventions that can have toxic and long-term consequences, patients input in decisions influencing outcomes are becoming increasingly important (Lipscomb et al., 2007). Combination of symptoms of disease and side effects of treatment can diminish the physical, social, and emotional function of patients with cancer and seriously impair the ability to perform normal daily activities. Although traditional outcome measures such as survival and progression-free survival are the key in cancer decision-making, there has been a growing recognition that patient-reported outcomes (PRO) measures such as symptom assessment and quality of life can provide additional important information that assesses effectiveness of interventions and overall burden of the disease (Lipscomb et al., 2007).

3.1 Assessment of PRO Using Validated Questionnaires

The field of clinical oncology has long accepted the need to improve patients' quality of life, and attend to cancer-related symptoms. Methods to ascertain symptom responses and QoL in clinical trials have been demonstrated in oncology and other clinical areas including respiratory, auto-immune deficiency, connective tissue, and neurologic disorders. In all of these therapeutic areas, the accepted method for symptom and QoL assessment is either the use of daily or weekly patient diaries or questionnaires developed and validated to address disease-specific symptoms and overall QoL. In oncology, symptom and QoL questionnaires have been developed that are either general to cancer or specific to a primary tumor site. ❷ *Table 169-2* provides type of questionnaires used in oncology clinical trials.

3.2 Evaluation of Change in Symptom Response/QoL

Evaluation of quality of life and cancer symptom responses to therapy may vary depending on the progressive nature of disease, and other related factors such as time from initial diagnosis,

◻ Table 169-2

Type of Questionnaires used to assess quality of life and disease-specific symptoms in cancer[a]

	Instrument
General QoL instruments	EuroQol-5D (EQ-5D)
	SF-36 Health Survey (SF-36)
Cancer-specific QoL instruments	European Organization for Research and Treatment of Cancer Core Questionnaire (EORTC QLQ-C30)
	Functional Assessment of Cancer Therapy-General (FACT-G)
	Brief Fatigue Inventory (BFI)
	Ferrans Quality of Life Index
	Functional Assessment of Chronic Illness Therapy (FACIT)-Fatigue
	Functional Living Index-Cancer (FLIC)
	Memorial Symptom Assessment Scale
	MD Anderson Symptom Inventory (MDASI)
	Nottingham Health Index
	Palliative Care Outcome Scale (POS)
	Q-tility Index (Q-tility)
	Quality of Life Index-Holmes (HQOLI)
	Quality of Life Index-Spitzer (QL-Index)
	Rotterdam Symptom Checklist
	Sickness Impact Profile
	Symptom Distress Scale (SyDS)
	Therapy Impact Questionnaire (TIQ)

List of general and cancer-specific questionnaires that have been used in oncology trials based on Medline search

[a]Based on Medline search

number and type of comorbidities, age and gender. For tumor types with typically slower progression, improvement in symptoms/QoL may be highly informative of treatment impact. In more progressive cancers, maintenance of QOL/symptom level can be viewed as beneficial based on the expectation of further deterioration over a short time period with less effective intervention. In either types of tumor we need to define the change in symptoms/QoL that will be considered clinically meaningful.

The magnitude of improvement in a PRO typically required for allocation as "response" has been referred to as the *minimally important difference (MID)* or ❷ *minimal clinically important difference (MCID)*. The MID, or MCID, is not a universal criteria as with RECIST, but is instrument specific. In other words, there will be a different MID assigned based on the instrument employed in the clinical trial.

By definition, the MID is the point at which an important detectable change in symptoms is noted. The MID can be based on the relationship of the PRO measure to other accepted efficacy endpoints (anchor approach), or on the distribution of responses to the instrument seen in multiple studies (distribution method). Before an instrument-specific MID can be specified, supportive evidence from several studies is required.

4 Quality of Life in Advanced RCC Patient

Patients with advanced RCC often have various sites of metastases. Symptoms due to the advanced disease along with the side-effects of available treatment options can affect multiple dimensions of patients' everyday lives and overall well-being (Gupta et al., 2008). Therefore the goal of treatments in advanced RCC should be not only to increase PFS and OS but also decrease symptom burden and overall quality of life.

Many different instruments have been used to assess the quality of life of patients with advanced RCC. These include generic health survey measures such as SF-12 and SF-36 and cancer specific measures such as Functional Assessment of Cancer Therapy (FACT) instruments or the European Organization for Research and Treatment of Cancer Quality of Life Questionnaire Core 30 (EORTC-QLQ-C30) (Gupta et al., 2008).

Recently a new instrument was developed to specifically assess kidney cancer-related symptoms and concerns. The functional Assessment of Cancer Therapy-Kidney Symptom Index (FKSI) is 15 item questionnaire which has been validated and has high internal consistency and reliability. This instrument has been demonstrated to provide clinically appropriate and precise evaluation of kidney cancer-related symptoms, and to be sensitive to disease changes including the impact of drug therapy. In addition a minimally important difference of 3–5 points was considered clinically meaningful to detect changes in symptom response (Cella et al., 2006).

The next section will review the quality of life of patients with advanced RCC treated with (1) non-targeted agents such cytokine therapy and others and (2) targeted agents such as multikinase inhibitors and mTOR inhibitors.

4.1 Effects of Cytokine Therapy and Other Non-Targeted Agents on Quality of Life

Cytokine therapy has been standard of care for treatment of advanced RCC for the past two decades. The recent arrival of targeted agents has led to shift in paradigm of treatment of advanced RCC. As a result a vast literature is available on the effect of cytokine therapy on quality of life of patients. ❷ *Table 169-3* summarizes different studies that assessed quality of life in patients treated IFN-α or IL-2. As seen from ❷ *Table 169-3* in most studies the use of cytokine therapy was associated with decrease in overall quality of life.

(Cole et al., 2003) conducted one of the largest prospective randomized study (n = 193) comparing combination of IL-2/IFN-α with high dose IL-2. The quality of life was assessed using EORTC-QLQ30. The results of this study showed that patients receiving IL-2/IFN-α combination noted diminished HRQoL on some symptom scales early in therapy, but experienced overall improved functional and symptomatic HRQoL during the course of treatment as compared to patients receiving subcutaneous high dose IL-2 (Cole et al., 2003). Another prospective randomized trial (n = 145) comparing IFN-α and combination of IFN-α with 13-cis-retinoic acid evaluated quality of life using FACT-biologic response modifier (FACT-BRM). QoL decreased during the first 8 weeks of treatment, and a partial recovery followed. Lower scores were associated with the combination therapy. Nevertheless the QoL decreased in both arms (Motzer et al., 2000).

Litwin and colleagues compared the quality of life of RCC patients with receiving immunotherapy with general population, population with other types of cancer and patients with

■ Table 169-3

Selected published prospective QoL studies in treatment of advanced RCC with IFN-α and IL-2

Author (year)	Study methodology	Treatments and sample size	HRQOL evaluation instruments and metrics	Outcomes, conclusions, and implications for burden of mRCC
Atzpodien et al. (2003)	Prospective, single arm trial	SC IL-2 + SC IFN-α-2a + oral CRA (n = 22)	–EORTC QLQ-C30	mRCC patients scored P77 in each of five functioning (physical, role, cognitive, emotional, social) scales before therapy while 3 weeks after therapy initiation there was a mean change in scores of P10 was found in all scales except cognitive. Therapeutic efficacy was associated with a rapid decline in functional HRQOL, suggesting HRQOL analysis might serve as an early indicator for immunotherapy response in mRCC
Bacik et al. (2000) Motzer et al. (2000)	Prospective, randomized trial	SC IFN-α-2a; SC IFN-α-2a + CRA (total n = 213) approximately 99% of patients had mRCC, the remainder had advanced RCC	–FACT-BRM	HRQOL decreased during the first 8 weeks for both treatment groups, though a partial recovery followed. Patients on the combination therapy had significantly lower scores than those on monotherapy at 8, 17 and 34 weeks
Cole et al. (2003)	Prospective, randomized trial	SC IL-2/IFN (n = 94); SC HD IL-2 (n = 99)	–EORTC QLQ-C30	Compared to SC IL-2/IFN, patients receiving SC HD IL-2 noted diminished HRQOL on some symptom scales early in therapy, but experienced overall improved functional and symptomatic HRQOL during the course of treatment
Heinzer et al. (1999)	Two prospective trials	Inhalational IL-2 (n = 15); IV IL-2 (n = 10)	–EORTC QLQ-C30	HRQOL deteriorated significantly (27% increase in QLQC30 score after treatment) in the IV group. For patients receiving inhalational IL-2 HRQOL decreased significantly (15% increase in QLQ-C30 score) after 1 month of treatment, but eventually (3, 6 and 9 months of treatment) returned to their baseline values
Kondagunta et al. (2006)	Prospective, single-arm trial	PEG-Intron (n = 32)	–FACT-BRM	Treatment resulted in an initial decrease in HRQOL at 2 weeks followed by a partial recovery

■ Table 169-3 (continued)

Author (year)	Study methodology	Treatments and sample size	HRQOL evaluation instruments and metrics	Outcomes, conclusions, and implications for burden of mRCC
Kroger et al. (1999)	Prospective, randomized trial	SC IFN-α-2a + SC IL-2 + IV, FU + oral isotretinoin + IV, vinblastine (n = 20)	–EORTC QLQ-C30	HRQOL decreased initially for all participants. HRQOL then improved for patients with stable disease or partial remission, but not for those with progressive disease (PD). Patients with PD had the highest fatigue score
Phan et al. (2002)	Prospective, randomized trial	HD IV IL-2 (n = 27); LD IV IL-2 (n = 30); SC IL-2 (n = 30)	– Questionnaires documenting employment status, activity and disability levels, symptoms, number of days hospitalized, and number of days affected by IL-2 therapy	Patient perception of symptoms and HRQOL measurements were similar among patients in all three treatment arms
Plasse et al. (1998)	Prospective, single-arm Trial	SC IL-2 + IFN-α + IV bolus FU (n = 46)	– EORTC QLQ-C30 – Symptom distress scale	HRQOL changes correlated with objective response, but not with worst toxicity grade; HRQOL decreased for all patients with progressive disease patients showing greater mean worsening in functional scale and symptom scores than those stable plus responded patients
Wong et al. (2002)	Prospective, single-arm trial	SC alpha-IFN-2a + oral CRA (n = 22)	–EORTC QLQ-C30	HRQOL worsened in the majority (65%) of patients

Different studies assessing the effect of cytokine therapy on quality of life (QoL) demonstrated that cytokine therapy is associated with decrease in overall QoL

Source: Reprinted from Cancer Treat Rev. 34 (3), Gupta K et al., Epidemiologic and socioeconomic burden of metastatic renal cell carcinoma (mRCC): A literature review, 193–205, Copyright (2008), with permission from Elsevier

CRA 13-cis-retinoic acid; EORTC QLQ-C30 European organization for research and treatment of cancer quality of life questionnaire core 30; FU 5-fluorouracil; HD high-dose; HRQOL health-related quality of life; IFN interferon; IL-2 interleukin-2; IPM irinotecan, cisplatin and mitomycin; C; IV intravenous; LD low-dose; mRCC metastatic renal cell carcinoma; RCC renal cell carcinoma; SC subcutaneous type 2 diabetes, hypertension and congestive heart failure. This study concluded that QoL for patients with advanced RCC was lower than general population but similar to other types of cancer including breast and prostate (❯ *Table 169-4*). In addition, the scores for patients with advanced RCC were comparable to those for patients with heart failure and type 2 diabetes (❯ *Table 169-5*); however, patients with advanced RCC scored significantly worse on two of the scales (social functioning and role limitations due to emotional problems) (Litwin et al., 1997).

4.2   Effect of Targeted Therapy on Quality of Life

4.2.1   Mutikinase Inhibitors

In phase III registration trial (n = 903), the impact of sorafenib versus placebo on renal cancer symptoms and quality of life was assessed. Symptoms were measured using FACT – Kidney Cancer Symptom Index (FKSI) and QoL was assessed by FACT-G (physical well-being domain). The questionnaires were administered at baseline and day 1 of each cycle. The results of this study demonstrated that over time there was no difference in the total score for symptoms as assessed by FKSI (p = 0.98) and QoL as assessed by FACT-G (p = 0.83) between sorafenib-treated patients and placebo. In addition FKSI single item analysis showed patients on sorafenib had fewer symptoms and concerns versus placebo. These symptoms that favored sorafenib included cough, fevers, shortness of breath, ability to enjoy life and worry the condition will get worse. The authors concluded that the soraefnib shows clinical benefit

◻ Table 169-4

Comparisons of HRQOL among patients with selected malignancies

Domain	Mean score[a]				
	Advanced renal cell Carcinoma	Breast cancer	Prostate cancer	Non-breast Female cancer	Non-prostate Male cancer
Physical function	1.32	1.57	1.54	1.83[b]	1.76[b]
Psychosocial function	1.12	1.63[b]	1.42	1.74[b]	1.54[b]
Medical function	0.38	0.88[b]	0.82[b]	0.90[b]	0.85[b]
Marital function	0.77	1.18	0.79	1.14	0.96[b]
Sexual function	1.70	1.41	1.88	1.62	1.63

The mean scores on CARES-SF is similar between advanced renal cell carcinoma treated with cytokine therapy and other tumor types

Source: Reprinted from Cancer Treat Rev. 34 (3), Gupta K et al., Epidemiologic and socioeconomic burden of metastatic renal cell carcinoma (mRCC): A literature review, 193–205, Copyright (2008), with permission from Elsevier

[a]Cancer rehabilitation evaluation system-short form (CARES-SF) scores, ranging from 0 (best) to 4 (worst)

[b]P < 0.05, compared to advanced renal cell carcinoma

◼ Table 169-5

HRQoL comparisons between Advanced Renal Cancer, general Population and other chronic illnesses

Domain	Mean score[a]				
	Advanced Renal cancer	General population	Type 2 diabetes	Hypertension	Congestive Heart failure
Physical function	65	84[b]	68	73	48[b]
Social function	69	83[b]	82[b]	87[b]	71
Bodily pain	70	75	69	72	63
Emotional well-being	74	75	77	78	75
Energy/fatigue	47	61[b]	56	58[b]	44
General health	52	72[b]	56	63[b]	47
Role limitations – physical	36	81[b]	57	62[b]	34
Role limitations – emotional	53	81[b]	76[b]	77[b]	64

The mean scores on SF-36 are lower for advanced renal cancer patients treated with cytokine therapy as compared to general population and comparable to other chronic condition such as diabetes and hypertension
Source: Reprinted from Cancer Treat Rev. 34 (3), Gupta K et al., Epidemiologic and socioeconomic burden of metastatic renal cell carcinoma (mRCC): A literature review, 193–205, Copyright (2008), with permission from Elsevier
[a]36-Item short form health survey (SF-36) scores, ranging from 0 (worst) to 100 (best)
[b]$p < 0.05$ compared to mRCC

without adversely impacting quality of life as measured by FACT-G and in fact having positive impact on some individual symptoms and concerns (Bukowski et al., 2007b).

The effects of sorafenib versus IFN-α on kidney cancer symptoms and QoL were assessed in phase II clinical trial (n = 189). FKSI and FACT-BRM were administered at baseline and day 1 of each cycle to assess kidney cancer symptoms and QoL. The results of this trial demonstrated a statistically significant (p = 0.015) and clinically meaningful improvement in kidney cancer symptoms in sorafenib treated patients as compared to IFN-α treated patients. Patients on sorafenib had higher scores on FACT-BRM and therefore clinically meaningful better QoL as compared to IFN-α (p = 0.073). Overall quality of life was better for patients on sorafenib as compared to IFN-α (Szczylik et al., 2007).

A similar result was observed when sunitinib was compared with IFN-α in a phase III multi-center trial (n = 750). Quality of life was assessed using FACT-G and kidney cancer symptoms were assessed using FKSI. The questionnaires were administered before randomization and day 1 and day 28 of each cycle. Patients on sunitinib had statistically significant and clinically meaningful better QoL (p < 0.001) and fewer kidney cancer symptoms (p < 0.001) as compared to IFN-α as reported in post-baseline assessments (Motzer et al., 2007).

The results of all these trials demonstrate that the quality of life of patients treated with newer multikinase inhibitors is much better than IFN-α and active therapy does not deteriorate QoL compared with palliative care.

4.2.2 Mammalian Target of Rapamycin (mTOR) Inhibitors

In a phase III, randomized, three-arm study of temsirolimus in the first-line treatment of patients with advanced RCC (n = 626), the OS of patients was value-weighted for their quality. Quality-adjusted survival was a pre-defined end-point. Quality-adjusted time without symptoms and toxicity (QTWiST) was estimated by partitioning overall survival into three distinct health states: time with serious toxicity, time with progression, and time without symptoms and toxicity (TWiST). Survival was value-weighted when patients completed quality of life questionnaires (EuroQoL – 5D (EQ-5D)) at weeks 12 and 32, when a grade 3 or 4 adverse event was reported, upon relapse or progression, or upon withdrawal from the study. The results of this study showed that patients receiving temsirolimus alone had 23% greater Q-TWiST than those receiving IFN-α alone (temsirolimus = 7.0 months vs. IFN-α = 5.7 months; p = 0.0015). There was no significant difference in Q-TWiST for the combination arm compared with IFN alone (IFN-α + temsirolimus = 6.1 months vs. IFN = 5.7 months, p = 0.3469). The authors concluded that patients receiving temsirolimus alone had significantly greater quality-adjusted survival than those receiving IFN-α alone (Parasuraman et al., 2007).

In phase III trial comparing everolimus with BSC post-TKIs, quality of life was assessed by EORTC-QLQ-C30 and disease related symptoms was assessed by FKSI questionnaire. The results have not been published as yet.

5 Conclusions

Renal cell carcinoma is the most common type of kidney cancer accounting for 90–95% of kidney cancers. The incidence of RCC is increasing steadily and represents a significant clinical burden. RCC is it asymptomatic and is often diagnosed at advanced stages creating challenges in treatment management.

Cytokine therapy such as IFN-α and IL-2 had been the main stay of treatment for advanced RCC for the past two decades. Both IL-2 and IFN-α are associated with significant toxicity and poor quality of life. Our review of studies where quality of life was assessed with cytokine therapy revealed that the quality of life was significantly lower for these patients. There were some cytokine regimens in which quality of life was lowered in early cycles of treatment and then patients later recovered. But this represents a small patient population. Given the limited efficacy of cytokine therapy in combination with deterioration of quality of life in patients with advanced RCC, cytokine therapy has limited use in management of RCC.

Newer targeted agents have shown greater or similar efficacy as cytokine therapies but much better quality of life than cytokine therapies. Both sorafenib and sunitinib demonstrated improved quality of life and fewer kidney cancer related symptoms as compared to IFN-α. Temsirolimus had a better quality adjusted survival than interferon. Even when compared to BSC, therapies such as sorafenib did not deteriorate quality of life and in fact showed improvement in certain kidney cancer related symptoms. The future of treatment of advanced RCC are these targeted agents which have shown much better efficacy and better quality of life as compared to traditional standard of care.

In metastatic diseases such as advanced RCC, the goal of therapy is to increase overall survival and relief of symptoms and maintenance of quality of life. Targeted agents are a significant improvement in the management of advanced RCC over traditional treatments. The future of treatment of advanced RCC is in combination of targeted agents with traditional therapies or other targeted agents with a fair balance between efficacy, toxicity and quality of life.

Summary Points

- Renal cell carcinoma is the most common type of kidney cancer and often diagnosed at advanced stages due to asymptomatic nature of disease.
- The goal of medical therapies in metastatic diseases such as advanced renal cell carcinoma is to prolong survival without adversely affecting quality of life and in fact improving quality of life relative to the previous standard of care.
- Cytokine therapy had been the treatment of choice for advanced renal cell carcinoma; however, quality of life of patients treated with cytokine therapy was very low with some recovery later for selected group of patients.
- Targeted agents have shown promising efficacy with similar or better overall QoL than cytokine therapy.
- Multikinase inhibitors such as sorafenib and sunitinib have shown clinically meaningful and statistically significant better quality of life as compared to interferon.
- Sorafenib has shown similar quality of life with improvement in some kidney cancer symptoms as compared to palliative care.
- Other targeted agents such as temsirolimus have also shown improve in quality-adjusted survival which is survival adjusted for quality of life.
- Targeted agents appear to be the future of treatment of advanced renal cell carcinoma. These agents control disease and maintain or improve quality of life.

Appendix

Notes on Renal Cell Carcinoma

- Renal Cell Carcinoma accounts for approximately 3% of adult malignancies and 90–95% of kidney cancers.
- The causes of RCC are largely unknown. Some of the known risk factors include smoking, obesity hypertension, diabetes, occupational exposure to petroleum, asbestos and other such materials. Genetic factors have also been studies but without any conclusions.
- RCC is often asymptomatic and rarely produces clinical signs and symptoms. Some of the signs include abdominal pain, blood in urine, fever, night sweats and weight loss. Most often it is diagnosed in advanced stages.
- The diagnosis of RCC is done through imaging techniques such as ultrasonography and computed tomography.
- Surgery is conducted in early stage renal cancer with curative intent.
- In advanced stage renal cancer cytokine therapy and more recently targeted agents have been used. These drugs do not cure but prolong survival by reducing the growth of cancer cells.

References

Aass N, De Mulder PH, Mickisch GH, Mulders P, van Oosterom AT, van Poppel H, Fossa SD, de aPrijck L, Sylvester RJ. (2005). J Clin Oncol. 23: 4172–4178.

Albers P. (2008). Eur Urol. Supplements 7: 36–45.

Atkins MB, Sparano J, Fisher RI, et al. (1993). J Clin Oncol. 11: 661–670.

Atzpodien J, Kuchler T, Wandert T, Reitz M. (2003). Br J Cancer. 89: 50–54.

American Cancer Society. (2006). http://www.cancer.org/downloads/STT/CAFF2006PWSecured.pdf (accessed Feb2008).

Bacik J, Fairclough D, Murphy B, Cella D, Mariani T, Mazumdar M, Motzer R. (2000). In: Paper presented at: ASCO Annual meeting Proceeding 2000; abstract 1377.

Bukowski RM, Eisen T, Szczylik C, Stadler WM, Simantov R, Shan M, Elting J, Pena C, Escudier B. (2007a). J Clin Oncol. 25: 5023.

Bukowski R, Cella D, Gondek K, Escudier B, Sorafenib TARGETs Clinical Trial Group. (2007b). Am J Clin Oncol. 30: 220–227.

Cella D, Yount S, Du H, Dhanda R, Gondek K, Langefeld K, George J, Bro WP, Kelly C, Bukowski R. (2006). J Support Oncol. 4: 191–199.

Cole BF, McDermott D, Parker R, Youmans A, Connolly C, Ernstoff M, Atkins MB, for the Cytokine Working Group. (2003). Proc Am Soc Clin Oncol. 22: (abstr 1555).

Coppin C, Porzsolt F, Awa A, Kumpf J, Coldman A, Wilt T. (2005). Cochrane Database Syst Rev. 1: CD001425.

Costa LJ, Drabkin HA. (2007). Oncologist. 12: 1404–1415.

Escudier B, Eisen T, Stadler WM, Szczylik C, Oudard S, Siebels M, Negrier S, Chevreau C, Solska E, Desai AA, Rolland F, Demkow T, Hutson TE, Gore M, Freeman S, Schwartz B, Shan M, Simantov R, Bukowski RM, TARGET Study Group. (2007). N Engl J Med. 356: 125–134.

Flanigan RC, Salmon SE, Blumenstein BA, Bearman SI, Roy V, McGrath PC, Caton JR Jr., Munshi N, Crawford ED. (2001). N Engl J Med. 345: 1655–1659.

Fyfe G, Fisher RI, Rosenberg SA, Sznol M, Parkinson DR, Louie AC. (1995). J Clin Oncol. 13: 688–696.

Gupta K, Miller JD, Li JZ, Russell MW, Charbonneau C. (2008). Cancer Treat Rev. 34: 193–205.

Heinzer H, Mir TS, Huland E, Huland H. (1999). J Clin Oncol. 17: 3612–3620.

Hudes G, Carducci M, Tomczak P, Dutcher J, Figlin R, Kapoor A, Staroslawska E, Sosman J, McDermott D, Bodrogi I, Kovacevic Z, Lesovoy V, Schmidt-Wolf IG, Barbarash O, Gokmen E, O'Toole T, Lustgarten S, Moore L, Motzer RJ, Global ARCC Trial. (2007). N Engl J Med. 356: 2271–2281.

Jemal A, Siegel R, Ward E, Murray T, Xu J, Smigal C, Thun MJ. (2006). Cancer J Clin. 56: 106–130.

Kondagunta G, Bacik J, Ishill N, Reuter V, Schwartz LH, Korkola J, Deluca J, Sweeney S, Chaganti RSK, Motzer RJ. (2006). In: Paper presented at: ASCO Annual Meeting Proceedings 2006; abstract 4528.

Kroger MJ, Menzel T, Gschwend JE, Bergmann L. (1999). Anticancer Res. 19: 1553–1555.

Lam JS, Leppert JT, Belldegrun AS, Figlin RA. (2005). World J Urol. 23: 202–212.

Lipscomb J, Gotay CC, Snyder CF. (2007). CA Cancer J Clin. 57: 278–300.

Litwin MS, Fine JT, Dorey F, Figlin RA, Belldegrun AS. (1997). J Urol. 157: 1608–1612.

McDermott DF, Regan MM, Clark JI, et al. (2005). J Clin Oncol. 23: 133–141.

Medical Research Council Renal Cancer Collaborators. (1999). Lancet. 353: 14–17.

Melichar B, Koralewski P, Ravaud A, Pluzanska A, Bracarda S, Szczylik C, Chevreau C, Filipek M, Delva R, Sevin E, Négrier S, McKendrick J, Santoro A, Pisa P, Escudier B. (2008). Ann Oncol. Apr 11 [Epub ahead of print].

Motzer RJ, Bander NH, Nanus DM. (1996). N Engl J Med. 335: 865–875.

Motzer RJ, Murphy BA, Bacik J, Schwartz LH, Nanus DM, Mariani T, Loehrer P, Wilding G, Fairclough DL, Cella D, Mazumdar M. (2000). J Clin Oncol. 18: 2972–2980.

Motzer RJ, Michaelson MD, Redman BG, Hudes GR, Wilding G, Figlin RA, Ginsberg MS, Kim ST, Baum CM, DePrimo SE, Li JZ, Bello CL, Theuer CP, George DJ, Rini BI. (2006a). J Clin Oncol. 24: 16–24.

Motzer RJ, Rini BI, Bukowski RM, Curti BD, George DJ, Hudes GR, Redman BG, Margolin KA, Merchan JR, Wilding G, Ginsberg MS, Bacik J, Kim ST, Baum CM, Michaelson MD. (2006b). JAMA. 295: 2516–2524.

Motzer RJ, Hutson TE, Tomczak P, Michaelson MD, Bukowski RM, Rixe O, Oudard S, Negrier S, Szczylik C, Kim ST, Chen I, Bycott PW, Baum CM, Figlin RA. (2007). N Engl J Med. 356: 115–124.

Motzer RJ, Escudier B, Oudard S, Porta C, Hutson TE, Bracarda S, Hollaender N, Urbanowitz G, Kay A, Ravaud A. (2008). J Clin Oncol. 26: abstr LBA5026.

Negrier S, Perol D, Ravaud A. (2006). J Clin Oncol. 24: 225s (abstr 4536).

Neidhart JA, Anderson SA, Harris JE, Rinehart JJ, Laszlo J, Dexeus FH, Einhorn LH, Trump DL,

Benedetto PW, Tuttle RL, Smalley RV. (1991). J Clin Oncol. 9: 832–836.

Parasuraman S, Hudes G, Levy D, Strahs A, Moore L, DeMarinis R, Zbrozek AS. (2007). J Clin Oncol. 25: Abstr 5049.

Parton M, Gore M, Eisen T. (2006). J Clin Oncol. 24: 5584–5592.

Phan G, Morton K, Liewehr D, Steinberg S, Rosenberg S, Yang J. (2002). In: Paper presented at: ASCO Annual Meeting Proceedings 2002; abstract 95.

Plasse T, Goss T, Dutcher J, Logan T, Gordon M, Clark J, Weiss G, Margolin K, Atkins M. (1998). In: Paper presented at: ASCO Annual Meeting Proceedings 1998; abstract 260.

Snow RM, Schellhammer PF. (1982). Urology. 20: 177–181.

Szczylik C, Demkow T, Staehler M, Rolland F, Negrier S, Hutson TE, Bukowski RM, Scheuring UJ, Burk K, Escudier B. (2007). J Clin Oncol. 25: 5025.

van Spronsen DJ, de Weijer KJ, Mulders PF, De Mulder PH. (2005). Anticancer Drugs. 16: 709–717.

Waters JS, Moss C, Pyle L, James M, Hackett S, A'hern R, Gore M, Eisen T. (2004). Br J Cancer. 91: 1453–1458.

Wong M, Goldstein D, Woo H, Testa G, Gurney H. (2002). Int Med J. 32: 158–162.

170 Quality of Life for Patients Receiving Cancer Chemotherapy: The Japanese Perspective

H. Uramoto · J. Tsukada

1 Introduction 2924

2 Current Developments in Cancer Treatment in Japan 2924

3 QOL Research Done in Japan 2925

4 Ongoing Studies 2929

5 Perspective 2929

  Summary Points 2931

Abstract: Measuring the quality of life (❷ QOL) can help the clinician and the patient to identify problems and to assess therapy. To our knowledge, few studies regarding the quality of life for patients receiving ❷ cancer chemotherapy have been conducted in Japan from a prospective viewpoint. The few studies have been pilot studies involved in a narrow area of cancer research. However, various aspects of cancer treatment in Japan have been rapidly and drastically altered by changes in the governmental, medical insurance, and patient environment. We herein present a review of the current developments concerning cancer treatment in Japan, review the QOL research performed within Japan, and discuss various perspectives regarding the quality of life for patients receiving cancer ❷ chemotherapy.

List of Abbreviations: *EORTC-QLQ,* European Organization for Research and Treatment of Cancer Core Questionnaire; *FACT-G,* functional assessment of cancer therapy scale-general; *FACT-L,* functional assessment of cancer therapy-lung; ❷ *MCID,* minimally clinically important differences; *NHP,* Nottingham health profile; *QALYs,* quality-adjusted life years; *QOL,* quality of life; *QOL-ACD,* quality of life questionnaire for cancer patients treated with anticancer drugs; ❷ *RCTs,* randomized controlled trials; *SIP,* sickness impact profile; *SF-8,* 8-short form health survey; *TOI,* trial outcome index; *WHO/QOL-26,* World Health Organization Quality Of Life Assessment Questionnaire

1   Introduction

Cancer is the leading cause of death in Japan, and more than 90% of cancer patients died in a hospital in 2005 (Statistics and information department, 2006). At present, the number of deaths is still increasing. However, current developments have rapidly and drastically altered the care of cancer patients in Japan, a result of changes in the governmental, medical insurance, and patient environment. In this chapter, we present the current developments concerning the treatment of cancer in Japan, review the QOL research done within the confines of the country, and discuss various perspectives regarding the quality of life for patients receiving cancer chemotherapy.

2   Current Developments in Cancer Treatment in Japan

Japanese government has addressed the issues by 10-year general strategy against cancer since 1983, new strategy against cancer to overcome since 1994, and the third 10-year comprehensive strategy against Cancer since 2004. Special law about cancer treatment, the Basic Act on Anti-Cancer Measures, has been established in 2006 suggesting that nation's trust might feel to be insufficient for previous activity. Thereafter the Basic Plan to Promote Anti-Cancer Measures, which included the opinions of patient, was initiated. The plan outlined general goals of a 20% reduction in the cancer death rate in the coming 10 years, alleviation of the degree of suffering for patients and their families, and improvement in the QOL during treatment and recuperation.

From the viewpoint of the medical specialist, the Japanese Board of Cancer Therapy has a plan to certify physicians to improve the standards for cancer treatment in clinical practice, in cooperation with the Japanese Society of Medical Oncology, which certifies medical specialists in the field of oncology.

Recently, a worldwide effort has been undertaken to reduce medical care costs, and a medical insurance revolution has also occurred in Japan. These forces have accelerated the transition from inpatient care to the outpatient clinic, due to consideration of the costs associated with hospital care. It is important to consider efficient medical management by shortening hospital stays and cutting the cost of inpatient services. In this context, outpatient chemotherapy deserves special notice because the discovery of new chemotherapeutic drugs without severe adverse effects allows for the more effective use of hospital beds, and improved overall medical cost-effectiveness (Uramoto et al., 2006a).

The cancer patient suffers from not only the major burden of the disease itself, with impairment of their physical and mental state, but also from the economic impact of their disease, through costs of care and reduced or lost income. Our questionnaire survey showed that 61.1% of patients wished to receive chemotherapy on an outpatient basis in comparison to merely 9.2% who desired inpatient treatment. The reasons for the preference of outpatient therapy included keeping in touch with family (45.5%), not wanting to be hospitalized (36.4%), a desire to work (24.2%), and the wish to continue hobbies (24.2%) (Uramoto et al., 2006b). In fact, Japanese patients seek emotional support from their familial relationships (Fumimoto et al., 2001).

Medical investigators have shown a great deal of interest in the physical, psychological, and social health of individuals suffering from disease and treatment-related toxicity (Buchanan et al., 2005; Gotay et al., 2004). These broad characteristics are generally grouped as QOL. The QOL is defined functionally by the patients' own perception of their performance in physical, occupational, psychological, social, financial, and somatic areas (Buchanan et al., 2005). Cancer research has produced numerous QOL studies (Maione et al., 2005; The Elderly Lung Cancer Vinorelbine Italian Study Group, 1999) and such assessment is an essential part of the cancer treatment process. One reason for this is that cancer treatments often involve such therapies as chemotherapy and radiation, which have high toxicities. Patients with late stage cancer are often symptomatic with specific problems that can cause extreme distress for the patient. Therefore, improvements in disease related symptoms and improvement in the QOL are the key desired outcomes of medical management. Furthermore, new pharmacological approaches such as molecularly-targeted therapy have recently been developed to improve the QOL with infrequent adverse events (Fukuoka et al., 2003; Kris et al., 2003; Shepherd et al., 2005), and they have sometimes caused lethal adverse effects (Ando et al., 2006; Cohen et al., 2007). With the rapid growth of symptom management trials, it is therefore timely and important to examine the contribution of the QOL assessment to this line of research (Shepherd et al., 2005). Therefore, the QOL should be evaluated scientifically in order to select the appropriate patients, regimens, and circumstances for treatment.

3   QOL Research Done in Japan

There has been not only a low absolute number of studies, but an even lower number of high quality studies (Naito et al., 2004; Shimozuma et al., 2002). Therefore, the current standards for analyzing the QOL and symptom control in randomized controlled trials (RCTs) are poor. There have been two approaches taken by Japanese researchers in the development of QOL questionnaires (Matsumoto et al., 2002). One was the translation of the Western questionnaire into Japanese. The other approach involves developing original QOL questionnaires based on the viewpoint of the Japanese patient (Kurihara et al., 1999). Research has primarily consisted

◼ Table 170-1

Literature regarding QOL studies in Japan

Type	Clinical setting	Intervention	Instrument	Outcomes	References
Non small cell lung cancer	Phase II	Gefitinib (epidermal growth factor tyrosine kinase inhibitor) 250 mg versus 500 mg	TOI and FACT-L	QOL improvement rate measured by TOI was 20.9% for the 250mg/d group and 17.8% for the 500mg/d group. QOL improvement rate measured by FACT-L was 23.9% for the 250mg/d group and 21.9% a t 250 and 500 mg/d, respectively	Fukuoka et al. (2003)
Non small cell lung cancer	Phase III	Docetaxel versus vinorelbine (anti-mitotic chemotherapy medication)	Face scale (QOL-ACD) and eight separate measures	No significant difference was observes between two arms in term of face scale. Docetaxel was associated with significantly better improvement in the overall symptom score than vinorelbine. The docetaxel arms showed significantly better improvement in anorexia and fatigue than vinorelbine arm	Kudoh et al. (2006)
Non small cell lung cancer	Phase III	Cisplatin plus irinotecan versus carboplatin plus paclitaxel, cisplatin plus gemcitabine, and cisplatin plus vinorelbine (cytotoxic anti-cancer drug)	FACT-L and QOL-ACD	No statistically significant difference in global QOL was observed among four treatment groups. Only the physical domain evaluated by QOL-ACD was significantly better in carboplatin plus paclitaxel, cisplatin plus gemcitabine, and cisplatin plus vinorelbine than in cisplatin plus irinotecan	Ohe et al. (2007)

◻ Table 170-1 (continued)

Type	Clinical setting	Intervention	Instrument	Outcomes	References
Colorectal cancer	Phase II	5-fluorouracil + low dose cisplatin versus 5-fluorouracil (antimetabolite chemotherapy drug)	QOL-ACD	No statistically significant differences between two arms were found, except for the intention to continue treatment at 4 weeks from randomization.	Nakata et al. (2007)
Breast cancer	Feasibility study	Intervention program for psychological distress	EORTC QLQ-Q30 andQLQ-BR23	The most QOL did not change significantly while appetite loss was significantly improved after 3 months	Akechi et al. (2007)
Epithelial ovarian cancer	Randomized comparative study	Docetaxel/carboplatin versus paclitaxel/carboplatin	FACT	Docetaxel/carboplatin was significantly superior to paclitaxel/carboplatin in regard to emotional wellbeing and FACT-G	Mori et al. (2007)
Various cancers	Double blind comparative study	Placebo versus tropisetron (serotonin 5-HT3 receptor antagonist)	QOL-emesis and vomiting in Japanese	Tropisetron group was significantly better than placebo group in physical wellbeing, mental wellbeing, functional wellbeing, global QOL scores	Kobayashi et al. (1999)
Esophageal ca	Pilot study	Concomitant S-1/nedaplatin radiotherapy	QOL-ACD	QOL was able to maintain	Inaba et al. (2005)
NSCLC	Pilot study	Outpatient vinorelbine therapy	QOL-ACD	Significant improvements indicating psychological wellbeing to be observed for outpatient vinorelbine therapy	Ishiura et al. (2007)

◻ Table 170-1 (continued)

Type	Clinical setting	Intervention	Instrument	Outcomes	References
Various cancers	Pilot study	Inpatients versus outpatients receiving cancer chemotherapy	SF-8 and QOL-ACD	No difference in the baseline scores of the SF-8 and QOL-ACD scales were observed in any of the analyzed domains	Uramoto et al. (2007)

Several studies regarding the quality of life for patients receiving cancer chemotherapy have been conducted in Japan from a prospective viewpoint. Phase II: early controlled clinical studies conducted on the effectiveness of the drug, Phase III: Effectiveness of the drug obtained in Phase II is intended to gather the additional information about effectiveness and safety, Randomized comparative study: a type of scientific experiment most commonly used in testing healthcare services involving the random allocation of different interventions to subjects, *TOI* Trial Outcome Index; *FACT-L* Functional Assessment of Cancer Therapy-Lung; *QOL-ACD* Quality of Life Questionnaire for Cancer Patients Treated with Anticancer Drugs; *EORTC QLQ-Q* European Organization for Research and Treatment of Cancer Core Questionnaire; *SF-8* 8-Short Form Health Survey

of sporadic pilot studies in very limited areas of cancer care, except for studies to confirm the validation and reliability (❷ *Table 170-1*).

For the patients with non-small cell lung cancer, the QOL improvement rate as measured by the TOI (Trial Outcome Index) was 20.9% for the 250 mg/d group and 17.8% for the 500 mg/d group. The QOL improvement rate as measured by the Functional Assessment of Cancer Therapy-Lung (FACT-L) was 23.9% for the 250 mg/d group and 21.9% at 250 mg/d and 500 mg/d, respectively. This study provided a unique demonstration of clinically significant improvement in disease-related symptoms, which was documented in both the patients with tumor progression and in those with stable disease in a Phase II trial. The median time to improvement for both doses was 29 days, the time of the first post-basal assessment (Fukuoka et al., 2003). Kudoh et al. reported that no significant difference was observed between the docetaxel and vinorelbine arms using the face scale for pain assessment (QOL-ACD) in a phase III trial. Docetaxel was associated with significantly better improvement in the overall symptom score than vinorelbine. The docetaxel arm showed significantly better improvement in anorexia and fatigue than did the vinorelbine arm (Kudoh et al., 2006). In another phase III trial, no statistically significant difference in global QOL was recorded among the four treatment groups (cisplatin plus irinotecan, carboplatin plus paclitaxel, cisplatin plus gemcitabine, and cisplatin plus vinorelbine) based on either the FACT-L or the QOL-ACD. Only the physical domain evaluated by QOL-ACD was significantly better in carboplatin plus paclitaxel, cisplatin plus gemcitabine, and cisplatin plus vinorelbine than in cisplatin plus irinotecan (Ohe et al., 2007). In the treatment of epithelial ovarian cancer, docetaxel/carboplatin was significantly superior to paclitaxel/carboplatin in regard to emotional wellbeing and FACT-General (physical wellbeing + social wellbeing + emotional wellbeing + functional wellbeing) (Mori et al., 2007). In colorectal cancer, no statistically significant differences between 5-Fu + low dose CDDP and 5-Fu arm were found, except for the intention to continue treatment at 4 weeks from randomization (Nakata et al., 2007).

Cytotoxic chemotherapy regimens are often associated with significant toxicity, which has a detrimental effect on the patient's QOL. Furthermore, such toxicity may result in a patient opting not to receive treatment. Tropisetron treatment was significantly better than the placebo group in physical wellbeing, mental wellbeing, and functional wellbeing in various cancers in a study to clarify the effectiveness of a specific 5-HT3 antagonist by delaying cisplatin-induced nausea and vomiting (Kobayashi et al., 1999).

The following study has several limitations such as sample size and an institutional bias. Despite the several limitations of the study, the findings suggest useful information for clinical practice in the near future. The intervention program was shown to be a feasible strategy for reducing clinically manifested psychological distress. Most of the QOL parameters did not change significantly while appetite loss was significantly improved after 3 months of intervention for the patients with breast cancer (Akechi et al., 2007). The QOL was able to be maintained for esophageal cancer patients receiving concomitant TS-1/CDGP radiotherapy (Inaba et al., 2005).

An increasing number of patients are undergoing outpatient chemotherapy as an alternative to inpatient chemotherapy. It is reported to be possible to transfer inpatients into alternative outpatient therapy without a decrease in the QOL-ACD indicating activity, physical condition, psychological condition, social relationship, and face scale. In fact, significant psychological improvements were observed for outpatient vinorelbine therapy (Ishiura et al., 2007). We previously reported that no differences in the baseline scores of the SF-8 and QOL-ACD scales were observed in any of the analyzed domains by a longitudinal study from admission to outpatient status on patients who were treated on an outpatient basis. These data suggest that these QOL measurement tools worked well for the outpatients evaluated, and that the QOL of outpatients after discharge is equal to that of inpatients receiving cancer chemotherapy (Uramoto et al., 2007).

4 Ongoing Studies

There are 23 QOL studies in ongoing clinical trials in Japan listed at the following the web site: UMIN-CTR (www.umin.ac.jp/ctr/index/htm) which has been accepted as a member site by the International Committee of Medical Journal Editors. These trials include one randomized comparative study of cisplatin, docetaxel, and irinotecan versus cisplatin and docetaxel for patients with stage IIIB or stage IV non-small cell lung cancer with the QOL evaluation as the primary outcome. The other 22 trials with QOL as the key secondary outcome encompass studies for lung (7), breast (5), urinary bladder (2), pancreatic (2), and gastric cancer (2), and 1 each involving hepatocellular carcinoma, ovarian cancer, esophageal cancer, glioblastoma, and prostate cancer. Assessments reflecting the QOL or symptom control should be included as major endpoints in most phase III trials for patients with advanced cancer. The cancer treatment may continue for a transitional period, in comparison with coronary disease treatment, in terms of quality-adjusted life years (QALYs) (Groeneveld et al., 2007) because most of the primary endpoints for cancer patients are the response rate or overall survival.

5 Perspective

Today, there are no researchers who deny the importance of a quality of life assessment for cancer patients, and cancer patients themselves may give priority to a high QOL rather than to survival (Matsumoto et al., 2002). However, it is often difficult to obtain serial measurements of QOL for cancer patients because of limited survival and other confounding factors in the practical clinical situation (Hollen et al., 1997). Furthermore, physicians may consistently underestimate the severity of physical symptoms (Stephens et al., 1997). There are a number of useful QOL assessment materials and instruments, Sickness Impact Profile (SIP), Nottingham Health Profile (NHP), World Health Organization Quality Of Life Assessment questionnaire (WHO/QOL-26), SF-36, and SF-8 for general QOL assessment, and the European Organization for Research and Treatment of Cancer Core Questionnaire (EORTC-QLQ), the Functional Assessment of Cancer Therapy Scale-General (FACT-G), and the QOL-ACD for disease-specific analysis (Cella et al., 1995; Hollen et al., 1994; Sprangers et al., 1998) due to complex and diverse causes. The QOL assessment is not necessarily meant to result in complete agreement or a unified course of action between the medical team and the patient, however the patients can use the assessment to note alterations in their living conditions. Nevertheless, QOL research reflects a growing appreciation of the need to evaluate cancer treatments more broadly than just that based on the tumor response or survival.

In phase III clinical trials, survival is generally the preferred end point. However, survival results can only be used for treatment selection recommendations, not for ongoing decisions. In that setting, physicians generally use objective response rates for the patients with complex medical histories and a myriad of comorbidities when making decisions regarding the continuation of chemotherapy (Gralla, 2004). Actually, there are cases with long term stable disease due to the effectiveness of chemotherapy that show a high level of QOL (Shepherd et al., 2005). Therefore, the key goals in the treatment of cancer are to improve both survival and QOL (❷ *Table 170-2*, because cancer patients typically have a limited survival (Uramoto et al., 2006c). Moreover, the symptoms correlate with the QOL and survival duration, providing further rationale for therapy selection based on these parameters (Gralla, 2004). The U.S. Food and Drug Administration and many European agencies recognize that end points other than survival may be important for evaluating the efficacy of new oncology products (Johnson JR et al., 2003; Chassany et al., 2002). The Health Services Research Committee of the American Society of Clinical Oncology also mentioned the usefulness of QOL assessment as one of the endpoints for cancer treatment (The Health Services Research Committee of The American Society of Clinical Oncology, 1996). Therefore, it is extremely important to judge the effects of cancer chemotherapy based not only on the medical examination but also on the patient's viewpoint, as an endpoint for research. The QOL assessment may facilitate the connection between patients and the medical staff because it is easy for both to understand. In general, if the QOL for outpatients in subgroup A is superior to

◻ Table 170-2

An expected therapeutic modality from the standpoint of relationships between survival benefit and QOL evaluation

QOL improvement	Survival benefit	Choice for treatment
–	–	Contraindication
+	–	Bridging proposal
–	+	
+	+	Ideal and standard therapy

The key goals in the treatment of cancer are to improve both survival and QOL that for subgroup B, then the decision to change to treatment A should be made whenever possible. When the QOL difference between subgroup A and B is negligible, then the patient's preference should be primarily considered in determining the course of action. Furthermore, measuring the QOL can help the clinician and the patient to identify problems and set priorities, and to assess therapy (Jacobsen et al., 2002). It appears that the QOL evaluation is an essential component, both for study in Phase II and III trails by effort to make clear minimally clinically important differences (MICD), and also to provide proactive clinical care of our cancer patients in years to come.

Ninety per cent of cancer patients are treated on an outpatient basis in the United States (Rubenstein, 1998), in comparison to just 60% in Japan (Ando and Saka, 2005). Recently, the discovery of new drugs and the advances in medical oncology have resulted in a dramatic increase in the outpatient treatment of cancer patients. In the near future, the number of patients who are able to continue working while receiving cancer chemotherapy is expected to increase greatly. Further study is still needed to determine the optimal therapies with the assistance of internationally accepted QOL assessment tools, and to provide the best possible care for cancer chemotherapy patients in Japan. While cooperation with other countries is essential, it should also be remembered that indispensable differences exist in various cultural practices and religious influences.

Summary Points

- There have so far been few studies conducted regarding the role of the QOL assessment, and few of these have been of a high quality.
- Changes in governmental policy, in the medical insurance industry, and in patients themselves have drastically and rapidly altered cancer care in Japan.
- An increasing number of patients are undergoing outpatient chemotherapy as an alternative to inpatient chemotherapy.
- There are a considerable number of QOL studies in ongoing clinical trial in Japan.
- The QOL evaluation should be included both as an endpoint in randomized controlled trials, and also as an essential element of a proactive approach to the clinical care of the cancer patient in the future.
- Further study is still needed to determine the optimal therapies with the assistance of internationally accepted QOL assessment tools, and to provide the best possible care for cancer chemotherapy patients in Japan. While cooperation with other countries is essential it should be remembered that there exist indispensable differences in cultural practices and religious influences.

References

Akechi T, Taniguchi K, Suzuki S, Okamura M, Minami H, Okuyama T, Furukawa TA, Uchitomi Y. (2007). Psychooncology. 16: 517–524.

Ando M, Saka H. (2005). Gan To Kagaku Ryoho. 32: 647–651.

Ando M, Okamoto I, Yamamoto N, Takeda K, Tamura K, Seto T, Ariyoshi Y, Fukuoka M. (2006). J Clin Oncol. 24: 2549–2556.

Buchanan DR, O'Mara AM, Kelaghan JW, Minasian LM. (2005). J Clin Oncol. 23: 591–598.

Cella DF, Bonomi AE, Lloyd SR, Tulsky DS, Kaplan E, Bonomi P. (1995). Lung Cancer. 12: 199–220.

Chassany O, Sagnier P, Marquis P. (2002). Drug Inf J. 36: 209–238.

Cohen MH, Gootenberg J, Keegan P, Pazdur R. (2007). Oncologist. 12: 713–718.

Fumimoto H, Kobayashi K, Chang CH, Eremenco S, Fujiki Y, Uemura S, Ohashi Y, Kudoh S. (2001). Qual Life Res. 10: 701–709.

Fukuoka M, Yano S, Giaccone G, Tamura T, Nakagawa K, Douillard JY, Nishiwaki Y, Vansteenkiste J, Kudoh S, Rischin D, Eek R, Horai T, Noda K, Takata I, Smit E, Averbuch S, Macleod A, Feyereislova A, Dong RP, Baselga J. (2003). J Clin Oncol. 21: 2237–2246.

Gotay CC, Isaacs P, Pagano I. (2004). Psychooncology. 13: 882–892.

Gralla RJ. (2004). Oncologist. 9 (Suppl. 6): 14–24.

Groeneveld PW, Suh JJ, Matta MA. (2007). J Interv Cardiol. 20: 1–9.

Hollen PJ, Gralla RJ, Cox C, Eberly SW, Kris MG. (1997). Lung Cancer. 18: 119–136.

Hollen PJ, Gralla RJ, Kris MG, Cox C. (1994). Cancer. 73: 2087–2098.

Inaba H, Miyazaki A, Tsuda T, Akasaka H, Kobayashi M, Okamoto M, Ogihara K, Yamauchi S, Koro T, Katoh N, Fujita K, Watanabe Y, Abiko R, Nakaya S, Kitajima S, Hoshikawa Y, Kimura M, Itoh F. (2005). Gan To Kagaku Ryoho. 32: 201–205.

Ishiura Y, Terasaki Y, Yamamoto H, Yokawa S, Fukushima W, Hirosawa H, Izumi R, Tanikawa F, Maruyama K, Ichihashi K, Miyazu M, Yoneda K, Kasahara K, Fujimura M. (2007). Gan To Kagaku Ryoho. 34: 1401–1404.

Jacobsen PB, Davis K, Cella D. (2002). Oncology. 16 (Suppl. 10): 133–139.

Johnson JR, Williams G, Pazdur R. (2003). J Clin Oncol. 21: 1404–1411.

Kris MG, Natale RB, Herbst RS, Lynch TJ Jr, Prager D, Belani CP, Schiller JH, Kelly K, Spiridonidis H, Sandler A, Albain KS, Cella D, Wolf MK, Averbuch SD, Ochs JJ, Kay AC. (2003). J Am Med Assoc. 290: 2149–2158.

Kurihara M, Shimizu H, Tsuboi K, Kobayashi K, Murakami M, Eguchi K, Shimozuma K. (1999). Psychooncology. 8: 355–363.

Kudoh S, Takeda K, Nakagawa K, Takada M, Katakami N, Matsui K, Shinkai T, Sawa T, Goto I, Semba H, Seto T, Ando M, Satoh T, Yoshimura N, Negoro S, Fukuoka M. (2006). J Clin Oncol. 24: 3657–3663.

Kobayashi K, Ishihara Y, Nukariya N, Niitani H, Furue H. (1999). Respirology. 4: 229–238.

Maione P, Perrone F, Gallo C, Manzione L, Piantedosi F, Barbera S, Cigolari S, Rosetti F, Piazza E, Robbiati SF, Bertetto O, Novello S, Migliorino MR, Favaretto A, Spatafora M, Ferraù F, Frontini L, Bearz A, Repetto L, Gridelli C, Barletta E, Barzelloni ML, Iaffaioli RV,

De Maio E, Di Maio M, De Feo G, Sigoriello G, Chiodini P, Cioffi A, Guardasole V, Angelini V, Rossi A, Bilancia D, Germano D, Lamberti A, Pontillo V, Brancaccio L, Renda F, Romano F, Esani G, Gambaro A, Vinante O, Azzarello G, Clerici M, Bollina R, Belloni P, Sannicolò M, Ciuffreda L, Parello G, Cabiddu M, Sacco C, Sibau A, Porcile G, Castiglione F, Ostellino O, Monfardini S, Stefani M, Scagliotti G, Selvaggi G, De Marinis F, Martelli O, Gasparini G, Morabito A, Gattuso D, Colucci G, Galetta D, Giotta F, Gebbia V, Borsellino N, Testa A, Malaponte E, Capuano MA, Angiolillo M, Sollitto F, Tirelli U, Spazzapan S, Adamo V, Altavilla G, Scimone A, Hopps MR, Tartamella F, Ianniello GP, Tinessa V, Failla G, Bordonaro R, Gebbia N, Valerio MR, D'Aprile M, Veltri E, Tonato M, Darwish S, Romito S, Carrozza F, Barni S, Ardizzoia A, Corradini GM, Pavia G, Belli M, Colantuoni G, Galligioni E, Caffo O, Labianca R, Quadri A, Cortesi E, D'Auria G, Fava S, Calcagno A, Luporini G, Locatelli MC, Di Costanzo F, Gasperoni S, Isa L, Candido P, Gaion F, Palazzolo G, Nettis G, Annamaria A, Rinaldi M, Lopez M, Felletti R, Di Negro GB, Rossi N, Calandriello A, Maiorino L, Mattioli R, Celano A, Schiavon S, Illiano A, Raucci CA, Caruso M, Foa P, Tonini G, Curcio C, Cazzaniga M. (2005). J Clin Oncol. 23: 6865–6872.

Matsumoto T, Ohashi Y, Morita S, Kobayashi K, Shibuya M, Yamaji Y, Eguchi K, Fukuoka M, Nagao K, Nishiwaki Y, Niitani H. (2002). Qual Life Res. 11: 483–493.

Mori T, Hosokawa K, Kinoshita Y, Watanabe A, Yamaguchi T, Kuroboshi H, Kato Y, Yasuda J, Fujita H, Nakata Y, Honjo H. (2007). Int J Clin Oncol. 12: 205–211.

Naito M, Nakayama T, Fukuhara S. (2004). Health Qual Life Outcomes. 2: 31.

Nakata B, Sowa M, Tsuji A, Kamano T, Sasaki K, Fukunaga Y, Takahashi M, Tsujitani S, Mikami Y, Mitachi Y, Nishimura S, Araki H, Yamamitsu S, Hirakawa K, Tominaga S, Shirasaka T, Inokuchi K. (2007). J Exp Clin Cancer Res. 26: 51–60.

Ohe Y, Ohashi Y, Kubota K, Tamura T, Nakagawa K, Negoro S, Nishiwaki Y, Saijo N, Ariyoshi Y, Fukuoka M. (2007). Ann Oncol. 18: 317–323.

Rubenstein EB. (1998). Curr Opin Oncol. 10: 297–301.

Shepherd FA, Rodrigues Pereira J, Ciuleanu T, Tan EH, Hirsh V, Thongprasert S, Campos D, Maoleekoonpiroj S, Smylie M, Martins R, van Kooten M, Dediu M, Findlay B, Tu D, Johnston D, Bezjak A, Clark G, Santabarbara P, Seymour L. (2005). N Engl J Med. 353: 123–132.

Shimozuma K, Okamoto T, Katsumata N, Koike M, Tanaka K, Osumi S, Saito M, Shikama N, Watanabe T, Mitsumori M, Yamauchi C, Hisashige A. (2002). Breast Cancer. 9: 196–202.

Stephens RJ, Hopwood P, Girling DJ, Machin D. (1997). Qual Life Res. 6: 225–236.

Sprangers MA, Cull A, Groenvold M, Bjordal K, Blazeby J, Aaronson. (1998). Qual Life Res. 7: 291–300.

Statistics and Information Department, Minister's Secretariat, Ministry of Health. (2006). Vital Statistics of Japan 2005. Ministry of Health, Labor and Welfare, Tokyo.

The Elderly Lung Cancer Vinorelbine Italian Study Group. (1999). J Natl Cancer Inst. 91: 66–72.

The health services research committee of American society of clinical oncology Outcomes of Cancer Treatment for Technology Assessment and Cancer Treatment Guidelines. (1996). J Clin Oncol. 14: 671–679.

Uramoto H, Iwashige A, Kagami S, Tsukada J. (2006a). J UOEH. 28: 209–215.

Uramoto H, Kabashima M, Yamazaki K, Kadota T, Narimatsu M, Iwashige A, Kagami S, Tsukada J. (2006b). Gan To Kagaku Ryoho. 33: 1681–1683.

Uramoto H, Kagami S, Iwashige A, Tsukada J. (2007). Anticancer Res. 27: 1127–1132.

Uramoto H, Sugio K, Oyama T, Ono K, Sugaya M, Yoshimatsu T, Hanagiri T, Morita M, Yasumoto K. (2006c). Lung Cancer. 51: 71–77.

171 Quality of Life Measures in Caregivers of Patients with Cancer

E. K. Grov · A. A. Dahl

1   Introduction: The Need for Caregiving *2936*

2   Definitions and Limitations *2937*
2.1 Quality of Life (QOL) 2937
2.2 Patients with Cancer 2937
2.3 Caregivers 2938

3   Becoming a Caregiver and the Caregiving Tasks *2938*

4   QOL Instrument Consideration *2939*

5   Psychometric Properties of Measures *2941*
5.1 Psychometric Measures 2941

6   Coverage and Format of Measures *2942*
6.1 The Caregiver Quality of Life Index-Cancer Scale (CQOLC) 2942
6.2 The Caregiver Reaction Assessment (CRA) 2942
6.3 Quality of Life in Life-Threatening Illness – Family Carer Version
    (QOLLTI-F) 2943
6.4 Measurement of Objective Burden (MOB) and of Subjective Burden (MSB) 2944
6.5 The Caregiver Strain Index (CSI) 2944
6.6 Bakas Caregiver Outcome Scale (BCOS) 2945

    Summary Points *2945*

Abstract: Many kinds of tasks and considerable responsibility are put on informal (family) caregivers when impaired cancer patients stay at home during their illness trajectory. The roles and functions of caregivers vary depending on the demands required from the patient and the family situation, but regularly the caregiver situation has five areas of challenge: physical, psychological, social, spiritual and financial. Caregivers' coping with these challenges in turn influences their quality of life (QOL). In this chapter we review measures that concern caregiving of adult patients, have been published in English, and that cover at least four of the five areas of challenge. We consider caregiver "burden" and "need" as aspects of QOL, and do not considered measures that focus only on "burden" or "need." Based on these selection criteria, we review six measures: The Caregiver Quality of Life Index – Cancer Scale, The Caregiver Reaction Assessment, The Quality of Life in Life-Threatening Illness – Family Carer Version, The Measurement of Objective Burden and of Subjective Burden, and Bakas Caregiving Outcomes Scale. The reliability and validity data of these scales are presented as well as data of their coverage, format and ❷ feasibility. The measures vary considerably in these regards, and all of them have their merits. The choice between these measures for the clinic or for research has to be guided by purpose, manpower and design considerations.

List of Abbreviations: ❷ *ADLs*, activities of daily living; *BCOS*, Bakas Caregiver Outcome Scale; *CQOLC*, The Cancer Quality of Life Index-Cancer Scale; *CRA*, The Caregiver Reaction Assessment; *CSI*, The Caregiver Strain Index; *MOB/MSB*, The Measurement of Objective Burden and of Subjective Burden; *QOL*, quality of life; *QOLLTI-F*, The Quality of life in life-threatening illness – Family carer version

1   Introduction: The Need for Caregiving

The trajectory of the cancer patient is characterized by various patterns of inpatient, outpatient, hospice, and at home status. Early discharge from hospital, and treatment and care at the lowest effective level are aims for modern health care. Home care provides a strong sense of familiarity for the patient and an environment that sustains relationship and values of importance for his/hers quality of life (QOL). Many cancer patients, particularly those with advanced illness, prefer to stay at home until treatment or care hospitalization.

Staying at home for severely ill cancer patients requires that they get help from health care professionals or lay helpers (formal, paid, secondary caregivers) and/or from family members or friends (informal, non-paid, primary caregivers).

A study from the United States of terminally ill patients (<6 months to live), among which half had cancer, showed that 96% were in a private residence while 4% were in an institution such as nursing home, residential hospice, or hospital. A need for assistance was reported by 87% of the patients and among the caregivers, 72% were women and 96% were family members (Emanuel et al., 1999).

The family's cancer journey may be characterized by four major dimensions: (1) *Life cycle stage of the family* – most cancer patients are middle aged or elderly and so are their eventual spouses; (2) *Cancer illness trajectory* – with varying time frames for diagnosis, treatment initiation, treatment completion, treatment failure, recurrence, decision to discontinue treatment, terminal illness and death; (3) *Family responses to cancer* – the impact of disease status and condition on the patient, his/her spouse and other family members close to him/her; (4) *Healthcare provider behavior* – the services offered by the specialist and general health care services and their availability (Kristjanson and Ashcroft, 1994).

The situation and challenges of ❷ informal caregivers of cancer patients has to be considered within these four dimensions, and many studies have shown that these caregivers can experience considerable stress within many ❷ domains of life during their task (Kitrungrote and Cohen, 2006).

2 Definitions and Limitations

2.1 Quality of Life (QOL)

There are two general approaches to QOL in the medical literature. QOL as a broad concept as exemplified by the definition of the World Health Organization: "Quality of life is defined as an individual's perception of his position in life in the context of the culture and value system in which he lives and in relation to his goals, expectations, standards, and concerns. It is a broad-ranging concept affected in a complex way by the person's physical health, psychological state, level of independence, social relationships, and their relationship to salient features of their environment" (World Health Organization, 1993).

And a narrower concept regularly called health-related QOL exemplified by Cella's definition: "the extent to which one's usual or expected physical, emotional or social well being are affected by a medical condition or its treatment" (Cella and Bonomi, 1995).

An important feature of valid measurements of QOL is that all relevant issues for the persons, situations and tasks involved are covered, and thus specific QOL measures for caregivers of patients with cancer have been developed.

A distinction has to be made between measures of "burden," "needs" and QOL of informal caregivers. Burden can be defined as "the extent to which the caregiver perceives that his or hers physical, social, mental, and spiritual status is suffering as a result of providing care for the family member" (Tebb, 1995). Need is defined as "a condition that is important to the subject and that is not being satisfied in the subject's present environment" (Hileman and Lackey, 1990). We consider QOL as the more comprehensive concept so that "burden" and "need" could be subsumed under the QOL heading, which also should cover the positive experiences associated with caregiving (Haley, 2003). Therefore measures focusing exclusively on "burden" and "need" will not be covered in this chapter (Deeken et al., 2003).

2.2 Patients with Cancer

Most cancer diseases are diagnosed in elderly adults, so this chapter will not cover caregiving to children or adolescents with cancer. The caregiver situations covered by this chapter are characterized by main responsibility for the patient by an informal caregiver usually at home and not by health care professionals or lay caregivers.

Collaboration between the informal caregiver and members of the primary and the specialist health care services is of crucial importance, but the care is mainly done by the informal caregiver eventually supported by other family members or close friends.

Cancer patients' need of care is determined by three factors: somatic symptom load (particularly pain and fatigue), mental distress (such as depression and anxiety) and reduced ability to carry out the basic and instrumental activities of daily living (ADLs) shown in ❷ Table 171-1 (Lawton and Brody, 1969).

◻ Table 171-1

Activities of daily living (ADLs)

Basic ADLs	Instrumental ADLs
Bathing	Ability to use telephone
Dressing	Shopping
Going to toilet	Food preparation
Transfer	Housekeeping
Continence	Laundry
Feeding	Mode of transportation
	Responsibility for own medication
	Ability to handle finances

Basic human, self-care demands necessary to be performed in order to function during the day

2.3   Caregivers

The cancer trajectories are variable, and most cancer patients will not be in need of special care from another person. However, a need for caregiving is manifested when the patient develop incapacitating somatic symptoms, considerable mental distress or reduced ability to carry out ADLs. So in our view a need for caregiving is not present, if patients have to retire, cannot travel or enjoy hobbies because of their cancer.

Close relationships between family members are characterized by a balance between the individual's needs and the fulfillment of these needs. Giving care to someone is an extension of caring about that person. Thus caregiving refers to particular kinds of actions triggered by the patient's condition which changes the relationship in a way where care becomes the dominant, overriding component of the relationship (Pearlin et al., 1990). Thus, just being married to a cancer patient, does not imply automatically becoming a caregiver, since a clear change in the roles of the relationship has to take place. "This care… goes beyond usual family activities that are a required part of daily life and can result in negative consequences to the caregiver's emotional and physical health" (Given and Sherwood, 2006).

Various reactions are appropriate when describing the role change and new functions of the caregiver, and their influence of the caring situation (Haley, 2003), which also will be influenced by the caregivers' somatic and mental health status as well as the quality of the pre-caregiver relationship with the patient (Andershed and Ternestedt, 1998; Given et al., 1993; Hoffmann and Mitchell, 1998).

3   Becoming a Caregiver and the Caregiving Tasks

Most informal caregivers have no professional competence in caregiving, and that has to be established and tried out through a process with several steps. The process begins at diagnosis or when the patient become symptomatic ill or debilitated, and continues several months after the person dies. According to Brown and Stetz (1999) this process has four phases: becoming a caregiver, taking care, midwifing the death, and taking the next step. (1) *Becoming a caregiver* – this phase covers acceptance and facing that a caregiver situation is coming up, choosing to take on the caregiver task, looking to future demands and development of caregiver competency. (2) *Taking care* – means managing the various caregiving tasks, facing and preparing for death, managing the environment, coming to know one's own strength, personal suffering, responding to family issues, and struggling with the health care system. (3) *Midwifing the death* – waiting and doing what is needed in relation to the death process of the patient. (4) *Taking the next step* – after the patient's death, the caregiver frequently will feel distress for a considerable amount of time processing experiencing relief, tying up loose ends, dealing with regrets, and moving ahead.

The tasks of the informal caregiver can be described under nine headings described in ❷ *Table 171-2* (Schumacher et al., 2000). Performing these tasks can have an impact on the informal caregiver in many ways, and they regularly have been classified under five areas of challenge: physical, psychological, social, spiritual, and financial (❷ *Table 171-3*) (Glajchen, 2004; Pearlin et al., 1990; Snyder, 2005).

4 QOL Instrument Consideration

Based on the major issues concerning QOL of informal caregivers for cancer patients covered so far, we defined the following inclusion criteria for measures under consideration:

1. Concerns QOL of caregiving of adult patients.
2. Have been published in English.
3. Cover at least four of the five areas of challenge: physical, psychological (positive and negative), social, spiritual, and financial.

We considered eight measures that fulfilled criterion 1–3. However, two of them:

The Functional Assessment of Cancer Therapy Scale – General Format (Cella et al., 1993) and the Brief Assessment Scale for Caregivers (Glajchen et al., 2005) did not pass criterion 3. An overview of the coverage of the six included measures is given in ❷ *Table 171-4*. All six

❏ Table 171-2
Caregiver tasks[a]

Monitoring (ensuring changes in the patient's condition have been noted)
Interpreting (making sense of what is observed
Making decisions (selecting a course of action)
Taking action (carrying out decisions and instructions)
Providing hands-on care (carrying out nursing and medical procedures)
Making adjustments (progressively refining caregiver's actions)
Accessing resources (obtaining what is needed)
Working together with the patient (sharing illness-related care in a way that is sensitive to the personalities and individuality of both patients and caregiver)
Negotiating the healthcare system (ensuring that patient's needs are adequately met)

Practical options performed by the informal caregiver in order to support the person in need of care
[a]According Schumacher et al. (2000)

◻ Table 171-3

Areas of challenge relevant for quality of life in informal caregivers[a]

Physical	Psychological	Social	Spiritual	Financial
Physical demands	Mental distress	Employment	Sense of peace and connectedness	Taking care of finances
Health problems	Helplessness	Role changes	Management of meaning	Economic strain
Sleep problems	Worry	Family function	Faith in God	
Overload	Anger	Relationship deprivation	Hope	
Fatigue	Resentment	Family conflict		
Patient behavior	Loss of self	Social support		
	Personal gain	Time constraints		
	Coping			

Conditions of significance when defining aspects related to quality of life among informal caregivers
[a]Based on Glajchen (2004), Pearlin et al. (1990), and Snyder (2005)

◻ Table 171-4

Areas of challenge covered by various caregiver measures

Measure	Physical	Negative emotions	Positive emotions	Social	Spiritual	Financial
The Caregiver Quality of Life Index-Cancer Scale	Yes	Yes	No	Yes	Yes	Yes
The Caregiver Reaction Assessment	Yes	Yes	Yes	Yes	No	Yes
Brief Assessment Scale for Caregivers	No	Yes	Yes	Yes	No	No
Quality of Life in Life-Threatening Illness – Family Carer Version	Yes	Yes	Yes	Yes	Yes	Yes
The Functional Assessment of Cancer Therapy Scale – General Format	Yes	Yes	No	Yes	No	No
Measurement of Objective Burden and of Subjective Burden	Yes	Yes	Yes	Yes	No	No
The Caregiver Strain Index	Yes	Yes	No	Yes	No	Yes
Bakas Caregiver Outcome Scale	Yes	Yes	Yes	Yes	No	Yes

Overview of elements of relevance for the considered measures, which of them that is met or not

measures cover the physical area of challenge, while the financial, spiritual and positive emotional areas were less well covered. The instruments are: The Caregiver Quality of Life Index-Cancer Scale (CQOLC) (Weitzner et al., 1999a); The Caregiver Reaction Assessment (CRA) (Given et al., 1992); Quality of Life in Life-Threatening Illness – Family carer version

(QOLLTI-F) (Cohen et al., 2006); Measurement of Objective and Subjective Burden (MOB/MSB) (Montgomery et al., 1985); The Caregiver Strain Index CSI (Robinson, 1983); Bakas Caregiver Outcome Scale (BCOS) (Bakas and Champion, 1999).

5 Psychometric Properties of Measures

Edwards and Ung (2002) reviewed the reliability and validity of four QOL measures for caregivers of patients with cancer, but only one of them were selected by our criteria, namely the Cancer Quality of Life Index-Cancer Scale (CQOLC). We therefore present the psychometric properties of our six measures here, but at the same time we recommend the paper by Edwards and Ung particularly because of its excellent definitions and structure. The various psychometric properties of our six selected measures are shown in ❯ *Table 171-5*.

❏ Table 171-5

Psychometric properties of selected measure for QOL in caregivers of cancer patients

	CQOLC[a]	CRA[b]	QOLLTI-F[c]	MOB/MSB[d]	CSI[e]	BCOS[f]
Factor analyses	–	Yes	Yes	–	–	Yes
Internal consistency	Yes	Yes	Yes	Yes	Yes	Yes
Test-retest reliability	Yes	–	Yes	–	–	–
Content validity	Yes	Yes	Yes	Yes	–	–
Convergent validity	Yes	Yes	Yes	Yes	Yes	Yes
Discriminant validity	Yes	Yes	–	–	Yes	–
Concurrent validity	–	Yes	–	Yes	–	Yes
Known group validity	Yes	–	–	–	–	–
Predictive validity	–	–	–	–	–	–

Presentation of satisfactorily key issues(yes) of the psychometric analyses for the six selected measures
[a]CQOLC The Caregiver Quality of Life Index-Cancer Scale (Weitzner et al., 1999a)
[b]CRA The Caregiver Reaction Assessment (Given et al., 1992)
[c]QOLLTI-F Quality of life in life-threatening illness – Family carer version (Cohen et al., 2006)
[d]MOB/MSB Measurement of Objective and Subjective Burden (Montgomery et al., 1985)
[e]CSI The Caregiver Strain Index (Robinson, 1983)
[f]BCOS Bakas Caregiver Outcome Scale (Bakas and Champion, 1999)

5.1 Psychometric Measures

Factor analyses: analyses of factor structure and item reduction due to low factor loading.
❯ *Internal consistency:* Average correlation between items.
❯ *Test-retest reliability:* Stability of scores from one administration time to another.
❯ *Content validity:* The measure offers an adequate sample of the construct, and has the ability to capture the content of what is wanted to be measured.
❯ *Convergent validity:* Different measures of the same construct provide similar results, and capture constructs that theoretically should be connected to each other.

❯ *Discriminant validity:* A measure of a construct can be differentiated from a different construct.

❯ *Known group validity:* Mean scale scores differ between groups in an expected manner.

❯ *Concurrent validity:* Scores are related to outcome criteria gather concurrently.

❯ *Predictive validity:* Scores are related to future events of medical significance.

Concerning reliability, internal consistencies have been tested for all six measures, while factor analyses and test-retest reliability only are reported by two measures. As to validity, convergent validity is reported by all measures, while data on content were reported for four measures, and convergent and discriminant validity for three. Predictive validity was not tested for any of the measures, although caregiving is associated with increased risk for morbidity and death (Braun et al., 2007; Schulz and Beach, 1999).

6   Coverage and Format of Measures

6.1   The Caregiver Quality of Life Index-Cancer Scale (CQOLC)

The aim of Weitzner et al. (1999a) was to develop an instrument for measurement of overall QOL in informal caregivers of cancer patients. The CQOLC is a questionnaire with 35 items. According to the list of items four domains are covered: burden, disruptiveness, positive adaptation, and financial concerns, and in addition eight single items cover sleep, sexual functioning, day-to-day focus, mental strain, information about illness, protection of patient, management of patient's pain, and family interest in caregiving. Weitzner et al. consider the CQOLC to be a unidimensional measure, but they have not published factor analytic data supporting that claim. The scoring is on a five point Liker scale from 0="extremely unimportant" to 4="extremely important" and the total score is the sum of the item scores with a scoring range from 0 to 140.

The 2 weeks test-retest correlation coefficient was 0.95. Internal consistency showed α 0.91. Content, convergent, discriminant and known-group validity has been demonstrated. The measure can be completed in 10 min. The measure is not included in the methodological paper (❯ *Table 171-6*).

Weitzner et al. (1999b) has also published a paper in which the CQOLC scores of the caregivers of curative and palliative patients were compared. It is unclear if any of the caregivers included in this study also participated in the methodological study.

6.2   The Caregiver Reaction Assessment (CRA)

In 1992 Given et al. (1992) stated: "Despite previous efforts in this area, there is still a need for valid, reliable measures for family members' reactions to caring for elderly relatives." To fulfill this purpose, the authors developed the CRA which consists of 24 items that cover five domains: self-esteem, lack of family support, impact on finance, impact on daily schedule, and impact on health. The domains are considered as subscales. Each item is rated on a five-point Likert scale from 1="strongly disagree" to 5="strongly agree." Each domain gets a mean sum score based on the summed item scores divided by the number of items, and the range of sum scores thus goes from 1.00 to 5.00. High scores on all subscales indicate

◻ Table 171-6

Coverage and format of selected measures for QOL in caregivers of cancer patients

	CQOLC[a]	CRA[b]	QOLLTI-F[c]	MOB/MSB[d]	CSI[e]	BCOS[f]
Format	Self-rating	Interview, Self-rating	Interview, Self-rating	Self-rating	Interview	Self-report
No of items	35	24	16	22	13	10
Dimensionality	Uni	Multi/Uni	Multi	Bidimensional	Uni	Uni
Domains	4	5	7	2	8	3
Scaling	Likert, 0–4	Likert, 0–5	Likert, 0–10	Likert, 0–5	Yes/No	Likert, −3–+3
Qualifications of the interviewer	NA	NG	NG	NA	NG	NA
Time frame	NG	NG	Last 2 days	NG	NG	NG
Time consumption	10 min	10 min	Median 12 min	NG	NG	NG
Feasibility	NG	Good	Good	NG	NG	NG

Overview of central descriptions and qualifications of the selected measures

NA not applicable; *NG* not given

[a]*CQOLC* The Caregiver Quality of Life Index-Cancer Scale (Weitzner et al., 1999a)

[b]*CRA* The Caregiver Reaction Assessment (Given et al., 1992)

[c]*QOLLTI-F* Quality of life in life-threatening illness – Family carer version (Cohen et al., 2006)

[d]*MOB/MSB* Measurement of Objective and Subjective Burden (Montgomery et al., 1985)

[e]*CSI* The Caregiver Strain Index (Robinson, 1983)

[f]*BCOS* Bakas Caregiver Outcome Scale (Bakas and Champion, 1999)

negative experiences with caregiving, except for self-esteem where a low score indicates negative experiences.

The original CRA did not provide a CRA total score, and Grov et al. (2006) introduced that scoring mode in order to reflect the total caregiver situation. For that purpose the self-esteem score was recoded.

Factor analyses have confirmed the five factor structure of the CRA (Given et al., 1992; Grov et al., 2006). The internal consistencies of the subscales of CRA were good in these two studies as well as the one by Nijboer et al. (1999).

The CRA has been used in several studies of caregivers of cancer patients (Given et al., 1993; McCorkle et al., 1993; Nijboer et al., 1999; Grov et al., 2006).

We finally mention that a version of the CRA with focus on post-caregiving reactions has been developed in Hebrew (Bachner et al., 2007).

6.3 Quality of Life in Life-Threatening Illness – Family Carer Version (QOLLTI-F)

Cohen et al. (2006) found after literature review that a QOL instrument for carers of patients with terminal cancer was needed. However, they did not define terminal cancer. The QOLLTI-F interview consists of 16 items covering seven domains: environment, patient condition, carer's own state, carer's outlook, relationships, quality of care and financial worries. Principal component analysis confirmed the seven domains. The response scale is 11-point numerical rating scale (range from 0 through 10), and the mean score of each domain is calculated. The time frame is the last two days. Internal consistency α was 0.86. The 16 items predicted 55% of the variance in a two-item global QOL measure, thus indicating content and convergent validity. Test-retest reliability was 0.80. We have found no other papers in which the QOLLTI-F has been tested in informal cancer caregivers except for the paper on the development of the measure. However, it was recently published. The measure is an appendix to that paper, and it is copyrighted by the authors.

6.4 Measurement of Objective Burden (MOB) and of Subjective Burden (MSB)

The MOB/MSB developed by Montgomery et al. (1985) was on the tradition that separates objective from subjective burden of caregivers. *Objective burden* is defined as the extent of disruption or changes in various aspects of the caregivers' life and household. The MOB is a nine-item measure designed to assess the extent to which caregiving behaviors have changed the caregivers' lives in nine areas: time for oneself, privacy, money, personal freedom, energy, recreational/social activities, relationship with other family members and health. The reported internal consistency of the MOB was α 0.85.

Subjective burden is defined as the caregivers' attitudes toward and emotional reactions to the caregiving experience. The MSB is a 13-item measure designed to assess emotional pain, distress, worry, guilt and reactions to negative behavior of the patient. The reported internal consistency of the MSB was α 0.86.

For both the MOB and the MSB scoring is on a five-point scale ranging from 1 to 5 (1 = rarely or never to 5 = most of the time), and scores are summed up to a total score on the MOB and the MSB separately. Content, convergent and concurrent validity has been demonstrated for the MOB/MSB. The measure is included in the paper by Montgomery et al., and there is no indication of copyright.

The MOB/MSB instrument has been used by Gaston-Johansson et al. in two studies of caregivers of patients who had bone marrow transplant for lymphomas (Foxall and Gaston-Johansson 1996) or breast cancer (Gaston-Johansson et al., 2004). These studies confirmed the internal consistencies and the validities reported by Montgomery et al.

6.5 The Caregiver Strain Index (CSI)

Strain is associated with problems that have a potential for arousing threat, and this meaning establishes strain and stressor as interchangeable concepts. Robinson's aim (1983) was to select and validate a series of questions for use as a screening interview instrument to identify strain in caregivers. The strain issues were identified by interviews of adult children caregivers of elderly parents recently hospitalized for a heart condition or for hip surgery. The 13 items cover eight domains: sleep disturbance, practical and work adjustment, family adjustments, change of plans, conflicting demands, emotional adjustments, upsetting changes in the patient, and financial strain.

The response alternatives are 1 = yes or 0 = no to each items, and the strain score is made by adding up the items scores giving a sum score from 0 to 13, higher score meaning poorer QOL (more strain). Internal consistency of the CSI was α 0.86 in Robinson's study. Convergent and divergent validities were tested and showed expected results. We have not found any papers in which the CSI has been tried out in informal cancer caregivers. The measure is included in the paper, and there is no indication of copyright.

6.6 Bakas Caregiver Outcome Scale (BCOS)

The BCOS was developed by Bakas and Champion (1999) as a self-rating instrument to measure changes in family caregiving in patients with stroke. Measurement of such changes could identify caregivers in need of support or interventions. The instrument covers three domains: social functioning, subjective well-being, and somatic health. The development of the instrument was based on data from two convenience samples of informal caregivers of stroke survivors.

The ten items are scored on a seven point Likert scale from −3 = "changed for the worst" to +3 = "changed for the best," and the scores on the ten items are added up with a score range from −30 to +30. Since the focus is on change, we presume that repeated measurements are a precondition for use of the BCOS. ❷ Factor analysis supported uni-dimensionality, and internal consistency of the BCOS was α 0.77. Convergent and divergent validity was tested and showed expected results. We have not found any papers in which the BCOS has been tested in informal cancer caregivers. The measure is not included in the paper, but can be derived from ❷ *Table 171-2* of the paper. We presume that the BCOS is copyrighted.

Summary Points

- There are many task and areas of challenge for informal caregivers of severely ill patients staying at home (Given et al., 2001).
- The impact of caregiving on the caregivers' QOL is obvious, and this has lead to instrument development and research.
- For review we have selected measures in English for caregivers of adult patients covering at least four of the five areas of challenge: physical, psychological, social, spiritual and financial.
- We have identified six measures which fulfilled our selection criteria, and they have been briefly presented.
- When considering coverage, format and feasibility they all have their merits as well as problems such as lack of psychometric parameters or lack of testing in caregivers of cancer patients.
- The choice between these measures for the clinic or for research has to be guided by purpose, manpower and design considerations.

References

Andershed B, Ternestedt BM. (1998). Cancer Nurs. 21: 106–116.

Bachner YG, O'Rourke N, Carmel S. (2007). J Palliat Care. 23: 80–86.

Bakas T, Champion V. (1999). Nurs Res. 48: 250–259.

Braun M, Mikulincer M, Rydall A, Walsh A, Rodin G. (2007). JCO. 25: 4829–4834.

Brown MA, Stetz K. (1999). Qual Health Res. 9: 182–197.

Cella DF, Tulsky DS, Gray G, Sarafian B, Linn E, Bonomi A, Silberman M, Yellen SB, Winicour P, Brannon J, Eckberg K, Lloyd S, Purl S, Blendowski C, Goodman M, Barnicle M, Stewart I, McHale M, Bonomi P, Kaplan E, Taylor IV S, Thomas jr CR, Harris J. (1993). JCO. 11: 570–579.

Cella DF, Bonomi AE. (1995). Oncology. 9: 47–60.

Cohen R, Leis AM, Kuhl D, Charbooeau C, Ritvo P, Ashbury FD. (2006). Palliat Med. 20: 755–767.

Deeken JF, Taylor KL, Mangan P, Yabroff KR, Ingham JM. (2003). J Pain Symptom Manage. 26: 922–953.

Edwards B, Ung L. (2002). Cancer Nurs. 25: 342–349.

Emanuel EJ, Fairclough DL, Slutsman J, Alpert H, Baldwin D, Emanuel LL. (1999). N Engl J Med. 341: 956–963.

Foxall MJ, Gaston-Johansson F. (1996). J Adv Nurs. 24: 915–923.

Gaston-Johansson F, Lachica EM, Fall-Dickson JM, Kennedy MJ. (2004). Oncol Nurs Forum. 31: 1161–1169.

Given B, Sherwood PR. (2006). Semin Oncol Nurs. 22: 43–50.

Given BA, Given CW, Kozachik S. (2001). CA Cancer J Clin. 51: 213–231.

Given CW, Given B, Stommel M, Collins C, King S, Franklin S. (1992). Res Nurs Health. 15: 271–283.

Given CW, Stommel M, Given B, Osuch J, Kurtz ME, Kurtz JC. (1993). Health Psychol. 12: 277–285.

Glajchen M. (2004). J Suppl Oncol. 2: 145–155.

Glajchen M, Kornblith A, Homel P, Fraidin L, Mauskop A, Portenoy RK. (2005). J Pain Symptom Manag. 29: 245–254.

Grov EK, Fossa SD, Tonnessen A, Dahl AA. (2006). Psychooncology. 15: 517–527.

Haley WE. (2003). J Suppl Oncol. 1: 25–29.

Hileman JW, Lackey NR. (1990). Oncol Nurs Forum. 17: 907–913.

Hoffmann RL, Mitchell AM. (1998). Nurs Forum. 33: 5–11.

Kitrungrote L, Cohen MZ. (2006). Oncol Nurs Forum. 33: 625–632.

Kristjanson LJ, Ashcroft T. (1994). Cancer Nurs. 17: 1–17.

Lawton MP, Brody EM. (1969). Gerontology. 9: 179–186.

McCorkle R, Yost LS, Jepson C, Malone D, Baird S, Lusk E. (1993). Psychooncology. 2: 21–32.

Montgomery RJ, Gonyea JG, Hooyman NR. (1985). Fam Relat. 34: 19–26.

Nijboer C, Triemstra M, Tempelaar R, Sanderman R, van den Bos GA. (1999). Soc Sci Med. 48: 1259–1269.

Pearlin LI, Mullan JT, Semple SJ, Skaff MM. (1990). Gerontology. 30: 583–594.

Robinson BG. (1983). J Gerontol. 38: 344–348.

Schulz R, Beach SR. (1999). JAMA. 282: 2215–2219.

Schumacher KL, Stewart BJ, Archbold PG, Dodd MJ, Dibble SL. (2000). Res Nurs Health. 23: 191–203.

Snyder C. (2005). In: Lipscomb J, Gotay CC, Snyder C (eds.) Outcomes Assessment in Cancer. Cambridge University Press, Cambridge, pp. 329–345.

Tebb S. (1995). Health Soc Work. 20: 87–92.

Weitzner MA, Jacobsen PB, Wagner H Jr, Friedland J, Cox C. (1999a). Qual Life Res. 8: 55–63.

Weitzner MA, McMillan SC, Jacobsen PB. (1999b). J Pain Symptom Manag. 17: 418–428.

World Health Organization. (1993). Qual Life Res. 2: 153–159.

172 Cancer: Influence of Nutrition on Quality of Life

M. M. Marín Caro · C. Pichard

1   *Introduction* *2948*

2   *Lifestyle and Cancer Risk* *2949*

3   *How Cancer Influences the Human Body* *2950*

4   *How Oncology Treatment Influences the Human Body* *2952*

5   *Impact of Cancer on Quality of Life* *2953*

6   *The Role of Nutritional Intervention* *2955*

7   *Assessment of the Nutritional Status* *2956*

8   *Types of Nutritional Intervention* *2957*

9   *Practical Approach to Improving the QOL with Nutritional*
      Intervention *2961*
9.1   What Is the Information Collected Until Now? 2961
9.2   What Does This Information Suggest and What Can Be Done? .. 2961
9.3   How Can We Apply All the Calculated Nutrients? 2961
9.4   What is the Following Step? 2962
9.5   What is Following After the Patient's Discharge? 2962

10 *Conclusion* *2962*

     Summary Points *2963*

Abstract: Cancer and its treatment result in a deterioration of patient's physical, psychological and social well-being. It has a direct impact on the metabolism resulting in an impaired use of the nutrients provided by the food intake. ❷ Malnutrition is typically found in oncology patients and results in a reduced response to the oncology treatment, increased morbidity and a decrease of quality of life (QoL). QoL is a concept for the evaluation of the patients' well being in all aspects of their life. Hence QoL can be used to assess the impact of the cancer treatment in terms of what matters to patients.

This chapter aims to show how nutritional treatment can improve the QoL. In order to promote this objective, nutritional care should be part of the oncology care. The optimal nutritional care is based on the balance between the patient's nutritional requirements and food intake. Nutritional care can be provided by different means: nutritional counseling, oral nutritional supplementation, enteral nutrition and parenteral nutrition. The focus of the nutritional care differs if the patient's undergo curative or palliative oncology treatment. In curative treatment, the nutritional intervention aims for an increased tolerance of and response to the treatment, increased immune function, decreased rate of complications and hence a decreased length of hospital stay. In palliative treatment, nutritional intervention is focused on the "management" of symptoms, delaying the loss of autonomy and improving their QoL. The evaluation of the QoL gives the possibility to integrate the patient's needs and expectations to the oncology care.

List of Abbreviations: *BIA,* Bioelectrical Impedance Analysis; *BMI,* ❷ Body Mass Index; *BW,* Body Weight; *EN,* Enteral Nutrition; *HPN,* Home Parenteral Nutrition; *ONS,* Oral Nutritional Supplements; *PEG,* Percutaneus Endoscopic Gastrostomy; *QoL,* Quality of life; *REE,* Resting Energy Expenditure; *SGA,* Subjective Global Assessment; *TPN,* Total Parenteral Nutrition

1   Introduction

Cancer takes place when abnormal growth of cells develops masses of tissue of malignant or cancerous origin. Cancer is not a single disease but a group of more than hundred of diseases denominated under this name. It is the second cause of death in developed countries. About 25 million people are living with cancer. Every year there are about ten million new cases and seven million cancer related deaths. Lung cancer is the most frequently diagnosed type of cancer accounting for 1.35 million new cases a year. This is followed by breast, colon, rectum, stomach and liver (Parkin et al., 2005).

Differences exist depending on the geographic zone in the world. Even when people emigrate, the cancer incidence changes with the possibility of acquiring the risk of suffering the type of cancer of the place where they have arrived. The so called "western lifestyle" is responsible for the majority of cancer cases in developed countries (e.g., colon, rectum, breast, prostate) (Parkin et al., 2005). On the other hand, cancer types frequently diagnosed in developing countries are liver, stomach and esophagus. Prognosis and survival depend a lot on the quality of the health care system. Good medical care facilitates an early detection of cancer and thus makes a more effective treatment possible. Generally, cancer survival and prognosis are better in developed countries (Parkin et al., 2005).

The strongest correlation between a type of cancer and a risk factor has been observed for lung cancer and a past exposure to tobacco smoking. About a third of cancer cases diagnosed in western countries and a fifth in developing countries have been associated with dietary habits. This indicates that through a promotion of a certain lifestyle with a balanced diet, physical activity, limited alcohol consumption and no smoking, the risk of cancer could be diminished by a large extent (Kushi et al., 2006). Nevertheless, many other risk factors remain such as environmental ones (e.g., carcinogens in foods, contact with chemical products, exposure to radiation, drugs, genetics and infectious agents (e.g., virus of *Hepatitis B* and *C*, *Helicobacter Pylori*)).

When people are affected by cancer, their health and QoL's are compromised. Their physical functions, psychological well-being and social life are altered. Health has been defined as not only the absence of disease but the positive balance between all dimensions which integrate the human well-being. Health related QoL is a person's well-being composed of its physical, psychological and social dimensions. In the last years, the concept of QoL has become being very important in oncology care. New lines of treatment have contributed to an increase of survival for many patients. Although total cure can often not be achieved, treatment can control or reduce the impact of the tumor on the patients. But alongside these benefits, oncology treatment has side effects causing an additional deterioration of the well-being. By measuring the QoL, the impact of the treatment can be evaluated in terms of what matters to the patient – his well-being.

Most of the patients with cancer suffer from nutritional problems (e.g., anorexia, nausea, vomiting, etc.) which interfere with their feeding and thus induce a weight loss (Ravasco et al., 2004). Complex mechanisms lead to the deterioration of the nutritional status triggered by substances produced by the tumor itself and the physiological response of the body to the tumor (Laviano et al., 2007). In addition, the location of the tumor might interfere directly with the food intake or digestion (e.g., esophagus cancer might cause swallowing problems, pancreas cancer decreases the fat absorption). This is further aggravated by the oncology treatment. During surgery, critical structures for food intake or digestion might have been resected (e.g., tongue, stomach). During chemotherapy, the drugs given to the patient to attack the tumoral cells will also affect healthy cells elsewhere in the body. Radiotherapy aims to affect only the tumoral region, but unfortunately harm to healthy tissue cannot be avoided. All three methods of cancer treatment produce metabolic stress and increase the demand for nutrients, resulting in a deterioration of the patient's nutritional status. This leads often to malnutrition which in turn diminishes the tolerance to the oncology treatment and increases the morbidity.

For patients with curative treatment, nutritional care accompanying all phases of the disease helps controlling cancer-related symptoms, improving the tolerance to oncology treatment, reducing morbidity, enhancing the immunometabolic host response and shortening the length of the hospital stay, thus increasing QoL. For patients who receive palliative treatment, the nutritional care is focused on the management of symptoms (e.g., anorexia, nausea, vomiting, early satiety, diarrhea), improving the performance status, delaying the loss of autonomy and consequently, increasing QoL (Marin Caro et al., 2007b).

2   Lifestyle and Cancer Risk

A large part of diagnosed cancer cases can be attributed to the lifestyle. One can reduce the personal cancer risk by a large factor by following some simple guidelines (Parkin et al., 2005). A balanced diet with at least five portions of vegetables and fruits a day, a low amount of saturated fat, few red meat and processed meats, limited use of sugar and more than 1.5 l of liquid a day is recommended. Further important ingredients for a healthy living are a frequent physical activity, limited consumption of alcoholic beverages and no smoking (Doyle et al., 2006) (see ❷ *Table 172-1*).

3   How Cancer Influences the Human Body

Cancer is associated with an inflammatory process activated by substances mediated by the tumor and the host immune activity (Bossola et al., 2007). In healthy people under normal conditions, the body corporal weight results from a balance between the energy intake and the energy expenditure. The metabolism of patients suffering from cancer is energetically inefficient. This is a direct consequence of the imbalance between the patient's nutritional needs, the energy consumption of the cancerous cells and the availability of nutrients in the body provided by the diet. The cancerous cells also produce energy from the available nutrients, but their investment of energy for that task is higher than the amount they produce.

❏ Table 172-1

Measures to help reducing the risk of specific types of cancer

Type of cancer	Measures to diminish the cancer risk
Esophagus	Avoid:
	• Drinking hot beverages
	• Deficiencies of micronutrients (e.g., selenium, calcium)
	• Pickled vegetables
	• Nitrosamine-rich foods
	• Mycotoxins
	• Alcohol
	• Smoking
	• Obesity
Stomach	Avoid:
	• High intakes of preserved salted foods
	• Salty foods in general
	• Smoked food
	Increase:
	• Fruits and vegetables
Breast, colon, rectum	Avoid:
	• Saturated fat
	• Obesity
	Increase:
	• Food rich in fiber (e.g., whole grain cereals, fruits, vegetables)
	• Water consumption
	Reduce:
	• Alcohol

Examples of specific measures which are considered to help decreasing the risk of cancer related to lifestyle habits

The organism suffers from an incapacity to use the nutrients suitably, and tumoral cells compete with healthy cells for the nutrients.

The sum of all these alterations can trigger what is denominated as cancer associated *anorexia-cachexia syndrome* (Laviano et al., 2005). It is a complex mechanism which has been related to malnutrition, increased morbidity and mortality and a decreased QoL. Some frequently observed symptoms of this syndrome are: anorexia (loss of appetite), early satiety, progressive weight loss, muscle and fat loss, anemia, asthenia, fatigue, oedema, immune dysfunction and decreased function skills. These symptoms are further aggravated by the oncology treatment and psychologic factors like depression and anxiety of the patients in face of their disease.

The anorexia-cachexia syndrome is responsible for about 20% of deaths of cancer patients (Delano and Moldawer, 2006). It causes alterations of the protein, carbohydrate and lipid metabolisms (e.g., ❷ hyperglycemia, ❷ hyperlipidemia, ❷ hypercholesterolemia). Although the level of glucose in the blood ("blood sugar") is increased, it cannot be well distributed to the organs and tissues of the body due to an abnormal insulin resistance. Hence, the body's overall energy supply is reduced. On the other hand, in most patients the resting energy expenditure (REE) is increased due to the cancer. This increased demand cannot be met by the metabolism which leads to a wasting of proteins and lipids in order to turn them to energy sources as an alternative. Consequently, body reserves are consumed but not restored (Argiles, 2005). In brief, cancer triggers "autocannibalism" (see ❷ *Figure 172-1*).

In general, uncomplicated starvation results in diminished use of glucose and mobilization of fat tissue triglycerides while muscular proteins are preserved as long as possible. The resting energy expenditure is decreased to reduce the energetic demand. In this case, refeeding restores a normal nutritional status, something which is not observed in cancer. For cancer patients,

■ Figure 172-1

Consequences of cancer. Cancer causes metabolic alterations aggravated by various symptoms including reduced food intake, ultimately leading to malnutrition and reduced quality of life

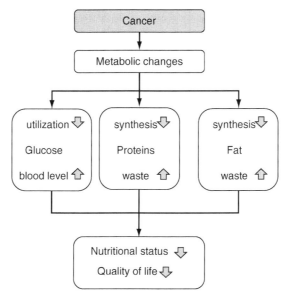

the anorexia-cachexia syndrome cannot be reverted once it has begun, although pharmaco-logic and nutritional measures exist to mitigate it (Argiles et al., 2001).

Besides the metabolic and physiological changes caused by cancer, the patients might face nutritional problems due to the cancer location (Van Cutsem and Arends, 2005). Patients with stomach or pancreas cancer have larger weight loss than breast cancer or lymphoma patients and have a higher probability of suffering from cachexia. Mouth and throat cancer interfere with mastication, salivation and swallowing. Gastrointestinal cancers (e.g., esophagus, stom-ach, pancreas, colon and rectum) may produce obstruction, early satiety if the gastric capacity is limited, or a malabsorption of nutrients.

4   How Oncology Treatment Influences the Human Body

Depending on type of oncology treatment (surgery, chemotherapy, radiotherapy) and the individual response to the treatment, the deleterious effects on nutritional status and QoL will be more or less pronounced (see ❷ *Figure 172-2*).

❑ Figure 172-2

Consequences of oncology treatment. Oncology treatment increases energy and protein requirements and causes symptoms which reduce food intake, deteriorate nutritional status and reduce quality of life

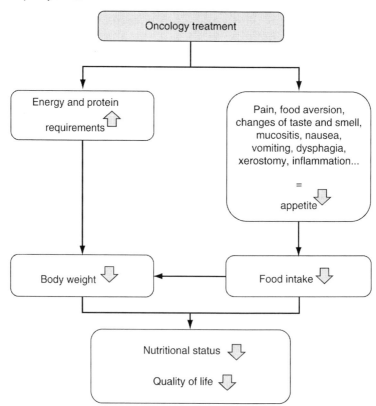

Surgery generates metabolic stress and increases the energy expenditure. Patients with head and neck surgery or esophagus cancer have problems related to their food intake (e.g., swallowing problems). Extensive gastric resections cause fat, proteins, vitamin B_{12} malabsorption and early satiety. Pancreatic resection results in glucose, fat, vitamins and minerals malabsorption, ❯ steatorrhea and hyperglycemia. Resections of the bowel lead to a malabsorption of nutrients (fat, proteins, vitamins, minerals) with diarrhea and loss of liquids (Capra et al., 2001).

Chemotherapy is an oncology treatment which affects all the cells of the organism. It has a direct effect on the cells of the gastrointestinal tract. The severity depends on the antineoplastic agents used (e.g., cisplatin, doxorubicin, fluorouracil, nitrogen mustard, dacarbazine), the dosage, the number of cycles, the treatment duration, other oncology treatments applied at the same time (e.g., radiotherapy) and the individual response. Severe gastrointestinal symptoms (e.g., anorexia, nausea, vomiting, diarrhea, constipation, abdominal pain, ❯ mucositis, taste and smell alterations) are induced with strong repercussion on the food intake through foods aversions and malabsorption of nutrients (Bergkvist and Wengstrom, 2006).

Radiotherapy is an oncology treatment with strong impact on nutritional aspects. In particular, food intake of patients undergoing radiotherapy is decreased and the assimilation of nutrients is reduced. The radiation affects both the malignant and the healthy cells as long as they are in the radiated zone. Acute or chronic complications (months or even years after irradiation therapy) can be observed. These side-effects depend on the tumoral zone, the administered radiation doses, the treatment time, the applied fractions at each treatment and other oncology treatments (e.g., chemotherapy) applied in the same time (Stone et al., 2003). The irradiation of tumors of head and neck cancer produce swallowing problems, mucositis, pain, ❯ dysphagia and changes of taste and smell (Grobbelaar et al., 2004). At thoracic level when the lung is irradiated, congestion, fever, chest pain or even pneumonitis can be caused. The irradiation of the esophagus can lead to esophagitis with pain and difficulty to swallow. Irradiation at abdominal or at pelvic level (e.g, stomach, pancreas, colon, rectum, prostate) can provoke diarrhea, malabsorption of nutrients, ulcerations, obstructions and inflammations of the small intestine, colon and anus.

5   Impact of Cancer on Quality of Life

"Health" means well-being in all dimensions (physical, mental, social). QoL is a concept designed to evaluate these dimensions to assess the impact of the illness and the treatment on the well-being of the patient.

QoL can be measured using questionnaires, generally filled in by the patient in some minutes. A large variety of tools for the measurement of QoL are available. The difference is their main focus such as symptoms, physical ability, emotional aspects, existential domains, treatment support, medical interaction, social interaction, and so on. Among the questionnaires frequently used in oncology are: (1) *The European organization for research and treatment of cancer quality of life core questionnaires (EORTC QLQ-C30)* (Aaronson et al., 1993) and (2) *The Functional Assessment of Cancer Therapy- General (FACT-G)* (Cella et al., 1993) which are cancer specific tools for assessing quality of life. Both come with modules specific to the cancer location (e.g., breast, head and neck, lung). Both have been extensively validated and are available in many languages. Other well known, but not cancer specific tools for assessing QoL are: The Medical Outcome Study 36 – Item Short Form (MOS SF-36) (Ware and Sherbourne, 1992) and the EuroQoL (EQ-5D) (Dolan, 1997).

The importance of measuring the QoL in oncology is the possibility to assess the impact of cancer and its treatment on the patient. For the patient, it means that all aspects of his well-being are taken into account (feelings, perceptions) (Siddiqui et al., 2006).

Cancer has a strong impact on patient's physical, psychological and social aspects. As discussed earlier, cancer and its treatment cause alterations all over the body. These factors contribute to a feeling of weakness and the loss of muscle strength. As a consequence, the performance status and mobility are decreased which results in an increase of the patient's dependence towards their relatives. Cancer also alters the psychological state of the patient. He feels stressed due to his disease, facing the diagnosis and his treatment. The patient also feels a constant preoccupation concerning his weight and loss of appetite. Stress, changes of humor and depression may affect his social relations and, results in anxiety and fear with further psychological and social implications. All these circumstances are affecting directly the patient's QoL (see ❷ *Figure 172-3*).

☐ Figure 172-3

Consequences of cancer and oncology treatment in the dimensions of quality of life. Deleterious effects of cancer and its treatment alter food intake and assimilation. Symptoms emerge which deteriorate the performance status, increase anxiety and emotional stress which, in turn negatively impact on physical, psychological and social dimensions of quality of life

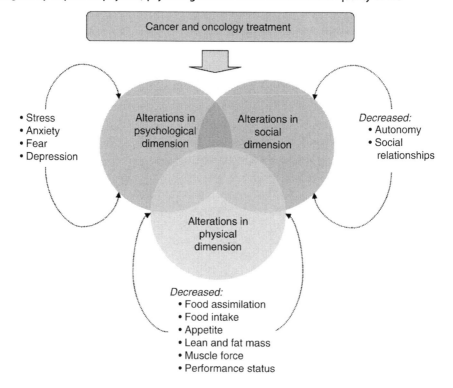

6   The Role of Nutritional Intervention

The absence of nutritional support reduces the ability to bear the oncology treatment and increases the probability to develop cancer-cachexia which in consequence reduces the chances in the fight against cancer. Therefore, it should be considered to integrate the nutritional intervention to the global oncology care. It has been shown that an early and regular nutritional assessment and support improves immune function and clinical outcomes, reduces infection rates (Braga et al., 2002b), reduces treatment toxicity (Odelli et al., 2005) and increases tolerance to the treatment (Grimble, 2005). This leads to an increased performance status, a decreased length of hospital stay and finally, an improvement of QoL (Marin Caro et al., 2007a). Nutritional intervention primarily aims at the prevention or reversal of malnutrition, and improvement of clinical outcomes and QoL. These goals can be obtained by balancing energy intake and energy expenditure using a balanced diet: *proteins (10–15%), carbohydrates (50–55%), fat (25–30%), vitamins, minerals and water according to the individual needs* (Doyle et al., 2006). *As a rough estimate, the needed amount of energy necessary for non-obese patients 25–30 kcal/kgBW/d can be taken for hospitalized patients and 30–35 kcal for ambulant patients. Approximately 1.2–2 g of proteins for every kilogram of corporal weight per day are necessary* (Arends et al., 2006).

The guideline for choosing the appropriate nutritional intervention is to use the most physiological way, that means, to use the gastrointestinal tract as much as possible. The decision of which nutritional measures are taken depends to a great extent on the type of oncology treatment (curative vs. palliative).

- *Curative oncology* treatment is generally very intensive and generates high risk of imbalance between energy expenditure and food intake, which in turn impairs the nutritional status. The nutritional intervention has to be focused on increasing both the tolerance and the response to the oncology treatment and decreasing the rate of complications. Optimal nutritional care should be part of the oncology care right from the diagnosis of cancer in order to prevent malnutrition. Such strategy allows to detect and treat nutritional disturbances early. Since nutritional intake accounts for about 20% of QoL (Ravasco et al., 2004), the attenuation of symptoms through an adequate diet affects QoL positively.

  Example: A patient has six cycles of chemotherapy and 30 sessions of radiotherapy scheduled. The treatment deteriorates his nutritional status to such an extent that the physician decides after the third cycle to suppress the fourth one. This gives the tumor the possibility to develop a resistance against the drugs.

  Example: A patient receiving radiotherapy feels that the amount of saliva is reduced compared to normal. The nutritionist advises the patient how to prepare the food with a creamier and juicier texture, and to reduce the intake of dry food (e.g., cookies, toasts).

  Example: A patient undergoing by chemotherapy feels changes of taste and smell. The nutritionist illustrates how to marinate the different types of meat with wine or fruit juice to prevent the patient from reducing the intake of meat. Discomfort related to metallic taste of cutlery is overcome by changing to plastics cutlery.

- *Palliative oncology treatment* is considered when the patient does not respond to curative treatment. In this case, the main focus of the nutritional intervention is to maintain/improve QoL. This means increasing the well being, sustaining the performance in every day life, controlling/alleviating the symptoms and trying to maintain the body weight and the body composition (lean and fat mass, balance of corporal water). It is important to consider the wishes of the patient and its family.

Example: A patient receives palliative chemotherapy and has early satiety and diarrhea. The nutritionist proposes 5–6 small meals a day and suggests to drink liquid in small sips apart from the meals. Another advice is to prefer energy dense food, and avoid energy-poor food such as salads and soups. Food should be prepared with little fat and if possible boiled. Warm food should be favored over cold one and spicy food should be omitted.

- For patients with *terminal cancer* (life expectancy less than one month), it is essential to maintain the hydratation status and to fulfill the patients needs of thirst or food preferences (Arends et al., 2006). The maintenance of the nutritional status is no more a priority.

7   Assessment of the Nutritional Status

The risk of suffering from malnutrition is determined by the type of cancer, its location and the oncology treatment. Validated and reliable tools to detect malnutrition are widely used (hospitals, home-care programs, nursing homes and so on). The main tools are: Malnutrition Universal Screening Tool (MUST), Nutritional Risk Screening (NRS-2002), Mini Nutritional Assessment (MNA) and The Subjective Global Assessment (SGA) (Kondrup et al., 2003). These instruments take into account the patient's weight and height for the body mass index (BMI), the weight change in the last 3–6 months, the changes in the food intake and further illnesses. Additionally, SGA takes into account gastrointestinal symptoms, functional capacity and physical examinations (muscle status, fat reserves, edema and ascitis) (Detsky et al., 1987).

These instruments classify the malnutrition in three levels of risk: (1) no or low risk, (2) moderate risk and (3) severe risk.

Independent of the mentioned screening methods – as a rule of thumb –, if a patient's weight loss is superior to 10–15% within the last six months, or the BMI is smaller than 18.5 kg m^{-2}, or the plasma ❯ albumin is lower than 30 g/L (with no evidence of hepatic or renal dysfunction), it is considered at severe nutritional risk (Weimann et al., 2006).

In absence of risk of malnutrition, some general nutritional recommendations should be given to the patient (e.g., types of nutrients, recommended quantities) and the screening should be repeated periodically. In case of moderate or severe risk, a complete nutritional assessment is necessary. The nutritionist measures fat and lean body mass (by measuring the triceps skinfold area and the mid-arm circumference area) and hydratation (with the bioelectrical impedance method BIA). The patient's dietary habits have to be analyzed qualitatively and quantitatively. Biochemical tests of inflammatory markers (e.g., C reactive protein) provide information about the patient's inflammation status and reflect the severity of the illness. If the patient has no renal or hepatic dysfunction, his albumin level is a marker for the risk of complications (specially in surgery) and of proteic malnutrition. With this knowledge about the nutritional problems and requirements of the patient, an adequate patient-specific nutritional intervention can be designed and monitored (see ❯ *Figure 172-4*).

❑ Figure 172-4

The implementation of nutritional care for curative and palliative oncology treatment for patients with moderate or severe nutritional risk. A comprehension nutritional assessment clarifies the patient's nutritional requirements. In order to tailor the optimal nutritional intervention to improve the nutritional status and quality of life (QoL)

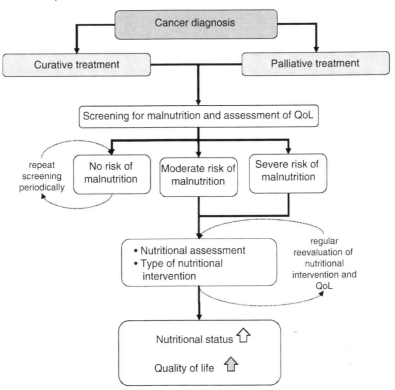

8   Types of Nutritional Intervention

There are four types of nutritional intervention: Counseling, Oral Nutritional Supplementation (ONS), Enteral Nutrition (EN) and Total Parenteral Nutrition (TPN) (Arends et al., 2006; Lochs et al., 2006).

(a) *Nutritional counseling:* A nutritionist organizes with the patient his food intake to ensure that the nutritional requirements of the patient are met. The patient has to be educated how to combine different ingredients for his meals such that his diet is balanced. The quantity and types of foods have to be calculated and selected by the nutritionist taking care about the patient's body composition. The diet has to be adapted to the specific needs and problems of the patient. General things which have to be taken into account are the cancer itself, the treatment and the nutritional status. However, very personal issues have to be considered as well such as additional

◘ Table 172-2

Symptoms related to cancer and oncology treatment and nutritional measures to alleviate them

Symptoms	Some measures for the nutritional symptoms management
Weight loss	• Choose food with little volume, but rich in nutrients
	Examples:
	• Enrich milk with powder milk (to increase the amount of protein), add dry fruits (e.g., nuts, hazelnuts), fruits and sugar or honey (to increase the amount of calories and to improve the flavor)
	• Prepare different types of purée: mix different foods like meat or eggs, vegetable, mashed potatoes and oil, butter or liquid cream
Decreased appetite	• Eat frequently small meals with high nutritional value
	• Modify the texture of foods to be easier masticable
	• Avoid the patient's favorite dishes during cancer treatment
Food aversion	Example:
	• The patient has an aversion against red meat: Mask the flavor of the meat with the marinate of aromatic spices (oregano, thyme) or wine. Or simply, replace the red meat by other sources of proteins (e.g., other types of meat, eggs)
	Avoid:
	• Strong flavors in the meals like fatty, spicy or sweet
Mucositis	If the mucositis has a degree that the patient can tolerate the food intake:
	• Change the feeding to a smooth, creamy, and homogenous texture
	Avoid:
	• Irritating foods like toasts or cakes
	• Irritating flavors like bitter or acetous
Dysphagia	• Choose smooth and homogeneous food. Give food which is easy to swallow and not irritating
	• Include complete purée in the mean meals or cooked foods easy to swallow, and mixtures of fruit, milk or yogurt between the meals
	• Chew the food well and eat slowly
	• In case of severe dysphagia, the patient requires a feeding tube
Nausea and vomiting	• Drink liquid outside the meals and drink in small sips
	• Food which is cold or at room temperature is better tolerated
	• Reinforce the carbohydrate intake in the main meals with better tolerated food (potatoes, rice, paste, bread)
	• Include small snacks between the meals with toasts or cakes with ham or cheese and juices of fruit
	Avoid:
	• Greasy or spicy food
	• Strong smells where the patient eats

■ Table 172-2 (continued)

Symptoms	Some measures for the nutritional symptoms management
❯ Xerostomy	• Drink sufficient liquid distributed during the day (like fruit juices, teas, broths)
	Avoid:
	• Eat dry foods and prepare food with palatable sauces
Diarrhea	• Replace the milk with liquids without lactose. Prefer to eat yogurt or cheese
	• Eat cooked vegetables and fruits
	• Maintain good hydratation during the day with fruit teas
	• Prepare cooked foods, like fish or chicken with rice or potatoes and vegetables
	Avoid:
	• Whole grain cereals
	• Greasy and very cold foods
Constipation	• Maintain an appropriate hydratation level throughout the day
	• Increase the fiber content of the diet: whole grain cereals, raw fruits with its skin

These symptoms might appear in acute or chronic form depending on the type of treatment (surgery, chemotherapy, radiotherapy), duration, frequency, doses and organs affected by the tumor. Alleviation can be achieved by nutritional counseling)

illnesses, allergies, medication and food habits or aversions. The patient has to be taught how to prepare his meal in terms of cooking (e.g., boiled), texture (e.g., creamy, juicy, puree) and optimizing the taste and smell (if the patient experiences changes of taste and smell). Furthermore, the patient might require general advice such as which foods are recommended or disadvised in his circumstances (see ❯ *Table 172-2*). He should be taught how many meals of which portion size he should eat at which times and how to have create comfortable ambience while eating. An advice for the patient should be to maintain some physical activity if possible.

Nutritional counseling has shown to improve QoL by increasing the nutritional intake and consequently improving the nutritional status (Ravasco et al., 2005).

(b) *Oral nutritional supplementation (ONS)* is chosen if the patient's nutritional requirements cannot be met with a diet only. The intention is to add the missing part with nutritional supplements. Nutritional supplements are available for all kind of nutritional deficiencies a patient can have (e.g., energy rich, protein rich). They are provided with different textures such that whenever oral intake is possible a suitable supplement can be found. The easy use of ONS for the patient and the gain on the level of nutritional status have a positive impact on the QoL (Fearon et al., 2003).

(c) *Enteral nutrition (EN)* is the nutritional supplementation by gastric or intestinal feeding tubes which can be chosen when the amount of food intake of the patient is very reduced or null (e.g., due to swallowing problems). With EN, the gut function can be maintained, thus contributing to the immune response of the body which reduces the risk of infections.

For some patients, EN is the only possibility to provide food which preserves the use of some part of the gastrointestinal tract. The loss of the ability to eat normally has typically a large negative influence on the patient's QoL. EN can at least provide the patient with the required nutrition and preserve some autonomy, thus avoid a further deterioration of the QoL.

When the use of EN is prolonged, the use of percutaneus endoscopic gastro-stomy (PEG) has to be considered. There, the necessary nutrients are fed directly to the stomach. PEG has shown to have a positive influence on patients' subjective personal image and increases the patient's independence through improved mobility (Loser et al., 2005).

(d) *Total parenteral nutrition (TPN)* has to be applied when it is not possible to use the gastrointestinal tract. There can be various reasons for that, such as an obstruction or an intestinal malabsorption. TPN is a complex technique to provide nutrients intravenously (e.g., by the jugular vein) with a catheter. The nutrients are administered in a form such that they can be assimilated easily by the organism (e.g., glucose, aminoacids, fatty acids). If TPN is applied to patients who stay at home, it is called home parenteral nutrition (HPN).

The disadvantages of TPN are a high risk of infection in the region where the indwelling catheter is placed and an increased hepatic workload (e.g., hyperglycemia). An example for the use of TPN is a patient who received bone marrow transplantation which makes food intake via the gastrointestinal tract impossible due a high degree mucositis and EN is excluded because of a high risk of infection and hemorrhage.

Due to the risks and the non-use of the gastrointestinal tract which reduces the immunologic function, TPN should be only the last choice. TPN reduces the patient's autonomy and impairs his social activity (Baxter et al., 2006). This obviously has negative implications on QoL, but not providing any food and leaving the patient to starvation is obviously not an option.

The role of *immunonutrition* in nutritional support: Immunonutrients have been extensively studied in the last years with promising results opening horizons for new lines of research for the future. There are nutrients with immunomodulating or anti-inflammatory prop-erties such as polyunsaturated fatty acids, arginine and nucleotides. Polyunsaturated fatty acids (eicosapentaenoic acid and docosahexaenoic acid) are commonly called n-3 fatty acids typically found in marine fish like salmon and sardine. Arginine is an amino-acid which is important for the growth of tissues and the synthesis of collagen. Nucleotides (RNA and DNA) have an important function in the transport and the liberation of energy within the cell. These substances play an important role in the reduction of the inflammatory response. They improve the immune function, the gut function and the oxygen metabolism (Braga et al., 2005). These nutrients are used as a part of artificial formulae provided for patients with cancer in order to mitigate the deleterious effects of the anorexia-cachexia syndrome and improve the QoL (Argiles, 2005). They have also shown to have positive results in gastrointestinal cancer patients undergoing surgery (Braga et al., 2002a). It enhances the immune competence leads to better clinical outcomes (e.g., reduced wound dehiscence, increased collagen synthesis, reduced infection rate, reduced length of antibiotic therapies and reduced length of stay) (Braga et al., 2002b; Gianotti et al., 2002). This might be extrapolated to the improvement of physical function, psychologic state and social well-being as surrogate markers which could influence the QoL. The use of these nutrients has been recommended for cancer patients undergoing gastrointestinal surgery (Weimann et al., 2006).

9 Practical Approach to Improving the QOL with Nutritional Intervention

We consider a hypothetical case of a 62 years old male patient who suffers from recently diagnosed larynx cancer. His physical activity level was moderate until three months ago when he started to have swallowing problems, dysphonia and progressive weight loss. An evaluation of the patient's QoL shows that the patient is very worried due to his fatigue, his altered humor and because he had to stop working. The oncologist discusses the therapeutic possibilities with the patient and proposes an intensive curative treatment started in one week (surgery, followed by chemotherapy and radiotherapy). Because of the patient's weight loss (>10% within the last three months) the oncologist requires a nutritional treatment.

9.1 What Is the Information Collected Until Now?

Actual body weight: 65 kg
Height: 1.75 m
BMI: 21.2 kg m^{-2}
Weight in the last 3–6 months: 72 kg (BMI: 23.5)
Usual body weight: 72 kg
Percentage of weight loss in the last three months: 10.7%
Problems related to the food intake: loss of appetite, swallowing problems, fatigue

9.2 What Does This Information Suggest and What Can Be Done?

Feeding problems have impaired the nutritional status, and further worsening is likely to occur once the oncology treatments starts. He is nutritionally evaluated in order to obtain more information about his nutritional status. Aside from the problems at food intake which the patient reports, the blood analysis shows that some vitamin, mineral and albumin levels are decreased. The bioelectrical impedance analysis shows that the patient has expended mainly his fat reserves, some of the muscular mass, and that his hydratation status is normal. The nutritionist calculates energy and protein requirements and tailors a diet which covers the patient's deficient nutrients.

9.3 How Can We Apply All the Calculated Nutrients?

It is important to involve the patient in his nutritional intervention. The nutritionist has to explain the function of different nutrients and why they are important to him to maintain an adequate nutritional status. The patient has to be conscious about the importance of his nutritional status for the tolerance and response to his oncology treatment and subsequently his QoL.

The objective of the nutritional intervention is the prevention of further weight loss and to prepare the patient for the treatment. For the design of the nutritional intervention, the nutritionist takes into account that there is about one week left before the start of the oncology treatment, which can be used for immunonutrition.

A diet plan with three meals a day is prepared. The food should have a creamy texture and be made of nutrients with little volume but dense in nutrients (see ❷ *Table 172-2*). Between the meals, the patient gets oral nutritional supplementation, rich in immunonutrients.

9.4   What is the Following Step?

Once the patient has passed the surgery, the surgeon has put a percutaneus endoscopic gastrostomy (PEG) access for the patient's feeding. This has been done because the patient is going to receive strong concomitant treatments which can repercute on his food intake and consequently, his nutritional status. As soon as possible, when the gastrointestinal tract can be used again, the nutritionist gives EN with a formula containing immunonutrients. This is continued for some days. The aim of nutritional intervention at that stage of oncology treatment is the reduction of postoperative complications (e.g., infections, bad wound healing, increased length of hospital stay). A couple of days later, the formula can be changed to another one without immunonutrients. When the patient's condition permits leaving the hospital, he is discharged by the physician. The patient has to be educated how, when and in what quantity he has to subminister his enteral nutrition formula.

9.5   What is Following After the Patient's Discharge?

The nutritional status of the patient has to be reevaluated periodically. If necessary (e.g., patient has symptoms like constipation or diarrhea), the formula or the quantity has to be changed. The nutritional intervention with PEG has to be maintained until the physician decides, that oral food intake is possible again. When oral food intake is started again, this will be done over a period in which the amount of food is increased step by step. The missing part to fulfill the patient's nutritional requirements is given with PEG. After the patient's oral food intake is stable and sufficient, the PEG can be removed. The nutritional intervention has to be maintained until the patient's nutritional status is stable and there is no further nutritional risk.

10   Conclusion

Cancer is a heavy burden for the patients, for their relatives and the society. Cancer and its treatment result in a deterioration of patient's physical, psychological and social well-being. This impact can be measured in terms of what is important to the person by assessing the QoL. Malnutrition typically found in oncology patients leads to a deterioration of QoL. Nutritional care should be integrated into the global oncology care. Depending on the type of oncology treatment (curative vs palliative), the priorities of the nutritional care are different. In curative treatment, the objective is to reduce the symptoms (e.g., dysphagia, vomiting), to increase the immune function, to decrease the infection rate, to reduce the length of hospital stay and to improve the tolerance to the treatment. In palliative treatment, the priorities are to control the symptoms, to delay the loss of autonomy and ultimately, to maintain or improve the QoL.

Summary Points

- Cancer is a heavy disease burden worldwide. It has deleterious effects on nutritional status and QoL.
- An appropriate nutritional intervention should be provided to improve or maintain nutritional status and to optimize clinical outcome and QoL.
- The correction of nutritional deficiencies in macro (proteins, carbohydrates and fat) and micronutrients (vitamins, minerals, electrolytes and mineral trace) intake can help to maintain the balance between the energy intake and expenditure. And thus contributing to maintain or even improve the nutritional status.
- The nutritional intervention should be integrated into the global oncology care. The patient should be nutritionally monitored during all the disease phase.
- The main focus of the nutritional intervention varies in case of curative versus palliative oncology treatment.

References

Aaronson NK, Ahmedzai S, Bergman B, Bullinger M, Cull A, Duez NJ, Filiberti A, Flechtner H, Fleishman SB, De Haes JC, et al. (1993). J Natl Cancer Inst. 85: 365–376.

Arends J, Bodoky G, Bozzetti F, Fearon K, Muscaritoli M, Selga G, Van Bokhorst-De, Van Der Schueren MA, Von Meyenfeldt M, Zurcher G, Fietkau R, Aulbert E, Frick B, Holm M, Kneba M, Mestrom HJ, Zander A. (2006). Clin Nutr. 25: 245–259.

Argiles JM. (2005). Eur J Oncol Nurs. 9(Suppl 2): S39–S50.

Argiles JM, Meijsing SH, Pallares-Trujillo J, Guirao X, Lopez-Soriano FJ. (2001). Med Res Rev. 21: 83–101.

Baxter JP, Fayers PM, Mckinlay AW. (2006). Clin Nutr. 25: 543–553.

Bergkvist K, Wengstrom Y. (2006). Eur J Oncol Nurs. 10: 21–29.

Bossola M, Pacelli F, Tortorelli A, Doglietto GB. (2007). Ann Surg Oncol. 14: 276–285.

Braga M, Gianotti L, Nespoli L, Radaelli G, Di Carlo V. (2002a). Arch Surg. 137: 174–180.

Braga M, Gianotti L, Vignali A, Carlo VD. (2002b). Surgery. 132: 805–814.

Braga M, Gianotti L, Vignali A, Schmid A, Nespoli L, Di Carlo V. (2005). Nutrition. 21: 1078–1086.

Capra S, Ferguson M, Ried K. (2001). Nutrition. 17: 769–772.

Cella DF, Tulsky DS, Gray G, Sarafian B, Linn E, Bonomi A, Silberman M, Yellen SB, Winicour P, Brannon J, et al. (1993). J Clin Oncol. 11: 570–579.

Delano MJ, Moldawer LL. (2006). Nutr Clin Pract. 21: 68–81.

Detsky AS, Mclaughin JR, Baker JP, Johnston N, Whittaker S, Mendelson RA, Jeejeebhoy KN. (1987). J Parenter Enteral Nutr. 11: 8–13.

Dolan P. (1997). Med Care. 35: 1095–1108.

Doyle C, Kushi LH, Byers T, Courneya KS, Demark-Wahnefried W, Grant B, Mctiernan A, Rock CL, Thompson C, Gansler T, Andrews KS. (2006). CA Cancer J Clin. 56: 323–353.

Fearon KC, Von Meyenfeldt MF, Moses AG, Van Geenen R, Roy A, Gouma DJ, Giacosa A, Van Gossum A, Bauer J, Barber MD, Aaronson NK, Voss AC, Tisdale MJ. (2003). Gut. 52: 1479–1486.

Gianotti L, Braga M, Nespoli L, Radaelli G, Beneduce A, Di Carlo V. (2002). Gastroenterology. 122: 1763–1770.

Grimble RF. (2005). Curr Opin Gastroenterol. 21: 216–222.

Grobbelaar EJ, Owen S, Torrance AD, Wilson JA. (2004). Clin Otolaryngol Allied Sci. 29: 307–313.

Kondrup J, Allison SP, Elia M, Vellas B, Plauth M. (2003). Clin Nutr. 22: 415–421.

Kushi LH, Byers T, Doyle C, Bandera EV, Mccullough M, Mctiernan A, Gansler T, Andrews KS, Thun MJ. (2006). CA Cancer J Clin. 56: 254–281.

Laviano A, Meguid MM, Inui A, Muscaritoli M, Rossi-Fanelli F. (2005). Nat Clin Pract Oncol. 2: 158–165.

Laviano A, Meguid MM, Preziosa I, Fanelli FR. (2007). Curr Opin Clin Nutr Metab Care. 10: 449–456.

Lochs H, Allison SP, Meier R, Pirlich M, Kondrup J, Schneider S, Van Den Berghe G, Pichard C. (2006). Clin Nutr. 25: 180–186.

Loser C, Aschl G, Hebuterne X, Mathus-Vliegen EM, Muscaritoli M, Niv Y, Rollins H, Singer P, Skelly RH. (2005). Clin Nutr. 24: 848–861.

Marin Caro MM, Laviano A, Pichard C. (2007a). Curr Opin Clin Nutr Metab Care. 10: 480–487.

Marin Caro MM, Laviano A, Pichard C. (2007b). Clin Nutr. 26: 289–301.

Odelli C, Burgess D, Bateman L, Hughes A, Ackland S, Gillies J, Collins CE. (2005). Clin Oncol (R Coll Radiol). 17: 639–645.

Parkin DM, Bray F, Ferlay J, Pisani P. (2005). CA Cancer J Clin. 55: 74–108.

Ravasco P, Monteiro-Grillo I, Marques Vidal P, Camilo ME. (2005). Head Neck. 27: 659–668.

Ravasco P, Monteiro-Grillo I, Vidal PM, Camilo ME. (2004). Support Care Cancer. 12: 246–252.

Siddiqui F, Kachnic LA, Movsas B. (2006). Hematol Oncol Clin North Am. 20: 165–185.

Stone HB, Coleman CN, Anscher MS, Mcbride WH. (2003). Lancet Oncol. 4: 529–536.

Van Cutsem E, Arends J. (2005). Eur J Oncol Nurs. 9(Suppl 2): S51–S63.

Ware JE Jr, Sherbourne CD. (1992). Med Care. 30: 473–483.

Weimann A, Braga M, Harsanyic L, Lavianod A, Ljungqvist O, Soeters P. (2006). Clin Nutr. 25: 224–244.